Fish Diseases and Medicine

Fish Diseases and Medicine

Edited by

STEPHEN A. SMITH

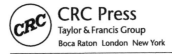

CRC Press
Taylor & Francis Group
Boca Raton London New York

CRC Press is an imprint of the
Taylor & Francis Group, an **informa** business

CRC Press
Taylor & Francis Group
6000 Broken Sound Parkway NW, Suite 300
Boca Raton, FL 33487-2742

© 2019 by Taylor & Francis Group, LLC
CRC Press is an imprint of Taylor & Francis Group, an Informa business

International Standard Book Number-13: 978-1-4987-2786-0 (Hardback)

Library of Congress Cataloging-in-Publication Data

Names: Smith, Stephen A., 1954- editor.
Title: Fish diseases and medicine / edited by Stephen Smith.
Description: Boca Raton, Florida : CRC Press, [2019] | Includes bibliographical references and index.
Identifiers: LCCN 2018051976| ISBN 9781498727860 (hardback : alk. paper) | ISBN 9781498727877 (e-book)
Subjects: LCSH: Fishes--Diseases.
Classification: LCC SH171 .F5625 2019 | DDC 571.9/517--dc23
LC record available at https://lccn.loc.gov/2018051976

Visit the Taylor & Francis Web site at
http://www.taylorandfrancis.com

and the CRC Press Web site at
http://www.crcpress.com

A special thanks to my parents, who provided me the opportunity of an education, my two daughters (Kestrel and Lanner) for their continued love and support, Dean Emeritus Dr. Peter Eyre for giving me the opportunity to develop the Aquatic Medicine Program, my long-time friend and colleague Dr. Lester Khoo for help in reviewing a number of chapters, and to the many colleagues, veterinary students and graduate students who have helped shape my career.

CONTENTS

PREFACE

With the ever-increasing global importance of fish to the welfare of this planet and its terrestrial and aquatic occupants, the health of both wild and captive fish populations is paramount to their survival. Over the past several decades, aquaculture has played an increasingly crucial role in feeding the world's growing population along with restoring depleted wild fish populations. Proliferation of aquaculture worldwide has not only seen an increased production of an expanding variety of fish species, including tropical, bait, ornamental and food fishes, but also the emergence of new pathogens and disease syndromes. This has necessitated a broader understanding of the basic biology of infectious and noninfectious diseases in fish, and resulted in the development of novel diagnostic techniques and innovative disease control methods.

This purpose of this book is to present the gross pathology of the most commonly encountered diseases and syndromes of fish in an organ-system–based approach. The book is not intended to include all diseases of fish, nor is it meant to replace the collection of a complete history, and the utilization of appropriate diagnostic assays and histopathology to reach a definitive diagnosis. The book provides the veterinarian, fish health professional, fisheries biologist and fish researcher with an understanding of anatomy, water quality, diagnostic methodology and basic clinical medicine of fish. Each organ system chapter provides an overview of the most common diseases or syndromes, followed by discussion of the etiological agent, route of transmission, typical host range, clinical presentation, possible differentials, most current means of diagnosis for that particular problem, and potential management and control methods. It is hoped this book will serve as a resource for the identification and control of fish diseases in a multitude of settings, from aquarium fish, to home ponds, to aquaculture species, to research fish and even to wild fish populations.

Stephen A. Smith, DVM, PhD

Dr. Stephen A. Smith is a professor of infectious diseases of aquatic, wildlife and exotic animals in the Department of Biomedical Sciences and Pathobiology in the Virginia-Maryland College of Veterinary Medicine at Virginia Tech.

Dr. Smith received his B.S., M.S. and D.V.M. from The Ohio State University and his Ph.D. from North Carolina State University. In addition to being an author of over 150 peer-reviewed journal articles and more than 35 book chapters on various subjects, he co-authored the book entitled *An Atlas of Avian Radiographic Anatomy* and served as an Editor and Issue Editor for several scientific journals. He has been a member of both the Aquatic Veterinary Medicine Committee and Animal Welfare Committee of the American Veterinary Medical Association, a member of the Institute for Laboratory Animal Research (ILAR) Committee of the National Academy of Sciences, and is a past president of the International Association for Aquatic Animal Medicine and a past president of the American Association of Fish Veterinarians. For the past 25 years, he has been the director of diagnostic and research activities of the VMCVM Aquatic Medicine Laboratory.

CONTRIBUTORS

Peter Bowyer, MSc, PhD
Aquaculture Consultant
Indianapolis, Indiana

Shane M. Boylan, DVM
South Carolina Aquarium
Mount Pleasant, South Carolina

David W. Bruno, BSc, PhD
Institute of Biological and Environmental Sciences
University of Aberdeen
Aberdeen, United Kingdom

Simon J. Davies, PhD
Department of Animal Production, Welfare
  and Veterinary Sciences
Harper Adams University
Newport, United Kingdom

Christine L. Densmore, DVM, PhD
U.S. Geological Survey
Leetown Science Center
Kearneysville, West Virginia

Diane G. Elliott, PhD
U.S. Geological Survey
Western Fisheries Research Center
Seattle, Washington

Richard G. Endris, MS, PhD
Endris Consulting, Inc.
Bridgewater, New Jersey

Salvatore Frasca Jr., VMD, PhD, Dipl ACVP
Department of Comparative, Diagnostic and
  Population Medicine
College of Veterinary Medicine
University of Florida
Gainesville, Florida

Jessica Gaskins, PharmD, FSVHP, DICVP
College of Pharmacy
Medical University of South Carolina
Charleston, South Carolina

Patricia S. Gaunt, DVM, PhD, Dipl ABVT
Department of Pathobiology and Population
  Medicine
College of Veterinary Medicine
Mississippi State University
Stoneville, Mississippi

Craig A. Harms, DVM, PhD, Dipl ACZM
Department of Clinical Sciences
College of Veterinary Medicine
North Carolina State University
Morehead City, North Carolina

Tharangani K. Herath, BVSc, PhD
Department of Animal Production, Welfare and
  Veterinary Sciences
Harper Adams University
Newport, United Kingdom

Grace A. Karreman, VMD, Adv Dip GIS App
Syndel Canada
Nanaimo, Canada

Lester Khoo, VMD, PhD
Thad Cochran National Warmwater
  Aquaculture Center
Delta Research and Extension Center
Stoneville, Mississippi

John S. Lumsden, DVM, PhD, Dipl ACVP
Department of Pathobiology
Ontario Veterinary College
University of Guelph
Guelph, Canada

Alisa L. Newton, VMD, Dipl ACVP
Wildlife Conservation Society
New York Aquarium
Brooklyn, New York

Trygve T. Poppe, DVM, PhD (retired)
Norwegian School of Veterinary Science
Oslo, Norway

Lysa Pam Posner, DVM, Dipl ACVAA
Department of Molecular Biomedical Sciences
College of Veterinary Medicine
North Carolina State University
Raleigh, North Carolina

Deborah B. Pouder, MAq
Tropical Aquaculture Laboratory
University of Florida
Ruskin, Florida

Nick Saint-Erne, DVM
PetSmart, Inc.
Phoenix, Arizona

Pedro A. Smith, DVM, MSc, DSc
Facultad de Ciencias Veterinarias y Pecuarias
Universidad de Chile
Santiago, Chile

Stephen A. Smith, DVM, PhD
Department of Biomedical Sciences and
   Pathobiology
Virginia–Maryland College of Veterinary Medicine
Virginia Polytechnic Institute and State University
Blacksburg, Virginia

Esteban Soto, DVM, PhD, Dipl ACVM
Department of Medicine and
   Epidemiology
School of Veterinary Medicine
University of California, Davis
Davis, California

Brittany Stevens, DVM
Department of Medicine and Epidemiology
School of Veterinary Medicine
University of California, Davis
Davis, California

Kuttichantran Subramaniam, PhD
Department of Infectious Diseases
   and Pathology
College of Veterinary Medicine
Gainesville, Florida

Thomas Waltzek, DVM, PhD
Department of Infectious Diseases
   and Pathology
College of Veterinary Medicine
Gainesville, Florida

Jeffrey C. Wolf, DVM, Dipl ACVP
Experimental Pathology Laboratories, Inc.
Sterling, Virginia

Roy P.E. Yanong, VMD
Tropical Aquaculture Laboratory
University of Florida
Ruskin, Florida

The editor gratefully acknowledges the following individuals, who contributed images to this book.

Dr. Stephen Atkinson
Oregon State University
Corvallis, Oregon

Mr. Craig Banner
Oregon Department of Fish and Wildlife
Salem, Oregon

Dr. Patricio Bustos
Aquatic Diagnostic Laboratory
Puerto Montt, Chile

Dr. Alvin C. Camus
College of Veterinary Medicine
University of Georgia
Athens, Georgia

Dr. Emily R. Cornwell
College of Veterinary Medicine
Cornell University
Ithaca, New York

Dr. Linden Craig
College of Veterinary Medicine
University of Tennessee
Knoxville, Tennessee

Dr. Ben Diggles
DigsFish Services Pty. Ltd.
Banksia Beach, Australia

Dr. John Drennan
Aquatic Animal Health Laboratory
Colorado Parks and Wildlife
Brush, Colorado

Dr. Hugh Ferguson (retired)
Fish Pathology Laboratory
University of Guelph
Guelph, Canada

Dr. Marcos Godoy
Centros de Investigaciones Biológicas Aplicadas
Puerto Montt, Chile

Dr. Andrew Goodwin
U.S. Fish and Wildlife Service
Portland, Oregon

Dr. Jennifer Haugland
Rollins Animal Disease Diagnostic Laboratory
North Carolina Veterinary Diagnostic Laboratory
    System
Raleigh, North Carolina

Dr. Kathy Heym
The Florida Aquarium
Tampa, Florida

Dr. Veronique LePage
University of Guelph
Guelph, Canada

Dr. Amedeo Manfrin
Istituto Zooprofilattico Sperimentale delle Venezie
Viale dell'Università
Adria, Italy

Mr. Andrew J. Mitchell (retired)
U.S. Department of Agriculture Agricultural
    Research Service
Stuttgart, Arkansas

Dr. Rich Moccia
University of Guelph
Guelph, Canada

Dr. Diane Morrison
Marine Harvest Canada
Campbell River, Canada

Ms. Emily Nadenbousch
U.S. Geological Survey
Leetown Science Center
Kearneysville, West Virginia

Dr. John Plumb (retired)
Auburn University
Auburn, Alabama

Dr. David Powell
Profishent, Inc.
Redmond, Washington

Dr. Mark D. Powell
University of Bergen
Bergen, Norway

Ms. Baileigh M. Reed-Grimmett
U.S. Geological Survey
Leetown Science Center
Kearneysville, West Virginia

Dr. Carlos Rodriguez
Disney's Animals, Science and Environment
Orlando, Florida

Dr. Spencer Russell
Vancouver Island University
Nanaimo, Canada

Dr. Johnny Shelley
Aquatic Animal Health Research Unit
U.S. Department of Agriculture Agricultural
 Research Service
Auburn, Alabama

Dr. Janek Simon
Institute of Inland Fisheries Potsdam-Sacrow
Potsdam, Germany

Dr. Andreas Thomsen
University of Freiburg
Freiburg, Germany

Thanks also to the Charleston Veterinary Referral Center, Michael Parks, Dr. David Sachs, and Dr. and Mrs. Rolf Gobien for their assistance with radiographic and endoscopic imaging.

CHAPTER 1

ANATOMICAL PHYSIOLOGY OF FISH

CHRISTINE L. DENSMORE

As veterinarians and animal health professionals, we are trained to deal with a very diverse group of creatures. We receive formal training in the life history, physiology and medicine specific to a wide variety of animals, and we address these differences by subdividing the field in a phylogenic approach that is largely species based. When approaching a case, we generally think in terms of canine, feline, equine, bovine, etc. medicine, and the differential diagnoses, diagnostic options, and therapeutic regimes and doses are recalled and considered based on those types of categorizations. Other groupings of animals may be approached by the typical veterinary practitioner with an even broader perspective. For instance, small mammal medicine incorporates many mammalian orders, including species of rodents, lagomorphs and mustelids, whereas avian medicine covers an entire class of the phylum Vertebrata. Given this perspective, piscine medicine can present even greater challenges in terms of physiological and morphological diversity among the subject matter and the patients. "Fish" span three classes of vertebrates and represent well over 33,000 individual species, more species than are contained in all the other classes of vertebrates combined. The life spans of fish can be measured in days in some instances or may exceed a century in others. The habitat of a fish may be an isolated pool of water in a desert climate or the deepest unexplored region of the ocean floor. Adult sizes among fish species range from less than 1 centimeter to approximately 15 meters in total length. Diversity among fish is truly amazing.

Looking up the word "fish" in a dictionary, one is likely to find a definition that describes a cold-blooded, limbless animal that is covered with scales, lives exclusively in water, and obtains oxygen from that water through its gills. Although this is generally accurate, there are a number of fish species that defy one or more of each of these descriptors. So how may we accurately define a fish? Taxonomically, they are members of the subphylum Vertebrata and one of three classes or superclasses of vertebrates: Agnatha (jawless fish like the lamprey), Chondrichtyes (cartilaginous fish including the sharks, skates, and rays, also known as elasmobranchs) or Osteichthyes (bony fish that include the majority of the more familiar species). They all have gills throughout their entire lives and generally live exclusively in (or at least rely heavily upon) an aqueous environment. Some like the arapaima, snakehead and some catfish actually do breathe air to the point that they may survive for a time out of water. Fish are generally motile, utilizing fins and lateral undulation to help with locomotion through water and, in rare cases with a few species, on land or other firm substrate. Most fish are ectothermic, or cold-blooded, with their body temperature solely dependent upon the environmental temperature. There are, however, noted exceptions that maintain their body temperature above environmental temperature including large pelagic species like the bluefin tuna (*Thunnus thynnus*) and deep-diving species like the opah (*Lampris* sp.).

This overview of anatomic physiology therefore cannot begin to cover the immense diversity of form and function that is found among fish. Instead, this chapter will endeavor to highlight the major consistencies and differences that are evident in the anatomy and physiology of those fish most likely to be encountered by the veterinarian or biologist working in the realm of aquatic animal health. The majority of this chapter will describe teleost fish, members of the infraclass Teleostei that includes bony fish with protrusible upper jaws, as these represent the majority of species commonly encountered in clinical or research settings. Attention will also be given to the more commonly encountered non-teleost fish including other bony fish like lungfish, sturgeons, and gars as well as the elasmobranchs.

EXTERNAL ANATOMY

Collectively, fish provide an excellent illustration of how in the biological sciences, form follows function. Size, body conformation and other external features that characterize a species are strongly linked to environmental demands. Like other vertebrate animals, fish display bilateral symmetry and their body contour is related to their life history (**Figures 1.1** through **1.3**). Pelagic fish that expend considerable energy swimming will tend to be fusiform in shape, schooling fish that turn and maneuver in tandem may tend to be more laterally compressed, and benthic dwellers will frequently exhibit dorsoventral compression. Morphological specialization with regard to ecological niche is highly evident among fish. The serpentine body form of eels, the torpedo-like shape that renders quick and agile movement to ambush predators like the pike, and even the bizarre but aesthetically pleasing appearance of syngnathids like seahorses and sea dragons are examples. In general, however, there are a number of external anatomical landmarks that are well conserved among

fish. Fish may be subdivided into three anatomical regions: head, body, and tail. Familiar landmarks on the fish's head include the mouth, nares and eyes. Many types of fish will also have special adaptive features evident on the head region, such as the barbels of catfish, sturgeon and cyprinids, or the extended spikey rostrum of sawfish (**Figure 1.4**). Separating the head from the body regions, most species will have bilaterally paired opercula, motile flaplike coverings that protect the gills beneath and function in the mechanics of respiration. Among the elasmobranchs, gill slits are present and opercula are not. Ventral and posterior on the body in some species is a cloaca, the chamber that receives duct outlets from the gastrointestinal, excretory and reproductive systems. Some species have separate distal openings to these organ systems that are grossly apparent, examples of which include the anus or urinary and genital pores/papillae. Behind the cloaca or pores, the body of most fish narrows into the caudal peduncle and the associated fin that forms the tail.

The fin of the fish is the familiar piscine appendage that primarily functions in locomotion. Like the fish themselves, fins come in a varied combination of presence, size, shape and location dependent on the species and their life history. Pectoral and pelvic

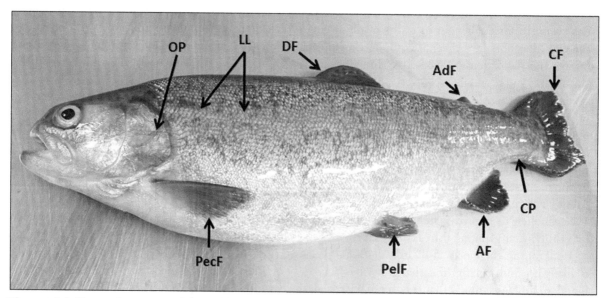

Figure 1.1 External anatomy of the rainbow trout (*Oncorhynchus mykiss*). OP, operculum; LL, lateral line; PecF, pectoral fin; PelF, pelvic fin; DF, dorsal fin; AF, anal fin; AdF, adipose fin; CF, caudal fin; CP, caudal peduncle. (Image courtesy of E. Nadenbousch.)

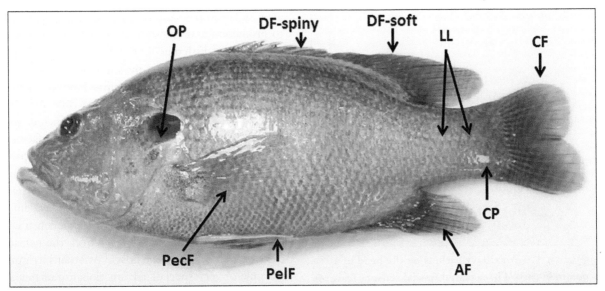

Figure 1.2 External anatomy of the green sunfish (*Lepomis cyanellus*). OP, operculum; LL, lateral line; PecF, pectoral fin; PelF, pelvic fin; DF, dorsal fin; AF, anal fin; CF, caudal fin; CP, caudal peduncle. (Image courtesy of E. Nadenbousch.)

fins are paired and located posterior to the opercula; generally, the pectoral fins are located laterally and pelvic fins ventrally. Further posterior and usually just behind the cloaca is the anal fin. The caudal fin, as the name implies, is comprised by the fish's tail and is categorized as protocercal (undifferentiated), heterocercal (differentiated into two unequally sized lobes), or homocercal (differentiated into two lobes of equal size). The dorsal fin or fins extend along the dorsal midline. Two distinct dorsal fins exist in some species. Also, in some fish, there is another smaller posterior dorsal fin known as the adipose fin. Among most of the bony fish, the fins are composed of integumentary tissue that is supported structurally by dermal fin rays, also known as lepidotrichia. In some fin structure, the lepidotrichia are fused into hard spines, a feature that distinguishes "spiny" from "soft" fins and spiny-rayed fish from soft-rayed fish. Oftentimes, in fish with two dorsal fins, the anterior fin is spiny and the posterior one is soft. Adipose fins are an exception, being fleshy and void of fin rays altogether.

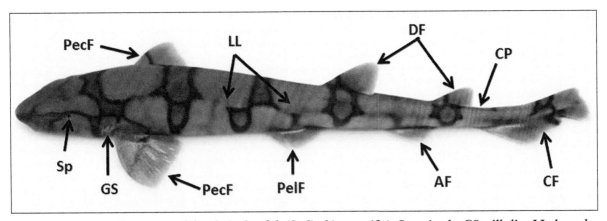

Figure 1.3 External anatomy of the chain dog fish (*Scyliorhinus rotifer*). Sp, spiracle; GS, gill slits; LL, lateral line; PecF, pectoral fin; PelF, pelvic fin; DF, dorsal fin; AF, anal fin; CF, caudal fin; CP, caudal peduncle. (Image courtesy of S. Boylan.)

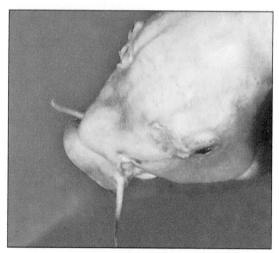

Figure 1.4 Maxillary barbels on the head of a common carp. These paired special sensory features are located near the mouth in some fish species and are associated with tactile and gustatory sensations. (Image courtesy of S.A. Smith.)

In many ways, the integument of fish is similar in general structure, composition and function to that of other animals. Skin covers the majority of the external body surface of fish with the exception of specialized areas like gills and sensory organs. Like the skin of terrestrial vertebrates, fish integument is composed of outer epidermal and underlying dermal layers. However, fish integument also exhibits some characteristically adaptive and distinguishing features. Most fish lack the outer keratinized, protective layer found in the skin of many other vertebrates. Instead, the epidermis contains an abundance of goblet cells that secrete a protective mucous layer covering the body surface of most fish (**Figure 1.5**). This slimy

exterior layer serves multiple functions largely related to protection and energy conservation in an aquatic environment. Fish mucous is composed largely of glycoproteins supplemented by a number of other bioactive substances such as immunoglobulins, lectins, enzymes and pheromones. Adaptive roles proposed for this outer mucous layer among fish include providing a physical barrier to protect skin surface and osmotic integrity, enhanced hydrodynamic capability, and enhanced disease resistance through first-line immune defense and toxin neutralization.[1] Species-specific adaptations of mucous are also evident; a prime example are some species of anemonefish with mucous that does not elicit stings from the nematocysts of their sea anemone hosts.[2] Another intriguing example of very specialized functionality of mucous occurs in some species of parrotfish and wrasses that produce nocturnal mucous cocoons that render protection against night-feeding ectoparasitic isopods.[3]

Another well-recognized feature of fish integument are the scales, the repeating platelike elements that originate in pockets of the dermis and cover the piscine body surface in various configurations (**Figures 1.6** and **1.7**). Scales are composed of bone, enamel, and dentin, and are covered by the epidermis. There is considerable diversity of scales among fish taxa related to their composition and appearance. There are the more subtle and toothlike placoid scales of sharks and other elasmobranchs, the large interlocking ganoid scales and bony scutes of some of the phylogenically lower bony fish like gars and sturgeon, and the elasmoid scales that may be

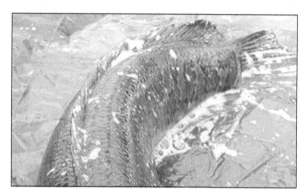

Figure 1.5 Mucous secretion from goblet cells of the skin of a northern snakehead fish (*Channa argus*).

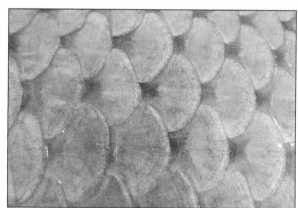

Figure 1.6 Large cycloid scales of an adult common carp (*Cyprinus carpio*).

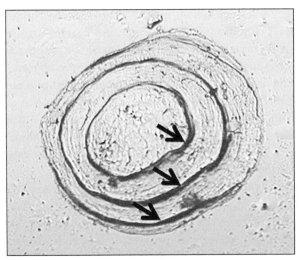

Figure 1.7 Single cycloid scale of a Chinook salmon (*Oncorhynchus tshawytscha*) fingerling. Note the "growth rings" that are often useful in age determination among scaled fish.

considered the typical fish scale.[4] Elasmoid scales are the most commonly present scale type among teleost fish, and they cover the body surfaces by partially overlapping in rows. Two subsets of elasmoid scales are cycloid scales with rounded posterior margins and ctenoid scales with toothlike posterior margins. Cosmoid scales, much like fused placoid scales, were present in some fossil fish species. Not all fish are equally scaly, however, and some species like the catfish lack scales altogether. Some other taxonomic groups like the seahorses and their kin (Syngnathids) are covered in bony plates instead of scales. Herring and anchovies among other groups may shed their scales, and scales in some species like the swordfish will disappear with age.[5] Modifications of scales are prominent and functional adaptations occur among many species. Examples would include the caudal fin spines of stingrays, the sharp caudal peduncle spines that are the namesake of the surgeonfish, and the erectable spikes that cover porcupinefish.

A unique hallmark of the skin of many fish is their coloration, resultant from the pigment cells, or chromatophores, contained in the dermis. Several types of chromatophores exist in fish skin, giving way to the potential for striking color patterns that serve aposematic (display) or cryptic functions for feeding, predator evasion, courtship, communication,

or other interactive aspects of their life history.[6] Chromatophores described in fish skin include melanophores (black), xanthophores (yellow), erythrophores (red), cyanophores (blue), leucophores (white, light scattering) and iridophores (silver, light reflecting). Chromatophores may also exhibit cellular motility in the integument, an adaptive feature that further enhances chromatic responses.[7] Development and change of coloration in piscine integument is a result of environmental cues creating neuroendocrine stimulation of the chromatophore populations.

SENSORY SYSTEMS

Sensory organs also may figure prominently among the external anatomy of fish. Like other vertebrates, most fish heavily utilize visual cues, and two eyes positioned laterally on the head are common features among most species. The anatomical and physiological principles of vision are largely the same among fish as for other animals, yet there are some unique aspects to fish ocular structure and function. Externally, most species do not have eyelids (although some sharks have nictitating membranes), and there is often a rostral indentation coupled by an elliptical shape to the eye that facilitates forward vision. The eyes of most fish also display adaptations related to enhanced visual acuity under water. As a general rule, the fish's cornea is relatively thinner than in terrestrial vertebrates and the lens is spherical rather than convex. These two adaptations serve to promote refractive power in the absence of an air–water interface at the cornea. Exceptions include some species of cartilaginous fish, as well as amphibious fish species with morphological adaptations of the cornea and lens suitable for visual acuity in both air and water. Photoreception among fish also displays notable differences both from terrestrial vertebrates, as well as among fish species dependent on visual cues in their environments. Both rods and cones exist in the fish retina, and the proportion and subtype of photoreceptor cells present depend largely on life history and typical aqueous light penetration to the habitat. For instance, deep sea and nocturnal fish will have a preponderance of rods for low visibility environments. Cones in fish also vary in their sensitivity to different wavelengths of light and, hence, color perception will also vary widely among species and is closely tied to both depth of habitat and the associated available electromagnetic spectrum of light.

Chemoreceptive ability is quite important among fish. As for other vertebrates, olfaction and gustation work in tandem in the fish for chemical perception of environmental cues. A pair of nares on the rostrum opens into the olfactory organs, which consist of olfactory epithelium intricately folded in rosettes and contained in blind-ended olfactory sacs. Olfactory cues are very common stimuli among fish for feeding, mating and homing behaviors. Taste buds containing gustatory receptor cells are sensory for taste. Among fish, the location of taste buds is variable and generally more extensive than among other animals. Fish taste buds are not restricted to the proximal alimentary tract, and generally do not exist on the tongue. They are usually distributed throughout the epithelial surfaces of the mouth (buccal cavity) and pharynx as well as in the opercular cavity along the gill rakers and arches and externally along fins and barbels. Some types of fish, including some catfish and cyprinids, have taste buds distributed all over the external body surface.[8,9] Chemical sensitivities through olfaction and gustation can be very keen among fish. For instance, amino acids may be detected at levels approaching 10^{-10} molar by many species.[10,11]

Auditory sensation in fish, while still based on the perception of sound waves, differs from that of terrestrial animals in many aspects. Fish have no external ears but rather rely on sound waves traveling through water and continuing through their tissues to reach the inner ear. In some fish, the swim bladder also plays a role in transmission of sound to the inner ear. Teleost fish with well-developed hearing (e.g., otophysans) have an intricate series of bones called the Weberian ossicles that conduct sound from the swim bladder to the inner ear, enhancing acoustical sensitivity. The inner ear of most fish contains three semicircular canals, each containing sensory hair cells and an otolith, or "ear stone." The otolith, the piscine equivalent to the mammalian otoconia, is composed mostly of calcium carbonate in an organic matrix.[12] Shape and size of otoliths vary both among species and with environmental parameters. Otoliths are widely used by fisheries biologists as a scientific tool to evaluate various aspects of life history including taxonomy, physiology, age determination, growth rates and environmental conditions.[13] Equilibrium and hearing are both functions of the relative motion of the otoliths and the mechanoreceptive hair cells. There appears to be considerable diversity in hearing ability among phylogenic groups, such as the ability to perceive and distinguish sounds at different frequencies; these are presumably closely related to differences in life history demands such as feeding and breeding behaviors.[14,15]

Another sensory organ based on mechanoreception and unique to fish and some amphibians is the lateral line system. The lateral line is a series of neuromasts, sensory units based on hair cells similar to those of the inner ear, embedded in a canal-like manner in the integument running bilaterally along the anteroposterior axis of the fish. In many of the more commonly encountered species, the lateral line is an apparent landmark running midway down the trunk in a relatively straight line. In some species, however, the lateral line may be more subtle or different in its shape or placement. Neuromasts may also be free-standing in fish skin independent of the lateral line formation or embedded in dermal bone of the fish's head.[15] Neuromasts function in sensory perception of hydrodynamically based stimuli, related to water movement over them in a unidirectional or oscillatory pattern. Neuromasts and the lateral line system represent key factors in how fish species interact with their surroundings through schooling behavior, response to prey or predators, and other environmental variables that are perceived as motion of water over the body surface.

Electroreception and magnetoreception are two other lessor known sensory attributes among some fish. Electroreception is noted among other groups of vertebrates including monotreme mammals and caudate amphibians as well as among many phylogeneic groups of fish. While sharks are widely recognized for their sensitivity to low-frequency electrical impulse detection of prey, many other species including catfish, sturgeons, lungfish, and ceolocanths similarly rely on electrical impulse detection.[16] Among fish with electrosensory perception, there are two general types of electroreceptors distributed in the skin of the head and trunk of fish.[17] Ampullary receptors detect low-frequency impulses produced by prey. The ampullae of Lorenzini, gel-filled canal-like organs in the skin open via pores and found on the snout of elasmobranchs, are examples. Tuberous receptors detect higher frequency alternating currents. These receptor organs are found in fish species like the infamous electric eel or the lesser known neotropical gymnotid fish that are capable of generating electrical impulses through electric organs that function in communication, defense or feeding behaviors.[16] Both types of electroreceptor organs contain groupings of sensory cells that respond to changes in electrical field with calcium ion flux across cell membranes activating sensory neurons.[15] Similarly, magnetoreception is postulated to occur among some species such as elasmobranchs, salmonid fish, and yellowfin tunas as a sensory adaptation useful for feeding, navigation, and homing behavior among some large pelagic fish. Although the physiology of magnetoreception among these species has not been definitively proven, electromagnetic and chemical-based mechanisms are theorized.[18]

RESPIRATORY SYSTEM

The gill, as the hallmark component of the piscine respiratory system is a defining feature of fish. Most fish species rely on a bilaterally paired set of gills to acquire oxygen from the water and remove carbon dioxide from the bloodstream in the respiratory process. The aqueous environment presents a challenge for oxygen acquisition as it contains roughly 30 times less oxygen compared to atmospheric air at sea level. The functional anatomy of the fish gill provides for efficient exchange of gases between water and circulating blood through two distinct mechanisms. First, the feather-like architecture of the gill provides substantial surface area for gas exchange. A fish weighing approximately a kilogram may have up to 18,000 cm^2 gill surface area for gas exchange.[19] Second, a countercurrent flow of water across the gill tissue with respect to direction of blood flow within the gill produces a consistent diffusion gradient that allows for maximal oxygen uptake from water and maximal CO_2 release into the water.

Gills are ubiquitous among fish species and are present throughout the entire life span of almost all species. Besides respiration, the gill has significant functions related to osmoregulation, ionoregulation and waste excretion among fish. Usually, the gills are located bilaterally on the posterior-most aspect of the head of a fish in a region known as the branchial chamber, or the opercular chamber. The branchial chambers are continuous with the mouth, or buccal chamber. In most species of bony fish, the exterior portion of the branchial chamber, through which ventilated water exits the body, is a flaplike cover known as the operculum. In other species, including most elasmobranchs, there is no operculum but rather a series of five to seven gill slits through which the effluent water passes. In these species, water is taken to the gill through either the mouth or the bilateral openings known as spiracles, located craniolaterally on pelagic species and dorsally on benthic species.[20] Most often, delivery of oxygenated water to gill capillaries relies on water flowing over the gill epithelium. Ram ventilation is used by some fast-swimming species, both elasmobranch and bony fish, to force water across the gill surfaces passively, rapidly, and sufficiently to ventilate them. Ram ventilation may be used only opportunistically by some species capable of it, or it may be used almost exclusively by some large pelagic predatory species like tuna and billfish.[21] More commonly, however, fish ventilate their gills by a coordinated expansion and contraction of the buccal and branchial chambers that pumps water across the gill surfaces.[22] Ventilation activity is often apparent in fish as bilateral opening and closing of the opercula, and respiratory rates of fish may be quantitatively evaluated through these opercular movements. Reversal of water flow across the gills may also be perceived as a "cough" that serves functionally to clear mucous and foreign matter from gill surfaces. Coughing behavior in fish may be useful as an indicator of disease or other physiological stress, as it is for terrestrial vertebrates.

Structurally, gill tissue is organized along bony or cartilaginous skeletal elements known as the gill arches. In most teleost fish species, there are four gill arches on each side of the head (**Figure 1.8**). The anterior side of the gill arch is formed of gill rakers, pointed protrusions that filter particulate matter from the water before it reaches the respiratory surfaces beyond. Gill rakers serve to protect the delicate gill tissue, and in some species, also may filter food items from the water column and direct them into

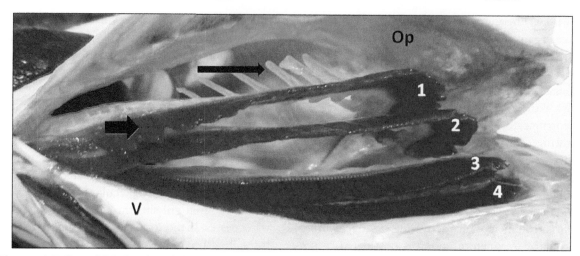

Figure 1.8 Branchial chamber (left side) of a rainbow trout. The four holobranchs associated with the four gill arches are numbered. The long arrow indicates the gill rakers on the leading or anterior side of the gill arch and the short arrow indicates the gill filaments on the trailing or posterior side. OP, operculum; V, ventral surface.

the alimentary canal. The posterior aspect of each gill arch supports two layers of gill filaments that orient perpendicularly to the long axis of the arch; each row is called a hemibranch and the two hemibranchs contained on a single arch are known as a holobranch (**Figure 1.9**). Branching from the gill filaments are the gill lamellae that represent the primary site of gas exchange. Gases diffusing through the thin epithelial layer of the lamellae are exchanged between the blood circulating through the lamellae and the water flowing through channels created by the interdigitating lamellar tissues. Numbers of lamellae present are not uniform among fish and will vary with species in relation to activity (oxygen demand) and the oxygen content of water in their habitat (oxygen supply). Most teleost fish also have a vestigial hemiarch known as the pseudobranch, which is located on the medial surface of the operculum in each branchial chamber and is morphologically divergent among species (**Figure 1.10**). Various physiological functions of the piscine pseudobranch

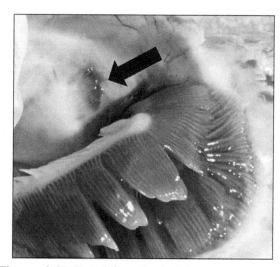

Figure 1.10 Pseudobranch of rainbow trout. Note the structural similarity between the pseudobranch on the medial aspect of the operculum (arrow) and the gill tissue in the branchial chamber. (Image courtesy of S.A. Smith.)

Figure 1.9 Individual holobranch removed from a rainbow trout gill. Gill rakers (white arrow), the gill arch (short black arrow), and the two hemibranchs (long arrows) are visible.

are postulated and include osmoregulatory, chemoregulatory, sensory and respiratory functions.[23] Provision of highly oxygenated blood to the choroid and retina of the eye is one of the more commonly theorized roles attributed to the pseudobranch.

Although the vast majority of piscine respiration is gill-dependent, there are taxa that acquire oxygen by other means. Cutaneous respiration occurs in many species of fish, especially in the larval stages.[24] Among some adult freshwater and marine teleosts, cutaneous respiration may still meet oxygen demands of the integumentary tissue. In others, such as the scaleless black bullhead catfish, the integument may additionally serve as a minor respiratory organ supplementing oxygen acquisition for the rest of the body as well.[25] Some fish species are also facultative or obligate air breathers. The lungfish, as the name implies, possess lungs homologous to those of tetrapods and are obligate air breathers. Other fish like gar, bowfin, and snakehead utilize the swim bladder and gulp air at the water's surface. In some species, such as the Asian catfish (*Pangasius hypothalamus*), a respiratory swim bladder functions as an air-breathing organ with alveolar-like architecture and associated vascularization for gas exchange (**Figure 1.11**).[26] Still other species like electric eels and some tropical catfish utilize other portions of the alimentary canal for oxygen uptake. In most of these species with specialization for oxygen extraction from air, carbon dioxide is still largely removed from circulating blood through gills.[24]

MUSCULOSKELETAL SYSTEM

The skeleton of fish, as for terrestrial vertebrates, provides structural support, protection of internal organs, and a basis for locomotor activity, albeit in an aqueous environment. In adult fish, skeletal elements are principally composed of either cartilage as in the elasmobranchs (class Chondrichthyes, also known as the cartilaginous fish) or bone in the class Osteichthyes, also known as the bony fish. Bone in fish, similar to bone in other animals, is mostly dermal or endochondral in origin. In some teleost species, the majority of the skeleton consists of acellular bone.[27] Persistence of the notochord in adults is another feature unique to some species; elasmobranchs, sturgeons and paddlefish are examples of fish that retain the notochord post embryonic development.[15]

The axial skeleton of fish includes the skull and vertebral column. Fish skulls are surprisingly complex and are comprised of a large number of individual bones that differ considerably among species.[28] For instance, the skull of the sea bream (*Sparus aurata*) is reported to contain 134 individual bones.[29] The neurocranium portion of the skull protects the brain, eyes, inner ears, and nares. The neurocranium anatomically includes four general subregions: the ethmoid, orbital, otic and basicranial regions, although the nomenclature varies.[15,28,30] The branchiocranium includes the mandibular region and the opercular and branchial skeletal elements that cover, protect, and mechanically support respiratory and other functions of the opercular chamber. The maxillary bones are uniquely structured to allow for upper jaw protrusion in feeding, a phylogenically distinguishing feature for teleost fish. Fish vertebrae are designated either precaudal or caudal, dependent on their location along the vertebral column. Generally, the precaudal vertebrae extend from the most proximal through the last rib-associated vertebrae, and the caudal vertebral segment immediately follows,

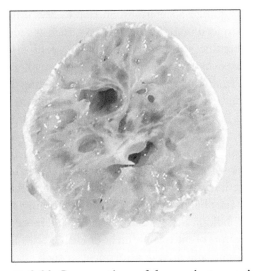

Figure 1.11 Cross sections of the respiratory swim bladder of the Asian catfish (*Pangasius hypothalamus*). Note the septate appearance and enhanced, alveolar-like surface area it provides as an adaptation for respiration. (Image of courtesy S.A. Smith.)

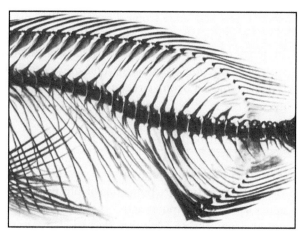

Figure 1.12 Whole fish (juvenile *Tilapia* sp.) stained with Alizarin Red and cleared with glycerin to show the typical separation of axial and appendicular skeletal elements among piscine species. (Image courtesy of S.A. Smith.)

extending distally to the tail. Besides ribs protecting the organs of the coelomic cavity, the axial skeleton of some teleost fish also includes intermuscular bones embedded in the myosepta of the body wall.[31] The last feature, figuratively and anatomically, of the piscine axial skeleton is the caudal complex, the modified caudal vertebrae and fin rays that provide structural support and oftentimes propulsive power to the fish's tail. The appendicular skeleton of a fish includes the pectoral and pelvic girdles that support the pectoral and pelvic fins. Unlike the appendicular skeletal elements of terrestrial vertebrates, these bones generally do not attach to the vertebral column of fish, although the pectoral girdle usually does attach to the skull through a posttemporal bone (**Figure 1.12**).[30] The position of the pelvic girdle is far more variable, as are the locations of the pelvic fins among fish species.

Muscle tissue of fish is categorized as skeletal, smooth, or cardiac, and performs the same general functions as described for other vertebrates. Skeletal muscle can also be further divided into white and red muscles that are biochemically suited for short bursts of activity or sustained activity, respectively. The majority of the muscle mass of fish is skeletal muscle located along the body wall supporting locomotor activity, most specifically related to propulsion through water. Skeletal muscle in most types of

fish is predominantly white muscle. White muscle is organized in discrete muscle bundles that are separated by connective tissue myosepta and divided into epaxial and hypaxial segments according to their location relative to the vertebrae on the horizontal axis (**Figure 1.13**). Between the epaxial and hypaxial musculature, there is also a smaller body of red muscle in many species. In some pelagic fish that perform sustained swimming activity such as the tuna or marlin, the red muscle is much more developed. Circulatory countercurrent exchange mechanisms for heat conservation in red muscle tissue are also noted among some of these pelagic species with highly metabolically active red muscle.[32]

GASTROINTESTINAL SYSTEM

Considerable diversity in foraging behavior and corresponding adaptations in the morphology and physiology of the digestive tract is evident among fish. Diet and foraging strategies among jawed fish species may be categorized in many ways, but may be summarized as four basic modes of food capture that include filter feeding, suction feeding, ram feeding, and biting.[33] Filter feeders like the anchovy, gizzard shad, or whale shark remove plankton or other small prey items from the water column by filtration through their gill rakers or similar adaptations. Suction feeders utilize suction to feed in many specific ways, such as vacuuming up benthic sediments, drawing in small organisms from rocky crevices, or slurping up a smaller pelagic fish from the water column. Ram feeding involves swimming open-mouthed through a concentration of food items or in pursuit of an individual larger prey item to be ingested whole. Biting to forage relies on singular or fused teeth for grabbing and tearing food items with bite force. Oftentimes, more than one of these mechanisms is utilized in a given species, and they may be quite intertwined in its feeding strategy. Morphologically, feeding strategies and more specific indicators of the trophic niche of a fish species are often apparent, and a large assortment of such adaptations may be noted among fish occupying a given habitat. For instance, the elongated proboscis of a butterflyfish allows for feeding among the nooks and crannies of a coral reef, whereas the beaklike mouth of a parrotfish is well suited for biting and scraping algae on

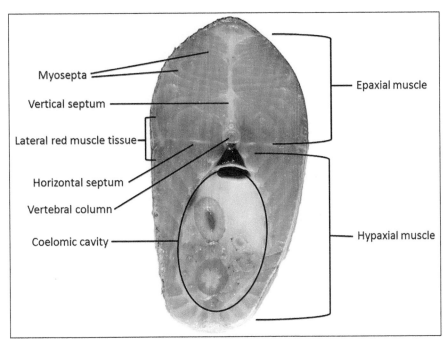

Figure 1.13 Transverse section of the trunk of a rainbow trout. Note the epaxial and hypaxial musculature and the myoseptal connective tissue surrounding and separating the muscle bundles.

the same reef. The familiar toothy grin of a barracuda or reef shark gives away its feeding behavior based on rapidly catching and biting down on prey, while the ventrally located mouth of goatfish is adaptive for benthic foraging. Teeth are present in many species and their presence, numbers, and morphology generally also reflect diet and foraging behavior. Besides the jaw, teeth may also be palatine (tongue), vomerine (roof of the mouth), or pharyngeal (pharynx) where they play an important part in crushing, shearing, and further subdividing prey items for digestion and directing them into the alimentary canal.

The foregut of fish consists of the esophagus and, in most species, the stomach. Generally, the esophagus is short, muscular, and highly pliable in species that swallow large prey items. Esophageal epithelium may also have an osmoregulatory role in euryhaline or marine species. Gastric morphology is more variable among fish, and many species such as some cyprinids lack a stomach altogether. A simple straight stomach is characteristic in a number of carnivorous species such as the pike and the halibut, yet other carnivores like the salmonid fish have a longer curving stomach shaped like a J or a U. Still other species, such as gizzard shad and surgeonfish, may

have a functional muscular "gizzard" in a portion of their stomach to aid in grinding action for digestion. Gastric mucosa secretes pepsin and hydrochloric acid to begin the digestion process in fish as for other vertebrates, and digesta passes through a pyloric sphincter into the intestine.

The intestine comprises the midgut and hindgut sections of the alimentary canal, yet there is little gross anatomical distinction between the two sections in most fish species other than a slightly greater diameter to the distal-most section. Unlike most vertebrates, there is no distinct anatomical or functional division into small and large intestine. Morphologically, the intestine is also highly variable among fish species. One of the more notable differences in this organ among fish is the overall length, ranging from approximately 20% to over 20 times the total body length.[34] Generally, carnivorous species have shorter intestines, whereas the intestine of herbivorous species may be quite long and convoluted (**Figures 1.14** and **1.15**). Looping of the midgut is common among fish with longer intestines, and patterns of intestinal coils can be taxonomically characteristic.[35] Functional aspects of the fish midgut and hindgut are similar to those of the intestine of other

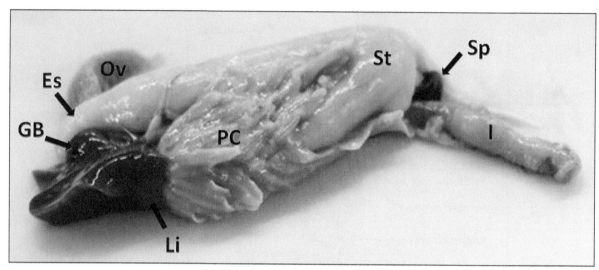

Figure 1.14 Gastrointestinal anatomy of the rainbow trout, a carnivorous fish with the characteristic J-shaped stomach and a short intestine with pyloric ceca. Es, esophagus; St, stomach; PC, pyloric ceca; I, intestine; Li, liver; GB, gallbladder; Ov, ovary; Sp, spleen.

vertebrates. Enzymatic digestion of chyme (partially digested food), absorption of nutrients, absorption of water and osmoregulation, and immunological defense are all important functions. Digestion and absorption in fish also rely on sufficient gut surface area through folding of intestinal mucosa into villi and the presence of microvilli on the enterocytes lining the gut lumen. Additional unique features that increase functional gut surface area among many fish species are the pyloric cecae, for example, blind-ended fingerlike pouches that originate from the proximal midgut. Pyloric ceca vary considerably in both number and appearance among species, and tend to be more developed in carnivorous fish with shorter guts.[36] Another unique feature of the gut among some fish is the spiral valve of the hindgut (**Figure 1.16**). Present in elasmobranchs and some of the bony fish including sturgeon and paddlefish, the

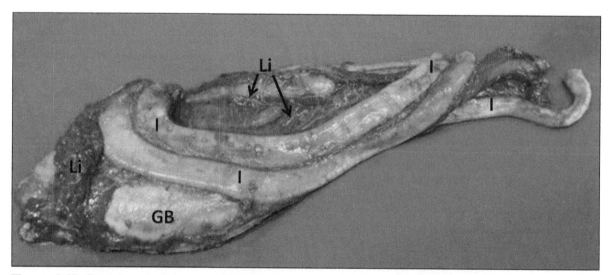

Figure 1.15 Gastrointestinal anatomy of the common carp, an herbivore. Its gastrointestinal tract is characterized by lack of a stomach and a comparatively long spiral intestine. I, intestine; Li, liver; GB, gallbladder.

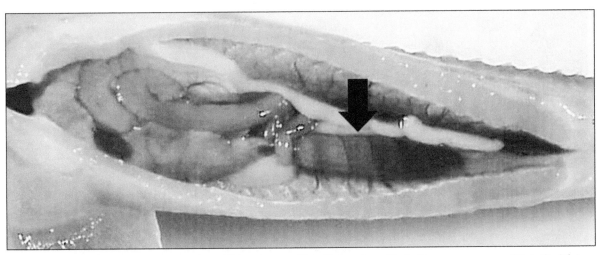

Figure 1.16 Spiral valve of a juvenile pallid sturgeon (*Scaphirhynchus albus*). (Image courtesy of S.A. Smith.)

spiral valve is a structural variation of the hindgut with a large diameter and an internal configuration of spiraling epithelium that effectively increases surface area for digestive processes.[37] The gastrointestinal tract of fish terminates in the cloacal or anal opening located caudoventrally in most species.

As in other vertebrate animals, the liver of fish is associated with digestion through the production of bile. Many species of fish also have a gallbladder that collects and holds bile from the hepatic tissues and transports it to the midgut through a bile duct. Likewise, the fish liver is also highly active metabolically and serves a number of other functions related to energy storage and regulation, metabolite biotransformation and cellular detoxification, and immunological response. Anatomically, the fish liver may vary considerably in appearance (**Figures 1.17** and **1.18**). In many species, it is large and multilobed, positioned in the anterior part of the coelomic cavity near the stomach and midgut. Many species have two distinct liver lobes, whereas in other species the liver is more diffusely located in the abdomen with multiple smaller hepatic tissue segments interdigitating with intestine, mesentery, and adipose tissue. Normal color, size and even texture of the liver are quite variable among species of fish, as well as within species and even potentially within the same individual animal over the course of its life. These characteristics are highly dependent on variables such as nutritional status, current levels of energy (i.e., glycogen and fat) stores, and other changing factors. Because of this

variability in "normal," a health assessment of the piscine liver may oftentimes be difficult to perform, grossly or histologically, without some additional frame of reference or basis for comparison.

The pancreas of fish has histologically distinguishable exocrine and endocrine components that perform the same general function as in other vertebrates through the production of digestive enzymes, insulin and glucagon. The pancreas is usually diffusely embedded in mesentery and adipose tissue, except in a few taxonomic groups like eels in which a distinct organ is grossly apparent.[33] In some fish, the exocrine pancreatic tissue is diffusely located within the liver tissue, and the organ though historically known as the hepatopancreas is more appropriately termed an intrahepatic pancreas.

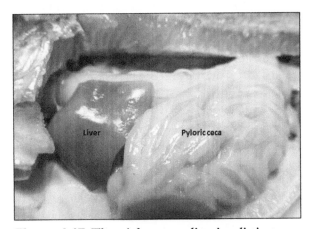

Figure 1.17 The rainbow trout liver is a distinct lobe in the anterior portion of the coelomic cavity. (Image courtesy of E. Nadenbousch.)

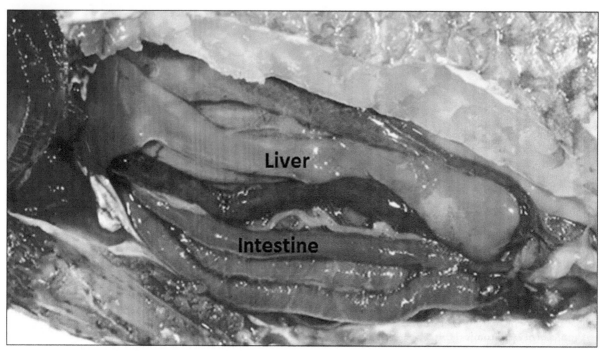

Figure 1.18 The elongated liver of the tilapia (hybrid *Tilapia* sp.). Comparatively, the common carp liver is more diffusely spread throughout the coelomic cavity, as seen in Figure 1.15. (Image courtesy of S.A. Smith.)

Many groups typically have an intrahepatic pancreas, including many species of catfish, tilapia, and cyprinids.

Another piscine organ of considerable importance, the swim bladder, is embryologically derived from the gastrointestinal tract yet does not function as a digestive organ but rather as a hydrostatic organ affecting buoyancy. The swim bladder, also known as the air bladder or gas bladder, is a gas-filled, balloon-like organ generally consisting of one large chamber or two interconnecting chambers located dorsally against the peritoneum of the coelomic cavity (**Figures 1.19** and **1.20**). This organ is not present in elasmobranch and some other groups, including many benthic species of bony fish. Carbon dioxide, oxygen and nitrogen gases largely make up the gas contents of the swim bladder, although they are not necessarily found in the same concentrations as in the environmental air.[15] Volumetric changes to the swim bladder allow for changes in buoyancy of the fish. There are two subtypes of swim bladder, physostomous and physoclistous, which differ physiologically in how the gas volume is adjusted. A physostomous swim bladder has a pneumatic duct that physically connects the chamber to the foregut, and gas is taken in or released through the alimentary canal and "air gulping" behavior. Most of the taxonomically higher teleost fish lose the patency of the pneumatic duct as adults, and swim bladder volume is controlled through vascular gas exchange in the physoclistous swim bladder. The physoclistous swim bladder also contains a gas gland and a rete mirabile that utilize pH-based gas solubility and countercurrent gas exchange principles to affect blood gases and their concentration within the chamber (**Figure 1.21**).[38]

CIRCULATORY SYSTEM

Fish have closed circulatory systems to circulate blood throughout the tissues for oxygenation and waste removal. Fish blood has much in common with that of other poikilothermic vertebrate species. It consists predominantly of plasma and mature, nucleated erythrocytes, and it also circulates the leukocytes and thrombocytes important to immune function and hemostasis. The oxygen-carrying capacity of fish blood is hemoglobin-based, as hemoglobin-bound O_2 is transported within the

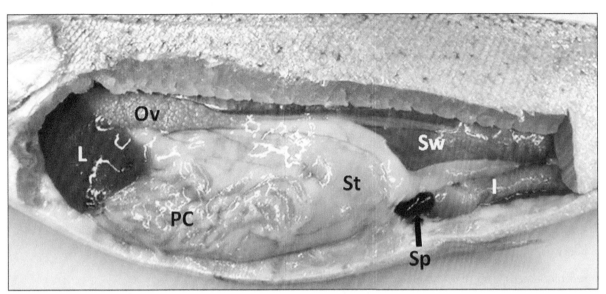

Figure 1.19 Typical morphology and location of the swim bladder and other coelomic organs of a rainbow trout. Although the swim bladder in most fish species is generally located along the dorsal extent of the coelomic cavity, anatomical differences exist among species, including the presence of one single chamber seen here in the trout as opposed to the two connected chambers found in some other species. SW, swim bladder; St, stomach; PC, pyloric ceca; I, intestine; L, liver; Ov, ovary; Sp, spleen.

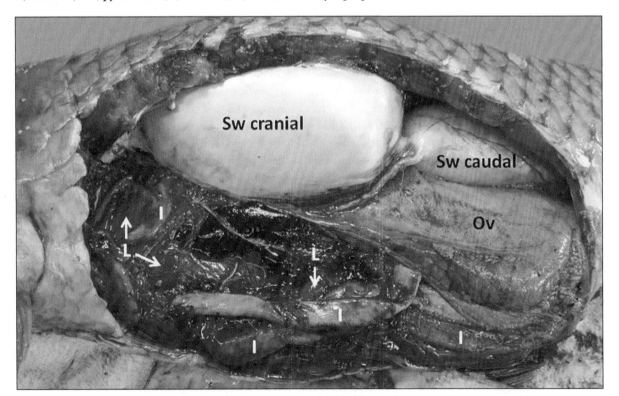

Figure 1.20 Typical morphology and location of the swim bladder and other coelomic organs of a common carp. Note the connected cranial and caudal chambers of the swim bladder present in this species. SW, swim bladder; I, intestine; L, liver; Ov, ovary.

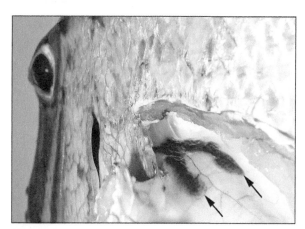

Figure 1.21 Rete mirabile in the swim bladder of a porgy (family Sparidae). (Image courtesy of S. Boylan.)

red blood cells, and to a lesser degree, as dissolved oxygen in the blood plasma. Carbon dioxide waste carried by blood from the tissues is largely transported in the form of the bicarbonate anion with a small portion remaining as dissolved CO_2 in plasma.

The vascular system of fish is a simple loop circuit with blood passing through the heart, directly through the gills for oxygenation, then through systemic circulation and returning to the heart. The heart serves as the principal pump to circulate blood, although accessory mechanisms like skeletal muscle compression of vessels are found in some species, particularly related to venous circulation.[39] Other species like the hagfish also have accessory hearts.[40] The size of a fish's heart as a function of total body mass is usually considerably smaller when compared to mammals and other vertebrates, but this is quite variable depending on life history demands of fish species. In particular, comparative ventricular mass varies greatly and may even approach that of some mammals for some highly active pelagic fish.[39] The fish heart rate is also generally lower than for endothermic vertebrates, although this too varies with life history and energy demands. Resting heart rates among fish are known to vary from the teens to nearly 100 beats per minute.[41]

A fish heart usually has two chambers, the atrium and ventricle in series, unlike the mammalian heart with four chambers in two parallel circuits (**Figure 1.22**). The sinus venosus is an additional thin-walled sac that receives venous blood from circulation. Blood from the sinus venosus passes into the atrium, a contractile chamber capable of holding a comparatively

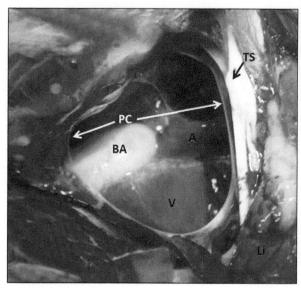

Figure 1.22 Heart and surrounding tissues in a common carp. PC, pericardium; BA, bulbous arteriosus; A, atrium; V, ventricle; TS, transverse septum; Li, liver.

large volume of blood.[41] Blood flows from the atrium into the ventricle, a comparably thick-walled chamber that is morphologically variable among fish (**Figure 1.23**). The ventricle consists of both spongy and compact myocardium, varying in presence and proportional amount among species. In most fish hearts, the last compartment in sequence is the bulbous arteriosus, an elasticized receiving cavity that dampens the blood pressure oscillations of the heart, resulting in a steadier continuous blood flow as opposed to the pulsed flow occurring in higher vertebrates.[39] Equivalent to the bulbous arteriosus, the conus arteriosus is the last compartment of the heart among elasmobranchs and some other species, differing in both its barrel-like shape and the presence of cardiac muscle (**Figure 1.24**).[15] Heart valves function among fish to support unidirectional blood flow throughout the heart.

From the heart, blood flows through the afferent branchial arteries to be oxygenated in the gills. Oxygenated blood leaves the gills via the efferent branchial arteries that merge to form the dorsal aorta, a vessel that runs nearly the length of the fish's body. From the dorsal aorta, circulating blood reaches the tissues through subdividing arteries, arterioles, and capillary networks. Blood, including CO_2 diffused

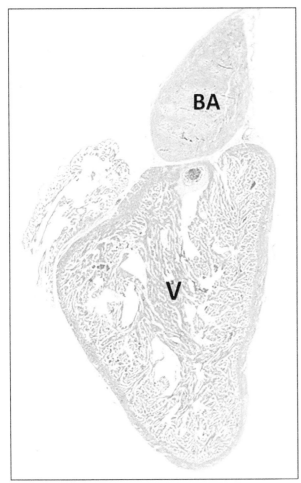

Figure 1.23 Transverse section of heart from a rainbow trout. Note the bulbous arteriosus (BA) and the spongy myocardium in the ventricle (V). H&E stain. (Image courtesy of S.A. Smith.)

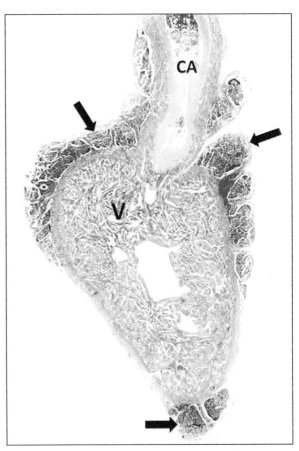

Figure 1.24 Transverse section of heart from a pallid sturgeon. Note the spongy myocardium in the ventricle (V), similar to the rainbow trout heart in Figure 1.22. In contrast, the sturgeon has a conus arteriosus (CA) as the last heart chamber. Also present along the epicardial surface of the sturgeon heart are aggregates of pericardial lymphoid tissue (arrows). H&E stain. (Image courtesy of S.A. Smith.)

from cells, returns to the heart through venous circulation reaching the postcardinal vein running parallel to the long axis of the fish and emptying into the sinus venosus. Two venous portal systems are present among most fish, including the renal portal and hepatic portal systems. Returning venous blood from the tail and posterior abdominal region of fish including integument and musculature passes through the renal portal system within the kidneys. Similarly, venous blood returning from the abdominal viscera flows through the hepatic portal vein and hepatic sinusoids in the liver before emptying into the duct of Cuvier (also known as the common cardinal vein) and the sinus venosus.

In some species, including the elasmobranchs, there exists a secondary circulatory system that functions to disseminate blood in parallel though vascular anastomoses. This secondary circulation through these vessels serves a number of tissues including integument and peritoneum. Blood circulating here differs from primary circulation with lower flow rates and lower hematocrit levels, although total secondary circulating volume may be greater.[19] Though its functional significance is not entirely clear, this secondary circulation may represent a progenitor stage of the lymphatic system of higher vertebrates.[42]

EXCRETORY AND IONOREGULATORY SYSTEMS

The excretion of metabolic wastes is a complex and varied process among fish species and is very closely linked with osmoregulation and ionoregulation. Most fish are not isosmotic with their surrounding aqueous environment. Osmoregulation is energetically expensive for fish, requiring up to half of the total energy output for some species.[19] Freshwater and seawater provide vastly different challenges for fish related to maintenance of body fluid and ion balances in the face of substantial environmental gradients, and the physiological mechanisms used to maintain these balances and excrete waste products vary accordingly. Typically, the gill and the kidney are the two most important organs of fish related to excretion and osmoregulation. Most fish produce ammonia as the predominant nitrogenous waste product, and this is excreted by diffusion across gill epithelium, and to a lesser extent through urine produced in the kidney. Fish also produce urea as nitrogenous waste, excreted through both gill and kidney to a lesser extent. Elasmobranchs are an exception in that urea is produced in relatively larger quantities and also serves an osmoregulatory function. Urea concentration in elasmobranch blood plasma is sufficiently high as to allow for osmoconformation with their saltwater environments.[43] The gill is also functionally critical to ionoregulation via ion transport (predominantly sodium, potassium, and chloride) between blood and water across its epithelial surface.

The kidney varies morphologically among species, but is generally a distinct organ located retroperitoneally (or, more correctly, retrocoelomically) along the dorsal aspect of the coelomic cavity just ventral to the vertebral column. Kidney (renal) tissue may appear divided into segments longitudinally (left and right) or transversely (cranial and caudal) depending on the species. There are three different gross morphologies seen in the freshwater fish kidney. Type I has the two sides of the kidney fused throughout its length with no distinctions between the anterior and posterior kidney; type II has a middle and posterior section of the kidney that are fused with a clear gross distinction between the

anterior and posterior kidney; and type III has only the posterior section that is fused with two separate branches of the anterior portion and a clear distinction between the anterior and posterior kidney. Marine fish have examples of the first three types of kidneys in various species with two additional morphologies: Type IV has only the distal portion of the posterior kidney fused with an anterior kidney that is not recognizable, and type V that has completely separate left and right kidneys.[44] Ontogenically, the kidney is divided into the cranial pronephros (e.g., anterior kidney), which in the adult fish serves as a lymphoid organ, and the caudal opisthonephros (e.g., posterior kidney), which largely maintains the excretory function. In some species, the two regions are physically distinct and in other species they are contiguous (**Figures 1.25** and **1.26**). A healthy kidney appears uniformly deep red in color. Scattered among the renal tissue of many species are the corpuscles of Stannius, or the Stannian corpuscles, appearing grossly as discrete, pale oval to irregular nodules (**Figure 1.27**). The corpuscles of Stannius are aggregates of endocrine tissue that function in calcium metabolism.[45]

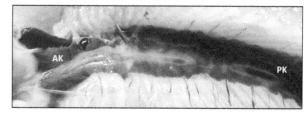

Figure 1.25 Anterior and posterior kidney tissues are contiguous in some species such as the rainbow trout. AK, anterior kidney; PK, posterior kidney.

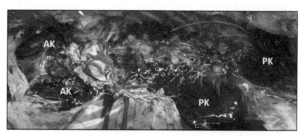

Figure 1.26 Anterior and posterior kidney tissues are discrete and separate in some species such as the common carp. AK, anterior kidney; PK, posterior kidney.

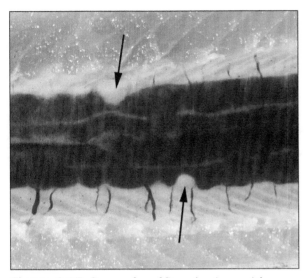

Figure 1.27 Corpuscles of Stannius (arrows) in a rainbow trout. (Image courtesy of S.A. Smith.)

Histologically, the functional unit of the excretory kidney of fish is the nephron. Although very similar in structure and function to the nephron of higher vertebrates, there are some distinguishing features of the fish nephron. First, there is no loop of Henle present, which limits the fish's capacity to hyperconcentrate urine, and as a result fish cannot produce urine hypertonic to their blood.[43] Second, the presence of glomeruli is not universal among species. Aglomerular kidneys are common among marine teleosts, functionally reducing the potential loss of water to the hypertonic environment. By contrast, a greater volume of urine is excreted among freshwater species, an adaptation to maintain fluid balance in a hypotonic environment. In most cases, the histological structure of the fish kidney is a function of its habitat; that is, freshwater fish have more elaborate, well-developed, multisegmental nephrons, whereas most marine fish have comparatively simple renal tubules. Marine sharks and skates have zonate kidneys with complicated countercurrent arrangements in their early and late nephrons to allow for the retention of urea.[46] Besides osmoregulation and nitrogenous waste excretion, the fish nephron is functionally important in ionoregulation of divalent cations such as calcium and magnesium.

Urine produced by kidneys is transported through ureters or mesonephric ducts. In many species, a widening of the distal mesonephric duct functions as a urinary bladder for urine storage prior to release.[47] The urinary bladder in some species may also have a role in osmoregulation as water, salts, and other substances may be resorbed through the epithelium to maintain fluid and ion balance.[43]

The integument and gastrointestinal system, with a vast surface area in contact with the external environment, also play an important role in osmoregulation and ionoregulation among fish. The rectal gland is a small organ that connects via a duct to the rectum distal to the spiral valve of elasmobranchs. It is a specialized secretory organ that produces sodium and chloride in concentrations significantly greater than both plasma and surrounding seawater to facilitate their elimination for fluid homeostasis.[48]

REPRODUCTIVE SYSTEM

Reproductive strategy among fish reflects species diversity and is quite wide-ranging. Although the majority of species are gonochoristic (separate sexes) and oviparous (females laying eggs to be externally fertilized by males), this strategy is not universal. There are many fish that are either synchronous or sequential hermaphrodites, reproduce via internal fertilization, and are live-bearing. Among most species, fecundity (eggs produced) is high and parental care of the young is minimal to absent. Still, there are many species of fish that provide parental care through behaviors such as nest building, guarding larva, or mouth brooding. Sexual dimorphism among reproducing adults is apparent among many fish, although far from universal. Among many species, there is no reliable way to grossly distinguish males from females, while in others, size and body conformation, coloration, or morphological differences that are externally evident will allow gender to be easily distinguished in mature fish (**Figures 1.28** and **1.29**). Oftentimes dimorphic features are only evident or become more striking when fish are reproductively mature or approaching spawning. Sexual dimorphism may be quite obvious among some species, such as the anal fin that functions as a gonopodium for mating in male livebearer fish

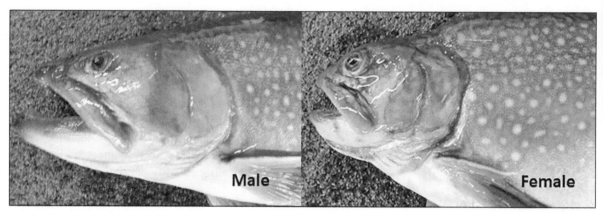

Figure 1.28 Sexual dimorphism among fish. Males and females of a given species may oftentimes be distinguished grossly based on one or more characteristics. In the brook trout (*Salvelinus fontinalis*), body conformation is a distinguishing feature. Note the elongated hooklike prominence known as a kype on the lower jaw of the male as compared to the female.

like guppies and swordtails. Among other species, dimorphism may be far more subtle, such as the more pointed dorsal fin among the males of most gourami species.[49]

The gonads that produce gametes among fish are equivalent to those of higher vertebrates. Likewise, gonadal development and function among fish is intricately related to the endocrine system and the regulatory effects of hormones, and largely parallels these effects in higher vertebrates. Ovaries of fish are usually paired and elongated, found in the posterior to mid-posterior area of the dorsal coelomic cavity (**Figures 1.30** and **1.31**). In some species, the paired ovaries fuse to form a single organ, or one ovary develops while the other does not to yield a single functional ovary. The ovaries appear clear to pale pink, yellow or orange, and developing ova are often grossly visible in the ovary, giving it a bumpy appearance. Ovary size is dependent on sexual maturity and the reproductive stage of development. The ovary of a mature, ripe female fish may represent over 50% of her total body weight (**Figure 1.32**).[50] Among most species of teleosts, the ovocoel, or ovarian lumen, will hold the ripe eggs until spawning, when they are released through the genital pore at the cloaca. Exceptions include the salmonid fish in which mature eggs are released freely into the abdominal cavity prior to spawning.

Testes of male fish are also internally located, usually in the caudodorsal portion of the coelomic cavity. They are generally paired, elongated, tubular and clear to white in color (**Figure 1.33**). Testes may be readily apparent among sexually mature male fish near spawning. Testes may also be hidden

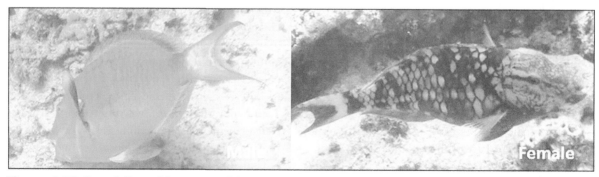

Figure 1.29 Sexual dimorphism among fish. Among some species like the stoplight parrotfish (*Sparisoma viride*), the color patterns may be distinctly different between males and females.

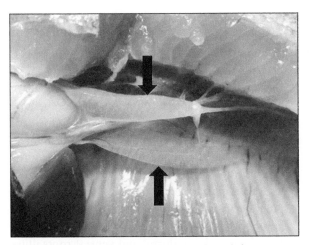

Figure 1.30 Immature ovaries of the rainbow trout.

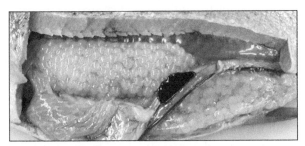

Figure 1.31 Mature ovarian tissue of the rainbow trout.

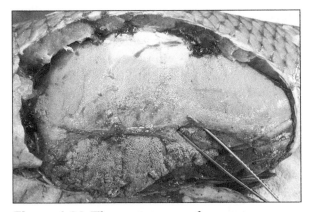

Figure 1.32 The mature ovary of a common carp.

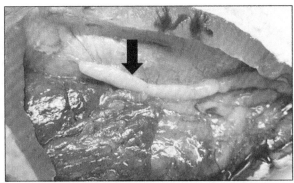

Figure 1.33 Mature testes of a largemouth bass (*Micropterus salmoides*).

cloaca. Again, salmonids are an example of an exception, and milt containing mature sperm is released into the abdominal cavity, then released externally at spawning through abdominal pores.[50]

Ovoviviparity and viviparity occur among groups of teleost fish, but to a far lesser degree among species. Less than 3% of teleost species are estimated to be live-bearing.[51] Among elasmobranchs, internal fertilization is the rule, occurring in roughly 60% of species.[51,52] This is reflected anatomically, as male elasmobranchs have tubular modifications of their pelvic fins called claspers that transfer sperm to the female oviduct. Internal fertilization may then be followed by oviparous development (external egg laying), or internal development of the offspring through either ovoviviparity (aplacental) or viviparity (placental). The female reproductive tract may be likewise modified to accommodate internal development among these species, including the presence of a uterus and cervix.[53]

NERVOUS SYSTEM

Piscine nervous systems are physiologically and morphologically consistent with those of other vertebrate animals, composed of central and peripheral subsystems that operate through neuronal activity. The central nervous system consists of the brain encased in the neurocranium, and the spinal cord is located in the neural canal of the vertebral column. In most species, the spinal cord extends from the caudal aspect of the brain and runs the length of the fish's body. Exceptions include the ocean sunfish

by visceral fat, and be subtle or difficult to identify among some species or among immature fish. In mature males that are pre-spawning, the testes may represent up to 10% of the total body weight.[50] Male gamete maturation takes place in the lobules of the testes. In most species, mature spermatozoa are carried through sperm ducts to the genital pore at the and the anglerfish in which the spinal cord is considerably reduced in length.[54] Also as in other vertebrates, the central nervous system is covered by meninges, although only a single meningeal layer is present in fish. The meningeal space and the ventricular system of the brain are continuous with the central canal of the spinal cord and contain cerebrospinal fluid.

The adult fish brain's relative size is smaller than the adult mammalian brain, although it is generally comparable to relative brain size for amphibians or reptiles.[19] Still, there is a considerable amount of difference in brain development relative to defined regions among fish, and these differences tend to mirror sensory and motor functional needs pertaining to life history.[55] On average, the elasmobranchs also tend to have comparatively larger brain size relative to body size when compared to teleost fish.

There are five distinct regions of the fish brain: telencephalon, diencephalon, mesencephalon, metencephalon and myelencephalon (**Figure 1.34**). The telencephalon, the most anterior portion of the fish brain, is the equivalent of the cerebrum in higher vertebrates. It is largely associated with the sense of olfaction, and a substantial portion of this region is comprised of the olfactory lobe in most species. The diencephalon is generally located posteriodorsally to the telencephalon. It contains the pineal body, which plays a prominent role in light detection related to many physiological and behavioral aspects of piscine life history, especially related to circadian rhythms

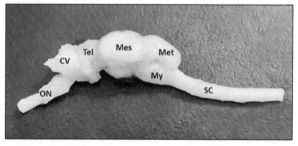

Figure 1.34 Brain of rainbow trout. Distinct regions of this brain (lateral view) are evident including the telencephalon (Tel), mesencephalon (Mes), metencephalon (Met), and myelencephalon (My). The optic nerve (ON) and proximal spinal cord (SC) are also visible, as well as a fragment of the cranial vault (CV) around the intact brain.

and endocrine functions.[56] The mesencephalon functions largely in processing of sensory input, especially optic input. The metencephalon contains the cerebellum, which functions in maintaining equilibrium and motor coordination. In some species that utilize electroreceptive sensation, the cerebellum is also specifically adapted to process this information as well. The myelencephalon is the brainstem, also known as the rhombencephalon, which is continuous with the spinal cord.

The peripheral nervous system is composed of the spinal nerves and the majority of the cranial nerves. Peripheral spinal nerves emerge from the spinal cord along its length via dorsal and ventral roots. There is variability among fish taxa regarding the number and functional significance of cranial nerves, yet in general terms, their functions parallel those of other vertebrates. There may be as many as 22 distinct cranial nerves in a fish with either a sensory, motor, or combined role.[57] Like other vertebrates, fish also possess an autonomic nervous system that controls the action of involuntary smooth muscles in viscera. Autonomic nerves of teleost fish also regulate color change through innervation of skin pigment cells.

ENDOCRINE SYSTEM

The piscine endocrine system is functionally very similar to those of other vertebrates with respect to the organs involved and the various hormones they produce. Still, there are some very unique aspects to piscine endocrinology. The hypothalamus and pituitary gland function in concert to produce a large number of hormones that regulate growth, metabolic, and reproductive development and function. Similarly, hormones produced by the thyroid gland, the pancreas, and the gonads largely mirror their physiological roles in higher vertebrates.

Although fish do not have adrenal glands per se, they do possess endocrine tissues that perform the equivalent functions. Interrenal tissue of fish is equivalent to the adrenal cortex of higher vertebrates. Located diffusely within the head kidney of teleosts, the interrenal tissue secretes steroids, mainly cortisol, in response to corticotropic action of ACTH and other stimulating hormones. Chromaffin cells are the equivalent of the adrenal medulla and secrete catecholamines. Among teleosts, the chromaffin tissue is generally closely associated with the interrenal cells in the head kidney. In elasmobranchs, the two tissues are physically separated. The interrenal gland is a distinct organ located dorsally between the two lateral lobes of kidney, and the chromaffin cells are located segmentally along the dorsal aspect of the kidney.[58] Both the corticosteroids and catecholamines serve equivalent functions among fish as compared to higher vertebrates, although cortisol in fish performs functions equivalent to those of both glucocorticoids and mineralocorticoids of other animals.[59]

Other endocrine organs of fish perform more unique or specialized functions not noted as extensively among other vertebrate species. The pineal gland, a neuroendocrine organ located dorsally on the diencephalon, is one such example that is found among most all fish species. Although present among all classes of vertebrates, the pineal gland seems to be of greater importance to circadian rhythm and associated functions among fish and the other classes as compared to mammals.[60] Also known as the pineal organ or the epiphysis, the pineal gland is photosensory and secretes melatonin that functions in circadian-based physiology. Locomotor activity, growth, thermal preference and skin pigmentation changes are among the physiological variables in fish that are potentially affected by the pineal gland's secretion of melatonin.[56,61]

The caudal neurosecretory system is a neuroendocrine organ unique to the jawed fish. It is located at the caudal aspect of the spinal cord and consists of neurosecretory cells known as Dahlgren cells that synthesize urotensin hormones. Among teleost species, the Dahlgren cells form a distinct neurohemal organ known as the urophysis. Urotensin 1 and urotensin 2, the two major hormones produced, appear to have physiological activity related to osmoregulation and saltwater adaptation, as well as influence upon smooth muscle activity of visceral organs, reproductive function, and other homeostatic mechanisms among fish.[62]

Fish also possess specialized endocrine organs related to calcium regulation. The ultimobranchial body is a glandular organ secreting calcitonin. It is derived from the last pair of pharyngeal bodies, and among adult fish the ultimobranchial bodies are located near the esophagus or heart. The corpuscles of Stannius, as previously noted, are distributed within or alongside the excretory kidney in teleost and holostean fish. The corpuscles of Stannius produce stanniocalcin, a hormone that regulates calcium uptake among fish, particularly teleosts. Stanniocalcin is a calcium channel blocker that reduces calcium uptake from the gill and gut among both freshwater and saltwater species of teleosts. Secretion of stanniocalcin appears to be regulated by the extracellular concentration of Ca^{2+}.[63] Calcitonin function among fish is not as definitively established, although a similar role in the down-regulation of calcium uptake by gills is probable.[64,65] Osteoblast activity and bone development as well as ovarian development and spawning have been associated with calcitonin production.[59,66]

IMMUNE SYSTEM

Functional immunology among fish is comparable to higher vertebrates in many respects. The piscine immune response is composed of both nonspecific and specific immunological responses, and involves both humoral and cell-mediated activities. Inflammatory responses to infection and injury as well as immunological hypersensitivity reactions also occur among fish. Many organs with a role in lymphoid function are known among elasmobranchs and bony fish. Fish possess neither bone marrow nor lymph nodes, yet a number of other organs fulfill the roles of lymphopoiesis and antigen presentation among other fish species.

A first line of immunological defense is represented by the epithelial surfaces of the skin and the mucosal surfaces of internal organs. More specifically, the mucus layer that coats these surfaces contains a number of immunologically active substances including immunoglobulins, complement, lectins and lysozymes that function protectively.[1] Additionally, mucosal-associated lymphoid tissue (MALT) and gut-associated lymphoid tissue (GALT) are lymphoid aggregates found along gut and other internal organ mucosal surfaces and play a role in antigen presentation and associated immune response.[19] A few species, including the sturgeon and paddlefish, have lymphomyeloid tissues associated with the heart as well.[67,68] Sturgeon pericardial lymphoid tissue consists of lymph node–like aggregates visible along the heart's epicardial surface (**Figure 1.24**).

The thymus, anterior kidney, and spleen all have a prominent role in immune function among teleost fish. The thymus is generally located dorsally under the operculum in the branchial chamber. It consists largely of lymphocytes, and its persistence and role in adult fish varies considerably with species, among other factors. The thymus involutes among adults of some species but is known to remain throughout their life span in others.[69] Renal tissue has a large role in immune function, and the anterior kidney in particular is composed largely of immunocytes and appears to be functionally equivalent to bone marrow among teleost fish. Besides hematopoiesis, antigen presentation and processing, cellular phagocytosis, and immunoglobulin production are all immune functions that occur in renal tissue. Among elasmobranchs, however, renal tissue does not appear to have a hematopoietic role beyond embryonic developmental stages. In these fish, two additional lymphoid organs known as the epigonal and Leydig's organ are found, with one or both of them present in a given species. The epigonal organ is located near the reproductive tissues, and Leydig's organ in the esophageal lining.[70]

The spleen is present among almost all species of bony fish and elasmobranchs, serving as a focus of hematopoiesis, antigen presentation and processing, lymphocyte proliferation and activation, and cellular phagocytosis. Located in the ventral coelomic cavity near the gastrointestinal tract, the spleen may be readily apparent, or encased and hidden by visceral adipose tissue. Among elasmobranchs, the spleen tends to be more elongated than among teleosts.[19] With a central role in immune function, its size and appearance are often good indicators of health and infection status among fish. A healthy spleen is usually grossly deep red in color and smooth in appearance. Splenic enlargement, nodular lesions, or color change may accompany many systemic infectious diseases in fish.

Blood represents another very important tissue with immunological function, as leukocytes and immunologically active molecules like immunoglobulin, complement, and cytokines among others are carried in the blood stream. Fish possess many types of leukocytes, including lymphocytes, granulocytes, monocytes/macrophages, and thrombocytes.[70] Subtypes of leukocytes as well as their morphology and functional significance vary considerably among species.[71]

REFERENCES

1. Shephard, K.L. Functions for fish mucus. *Reviews in Fish Biology and Fisheries* 1994;4:401–429.
2. Mebs, D. Chemical biology of the mutualistic relationships of sea anemones with fish and crustaceans. *Toxicon* 2009;54:1071–1074.
3. Grutter, A.S., Rumney, J.G., Sinclair-Taylor, T., Waldie, P. and Franklin, C.E. Fish mucous cocoons: The "mosquito nets" of the sea. *Biology Letters* 2011;7:292–294.
4. Sire, J. and Akimenko, M. Scale development in fish: A review, with description of *sonic hedgehog (shh)* expression in the zebrafish (*Danio rerio*). *International Journal of Developmental Biology* 2004;48:233–247.
5. Nakamura, I. *FAO Species Catalogue, Vol. 5. Billfishes of the World: An Annotated and Illustrated Catalogue of Marine Sailfishes, Spearfishes and Swordfishes Known to Date.* FAO Fisheries Synopsis No. 125, 1985.
6. Fujii, R. and Oshima, N. Factors influencing motile activities of fish chromatophores. In: *Advances in Comparative and Environmental Physiology 20*. R. Gilles, ed. Springer-Verlag, Berlin, 1994; pp. 1–54.
7. Fujii, R. The regulation of motile activity in fish chromatophores. *Pigment Cell Research* 2000;13:300–309.
8. Caprio, J., Brand, J.G., Teeter, J.H., Valentincic, T., Kalinoski, D.L., Kohbara, J., Kumazawa, T. and Wegert, S. The taste system of the channel catfish: From biophysics to behavior. *Trends in Neurosciences* 1993;16:192–197.
9. Gomahr, A., Palzenberger, M., Kotrschal, K. Density and distribution of external taste buds in cyprinids. *Environmental Biology of Fishes* 1992;33:125–134.
10. Caprio, J. High sensitivity of catfish taste receptors to amino acids. *Comparative Biochemistry and Physiology Part A: Physiology* 1975;52:247–251.
11. Hara, T.J. The diversity of chemical stimulation in fish olfaction and gustation. *Reviews in Fish Biology and Fisheries* 1994;4:1–35.
12. Campana, S.E. Chemistry and composition of fish otoliths: Pathways, mechanism, and applications. *Marine Ecology Progress Series* 1999;188:263–297.
13. Campana, S.E. Otolith science entering the 21st century. *Marine and Freshwater Research* 2005;56:485–495.
14. Popper, A.N. and Fay, R.R. Sound detection and processing by fish: Critical review and major research questions (part 2 of 2). *Brain, Behavior and Evolution* 1993;41:26–38.

15. Helfman, G.S., Collette, B.B. and Facey D.E. *The Diversity of Fishes*. Blackwell Sciences Inc., Malden, MA, 1997.

16. Albert, J.S., Crampton, W.G.R. and Evans, D.H. Electroreception and electrogenesis. In: *The Physiology of Fishes*, 3rd ed. J.B. Claiborne, ed. CRC Press, Boca Raton, FL, 2006; pp. 429–470.

17. Carr, C.E., Maler, L. and Sas, E. Peripheral organization and central projections of the electrosensory nerves in gymnotiform fish. *Journal of Comparative Neurology* 1982;211:139–153.

18. Johnsen, S. and Lohmann, K.J. The physics and neurobiology of magnetoreception. *Nature Reviews Neuroscience* 2005;6(9):703–712.

19. Bone, Q. and Moore, R.H. *Biology of Fishes*, 3rd ed. Taylor & Francis Group, New York, 2008.

20. Grigg, G.C. Use of the first gill slits for water intake in a shark. *Journal of Experimental Biology* 1970;52:569–574.

21. Wegner, N.C., Sepulveda, C.A., Bull, K.B. and Graham, J.B. Gill morphometrics in relation to gas transfer and ram ventilation in high-energy demand teleosts: Scombrids and billfishes. *Journal of Morphology* 2010;271:36.

22. Shelton, G. The regulation of breathing. In: *Fish Physiology IV*. W.S. Hoar and D.J. Randall, eds. Academic Press, San Diego, CA, 1970; pp. 293–359.

23. Graham, J.B. Aquatic and aerial respiration. In: *The Physiology of Fishes*, 3rd ed., D.H. Evans and J.B. Claiborne, eds. CRC Press, Boca Raton, FL, 2006; pp. 85–117.

24. Moyle, P.B. and Cech Jr., J.J. *Fishes: An Introduction to Ichthyology*, 2nd ed. Prentice-Hall, Englewood Cliffs, NJ, 1988.

25. Nonotte, G. Cutaneous respiration in six freshwater teleosts. *Comparative Biochemistry and Physiology*. 1981;A70:541–543.

26. Podkowa, D. and Goniakowska-Witalinska, L. The structure of the airbladder of the *catfish Pangasius hypophthalmus* Roberts and Vidthayanon 1991 (previously *P. sutchi* Fowler 1937). *Folia Biologica-Krakow* 1998;46:189–196.

27. Horton, J.M. and Summers, A.P. The material properties of acellular bone in a teleost fish. *The Journal of Experimental Biology* 2009;212:1413–1420.

28. Gregory, W.K. Fish skulls, a study of the evolution of natural mechanisms. *Transactions of the American Philosphical Society* 1933;23:481.

29. Faustino, M. and Power, D.M. Osteologic development of the viscerocranial skeleton in sea bream: Alternative ossification strategies in teleost fish. *Journal of Fish Biology* 2001;58:537–572.

30. Stiassny, M.L. Skeletal system. In: *The Laboratory Fish*. G.K. Ostrander, ed. Academic Press, San Diego, CA, 2000; pp. 109–118.

31. Danos, N. and Ward, A.B. The homology and origin of intermuscular bones in fishes: Phylogeny or biomechanical determinants? *Biological Journal of the Linnean Society* 2012;106:607–622.

32. Carey, F.G. and Teal, J.M. Heat conservation in tuna fish muscle. *Zoology* 1966;56:1464–1469.

33. Clements, K.D. and Raubenheimer, D. Feeding and nutrition. In: *The Physiology of Fishes*, 3rd ed. D.H. Evans and J.B. Claiborne, eds. CRC Press, Boca Raton, FL, 2006; pp. 47–82.

34. Buddington, R.K. and Kuz'mina, V. Digestive system. In: *The Laboratory Fish*. G.K. Ostrander, ed. Academic Press, San Diego, CA, 2000; pp. 173–179.

35. Al-Hussaini, A.H. On the functional morphology of the alimentary tract of some fish in relation to differences in their feeding habits: Anatomy and histology. *Quarterly Journal of Microscopical Science* 1949;3(10):109–139.

36. Buddington, R.K. and Diamond, J.M. Pyloric ceca of fish: A "new" absorptive organ. *American Journal of Physiology—Gastrointestinal and Liver Physiology* 1987; 252:G65–G76.

37. Buddington, R.K. and Christofferson, J.P. Digestive and feeding characteristics of the chondrosteans. *Environmental Biology of Fishes* 1985;14:31–41.

38. Fänge, R. Gas exchange in fish swim bladder. *Reviews of Physiology, Biochemistry and Pharmacology* 1983;97: 111–158.

39. Olson, K.R. and Farrell, A.P. The cardiovascular system. In: *The Physiology of Fishes*, 3rd ed. D.H. Evans and J.B. Claiborne, eds. CRC Press, Boca Raton, FL, 2006; pp. 119–152.

40. Randall, D.J. Functional morphology of the heart in fishes. *American Zoologist* 1968;8:179–189.

41. Farrell, A.P. From hagfish to tuna: A perspective on cardiac function in fish. *Physiological Zoology* 1991;64:1137–1164.

42. Olson, K.R. Circulatory system. In: *The Laboratory Fish*. G.K. Ostrander, ed. Academic Press, San Diego, CA, 2000; pp. 161–171.

43. Marshall, W.S. and Grosell, M. Ion transport, osmoregulation, and acid-base balance. In: *The Physiology of Fishes*, 3rd ed. D.H. Evans and J.B. Claiborne, eds. CRC Press, Boca Raton, FL, 2006; pp. 177–230.

44. Ogawa, M. Comparative study of the external shape of the teleostean kidney with relation to phylogeny. *Science Reports of the Tokyo Kyoiku Daigaku. Section B* 1961;10(149):61–68.

45. Bonga, S.W. and Pang, P.K.T. Stannius corpuscles. *Vertebrate Endocrinology: Fundamentals and Biomedical Implications* 2012;1:439–464.

46. Hentschel H., Eiger, M., Dawson, M. and Renfro, J.L. *Urinary Tract in the Laboratory Fish*. G.K. Ostrander, ed. Elsevier, Academic Press, San Diego, CA, 2000; pp. 181–187.

47. Curtis, B.J. and Wood, C.M. The function of the urinary bladder *in vivo* in the freshwater rainbow trout. *Journal of Experimental Biology* 1991;155:567–583.

48. Burger, J.W. and Hess, W.N. Function of the rectal gland in the spiny dogfish. *Science* 1960;131(3401): 670–671.

49. Saurabh, S., Sridhar, N., Barlya, G., Hemaprasanth, Raghavendra, C.H., Ragunath, M.R. and Jayasankari, P. Sexual dimorphism in fishes. *Aqua International* November 2013:30–32.

50. Redding, J.M. and Patino, R. Reproductive system. In: *The Laboratory Fish*. G.K. Ostrander, ed. Academic Press, San Diego, CA, 2000; pp. 261–267.

51. Goodwin, N.B., Dulvy, N.K. and Reynolds, J.D. Life-history correlates of the evolution of live bearing in fishes. *Philosophical Transactions of the Royal Society of London B* 2002;357:259–267.

52. Wourms, J.P. and Lombardi, J. Reflections on the evolution of piscine viviparity. *American Zoologist* 1992;32: 276–293.

53. McMillan, D.B. *Fish Histology: Female Reproductive Systems*. Springer Science & Business Media, Dordrecht, The Netherlands, 2007.

54. Chanet, B., Guintard, C., Betti, E., Gallut, C., Dettai, A. and Lecointre, G. Evidence for a close phylogenic relationship between the teleost orders Tetraodontiformes and Lophiiformes based on an analysis of soft anatomy. *Cybium* 2013;37:179–198.

55. Lisney, T.J. and Collin, S.P. Brain morphology in large pelagic fishes: A comparison between sharks and teleosts. *Journal of Fish Biology* 2006;68:532–554.

56. Ekstrom, P. and Meissl, H. The pineal organ of teleost fishes. *Reviews in Fish Biology and Fisheries* 1997;7: 199–284.

57. Butler, A.B. Nervous system. In: *The Laboratory Fish*. G.K. Ostrander, ed. Academic Press, San Diego, CA, 2000; pp. 129–150.

58. Takei, Y. and Loretz, C.A. Endocrinology. In: *The Physiology of Fishes*, 3rd ed. D.H. Evans and J.B. Claiborne, eds. CRC Press, Boca Raton, FL, 2006; pp. 271–318.

59. Janz, D.M. Endocrine system. In: *The Laboratory Fish*. G.K. Ostrander, ed. Academic Press, San Diego, CA, 2000; pp. 189–217.

60. Arendt, J. Melatonin and the pineal gland: Influence on mammalian seasonal and circadian physiology. *Reviews of Reproduction* 1998;3:13–22.

61. Falcon, J., Besseau, L., Sauzet, S. and Boeuf, G. Melatonin effects on the hypothalamo-pituitary axis in fish. *Trends in Endocrinology and Metabolism* 2007;18: 81–88.

62. Winter, M.J., Ashworth, A., Bond, H., Brierley, M.J., McCrohan, C.R. and Balment, R.J. The caudal neuro-secretory system: Control and function of a novel neuroendocrine system in fish. *Biochemistry and Cell Biology* 2000;78:193–203.

63. Barlet, J.P., Gaumet, N., Coxam, V. and Davicco, M.J. Calcitonin and stanniocalcin: Particular aspects of the endocrine regulation of phospho-calcium metabolism in mammals and fish. *Annales D'endocrinologie* 1998;59: 281–290.

64. Milhaud, G., Bolis, L. and Benson, A.A. Calcitonin, a major gill hormone. *Proceedings of the National Academy of Science USA* 1980;77:6935–6936.

65. Milhaud, G., Rankin, J.C., Bolis, L. and Benson, A.A. Calcitonin: Its hormonal action on the gill. *Proceedings of the National Academy of Science USA* 1977;74:4693–4696.

66. Fenwick, J.C. Calcium exchange across fish gills. *Vertebrate Endocrinology: Fundamentals and Biomedical Implications* 1989;3:319–342.

67. Fänge, R. Lymphoid organs in sturgeon (Acipenseridae). *Veterinary Immunology and Immunopathology* 1986;12: 153–161.

68. Peterman, A.E. and Petrie-Hanson, L. Ontogeny of American paddlefish lymphoid tissues. *Journal of Fish Biology* 2006;69:72–88.

69. Chilmonczyk, S. The thymus in fish: Development and possible function in the immune response. *Annual Review of Fish Diseases* 1992;2:181–200.

70. Fänge, R. Blood cells, hemopoiesis, and lympho-myeloid tissues in fish. *Fish and Shellfish Immunology* 1994;4:405–411.

71. Hrubec, T.C. and Smith, S.A. Chapter 126 hematology of fish. In: *Schalm's Veterinary Hematology*, 6th ed. D.J. Weiss and K.J. Waldrop, eds. Wiley-Blackwell, Hoboken, NJ, 2010; pp. 995–1004.

CHAPTER 2

WATER QUALITY AND ENVIRONMENTAL ISSUES

DEBORAH B. POUDER AND STEPHEN A. SMITH

Water quality is one of the most important aspects of fish keeping, production, and health. Unfortunately, it is also often the most neglected and least understood concept. The health of a fish is directly related to the quality of its aquatic environment. Poor water quality probably kills more fish than infectious agents and other disease syndromes, and mortalities may be due to either acute or chronic water problems. Maintaining proper water quality relies on knowledge of the water source, regular testing of source and system water, recording and analyzing the data, and keen observations of the health of a population of fish in the system. Failure to provide timely intervention and correction of poor environmental conditions can result in catastrophic losses, which can have devastating financial and/or emotional effects on the owner of the fish.

One absolute is that water quality changes with time. Some parameters, such as dissolved oxygen or pH, change throughout a single day in certain systems, while other parameters, such as alkalinity and hardness, may change over weeks or months. In addition to these expected cycles, events such as a biofilter failure or chemical treatment may greatly alter water quality. Because of these expected and unexpected changes, it is important to evaluate system water quality on a regular basis. These tests will assure that the water is of good quality and will also provide a baseline for which to compare future measurements. If fish suddenly stop eating or exhibit behavioral changes or other signs of disease, water quality testing of all pertinent parameters should be performed on the system water as quickly as possible.

GENERAL TESTING CONSIDERATIONS

In addition to higher-end laboratory testing equipment and standard methods of measurement, a wide variety of single-parameter and multiparameter test kits as well as portable meters are available for field or tank-side use. For most parameters, kits are a cost-effective, portable and convenient method of testing. Kits or test strips such as those sold at pet stores can be a good choice for hobbyists (**Figures 2.1** and **2.2**). However, test kits designed for aquaculture production or a spectrophotometer may be better suited for fish farmers, professional aquarists, wholesalers and retailers, fish health specialists, and veterinarians (**Figures 2.3** and **2.4**). When evaluating a kit, it is important to not only consider the parameter detection limits but also the precision of the test. Although some kits may have a broad detection range, they may not be as sensitive. If readings are at or above the detection range of a test, dilutions with distilled water may be performed to allow a reading. However, even minor deviations from directions or an inaccuracy in methodology can magnify errors in testing. With the exception of temperature and pH, most water chemistry parameters of concern are measured in milligrams per liter (mg/L), which is equivalent to parts per million (ppm).

For tests using color as an indicator, results may be affected by color of the water sample whether by a natural (e.g., phytoplankton bloom, clay turbidity) or an artificial (e.g., chemical treatment) process. A blank (i.e., identical water sample without addition of testing reagents) should be used when making a color comparison (**Figure 2.5**). It may be difficult or impossible to accurately measure significantly colored water by a colorimetric method. In addition, some naturally occurring compounds as well as chemical treatments may interfere with certain test reagents providing inaccurate results.

Meters and other hand-held measuring devices, although more costly, are often simpler and more time-efficient for testing some parameters

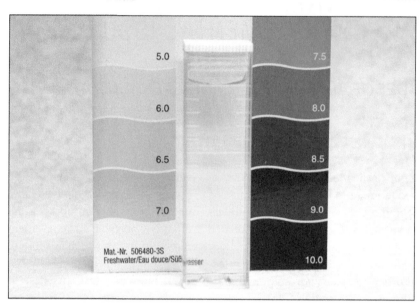

Figure 2.1 Water sample tube (center) with pH color comparator chart. (TetraTest, Spectrum Brands, Blacksburg, VA.)

(**Figure 2.6**). However, meters require regular calibration and maintenance to ensure accuracy. In many cases, low-cost meters have an attractive price but may not provide the necessary durability and reliability needed for professional use. Initial and regular testing with calibration standards is crucial to ensure best results.

When collecting a sample of water for testing, disturbing sediments or detritus as well as the water surface should be avoided. A water sample containing

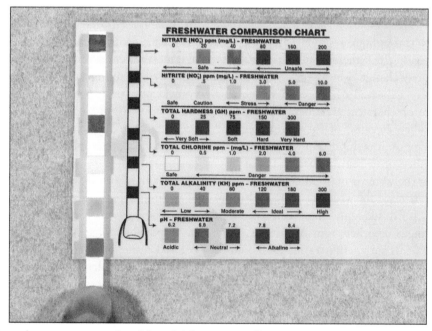

Figure 2.2 Aquarium water test strip with multiple water quality parameters. (Quick Dip Jungle Test Strips, Spectrum Brands, Blacksburg, VA.)

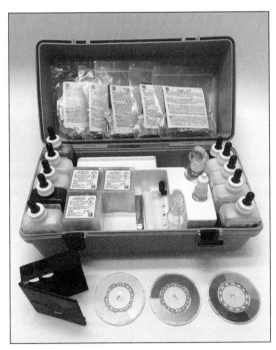

Figure 2.3 Water quality test kit for commercial aquaculture. (HACH Company, Loveland, CO.)

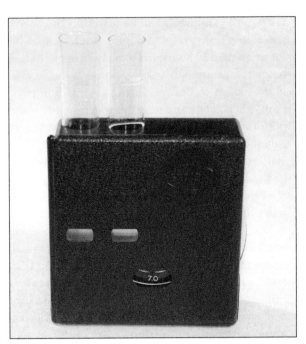

Figure 2.5 Standard blank (right tube) and test sample (left tube) color comparison method with pH color disk. (HACH Company, Loveland, CO.)

fish (i.e., fish transport water) is not suitable for testing. Thus, an additional sample of water should be available for evaluation. It is important to test the water sample as soon after collection as possible. If water samples must be transported or held prior to testing, a clean container with a tight-sealing lid should be used. If the sample must be held prior to

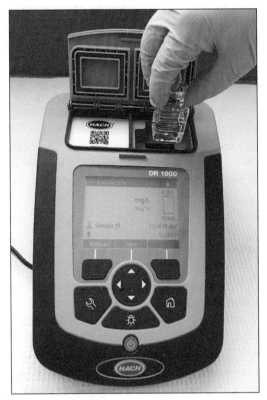

Figure 2.4 Spectrophotometer for water analysis. (HACH Company, Loveland, CO.)

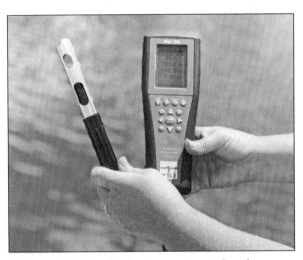

Figure 2.6 Dissolved oxygen meter and probe. (YSI Inc., Yellow Springs, OH.)

testing, the sample should be placed in the dark on ice or in a refrigerator. Samples should not be held for more than 24 hours and must be brought to room temperature prior to testing. Some parameters are more subject to change during the holding period than others. For more sensitive water quality testing performed by a laboratory, the lab should be consulted prior to water collection to determine if special collection containers and methodology should be used to prevent degradation or interferences.

Regardless of testing method, the key to good water quality management is regular testing and record keeping. Many water quality and subsequent fish health problems can be avoided by regularly reviewing testing data and evaluating trends. Water quality test results may also be requested in cases of litigation making record keeping, testing accuracy and interpretation of the results crucial. Although water quality testing may be costly and time-consuming, the benefits of increased fish health and, very often, the reduced need for therapeutants to treat an infectious disease initiated or exacerbated by water quality problems far outweigh these disadvantages.

SOURCE WATER AND TREATED WATER

Municipal/city water

Municipal (i.e., tap) water can be a good option for use in small systems if some precaution is taken to first remove disinfectants. However, the higher cost of this water source usually precludes its use in large systems or commercial production. Most municipalities treat drinking water with either chlorine or chloramine for disinfection purposes. As both chemicals are extremely toxic to fish, they must be completely removed or neutralized before the water comes in contact with fish. Since municipal water has been treated for most pathogens and does not contain living organisms such as insects or wild fish, this type of water is generally a good choice from a biosecurity perspective.

Ground water (well water or spring)

Though some generalizations can be made, ground water can vary greatly from location to location. Although commercial laboratory testing may deem well water safe for drinking, it may or may not be suitable for fish, so additional water quality testing for fish-pertinent parameters (e.g., ammonia, nitrite, pH, alkalinity, hardness and various gases) should be conducted. Well water usually has little or no dissolved oxygen but may contain high levels of dissolved nitrogen or carbon dioxide. As such, well water should always be degassed and aerated thoroughly before coming in contact with fish. Some wells contain high levels of hydrogen sulfide or iron, both of which are detrimental to fish. Degassing or aeration can help remove hydrogen sulfide and will allow dissolved iron to settle out as rust, which can then be separated from the water. If ammonia is present in the water, biofiltration may be necessary before the water is used for fish. Like water from wells, spring water may be low in dissolved oxygen and high in other dissolved gases. Springs may also contain fish, insects, and pathogens, which are a biosecurity concern.

Surface water

Some aquarists and commercial fish facilities have access to water from streams, rivers, ponds, reservoirs, lakes, bays or oceans. Water quality for these sources can vary greatly depending on location, human usage, and environmental factors, and in some cases, there may be legal issues associated with its use. Wild fish, insects, pathogens, environmental contamination and toxic algal blooms are biosecurity concerns in these water sources. Use of water from any of these sources should be carefully monitored, and it may be necessary to treat incoming water to reduce or eliminate pathogens, toxins, or contaminants.

Reverse osmosis (RO) water treatment

Reverse osmosis (RO) is a method by which water is forced through a semipermeable membrane to remove many of the impurities (e.g., heavy metals, minerals, phosphates, nitrates and other dissolved solids) from the water. RO water can be a good choice for makeup water for evaporation in some systems, but not for initial startup or large water changes in freshwater systems because it lacks important ions that fish require for life. RO water is also commonly mixed with synthetic sea salt, which contains minerals and ions meant to replicate levels found in natural seawater, for marine systems. Its use makes marine fish keeping and production possible at inland locations; however, it is expensive and may be cost-prohibitive on a large scale.

Softened water treatment

Softened water has had the calcium and magnesium, which accounts for the water's "hardness," replaced by sodium ions. Putting water through a water softener does not appreciably decrease the total dissolved solids since ions have simply been replaced, not removed. For fish that do not tolerate hard water, softened water may be an acceptable option. However, because of the ion replacement, the sodium in the water may be higher, which may not be tolerated by some fish species.

SPECIFIC WATER QUALITY PARAMETERS

Temperature

Water temperature plays a vital role in the survival, growth and reproduction of fish. Each species of fish has a preferred temperature range for survival and a narrower range at which fish will reproduce or exhibit optimal growth. Because most fish are poikilothermic, their metabolism is directly affected by water temperature; however, a few species of fish, such as tunas and lamnid sharks, are regional endotherms capable of maintaining portions of their bodies at stable temperatures not influenced by the environment.

The immune and metabolic systems of fish are designed to work best within a species' optimal temperature range. When outside that range, fish can become stressed and more susceptible to disease. Some clinical diseases may manifest only within a specific temperature range, whereas in others temperature may have a direct effect on the rate and duration of a pathogen's progression. In addition to the direct effect on fish, temperature also plays a major role in environmental conditions. Water quality parameters (e.g., un-ionized ammonia, dissolved oxygen), solubility of gases, biological oxygen demand, decay of organic material, and rates of chemical dissolution are all affected by temperature. Therefore, temperature should be

regularly monitored and noted especially in any disease event.

Rapid temperature changes can have a detrimental effect on fish. This change often comes into play when moving or stocking fish. A temperature change as little as 3°C–4°C can stress or kill fish, so fish should be acclimated to changes in temperature.[1] Because of species differences, there is no single time to temperature change ratio for acclimation that is suitable for all fish. There is evidence that some fish acclimate more quickly when going from higher temperatures to lower temperatures than when going from lower to higher temperatures and that the detrimental effects of moving fish are more pronounced when moving fish from lower to higher temperatures.[1,2] Regardless, temperature changes should be made as slowly as possible to limit the impact on fish health.

Dissolved oxygen

Dissolved oxygen (DO) refers to the amount of oxygen gas that is dissolved in water. Fish absorb dissolved oxygen directly from the water across the gill membrane into their bloodstream. Although some species, such as bettas and gouramis, are capable of breathing atmospheric air, sufficient oxygen levels should always be maintained in the water even for these fish. In addition to oxygen demands of fish, nitrifying bacteria require and consume oxygen.

Whereas air consists of almost 210,000 mg/L (21%) oxygen, most water conducive for fish in culture or captivity contains less than 11 mg/L at saturation. Where air and water are in contact, oxygen will continue to enter the water until the pressure of oxygen in the water is equal to the pressure of oxygen in the atmosphere. When these two pressures are equal, the water is said to be saturated with oxygen. Although the pressures will always attempt to equalize, it is still possible for oxygen to be below saturation because fish, decaying organic material, bacteria and other living organisms constantly consume oxygen. The larger the surface area of a body of water, the greater the area of diffusion. In addition, the solubility of oxygen in water is dependent on temperature, salinity, and pressure. As water temperature increases, the amount of oxygen the water can hold decreases. Likewise, as salinity increases, less oxygen can be dissolved into the water. Conversely, as pressure increases, solubility increases. While pressure changes for a given location have a fairly negligible effect on saturation, the differences in barometric pressure due to elevation can be significant.[1] For instance, at the same temperature and salinity, oxygen solubility would be higher at sea level than in the mountains.

In ponds with a phytoplankton bloom, the greatest contribution of oxygen to the system is from photosynthesis. Plants produce oxygen as a byproduct of photosynthesis, a process by which plants use light energy to produce food from carbon dioxide and water and produce oxygen. In the absence of light, the fish, plants, bacteria, and other organisms in the water continue to respire (i.e., consuming oxygen and producing carbon dioxide), but no oxygen is produced. With this diel cycle, oxygen levels are lowest in the early morning near dawn and highest late in the afternoon. Heavy phytoplankton blooms can cause large swings in oxygen levels, which must be closely monitored to prevent catastrophically low levels of oxygen in the overnight and early morning hours. Cloudy weather will also contribute to lower oxygen production due to reduced light levels. Aeration is crucial for fish survival and health during low-level periods. Conversely, with heavy phytoplankton blooms, dissolved oxygen levels in the afternoon may become supersaturated and can exceed 25 mg/L in some ponds.

Mechanical aeration or oxygen supplementation is crucial for providing sufficient oxygen in any fish culture or display system. Aerators work by increasing the contact between air and water, circulating the water, and, particularly in outdoor systems, reducing temperature and oxygen stratification. In a tank system, an aeration system often consists of an air pump or blower, air tubing, and one or more air stones, depending on the system size. The efficiency with which an air system can put oxygen into the water is a function of the size of the air bubbles created and the length of time those air bubbles are in contact with the water. Very small air bubbles, like those from a fine pore stone, that travel slowly from the bottom to the top of the tank are more efficient in adding oxygen to the water than large air bubbles that boil the water or airstones that sit near the water

surface. Oxygenation, as opposed to aeration, relies on adding pure gaseous or liquid oxygen to the water through cones or other types of saturators or via micropore stones. Oxygenation is most commonly used in intensive recirculating systems and when hauling or shipping fish.

For optimal fish health, dissolved oxygen levels for warm-water fish should be maintained at 5 mg/L or higher, whereas cold-water fish should have dissolved oxygen levels that are even higher. In heavily stocked production systems (e.g., recirculation systems or ponds with heavy phytoplankton blooms), maintaining these ideal levels can be a significant challenge. Oxygen levels below 1.5 mg/L can result in death of warm-water fish especially if exposure is prolonged.[3] Although some fish may survive oxygen levels down to 1.5 mg/L for short periods of time, growth will be slowed, and the fish's immune system will be compromised leaving them susceptible to disease even several weeks after the low DO event.[3] Because of their higher oxygen requirement, large fish will typically succumb to low dissolved oxygen levels before small fish (**Figure 2.7**).

Some sources of water, such as wells, commonly have very little to no oxygen. Aerating this water before it comes in contact with fish is critical to ensure fish health. Additionally, some chemicals also have adverse effects on dissolved oxygen. For instance, formalin will chemically remove oxygen from water at a rate of 1 mg/L oxygen for every 5 mg/L formalin, while copper sulfate, an algaecide used to kill undesired plants or reduce heavy

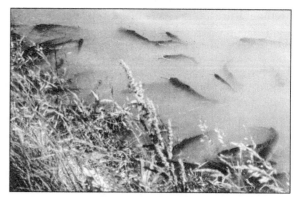

Figure 2.7 Oxygen deprivation in channel catfish (*Ictalurus punctatus*). (Image courtesy A. Mitchell.)

phytoplankton blooms, generally results in a reduction in oxygen production and an increased oxygen demand as the dead plant material decays.

Although test kits for dissolved oxygen are commercially available, most are time-consuming and must be performed with precision to prevent error. For the frequency that dissolved oxygen should be tested in production or other large-scale managed systems, a dissolved oxygen meter or ampule system is often the most efficient testing method (**Figures 2.6** and **2.8**). When working with outdoor systems influenced by photosynthesis, dissolved oxygen should be tested just prior to or at dawn to determine the lowest level. In heavily stocked ponds, dissolved oxygen is often checked throughout the night to allow most efficient use of aeration and to prevent catastrophic losses. Even in a planted decorative ornamental pond or planted aquarium with appropriate lighting, diel variations can occur. However, in an indoor recirculating or flow-through system void of plant life, time of day for testing is less critical. Dissolved oxygen is best tested pond- or tankside to avoid changes due to sampling, holding, or transporting.

Carbon dioxide

Carbon dioxide (CO_2) is the byproduct of respiration of fish, plants, bacteria and other organisms. In systems influenced by photosynthesis (e.g., ponds, planted tanks), carbon dioxide exhibits a diel curve opposite that of dissolved oxygen with CO_2 levels being highest near dawn and decreasing throughout the day as it is consumed by plants for photosynthesis (**Figure 2.9**). As carbon dioxide forms carbonic acid in water, it directly affects pH. The higher the CO_2 level, the lower, or more acidic, the pH of the water. Plants, including phytoplankton, in a system take up carbon dioxide for use in photosynthesis during the day when light is available. With the absence of light, photosynthesis and, thus, the uptake of carbon dioxide by plants ceases while production of CO_2 by plants and other organisms in the water continues. Therefore, carbon dioxide levels are highest early in the morning. Throughout the day, carbon dioxide levels decrease as plants consume carbon dioxide for photosynthesis resulting in the lowest CO_2 level in the late afternoon.

Well water and spring water may contain supersaturated levels of carbon dioxide. The use of

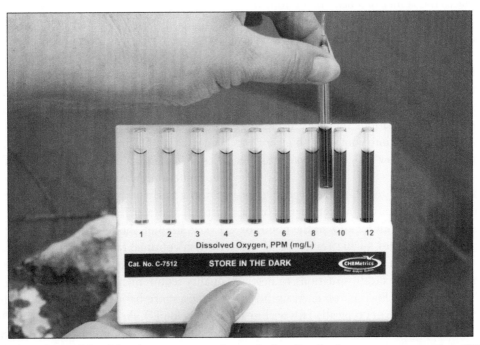

Figure 2.8 Sample ampule with color comparator for analyzing dissolved oxygen concentration. (CHEMetrics Inc., Midland, VA.)

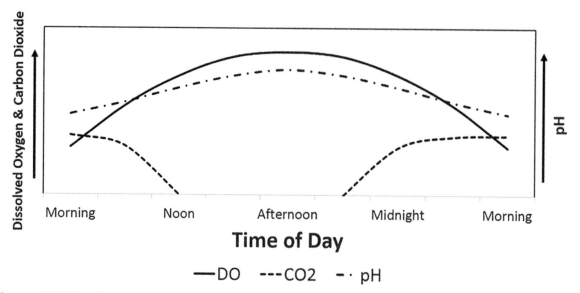

Figure 2.9 Diurnal (i.e., daily) trends of dissolved oxygen, carbon dioxide, and pH in a pond with a moderate phytoplankton bloom. (Adapted from Boyd, C.E., *Water Quality: An Introduction*, 2nd ed., Springer International, New York, 2015.)

oxygenation instead of aeration in intensive recirculating systems can also contribute to elevated CO_2 levels because there may be little to no surface agitation of the water. High levels of carbon dioxide in the water can be detrimental to fish health because the gas reduces the ability of a fish's blood to transport oxygen. Fish in water with high carbon dioxide concentrations (>10 mg/L for some fish species) can suffocate even if dissolved oxygen levels are high, and low dissolved oxygen levels will compound the adverse effects of CO_2. Although highly soluble in water, excess carbon dioxide can be easily removed from water in these situations by either degassing the water before coming into contact with fish or by agitating the water to allow CO_2 to dissipate into the atmosphere.

Commercial titration test kits are available for testing carbon dioxide levels. However, as with other gases, it is important to test for CO_2 at the pond- or tank-side to avoid changes during transport of the water. In the absence of a CO_2 test kit, pH measurements may be useful in certain situations to determine if CO_2 is present. This is particularly useful in marine systems where the pH typically falls within a narrow range of approximately 8.0–8.5. A lower pH may be an indication of elevated CO_2 in the system. To determine the potential presence of CO_2, the pH

of the water in the system is tested first. Then, some of the water is placed in an open-topped container (e.g., bucket) and aerated heavily for 1–2 hours. If the pH of the water in the container after agitation is higher than that of the system, it is an indication that CO_2 levels may be elevated in the system.

pH

The pH is the inverse logarithm of the hydrogen ion (H^+) activity, but more practically it is the measure of acid or base measured on a scale of 1–14. A pH below 7 is acidic and a pH above 7 is basic, while a pH of 7 is neutral. Although many freshwater fish can tolerate pH in the range of 6.5–8.0, each species of fish has an optimal pH range for growth and reproduction. Marine fish typically live at a higher pH in a fairly narrow range, typically 8.0–8.5, with natural seawater having a pH of approximately 8.2. Every attempt should be made to keep pH within the fish's optimal range. For this reason, mixing species of fish that have significantly differently water quality requirements, such as African cichlids (which prefer a more basic pH) and discus (which prefer a more acid pH), should be discouraged. Although pH outside of the optimum range may not kill fish, it is a constant stressor that can lower the immune system, making fish more susceptible to disease. Nitrifying bacteria also have specific pH requirements with many nitrifying bacteria inhibited below a pH of 6 resulting in an accumulation of ammonia and nitrite in the system.

In systems containing phytoplankton or other aquatic plants, photosynthesis plays a large role in the changes of pH of the water throughout the day. At night, all living organisms (e.g., fish, bacteria, aquatic plants) in a body of water respire, releasing carbon dioxide. Because carbon dioxide is an acid in water, the pH decreases as the carbon dioxide levels increase. Once the sun rises or appropriate lighting is turned on, plants begin to photosynthesize, utilizing carbon dioxide, which increases pH. In ponds with heavy phytoplankton blooms, the water may exceed a pH of 10 in late afternoon, especially in waters with low total alkalinity. Because of this photosynthetic cycle, the pH is lowest in the early morning when carbon dioxide levels are highest and highest in the afternoon when carbon dioxide levels are lowest. In a pond or a planted system, the pH should be tested at dawn to determine the lowest pH and again in late afternoon to determine the highest pH. The time of day for testing pH of water in an indoor recirculating system or non-planted aquarium is generally not a concern.

Many methods are available for testing pH including test strips, colorimetric kits, handheld meters or pens, and benchtop laboratory-grade meters. Colorimetric kits and test strips are easy methods for many management needs; however, more precise measurements may be needed in some cases, such as for spawning certain species of fish. When using pH pens or meters, it is crucial to calibrate the equipment regularly using standard pH calibration solutions (i.e., pH 4.0, 7.0, and 10.0). Calibration solutions that are past the expiration date or have been exposed repeatedly to ambient air or extreme temperatures can alter the pH of the buffers and cause incorrect readings. Used calibration solutions should be discarded and never placed back into the original bottle.

Because pH is measured on a logarithmic scale, a 1.0 unit change in pH is actually a 10-fold increase or decrease in hydrogen ion activity, whereas a 2.0 unit change in pH is a 100-fold increase or decrease in hydrogen ion activity. Rapid changes of even 1 or 2 units of pH can be very detrimental to fish. Therefore, care should be taken to avoid large pH changes, particularly when moving fish from transport water, introducing fish into a new system or making large water changes. Fish should be acclimated to new water conditions slowly to ensure their bodies can compensate for the pH change.

Nitrogenous compounds and the nitrogen cycle

The nitrogen cycle is a microbiological process that converts ammonia, the primary waste product of fish, to less toxic nitrate via a series of steps. Nitrate is then removed by plants and phytoplankton, water changes, or through anaerobic denitrification. The nitrogen cycle is an aerobic process and creates free hydrogen (H^+) ions, reducing the pH of a system over time unless adequate buffers are present in the water. A number of bacteria are involved in the nitrogen cycle with the genera *Nitrosomonas*, *Nitrosococcus*, *Nitrosospira*, *Nitrosolobus* and *Nitrosovibrio* associated with ammonia reduction to nitrite, and the genera of *Nitrobacter*, *Nitrococcus*, *Nitrospira* and *Nitrospina* associated with nitrite oxidation to nitrate.[4–7] In ponds, the nitrifying bacteria colonize the substrate as well as macrophytes and other structures, while in an aquarium or other recirculating system, the bacteria colonize the substrate and biological filter material. A new biofilter may require 6 to 8 weeks to colonize sufficient bacteria to effectively oxidize ammonia to nitrite and nitrite to nitrate.

Nitrifying bacteria require both oxygen and alkalinity to function. If oxygen levels are insufficient, the nitrifying bacteria may cease to function or die, resulting in elevated ammonia and nitrite levels. Because alkalinity is consumed during nitrification, this parameter must also be monitored and supplemented over time. If alkalinity is depleted, a sudden, catastrophic decrease in pH may occur, which can result in the acute mortality of fish as well as bacteria in the substrate or biofilter.

Ammonia

Ammonia is the primary final product of nitrogen catabolism. In aquaculture or aquarium systems, feed and fertilizers contribute a large portion of this nitrogen. Feed protein in excess of that necessary for growth or maintenance of fish is catabolized into ammonia and eliminated primarily by diffusion through the gills into the water. Urea is produced in much smaller amounts and is eliminated via the gills and kidney.[8] Decomposing feed, feces and dead organic material also contribute to the overall concentration of ammonia in a system.

In water, ammonia exists in two forms in equilibrium: un-ionized ammonia (NH_3) and ionized ammonium (NH_4^+). The combined concentration of the two is referred to as total ammonia. The portion of total ammonia in the un-ionized or ionized form is primarily a factor of pH and temperature and, to much less extent, salinity.[9] Un-ionized ammonia increases with increasing pH and temperature but decreases slightly with higher salinity.[9,10] In most freshwater fish species, the majority of ammonia is excreted as NH_3 by passive diffusion across the gills down a partial pressure gradient, whereas marine fish may also excrete NH_4^+.[11,12] Because un-ionized ammonia is uncharged and lipid-soluble, it can easily diffuse into the gills making it much more toxic than ionized ammonia. The gills of some fish may be 100 times more permeable to NH_3 than to NH_4^+.[13] High environmental ammonia levels decrease the rate of diffusion from the gills, resulting in elevated blood and tissue ammonia levels.[11]

Ammonia is being continuously produced in aquaculture and aquarium systems, thus methods must be incorporated to eliminate it before it can accumulate to levels harmful to fish. Ammonia toxicity is one of the most common water quality problems affecting fish in closed systems and can cause acute mortality or chronic, sublethal tissue damage and stress. Significant changes in water temperature or dissolved oxygen levels can compound these effects.[8] Damage to fish may occur at un-ionized ammonia levels as low as 0.05 mg/L. Detectable ammonia levels above baseline metabolic levels in the system might indicate a problem, and corrective management measures should be undertaken immediately.

Ammonia is colorless and, even at levels toxic to fish, odorless, so testing is necessary to determine if it is present in water. Although handheld meters for measuring NH_3 and NH_4^+ are available, they have a high initial investment cost and have been shown to give higher mean concentrations of total ammonia

than standard methods.[14] On the other hand, colorimetric test kits can be useful in efficiently and affordably monitoring ammonia for management purposes.

There are two types of colorimetric ammonia test kits. One kit uses the Nessler method and the other uses the ammonia salicylate method. The Nessler method is often cheaper and quicker to perform than the ammonia salicylate method; however, it has many disadvantages. When testing seawater, even after necessary pretreatment to reduce interferences, the sensitivity of the test is reduced and, therefore, this test method is not recommended for saltwater.[15] If formalin, formalin-containing products, or ammonia-binding products have been recently used (up to 72 hours or more) in the water, the Nessler method will result in a falsely elevated ammonia result. Chlorine, high hardness (>500 mg/L $CaCO_3$), iron, and sulfide also interfere with this method.[15,16] The Nessler method in some kits has been shown to have low accuracy and precision except at high levels of total ammonia (>0.8 mg/L).[14] Finally, because Nessler reagent contains mercury, the reagent and test sample must be disposed as hazardous waste. Conversely, the salicylate method has greater precision and accuracy, is not affected by formalin or ammonia-binding products, can be used to accurately test saltwater, and does not require special disposal methods. Excessive levels of calcium (>1000 mg/L $CaCO_3$), magnesium (>6000 mg/L $CaCO_3$), nitrate (>100 mg/L NO_3^--N), nitrite (>12 mg/L NO_2^--N), phosphate (>100 mg/L PO_4^{3-}-P), and sulfate (>300 mg/L SO_4^{2-}) will interfere with the salicylate method.[15] Monochloramine in chloraminated municipal water interferes at all levels and will cause a false high reading.[15]

When using a test kit to measure ammonia, the result is given in total ammonia or total ammonia nitrogen. To determine the portion of total ammonia in the more toxic un-ionized form (NH_3), the pH and temperature must also be known. Once all three parameters are known, a table can be used to determine the un-ionized fraction of ammonia (NH_3) at the applicable pH and temperature (**Tables 2.1** and **2.2**, Equation 1). If temperature or pH falls between values on the table, the next highest value is used to determine the worst case scenario because

Table 2.1 **Fraction of un-ionized ammonia in aqueous solution at different pH values and temperatures**

	TEMPERATURE													
	°F													
	42.0	46.4	50.0	53.6	57.2	60.8	64.4	68.0	71.6	75.2	78.8	82.4	86.0	89.6
	°C													
PH	6	8	10	12	14	16	18	20	22	24	26	28	30	32
7.0	0.0013	0.0016	0.0018	0.0022	0.0025	0.0029	0.0034	0.0039	0.0046	0.0052	0.0060	0.0069	0.0080	0.0093
7.2	0.0021	0.0025	0.0029	0.0034	0.0040	0.0046	0.0054	0.0062	0.0072	0.0083	0.0096	0.0110	0.0126	0.0150
7.4	0.0034	0.0040	0.0046	0.0054	0.0063	0.0073	0.0085	0.0098	0.0114	0.0131	0.0150	0.0173	0.0198	0.0236
7.6	0.0053	0.0063	0.0073	0.0086	0.0100	0.0116	0.0134	0.0155	0.0179	0.0206	0.0236	0.0271	0.0310	0.0369
7.8	0.0084	0.0099	0.0116	0.0135	0.0157	0.0182	0.0211	0.0244	0.0281	0.0322	0.0370	0.0423	0.0482	0.0572
8.0	0.0133	0.0156	0.0182	0.0212	0.0247	0.0286	0.0330	0.0381	0.0438	0.0502	0.0574	0.0654	0.0743	0.0877
8.2	0.0210	0.0245	0.0286	0.0332	0.0385	0.0445	0.0514	0.0590	0.0676	0.0772	0.0880	0.0998	0.1129	0.1322
8.4	0.0328	0.0383	0.0445	0.0517	0.0597	0.0688	0.0790	0.0904	0.1031	0.1171	0.1326	0.1495	0.1678	0.1948
8.6	0.0510	0.0593	0.0688	0.0795	0.0914	0.1048	0.1197	0.1361	0.1541	0.1737	0.1950	0.2178	0.2422	0.2768
8.8	0.0785	0.0909	0.1048	0.1204	0.1376	0.1566	0.1773	0.1998	0.2241	0.2500	0.2774	0.3062	0.3362	0.3776
9.0	0.1190	0.1368	0.1565	0.1782	0.2018	0.2273	0.2546	0.2836	0.3140	0.3456	0.3783	0.4116	0.4453	0.4902
9.2	0.1763	0.2008	0.2273	0.2558	0.2861	0.3180	0.3512	0.3855	0.4204	0.4557	0.4909	0.5258	0.5599	0.6038
9.4	0.2533	0.2847	0.3180	0.3526	0.3884	0.4249	0.4618	0.4985	0.5348	0.5702	0.6045	0.6373	0.6685	0.7072
9.6	0.3496	0.3868	0.4249	0.4633	0.5016	0.5394	0.5762	0.6117	0.6456	0.6777	0.7078	0.7358	0.7617	0.7929
9.8	0.4600	0.5000	0.5394	0.5778	0.6147	0.6499	0.6831	0.7140	0.7428	0.7692	0.7933	0.8153	0.8351	0.8585
10.0	0.5745	0.6131	0.6498	0.6844	0.7166	0.7463	0.7735	0.7983	0.8207	0.8408	0.8588	0.8749	0.8892	0.9058
10.2	0.6815	0.7152	0.7463	0.7746	0.8003	0.8234	0.8441	0.8625	0.8788	0.8933	0.9060	0.9173	0.9271	0.9389

Source: Based on Emerson, K. et al. *Journal of the Fisheries Research Board of Canada* 1975;32:2379–2383.

Table 2.2 **Summary of water quality equations**

Equation 1: Un-ionized ammonia (NH_3) from total ammonia ($NH_3 + NH_4^+$)
Total ammonia (from test) × fraction of un-ionized ammonia (from **Table 2.1**) = NH_3

Equation 2: Un-ionized ammonia (NH_3) from total ammonia nitrogen ($NH_3^- -N + NH_4^+ -N$)
Total ammonia nitrogen (from test) × fraction of un-ionized ammonia (from **Table 2.1**) × 1.2 = NH_3

Equation 3: Nitrite-nitrogen ($NO_2^- -N$) to nitrite (NO_2^-)
$NO_2^- -N × 3.3 = NO_2^-$

Equation 4: Nitrate-nitrogen ($NO_3^- -N$) to nitrate (NO_3^-)
$NO_3^- -N × 4.4 = NO_3^-$

Equation 5: Equivalency of gr/gal to mg/L
1 gr/gal = 64.79891 mg/gal ÷ 3.785 L/gal = 17.1 mg/L

Equation 6: Total alkalinity in gr/gal (drops) to mg/L
Drops of titrant (= gr/gal) × 17.1 = Total alkalinity in mg/L

Equation 7: Total alkalinity in dKH to mg/L
Drops of titrant (= dKH) × 17.86 = Total alkalinity in mg/L

Equation 8: Total hardness in gr/gal (drops) to mg/L
Drops of titrant (= gr/gal) × 17.1 = Total hardness in mg/L

Equation 9: Total hardness in dGH to mg/L
Drops of titrant (= dGH) × 17.86 = Total hardness in mg/L

Equation 10: Calculation of % N_2
%N_2 = [%TGP − (%DO × 0.2095)] ÷ 0.7808

higher pH and temperature result in more NH_3. The fraction is multiplied by the total ammonia reading.

Example:

- Total ammonia reading = 0.9 mg/L
- Temperature = 75°F
- pH = 8.0
- Fraction of NH_3 from **Table 2.1** = 0.0502
- NH_3 = 0.9 mg/L × 0.0502 = 0.0452 mg/L

Some ammonia test kits report total ammonia as total ammonia nitrogen (TAN) (i.e., NH_3-N + NH_4^+-N), which accounts for only the weight of the nitrogen atom and does not include the weight of the hydrogen atoms. In this case, the preceding example would calculate NH_3-N. To convert NH_3-N to NH_3, multiply by 1.2 (e.g., 0.0452 mg/L NH_3-N × 1.2 = 0.054 mg/L NH_3) (**Table 2.2**, Equation 2). Ammonia may be tested at any time during the day; however, if diel fluctuations affect the pH and temperature of the system water, those two parameters should be measured at the time of day when they are highest to determine the highest un-ionized ammonia level.

Nitrite

Nitrite (NO_2^-) is the intermediate product of the oxidation of ammonia to nitrate. In the absence of sufficient nitrite-oxidizing bacteria, nitrite levels will increase in a system. The bacteria that oxidize nitrite to nitrate also tend to grow more slowly than ammonia oxidizing bacteria, which can result in extended nitrite exposure in new or insufficient biofilters, or those damaged by events such as chemical treatments or low oxygen.[17] In freshwater fish, nitrite is actively transported across gill membranes by the chloride transport mechanism.[18] Intestinal uptake of nitrite also plays a significant role in marine fish, which actively drink seawater.[19] Once in the blood, nitrite oxidizes hemoglobin to methemoglobin, which is unable to carry oxygen through the body, resulting in functional anemia and hypoxia.[20] If enough methemoglobin is present, it will cause the blood to appear tan or brown instead of red. Consequently, methemoglobinemia caused by nitrite toxicity is often called "brown blood disease" (**Figure 2.10**).

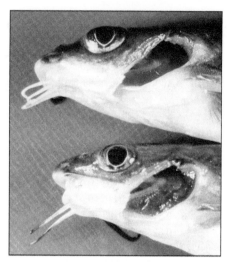

Figure 2.10 Nitrite toxicity in channel catfish (*Ictalurus punctatus*) showing darker discoloration of gill tissue in affected fish (lower) compared to red gill tissue of normal fish (upper). (Image courtesy A. Mitchell.)

Sensitivity to nitrite toxicity is species-specific. Some fish, such as salmonids, channel catfish, and tilapia concentrate nitrite in their blood plasma higher than environmental levels, producing elevated levels of methemoglobin.[21] However, centrarchids, such as largemouth bass, are relatively insensitive to nitrite toxicity because they do not concentrate nitrite above ambient levels.[21]

Because nitrite is actively transported across the gill membranes by the chloride transport mechanism, increased levels of chloride (Cl^-) in the water can help competitively inhibit the uptake of nitrite in some fish and provide protection from the formation of methemoglobin. However, increasing chloride levels does not decrease environmental nitrite levels, and management adjustments must be made to remove nitrite from system water. Although chloride levels are extremely high in seawater, some marine and estuarine animals may still be vulnerable to nitrite toxicity.[20] Methemoglobinemia may be only one toxic mechanism of elevated nitrite. Damage to gills, liver, and brain and numerous physiological disturbances have also been reported.[17,21–23]

Many nitrite test kits and spectrophotometer default settings report nitrite as nitrite-nitrogen (NO_2^--N). The annotation NO_2^--N means "nitrite as nitrogen" and accounts for only the weight of the nitrogen atom instead of the entire nitrite ion, which also includes the two oxygen atoms. Because references levels for fish are often given as nitrite, a reading of nitrite-nitrogen must be converted to nitrite. To convert nitrite-nitrogen to nitrite, multiply the NO_2^--N by 3.3 (**Table 2.2**, Equation 3).

Example:

$$0.05 \text{ mg/L } NO_2^-\text{-N} \times 3.3 = 0.165 \text{ mg/L } NO_2^-$$

Nitrate

Nitrate (NO_3^-) is the final product of the nitrification cycle. Traditionally, nitrate has been considered non-toxic to fish.[24] Although fish are able to tolerate much higher levels of nitrate than either ammonia or nitrite, research has shown hematological and biochemical changes in response to nitrate exposure, and toxicity may increase with exposure time.[25,26] In many cases, eggs, fry, and juveniles appear to be more sensitive than adults to nitrate toxicity; however, the opposite has also been demonstrated for some species.[27]

In a pond, plants can uptake nitrate, and high levels of nitrates can encourage phytoplankton blooms. In tank systems, nitrate removal is dependent upon water changes or a separate, anaerobic denitrification system. In warm water production ponds, nitrate levels usually do not exceed 5 mg/L, even in colder months.[28] However, nitrate levels in intensive recirculating systems with little to no water exchange may exceed 200 mg/L.[25] With increased focus on intensifying production and reducing or eliminating water discharge in commercial aquaculture, nitrate monitoring becomes more important. In general, levels of nitrate should be maintained below 50 mg/L.

Many nitrate test kits and spectrophotometer default settings report nitrate as nitrate-nitrogen (NO_3^--N), which accounts for only the weight of the nitrogen atom instead of the entire nitrate ion that also includes the three oxygen atoms. As references values for fish are often given as nitrate, a measurement of nitrate-nitrogen must be converted to nitrate. To convert nitrate-nitrogen to nitrate, multiply NO_3^--N by 4.4 (**Table 2.2**, Equation 4).

Example:

$$40 \text{ mg/L } NO_3^-\text{-N} \times 4.4 = 176 \text{ mg/L } NO_3^-$$

It is noteworthy that comparison of several strips and test kits for testing nitrate have shown poor agreement with standard methods for nitrate, and caution should be used in making management decisions based on these results.[29]

Total alkalinity

Total alkalinity is the measurement of all titratable bases in the water expressed as milligrams per liter (mg/L) of calcium carbonate ($CaCO_3$). Total alkalinity is the buffering capacity of water or its ability to resist change in pH by neutralizing hydrogen ions (H^+). Total alkalinity and pH are closely related, with lower alkalinity generally associated with lower pH (**Table 2.3**).

Total alkalinity in natural water may range from 0 mg/L to greater than 500 mg/L, though 10–300 mg/L is more common.[3] Limestone is the major source of alkalinity in many water sources. Water in areas with sandy or organic soils usually have low total alkalinity (<50 mg/L). Moderate alkalinity (50–150 mg/L) is common in humid regions with ample limestone, whereas moderate to high alkalinity (50–300 mg/L) is common in semiarid or arid regions.[3] The average total alkalinity of seawater is 116 mg/L.[3]

In ponds, total alkalinity plays a large role in the extent of diel fluctuations of pH attributed to photosynthesis. Ponds with low to moderate total alkalinity and heavy phytoplankton blooms may have pH levels exceeding 9 during the late afternoon. Early morning pH in the same pond may be 7 or lower. Ponds with high alkalinity levels will have smaller diel fluctuations.

Table 2.3 **General relationship of total alkalinity to pH in water**

TOTAL ALKALINITY	PH
0 mg/L	<5.0
<50 mg/L (low)	5.0–7.0
50–300 mg/L (moderate to high)	7.0–8.5
>300 mg/L (very high)	>9.0

Source: Modified from Boyd, C.E., *Water Quality: An Introduction*, 2nd ed., Springer International, New York, 2015.

Hydrogen ions are produced when carbon dioxide forms carbonic acid in water and when ammonia is converted to nitrite and then nitrate in a biofilter. These hydrogen ions combine with carbonates, bicarbonates, and hydroxides thus consuming alkalinity. If alkalinity is depleted over time, the pH of water can drop drastically (sometimes to 4 or lower) in the matter of hours. This condition is known as "old tank syndrome" (although it may occur in a short period of time in naturally low alkalinity waters), and fish can be killed because of the large, rapid drop in pH. Additionally, the nitrifying bacteria within a biofilter will not be able to function at these low pHs and without bicarbonates. Alkalinity can be replenished in a recirculating system by periodically exchanging a portion of the tank water with new water with a moderate total alkalinity or by adding chemical buffers, such as agricultural limestone or sodium bicarbonate (i.e., baking soda), to the water. Although sodium bicarbonate will quickly add to the alkalinity of the water, it will also be consumed fairly quickly. Agricultural limestone, dolomite, and some other sources of alkalinity are slower reacting but longer lasting, resulting in less need for frequent additions. Agricultural limestone and dolomite are commonly used to increase alkalinity in ponds.

Test kits measure total alkalinity by titration, adding one drop of titrant at a time until a specified color change occurs. For many of these kits, each drop of titrant is equal to 1 grain per gallon (1 drop = 1 gr/gal). One grain equals 64.79891 milligrams, so after converting gallons to liters, 1 gr/gal is equal to 17.1 mg/L as follows (**Table 2.2**, Equation 5):

$$1 \text{ gr/gal} = 64.79891 \text{ mg/gal} \div 3.785 \text{ L/gal} = 17.1 \text{ mg/L}$$

To convert total alkalinity in grains per gallon to milligrams per liter, multiply by 17.1 (**Table 2.2**, Equation 6).

Example:
- Eight drops of titrant = 8 gr/gal
- $8 \text{ gr/gal} \times 17.1 \text{ mg/L} = 136.8 \text{ mg/L}$

Some test kits (particularly those geared toward hobbyists) refer to total alkalinity as "carbonate hardness" or "KH," which is often measured in degrees (dKH) rather than in grains per gallon or milligrams per liter. dKH is equal to 17.86 mg/L. To convert total alkalinity in dKH to milligrams per liter, multiply by 17.86 (**Table 2.2**, Equation 7).

Example:

$$8 \text{ dKH} \times 17.86 = 142.88 \text{ mg/L}$$

Total alkalinity should be tested at least once a month in ponds and more frequently in recirculating systems to ensure levels are sufficient for productivity and biofiltration. More frequent weekly measurements may be necessary if alkalinity is less than 50 mg/L or stocking density or feeding rates are high.

Total hardness

Total hardness is the measurement of divalent cations, primarily calcium and magnesium, in the water, and, like total alkalinity, is expressed as milligrams per liter (mg/L) or parts per million (ppm) of calcium carbonate ($CaCO_3$). Total hardness and total alkalinity may have similar concentrations in a given water source since bicarbonate and carbonate in water are often derived from limestone or dolomite, which also contain calcium and magnesium. Total hardness is particularly important when spawning fish and raising fry because calcium is critical to egg, bone, and tissue development. However, some species that originate in areas with extremely soft water might require low hardness water to spawn and develop, so it is important to know the specific requirements for each species that will be spawned or maintained.

Test kits measure total hardness by titration, adding one drop of titrant at a time until a specified color change occurs. For many of these kits, each drop of titrant is equal to 1 grain per gallon (1 drop = 1 gr/gal). One grain equals 64.79891 milligrams so, after converting gallons to liters, 1 gr/gal is equal to 17.1 mg/L as follows (**Table 2.2**, Equation 5):

$$1 \text{ gr/gal} = 64.79891 \text{ mg/gal} \div 3.785 \text{ L/gal} = 17.1 \text{ mg/L}$$

To convert total hardness in gr/gal to mg/L, multiply by 17.1 (**Table 2.2**, Equation 8).

Example:
- 8 drops of titrant = 8 gr/gal
- 8 gr/gal × 17.1 mg/L = 136.8 mg/L $CaCO_3$

Some test kits (particularly those geared towards hobbyists) refer to total hardness as "general hardness" or "GH," which is often measured in degrees (dGH) rather gr/gal or mg/L. dGH is equal to 17.86 mg/L. To convert total alkalinity in dGH to milligrams per liter, multiply by 17.86 (**Table 2.2**, Equation 9).

Example:

8 dGH × 17.86 = 142.88 mg/L $CaCO_3$

Total hardness should be tested once a month in most systems. However, if breeding fish or raising fry, total hardness should be tested more frequently to ensure adequate levels for egg and fry development.

Chlorine and chloramine

Chlorine is frequently used as a disinfectant in municipal water sources, and for cleaning and disinfection of fish systems. Because chlorine easily volatilizes from water, some municipalities use chloramine, a combination of chlorine and ammonia, which provides more stable and longer-lasting disinfection. Chloramine also results in fewer disinfection by-products than chlorine.[30]

No level of chlorine or chloramine is considered safe for fish. Both chlorine and chloramine are extremely toxic to fish and must be completely removed before the water comes in contact with fish. Chlorine can be removed from water by aeration, activated carbon, or chemical addition. For activated carbon, it is important to have sufficient contact time to remove all chlorine. Activated carbon must be changed over time as the surface area becomes saturated with chlorine and other contaminants in the water. Sodium thiosulfate is a chemical commonly used for dechlorination of water prior to use for fish. The amount of sodium thiosulfate needed to remove chlorine can vary depending on pH, but a range of 2–7 mg/L sodium sulfate per 1 mg/L chlorine has been suggested for dechlorination.[31]

Because of the stability of chloramine, vigorous aeration will not remove it from water. Instead, activated carbon or chemical methods of removal must be used. Sodium thiosulfate will remove the chlorine from chloramine, but ammonia will remain in the water. A mature biological filter will reduce this ammonia level. Many commercial dechlorinators will break the chlorine-ammonia bond and remove the chlorine. Some of these products will bind the remaining ammonia to produce a non-toxic substance, whereas others will simply cause an ammonia test to read negative, although the ammonia is still present and toxic. Regardless of removal method and initial chlorine form (i.e., free chlorine or chloramine), chlorine levels should always be measured after dechlorination to ensure that no residual chlorine remains in the water.

Chlorine test kits are available that will test over various ranges. Pool chlorine test kits may be more accessible in an emergency situation if chlorine toxicity is suspected. Because chlorine is easily volatilized from water, levels must be checked as soon as a problem is suspected.

Hydrogen sulfide

Hydrogen sulfide (H_2S) is an odiferous, flammable gas that is highly toxic to fish and other animals including humans. It is produced as sulfur-reducing bacteria decompose organic matter under anaerobic conditions such as in the sediment layers of fishponds, deep gravel or sand beds of aquaria, in pipes and hoses that have not been used regularly, or underground water sources. Disturbing these anaerobic layers, such as when harvesting a fishpond or when vigorously cleaning a tank after long-neglected maintenance, can release the gas into the water column. Because the decomposition process also occurs underground, wells and springs in certain areas may contain hydrogen sulfide, resulting in the need for degassing of the water before use in fish systems.

Hydrogen sulfide is lipid soluble and is able to pass through biological membranes.[32] Concentrations of hydrogen sulfide as low as 0.01 mg/L may be lethal to certain aquatic organisms.[1] Decreased pH and increased temperature result in higher proportions of hydrogen sulfide in the more toxic un-ionized form.

Hydrogen sulfide has a distinctive "rotten egg" smell that can be noted at levels as low as 0.003 mg/L.[33] If the smell is detected, concentrations should be immediately tested in the water. Any detectable level should be considered detrimental. In well-ventilated areas, hydrogen sulfide may not be detected by smell but may still be present at problematic levels. Water sources, such as wells and springs, and systems with high organic loads should be regularly tested for hydrogen sulfide.

Occupational exposure to hydrogen sulfide is also of significant concern.[34] Respiratory and eye irritation, nervous system depression, loss of consciousness, and death in humans have been reported at progressively increased exposure levels. At concentrations of 100 mg/L or more, olfactory fatigue or paralysis can occur, resulting in no noticeable smell by humans, which can result in a false sense of safety.

As with other dissolved gases, hydrogen sulfide is most accurately tested on-site. Ensure water is not agitated while collecting the sample because this will help degas the hydrogen sulfide from the water. When testing a water source (e.g., well), the water should be run sufficiently to clear any potential contaminants from the piping.

Nitrogen gas (N$_2$)

Nitrogen is the most prevalent gas in the atmosphere, accounting for 78.08% of all gases. Like dissolved oxygen, its solubility in water is influenced by pressure and temperature. Solubility of N$_2$ increases as pressure increases and/or water temperature decreases. As long as levels do not exceed 100% saturation in water, nitrogen gas is considered inconsequential for fish. However, when the saturation of N$_2$ exceeds 100% in the water, then supersaturation occurs. As a result, gas emboli may form in various fish tissues (i.e., gas bubble disease), causing acute or chronic disease or death (**Figure 2.11**).

Nitrogen may become supersaturated in water through both natural and man-made circumstances. Source waters such as springs and wells may contain high concentrations of N$_2$ under pressure. As the water rises or is brought to the surface and pressure is reduced, water may become supersaturated with N$_2$. If water temperature rapidly rises, a similar effect may be seen. In addition, supersaturation may also occur at the base of waterfalls or dams where overflowing water is forced into deep plunge basins.

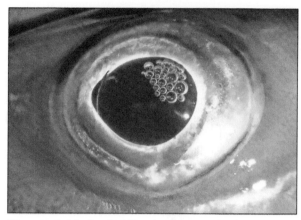

Figure 2.11 Gas bubbles in anterior chamber of the eye of an amberjack (*Seriola* sp.) due to "gas bubble disease" or nitrogen supersaturation of the water column in a recirculation system.

System design or failure may also cause supersaturation if air is allowed to be drawn into the water through small holes or cracks in piping or leaks in pumps or other system components. Air sucked into a water intake may also cause supersaturation as the nitrogen-rich air mixes with the water.

Saturation of N$_2$ can be calculated after testing percent total gas pressure (TGP) with a saturometer and percent saturation of dissolved oxygen (DO) with a dissolved oxygen meter (**Figure 2.12**). If carbon dioxide and argon are considered negligible, the following equation may be used to determine the saturation of N$_2$ in water, where 0.2095 is the percentage of O$_2$ and 0.7808 is the percentage of N$_2$ in the atmosphere (**Table 2.2**, Equation 10):

$$\%N_2 = \frac{\%TGP - (\%DO \times 0.2095)}{0.7808}$$

Example:

- Total gas pressure (TGP) measurement from saturometer: 130%
- Dissolved oxygen (DO) measurement from DO meter: 95%

$$\%N_2 = \frac{130 - (95 \times 0.2095)}{0.7808}$$

$$\%N_2 = 141\%$$

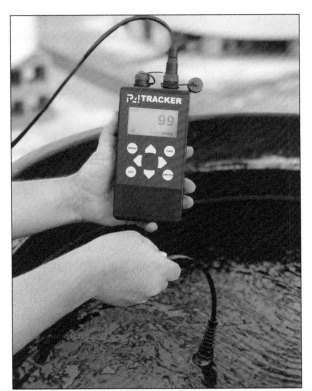

Figure 2.12 Saturometer and probe. (Point Four Systems, Inc. Pentair Aquatic Eco-Systems, Apopka, FL.)

CLINICAL SIGNS AND MANAGEMENT

Water quality parameters for the immense diversity of fish will vary depending on the species, life stage and habitat they live in (**Table 2.4**). However clinical signs associated with water quality problems are generally nonspecific in nature and may include an increased opercular rate (i.e., respiratory rate) or "gilling," gasping, or "piping" at the surface, congregating in higher oxygenated areas and other behavioral signs of respiratory distress.[35] Fish may also display clamped fins, increased mucus production of the skin and gills, skin lesions, corneal edema, secondary opportunistic infections, lethargy, anorexia, and poor growth.[35] The mechanism(s) of toxicity associated with poor water quality are usually multifaceted and may involve increased levels of toxic metabolites in the blood and tissues, changes in blood pH, osmoregulatory disturbances, irritation of the skin and gills, altered immune system function, decreased transport of oxygen into the capillaries of the gill from the water, and decreased transport of CO_2 and NH_3 out of the capillaries into the water.[20,35,36] Depending on the cause and magnitude of the water quality issue, fish may experience either acute death or chronic mortality. Fish that die

Table 2.4 **Summary of general ranges recommended for water chemistry parameters for freshwater and marine fish**

WATER PARAMETER	RECOMMENDED RANGE FOR FRESHWATER FISH	RECOMMENDED RANGE FOR MARINE FISH
Temperature	Species dependent	Species dependent
Dissolved oxygen	5–15 mg/L	5–15 mg/L
Carbon dioxide	<20 mg/L	<20 mg/L
pH	6.5–9.5	8.0–8.5
Total alkalinity	50–200 mg/L	100–200 mg/L
Total hardness	50–200 mg/L	Not applicable
Un-ionized ammonia	<0.05 mg/L	<0.05 mg/L
Nitrite	<0.05 mg/L	<0.05 mg/L
Chlorine	0 mg/L	0 mg/L
Hydrogen sulfide	0 mg/L	0 mg/L
Nitrogen gas	<100% saturation	<100% saturation

Note: Optimal recommendations will vary depending on species.

acutely of poor water quality issues may have no histological evidence of pathology, whereas those that exhibit chronic mortality will generally only show nonspecific histological alterations of hyperplasia, lamellar fusion and telangiectasia of the gill tissues.[35]

For the most part it is difficult to distinguish between ammonia toxicity, nitrite toxicity, or other water quality toxicities based on clinical signs alone. There are, however, a couple of notable exceptions to this general rule where clinical sings may lead one to suspect a certain toxicity. For instance, in nitrite toxicity the gills can appear pale or tan in color, and in severe cases the gills and blood may exhibit a dark brown discoloration.[25,36,37] In cases of water supersaturation, there may be small air bubbles in the capillaries of the gills, fins and tail, anterior chamber of the eye, or in the subcutis. And in hydrogen sulfide toxicity, there may be a sulfur or rotten egg smell to the water. However, in general, it is essential to have a good clinical history and water quality analysis to determine the cause of most water quality problems.

Correction of most water quality problems is primarily aimed at rapidly eliminating or reducing the offending toxicity. For metabolic waste (i.e., ammonia, nitrite, and nitrate) toxicities, this usually involves multiple partial water changes, temporary cessation or reduction of feeding, removal of excess organic debris, increased oxygenation, and/or reduction in populations numbers (i.e., stocking density) if feasible.[35,36,38] In addition, there are several commercial ammonia-binding agents available for reducing elevated ammonia levels in the water. In nitrite toxicity, nitrite is actively transported from the water by way of the chloride cells of the gills. Thus, in freshwater fish the addition of sodium chloride to the water can competitively inhibit the uptake of nitrite thereby, reducing the effect of elevated nitrite levels on the fish. Though still vulnerable, marine fish are less likely to be affected by nitrite toxicity since seawater already has increased levels of chloride, which reduces the uptake of nitrite by the chloride cells. Adjustment of water pH abnormalities generally involves improving the buffering capacity of the water.[36,39] Several buffering compounds are available for adjusting the pH of the water. Sodium bicarbonate can be added to the system to improve the buffering capacity (i.e., alkalinity) of the water, though this is generally only a temporary solution.[36] Crushed coral, crushed oyster shell, or limestone can be added as a substrate or filtration component for long-term management of alkalinity problems in a system.[36]

Another water quality toxicity that commonly occurs in aquatic systems is the presence of chlorine or chloramine in the source water. Chlorine can be removed from water with a dechlorinator such as sodium thiosulfate or by aeration of water for 24 hours before using. Unfortunately, sodium thiosulfate does not remove chloramines intact from the water and leaves ammonia behind. The most common methods of removing chloramine from water is by passing the water slowly through granular activated carbon, which binds the chloramine, or by using a commercial product such as Amquel® (i.e., sodium hydroxymethanesulfonate), which removes ammonia, chlorine, and chloramine. Supersaturation of water with elevated pressures of atmospheric gases can be corrected with agitation (i.e., aeration) of the water or degassing columns where the water flow is broken up releasing freed gases to the atmosphere before reaching the fish. And finally, the presence of hydrogen sulfide in a system, filter, or hoses needs to be aggressively managed by water agitation, increased aeration, or degassing columns all of which are aimed at making the system aerobic.

REFERENCES

1. Boyd, C.E. *Water Quality for Pond Aquaculture. Research and Development Series No. 43.* Auburn University, Auburn, AL, 1998.
2. Roots, B.I. and Prosser, C.L. Temperature acclimation and the nervous system in fish. *Journal of Experimental Biology* 1962;39:617–629.
3. Boyd, C.E. *Water Quality: An Introduction*, 2nd ed. Springer International, New York, 2015.
4. Burrell, P.C., Phalen, C.M. and Hovanec, T.A. Identification of bacteria responsible for ammonia oxidation in freshwater aquaria. *Applied and Environmental Microbiology* 2001;67:5791–5800.
5. Sauder, L.A., Engel, K., Stearns, J.C., Masella, A.P., Pawliszyn, R. and Neufeld, J.D. Aquarium nitrification revisited: *Thaumarchaeota* are the dominant ammonia oxidizers in freshwater aquarium biofilters. *PLOS ONE* 2011;6(8):e23281.
6. Hagopian, D.S. and Riley, J.G. A closer look at the bacteriology of nitrification. *Aquacultural Engineering* 1998;18:223–244.

7. Hovanec, T.A., Taylor, L.T., Blakis, A. and Delong, E.F. *Nitrospira*-like bacteria associated with nitrite oxidation in freshwater aquaria. *Applied and Environmental Microbiology* 1998;64:258–264.

8. Smutna, M., Vorlova, L. and Svobodova, Z. Pathobiochemistry of ammonia in the internal environment of fish (review). *Acta Veterinaria Brno* 2002;71:169–181.

9. Bower, C.E. and Bidwell, J.P. Ionization of ammonia in seawater: Effects of temperature, pH, and salinity. *Journal of the Fisheries Research Board of Canada* 1978;35:1012–1016.

10. Emerson, K., Russo, R.C., Lund, R.E. and Thurston, R.V. Aqueous ammonia equilibrium calculations: Effect of pH and temperature. *Journal of the Fisheries Research Board of Canada* 1975;32:2379–2383.

11. Wilkie, M.P. Mechanisms of ammonia excretion across fish gills. *Comparative Biochemistry and Physiology* 1997;118A:39–50.

12. Randall, D.J. and Wright, P.A. Ammonia distribution and excretion in fish. *Fish Physiology and Biochemistry* 1987;3:107–120.

13. Evans, D.H., More, K.J. and Robbins, S.L. Modes of ammonia transport across the gill epithelium of the marine teleost fish *Opsanus beta*. *Journal of Experimental Biology* 1989;144:339–356.

14. Zhou, L. Comparison of Nessler, phenate, salicylate and ion selective electrode procedures for determination of total ammonia nitrogen in aquaculture. *Aquaculture* 2015;450:187–193.

15. Hach Spec Manual. *Hach fact sheet: Nitrogen, ammonia*. Hach Company, Loveland, CO, 2007.

16. Le, P.T.T. and Boyd, C.D. Comparison of phenate and salicylate methods for determination of total ammonia nitrogen in freshwater and saline water. *Journal of the World Aquaculture Society* 2012;43:885–889.

17. Jensen, F.B. Uptake and effects of nitrite and nitrate in animals. In: *Nitrogen Metabolism and Excretion*. P.J. Walsh and P.A. Wright, eds. CRC Press, Boca Raton, FL, 1995; pp. 289–304.

18. Perrone, S.J. and Meade, T.L. Protective effect of chloride on nitrite toxicity to Coho salmon (*Oncorhynchus kisutch*). *Journal of the Fisheries Research Board of Canada* 1977;34:486–492.

19. Grosell, M. and Jensen, F.B. Uptake and effects of nitrite in the marine teleost fish *Platichthys flesus*. *Aquatic Toxicology* 2000;50:97–107.

20. Tomasso, J.R. Toxicity of nitrogenous wastes to aquaculture animals. *Reviews in Fisheries Science* 1994;2:291–314.

21. Palachek, R.M. and Tomasso, J.R. Toxicity of nitrite to channel catfish (*Ictalurus punctatus*), tilapia (*Tilapia aurea*), and largemouth bass (*Micropterus salmoides*): Evidence for a nitrite exclusion mechanism. *Canadian Journal of Fisheries and Aquatic Sciences* 1984;41:1739–1744.

22. Margiocco, C., Arillo, A., Mensi, P. and Schenone, G. Nitrite bioaccumulation in *Salmo gairdneri* Rich. and hematological consequences. *Aquatic Toxicology* 1983;3:261–270.

23. Jensen, F.B. Nitrite disrupts multiple physiological functions in aquatic animals. *Comparative Biochemistry and Physiology Part A: Molecular & Integrative Physiology* 2003;135:9–24.

24. Bromage, N.R., Shepherd, C.J. and Roberts, J. Farming systems and husbandry practice. In: *Intensive Fish Farming*. C.J. Shepherd and N.R. Bromage, eds. BSP Professional, Oxford, 1988; pp. 94–95.

25. Hrubec, T.C., Smith, S.A. and Robertson, J.L. Nitrate toxicity: A potential problem of recirculating systems. *Successes and Failures in Commercial Recirculating Aquaculture* 1996;1:41–48.

26. Camargo, J.A., Alonso, A. and Salamanca, A. Nitrate toxicity to aquatic animals: A review with new data for freshwater invertebrates. *Chemosphere* 2005;58:1255–1267.

27. Hamlin, H.J. Nitrate toxicity in Siberian sturgeon (*Acipenser baeri*). *Aquaculture* 2006;253:688–693.

28. Boyd, C.E. and Tucker, C.S. *Pond Aquaculture Water Quality Management*. Springer Science and Business Media, New York, 1998.

29. Naigaga S. Assessing the reliability of water test kits for use in small-scale aquaculture. Auburn University, MS thesis. 2015, http://etd.auburn.edu/handle/10415/4974.

30. CDC Chloramine website. Disinfection with chloramine. http://www.cdc.gov/healthywater/drinking/public/chloramine-disinfection.html (accessed 13 March 2018).

31. MacQuarrie, C. and Wilton, S. The ins and outs of dechlorination. *Hatchery International* 2002;September/October 2002:26–28.

32. Torrans, E.L. and Clemens, H.P. Physiological and biochemical effects of acute exposure of fish to hydrogen sulfide. *Comparative Biochemistry and Physiology Part C: Comparative Pharmacology* 1982;71:183–190.

33. Reiffenstein, R.J., Hulbert, W.C. and Roth, S.H. Toxicology of hydrogen sulfide. *Annual Review of Pharmacology and Toxicology* 1991;32:109–134.

34. Nikkanen, H.E. and Burns, M.M. Severe hydrogen sulfide exposure in a working adolescent. *Pediatrics* 2004;113:927–929.

35. Roberts, H.E. and Smith, S.A. Disorders of the respiratory system in pet and ornamental fish. *The Veterinary Clinics of North America: Exotic Animal Practice* 2011;14:179–206.

36. Roberts, H. and Palmeiro, B. Toxicology of aquarium fish. *The Veterinary Clinics of North America: Exotic Animal Practice* 2008;11:359–374.

37. Lewis, W.M. and Morris, D.P. Toxicity of nitrite to fish: A review. *T Am Fish Soc* 1986;115:183–195.

38. Hadfield, C.A., Whitaker, B.R. and Clayton, L.A. Emergency and critical care of fish. *The Veterinary Clinics of North America: Exotic Animal Practice* 2007;10:647–655.

39. Boyd, C.E., Tucker, C.S. and Somridhivej, B. Alkalinity and hardness: Critical but elusive concepts in aquaculture. *Journal of the World Aquaculture Society* 2016;47:6–41.

DIAGNOSIS OF FISH DISEASES

*ESTEBAN SOTO, SHANE M. BOYLAN, BRITTANY STEVENS,
STEPHEN A. SMITH, ROY P.E. YANONG, KUTTICHANTRAN
SUBRAMANIAM, AND THOMAS WALTZEK*

HISTORY

As in any other species, obtaining a thorough history for fish patients is of vital importance.[1-3] Information gathered in the history helps to direct and focus the physical examination and can aid in the selection of additional pertinent diagnostics. Oftentimes, simply by gathering a thorough clinical history, a preliminary diagnosis can be reached. It is important to realize that fish clients can vary tremendously in their relationships to the patient as well as in their knowledge of proper fish husbandry and health. The fish practitioner may encounter a new fish owner who brings their pet to the veterinary office as a beloved member of the family or a client with an ornamental backyard fishpond. Alternatively, the practitioner may be called upon to visit a large-scale aquaculture facility where the focus is on the maintenance of population (e.g., herd) health rather than the individual animal. The history should be tailored to take into account the knowledge level of the client and should address the specific needs and concerns of each client.

The general history should focus on determining what species are affected, what clinical signs have been appreciated by the client and the time course of the disease.[1-3] It is also important to note that prior to seeking an examination and treatment with a veterinarian, it is quite common for fish clients to seek out information regarding fish diseases and treatments from a wide variety of sources including the Internet, husbandry manuals and advice from hobbyists or other fish keepers. Prior to being seen by a veterinarian, the patient may have already been treated with a wide variety of environmental

adjustments or any of the numerous readily available over-the-counter therapeutics aimed at treating fish disease. The client should be questioned about what treatments have been attempted and the success or failure of these treatment endeavors. Specifically, clients should be asked about the application of any chemicals, antimicrobials, antiparasitics or supplements to the water or the feed. Similarly, the client should be questioned whether any environmental alterations have been attempted, such as adjusting the water temperature or salinity. To help aid the clinician in the determination of the active ingredients and dosages of therapeutics used, it can be helpful for the client to provide the packaging or bring pictures of the labels for products that were used.

As compared to land-dwelling animals, fish patients have the added challenge that their water environment plays a critical role in their health.[4] Therefore, questions regarding the environment and water quality must be investigated as thoroughly as questions regarding the fish patient itself. A current water quality analysis should be performed as part of any clinical examination and details regarding historical water quality results and trends should be obtained. Performing a field call or home visit to inspect the patient's living environment and the life support systems (i.e., filtration, ultraviolet [UV], ozone) can greatly aid in the diagnosis of environmental problems. In lieu of visiting the site, it can be beneficial for the owner to provide pictures or video of the patient's living environment and life support system and equipment. General questions to ask during the client account of the clinical history are presented in **Tables 3.1** and **3.2**.

Table 3.1 **General history questions**

- Common name and genus/species of the patient
- Age of the patient, or how long has the owner had the patient?
- Origin: Captive bred, wild-caught/imported, unknown
- Source: Pet store, breeder, farm, wild-caught, etc.
- What other species are present in pond/raceway/cage/tank?
- What clinical signs has the owner appreciated?
- Duration of problem(s)?
- What species are affected?
- Any mortalities?
- Any changes in behavior noted?
- Any changes in appetite noted?
- Is a quarantine system in place? For fish, invertebrates, plants? Any prophylactic treatments routinely performed?
- When was the last introduction of fish, invertebrates, plants?
- Does tank/pond/facility have history of previous disease(s)?
- Have any treatments for the disease been attempted?
- Name, dosage and frequency of any chemicals, antibiotics, anti-parasitics or supplements that have been used to treat the fish
- Have any adjustments to water temperature, salinity or other water quality parameters been made?

SAMPLE SELECTION

Good sample selection, especially in population health–type evaluations where disease prevalence can be low, is critical.[2,5] Strictly random sampling in a population with low-level mortalities may lead to evaluation of healthy fish. The clinician should select moribund fish showing typical disease signs, along with a healthy individual for comparison, especially in species that the clinician is unfamiliar with. If possible, multiple fish should be chosen at different stages of disease, including at least one or more with early-stage disease, as secondary complications that mask initiating causes are often seen in much later stages of disease.

Evaluation of freshly dead fish, although not ideal, can also be helpful, especially if disease prevalence is low, samples examined to date reveal no significant findings, and environmental and management factors have been carefully evaluated and ruled out.[2,5] Selection of freshly dead (i.e., collected immediately after death) fish for evaluation will help to avoid postmortem artifact and a subsequent misdiagnosis. Although dead fish may have lesions that make assessment of "freshness" more challenging, freshly dead fish should have relatively clear eyes, good coloration, red to pink gills, and should not have a bad odor. Dead fish are often cannibalized, undergo rapid autolysis, and/or become overrun by

Table 3.2 **Environmental and husbandry questions**

- Pond/raceway/cage/tank size, shape, number of gallons?
- What is the source of the water?
- What water conditioners, salt, buffers, etc. are used on a routine basis?
- How often are water changes performed? What percentage of water is changed?
- What life support equipment is in place (biofiltration, mechanical filtration, chemical filtration, UV, ozone, protein skimmer, degassing towers, etc.)? How often is life support equipment cleaned or changed?
- Is supplemental aeration or oxygenation applied?
- What structures or decorations are present, including substrate and plants?
- What type of lighting is provided (natural, artificial, bulb type, light cycle, frequency of changing of bulbs)?
- What water quality parameters are measured and how frequently? What are the latest water quality results?
- What is the cleaning routine for the pond/raceway/cage/tank? Are cleaning tools specific for each pond/raceway/cage/tank? What disinfection agents are used?
- What type of food is fed? How much and how frequently? Are fish fed consistently all year round or does feeding routine change seasonally? How old is the food? Does food have a known expiration date? How is the food stored?

secondary postmortem organisms such as fungi, bacteria, and parasites, including opportunistic histophagous ciliates of the genera *Tetrahymena* or *Uronema*. For this reason, the relevance of wet mount findings from lesions on dead fish must be interpreted with caution.

Although fish demonstrating clinical signs of disease are ideal specimens for antemortem diagnostics and necropsy, freshly dead, frozen, and formalin-fixed specimens may have diagnostic value.[2,5] Freshly dead fish examined immediately or kept in a plastic bag in the refrigerator or on ice for 6–12 hours can provide almost as much information as moribund fish, whereas frozen and formalin-fixed fish are much less informative. Common external parasites (e.g., protozoans and monogeneans) often die or leave a dead host, and bacterial cultures collected from fish that have been dead for as little as 30 to 60 minutes may be contaminated due to rapid autolysis of the organs.

APPROACHES TO DISEASE DIAGNOSTICS

Numerous factors will guide the clinician's approach to disease diagnostics for each case. If the affected animal is considered too valuable to sacrifice for financial or personal reasons (e.g., brood stock, rare or endangered species, strong human–animal bond), antemortem, nonlethal diagnostics can be performed. If the outbreak involves a population health scenario (aquaculture/production or less valuable fish in a large display system), a full necropsy of representative fish is a much more informative option. Other factors include size limitations, client budget, logistics (i.e., time, location, and resources), available equipment and supplies, and the rapidity and severity of the disease progression.

PHYSICAL EXAM

Observational examination

An observational examination of the patient in the water should be performed as part of every routine examination.[1–6] This observational examination allows the practitioner to study the behavior of the patient in a manner that is less compromised by the stress of capture/handling or the sedative effects of anesthetics. Ideally the patient would be observed in its home tank, pond environment or aquaculture setting. This allows for observation of the patient's interactions with other tank mates if present and will allow for a more thorough assessment of the patient's behaviors as compared to simply observing the fish in a small transport container. A site visit to the patient's living environment will also allow for inspection of the patient's living quarters and life support systems, which can be very useful in detecting environmental problems.

During the observational examination, the patient's swimming patterns and position in the water column should be noted.[1–3] If possible, a normal conspecific's behavior and swimming patterns should be observed for comparative purposes. Sick fish may congregate together away from the remainder of the group or may isolate themselves from other fish. Absence of normal schooling behavior in a schooling species is cause for concern. Weak or moribund fish may be found at the water outlet (e.g., raceway screens) or trapped at the aquarium skimmer or filter water intake tube (**Figure 3.1**). Fish with respiratory compromise may be found congregating at the water's surface or at areas of relatively higher oxygen content such as inflow pipes, aerators or waterfalls. Aberrant or whirling swimming patterns can be indicative of neurological disease. Inappropriate position in the water column (e.g., bottom sitting or floating at the surface), inappropriate recumbency (e.g., dorsal/lateral), abnormal listing (e.g., tilting to the right or left) or abnormal pitching (e.g., not

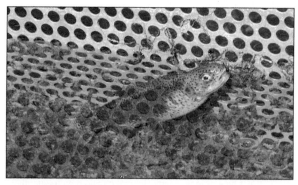

Figure 3.1 Moribund rainbow trout (*O. mykiss*) on lower screen of raceway.

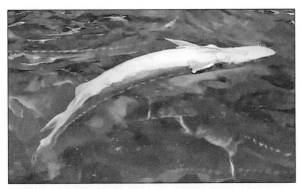

Figure 3.2 **Abnormal positive buoyancy in a white sturgeon (*Acipenser transmontanus*).**

remaining horizontal in the water column) can be signs of a buoyancy disorder (**Figure 3.2**).

Fish may also exhibit other characteristic signs of disease.[6] "Flashing" or scraping along the bottom or sides of an enclosure is commonly seen when fish are affected by external parasites. Fish with respiratory disease will often have an increased opercular rate with exaggerated flaring of the operculum. "Piping" behavior, where fish repeatedly gape at the water's surface, can also be seen in fish with respiratory compromise. Holding the fins close or clamped to the body wall is another nonspecific behavior that fish will exhibit when affected by a variety of ailments. In addition to abnormal behaviors and color changes, any obvious lesions or physical abnormalities should also be documented during the observational examination with the intent of performing further inspection of these abnormalities during the physical portion of the examination.

Direct examination

Following the completion of the observational examination, a direct or "hands-on" physical examination is generally necessary for a closer assessment of any abnormalities noted during the observational examination, a systematic inspection of all body systems and procurement of necessary diagnostic samples. Although it is possible to examine fish and perform certain procedures under manual restraint alone, this is generally restricted to only very rapid procedures or for animals that are too weak/ill to undergo general anesthesia. Several studies have shown that general anesthesia significantly reduces handling stress in fish patients.[7-12] Therefore, when performing the direct examination of the patient, general anesthesia is usually recommended to minimize stress and potential harm to the patient. General anesthesia is also indicated to help protect the practitioner from harm when dealing with species that have the potential to be injurious.[1-3] Scorpaenidae (i.e., lionfish, scorpionfish, stonefish) and certain catfish species have venomous barbs or spines along their fins that can cause considerable pain or even death upon envenomation. Several species of fish including eels, triggerfish, surgeonfish, pufferfish and most species of elasmobranchs have teeth, barbs, modified scales or spines that can inflict injury to the handler. Other species such as electric eels, electric catfish and torpedo rays can produce strong electrical currents and must be handled with rubber gloves and appropriate precautions. Finally, large species, such as species of *Arapaima*, have the ability to inflict damage to the handler when trying to evade capture or restraint simply as a result of their large size and ample muscle mass. For a full discussion of fish sedation and anesthesia, see Chapter 17.

Prior to examining the fish patient, all necessary equipment for the procedure should be gathered and readied. A list of suggested equipment, supplies and chemicals for a fish examination either in the clinic or while on a field visit can be found in **Table 3.3**.

While handing fish patients it is important to minimize trauma to their skin. Fish have a protective mucous layer that covers the epidermis, which provides an important line of defense against external pathogens. Preserving this mucous layer and avoiding epidermal abrasion/ulceration should therefore be paramount during the examination. Handlers should wear powder-free latex or nitrile examination gloves, both to help protect the fish's skin and to help protect the handler from possible zoonotic pathogens.[13] If the fish needs to be placed on a surface for examination, the surface should be covered in a nonabrasive material (e.g., synthetic chamois, plastic drapes or bubble wrap) to protect the fish. Absorptive materials such as paper or cloth towels are generally not recommended, as these materials may wick moisture from the mucous layer and have the potential to cause microabrasions on the skin of the fish patient. It should be noted that fish patients

Table 3.3 **Diagnostic fish health equipment**
• Appropriately sized containers for anesthetizing/recovering the patient
• Appropriately sized nets
• Tricaine methanesulfonate (MS-222) or other appropriate anesthetic
• Sodium bicarbonate (for buffering MS-222)
• Glass slides and coverslips
• Compound and dissecting microscopes
• Portable air pump
• Aquarium tubing
• Air stone
• Powder-free gloves
• Chamois or other nonabrasive material
• Small suture scissors or iris scissors, forceps
• Tape measure and calipers
• Gram scale for measuring MS-222 and small patients
• Larger scale for weighing larger patients
• Ophthalmoscope
• Doppler
• Various sized syringes and needles
• Blood collection tubes
• Bacterial and fungal culture media, viral transport media
• Sterile swabs/culturettes
• Variously sized punch biopsies
• 10% neutral buffered formalin or other fixative(s)
• Containers for preserved tissues and tissue cassettes
• Water dechlorination product (i.e., sodium thiosulfate)
• Bottles for water sample collection
• Water quality analysis equipment or kit

are quite slippery when handled in exam gloves and when placed on nonabrasive surfaces.

The examination of the fish patient should be conducted in an organized and thorough manner and follow the same routine each time so that nothing is missed. A standardized "head-to-tail" approach when performing the physical examination is generally recommended.

General appearance

The general appearance and overall body condition of each patient should be assessed as part of the routine examination. A 1–5/5 scale when judging body condition can be used, with 3/5 being the ideal body condition, 1/5 being emaciated and 5/5 being obese. It is quite common for fish with chronic disease to become emaciated. Emaciation can be distinguished by loss of muscle mass along the epaxial muscles resulting in a more triangular "pinched" appearance to the dorsum of the fish. A concave abdomen and sunken eyes can also be indicative of emaciation. Conversely, when fish become overconditioned they begin to lose their typical fusiform shape and tend to take on a more rounded or football-shaped appearance. In some species, they will also develop a more noticeable raised area just caudal to the skull as fat is commonly deposited in this area.

Neurologic examination

An assessment of the patient's neurological status should be performed prior to induction of anesthesia. The patient's general attitude and response to stimuli should be observed. Similar to other veterinary patients, if the fish exhibits normal behaviors and appears alert, the designation of "bright, alert, responsive" may be applied to the fish patient. Other assessments of attitude can include: "quiet, alert, responsive," decreased responsiveness to stimuli/ obtunded or moribund/stuporous. Knowledge of the species' normal behavior or ability to observe normal conspecifics is again quite useful in assessing the neurologic status of the patient and its response to stimuli. For example, a benthic species that relies on camouflage as part of its natural history strategy may need a more aggressive stimulus to incite a reaction as compared to another species that spends the majority of its time in the water column. The presence or absence of aberrant swimming patterns such as whirling, lethargic swimming, running into objects, repetitive movements or arching of the spine should also be noted.

Once the fish is appropriately anesthetized, general morphometrics and a weight of the patient should be obtained. Fish should be weighed to the nearest gram on an appropriately sized scale and the weight should be recorded. Standard measurements of total length (longest length of the fish from rostrum to tip of caudal fin), fork length (length from the rostrum to the fork of caudal fin) and girth (obtained at

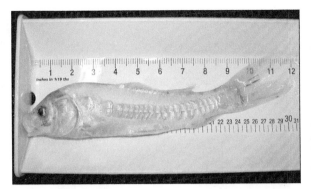

Figure 3.3 Severely emaciated koi on a commercial measuring board to obtain standard measurements.

widest portion of the fish) can also be obtained during the examination (**Figure 3.3**). Trends of change in weight and morphometrics can be useful to help give a more complete picture of patient growth over time or changes due to disease (e.g., coelomic distension, weight loss). Accurate patient weights are also necessary for calculating appropriate drug dosages should the patient require medication.

Mouth

The mouth of each patient should be opened and examined with a light source. Trauma to the most rostral portion of the mouth or nose from contacting structures, aquarium decorations, enclosure walls or substrate is commonly observed. Traumatic wounds from food/prey items or altercations with tank mates may also be present. The jaw mechanism of the fish should open and close smoothly without signs of stiffness or crepitus. The interior of the mouth should also be inspected for the presence of any lesions, masses, parasites or foreign objects such as rocks or tank decor (**Figures 3.4** to **3.6**). If present, the teeth of the fish should also be inspected for any signs of lesions or trauma. In certain species of diodontids (i.e., burrfishes) and tetradontids (i.e., pufferfish), malocclusion of the teeth plates or improper wear due to lack of appropriate food sources may be present and require attention. Many species also possess pharyngeal teeth, which can be seen or palpated at the back of the throat region. In eel species these pharyngeal teeth and jaws are well ossified and can be readily appreciated on radiographs.[14]

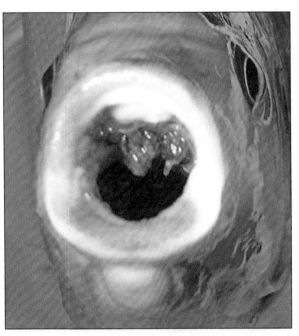

Figure 3.4 Leeches in the oral cavity of a tilapia (*Oreochromis* sp.).

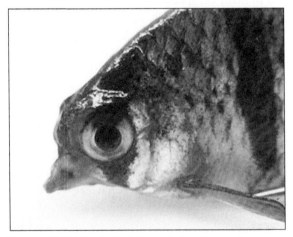

Figure 3.5 *Erysipelothrix* sp. infection causing stomatitis in longfin tiger barb (*Puntigrus tetrazona*). (Image courtesy of J. Shelley.)

Nostrils

Most fish species possess paired nostrils at the rostral aspect of the head. The paired nostrils usually contain both an incurrent and an excurrent opening for water to flow in a unidirectional manner over the olfactory epithelium. The anterior and posterior nostril openings may be separated by a small flap of tissue as in the cyprinids or may be widely separated

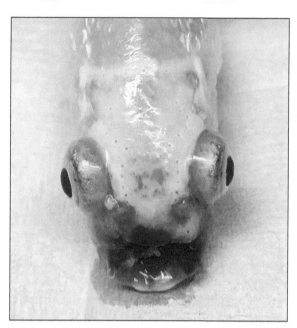

Figure 3.6 Atypical *Aeromonas salmonicida* infection causing stomatitis in a koi.

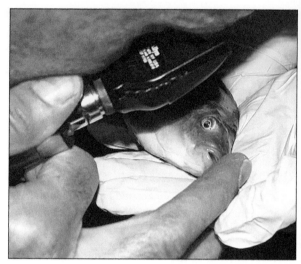

Figure 3.7 Ophthalmoscopic examination of the eye of a tilapia.

as in many eel species. The nostrils of a fish patient should be examined for any signs of occlusion, ulceration, hemorrhage, edema or for the presence of any masses. Fish use the sense of olfaction for a wide variety of purposes including the recognition of conspecifics (i.e., important in schooling species), location of prey or potential mates, avoidance of predators, or for navigation as in salmonids that primarily use olfaction to navigate back to their natal streams during spawning.[15] Therefore, damage to the nostrils or the olfactory epithelium may impair a fish's ability to adequately perform normal behaviors.

Eyes

The approach to the teleost ocular examination is performed in a manner similar to other veterinary patients.[14,16,17] An ophthalmoscope can be used to inspect the periocular tissues, the cornea and the intraocular structures of the eye (**Figure 3.7**). If further detail is needed, a slit lamp can be used to provide better magnification of the eye, while indirect ophthalmoscopy with an ophthalmic lens can be performed to provide better detail of the retina (**Figure 3.8**). Other more advanced equipment such as a tonometer or ultrasound can also be used to further investigate causes of ocular disease.

The globes should be examined for symmetry of size and shape, and any exophthalmia, endophthalmia or buphthalmia should be noted. Unlike other vertebrate species, the condition of exophthalmia is seen quite commonly in fish patients as a response to a variety of etiologies such as bacterial, viral, fungal or parasitic infections; gas bubble disease; osmotic derangements; rapid changes in pressure; or neoplasia (**Figures 3.9** and **3.10**). There is considerable variation in the ocular structures of fish and some breeds have even been specifically bred

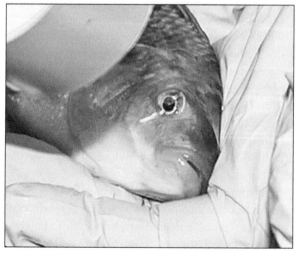

Figure 3.8 Slit-lamp examination of the eye of a tilapia.

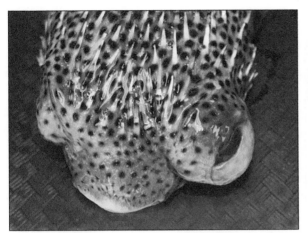

Figure 3.9 Exophthalmia in a porcupinefish caused by *Metabronema* sp. (Nematoda) infection.

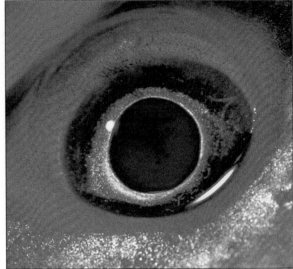

Figure 3.11 Normal eye of tilapia stained with fluorescein dye.

to display unusual ocular conformations such as the "bubble eye" and "telescope eye" goldfish breeds.[18] Therefore, knowledge of normal anatomy for that species is essential to prevent misdiagnosis.

The cornea should be clear and free of opacities or ulceration. Common causes of corneal opacities in fish patients include physical trauma, scarring, bacterial, fungal or parasitic infection, or keratitis secondary to poor water quality, toxicants or riboflavin, thiamine or vitamin A deficiency.[19] Fluorescein dye can be used to highlight active ulcerations of the cornea if present (**Figures 3.11** and **3.12**). The anterior chamber should be clear

and free from conditions such as hyphema, hypopyon, parasites or gas bubbles (**Figure 3.13**). Gas bubbles can be seen commonly in this location secondary to gas supersaturation disease. Cataracts are another common occurrence in many species of fish (**Figure 3.14**). Possible causes include nutritional deficiencies, ocular trauma, infections, parasitic infestations (i.e., larval *Diplostonum* sp.), toxic insult or transient changes due to rapid osmotic shifts.[14,20]

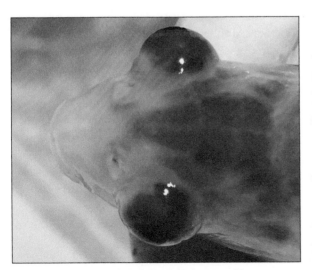

Figure 3.10 Exophthalmia in fish caused by a systemic bacterial infection.

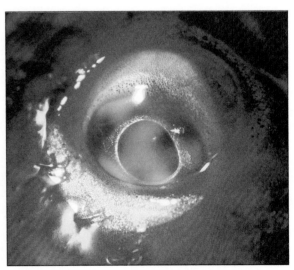

Figure 3.12 Eye of tilapia with ulcerative lesion stained with fluorescein dye.

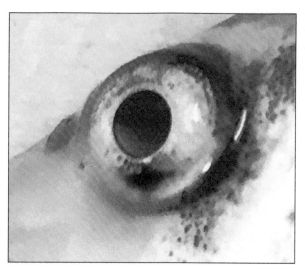

Figure 3.13 Hyphema in the eye of koi.

Opercular cavity and gills

The respiratory rate of the fish can be obtained by observing and counting the movements of the opercula per minute. It is ideal to obtain an opercular rate prior to handling or anesthetizing the fish, as stress, exertion or the effects of anesthetic drugs will artifactually alter the rate. While observing opercular movements it is also useful to note the level of respiratory effort. Fish that have respiratory compromise will often open their mouths wider and more forcefully expel water from the opercular cavity in an effort to increase water flow over the gills.

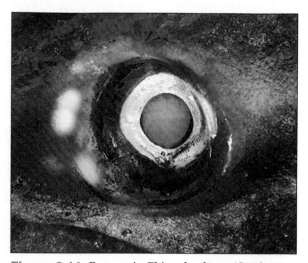

Figure 3.14 Cataract in Chinook salmon (*O. tshawytscha*) due to encysted digenetic trematode infection.

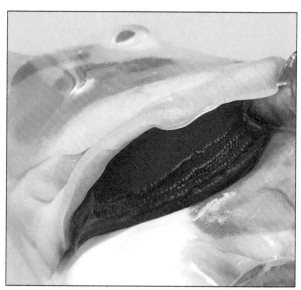

Figure 3.15 Examination of opercular cavity and gills by lifting operculum.

The opercula on each side of the fish should be gently lifted to allow for visual inspection of the opercular cavity and the gills (**Figure 3.15**). In species, such as eels, pufferfish and seahorses, that have small opercular openings, an otoscope or small endoscope may be introduced through the opercular opening to allow for examination the gills. Each operculum should be examined for completeness and for signs of trauma or lesions. It should be noted that males of the cyprinid family develop white spots or bumps along the opercula and along the pectoral fins during breeding season. These are referred to as "nuptial tubercles" and should not be confused for lesions caused by other common infectious etiologies (e.g., *Ichthyophthirius multifiliis* or lymphocystis virus). The pseudobranch can be appreciated on the dorsal medial aspect of the operculum in many species. The condition of goiter can also sometimes be detected during the examination of the opercular cavity. In teleosts, abnormal proliferation of the thyroid tissue appears as a red fleshy mass at the ventral aspect of the opercular cavity (**Figure 3.16**). In elasmobranchs the condition of goiter can usually be detected as a visible or palpable swelling in the submandibular space (**Figure 3.17**).

Contained within the opercular cavity, most fish species possess four paired gill arches.[21] Cartilaginous gill rakers can be seen at the leading edge of the gill

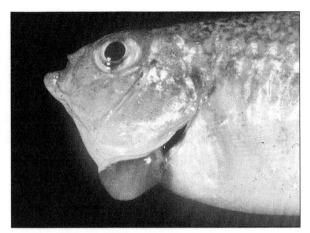

Figure 3.16 Goiter in a sheepshead minnow, *Cyprinodon variegatus.* (Image courtesy of A. Camus.)

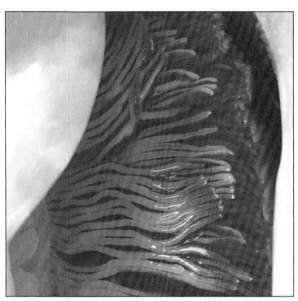

Figure 3.18 Paler appearance of gills due to excessive mucus.

arches and their function is primarily in the sifting of food particles. The primary gill filaments extend from the gill arches and should be dark pink to red in coloration (**Figure 3.15**). Generalized pallor of the gills may indicate anemia or an excessive mucous coating, whereas hyperemia may be suggestive of inflammation (**Figures 3.18** and **3.19**). Brown discoloration of the gills can be indicative of elevated environmental (i.e., water) nitrite levels, which can result in the blood disorder of methemoglobinemia (**Figure 3.20**).[22] The gills should also be inspected for external metazoan parasites and any areas of hemorrhage, discoloration, necrosis, fraying or clumping (**Figure 3.21**). Obtaining a small 2–3 mm gill biopsy of the distal tips of several primary lamellae and

examination under the microscope is recommended as part of every routine examination.

Musculoskeletal system

The fish patient should be examined for any grossly visible signs of skeletal dissymmetry or deformity such as scoliosis, kyphosis, or lordosis (**Figure 3.22**). The axial and appendicular skeleton of the fish should be palpated and flexed, feeling for stiffness

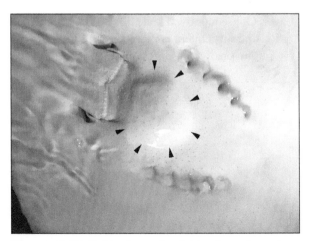

Figure 3.17 Goiter (arrowheads) in elasmobranch (ray).

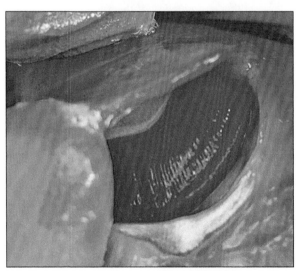

Figure 3.19 Hyperemia of gills suggesting inflammation.

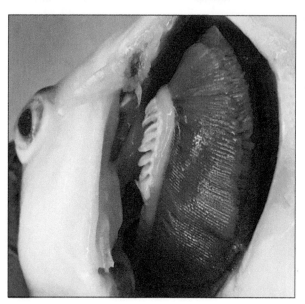

Figure 3.20 Darker appearance of gills due to methemoglobinemia.

or crepitus, masses, bony protrusions (i.e., possible indicator of cachexia), or indications of decalcification (e.g., "softening" of skull). Skeletal deformities, especially those involving the spine, have been implicated to be caused by a wide variety of factors such as trauma, parasitic infection, electric current,

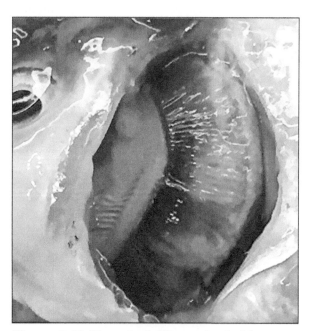

Figure 3.21 Necrosis of gills associated with *Flavobacterium columnare* infection.

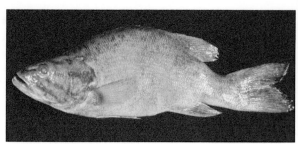

Figure 3.22 Skeletal deformity in a smallmouth bass (*Micropterus dolomieu*).

hereditary factors, defective embryonic development, unsuitable water temperature or enclosure design, salinity fluctuation, environmental hypoxia, ultraviolet radiation, vitamin and/or mineral deficiency in the diet, and numerous toxins.[23–25]

Integument

The skin of the fish should be examined for any areas of discoloration, ulceration, hemorrhage, masses/nodules, missing scales, edema or trauma (**Figures 3.23** and **3.24**). On palpation, the skin should have a uniform and smooth texture. Focal areas of roughened skin (i.e., "sandpaper" texture) are areas where inadequate mucous covering is present and likely represent areas of superficial ulceration. Fluorescein dye can be used as an additional diagnostic tool to detect superficial ulcers of the integument. In scaled species, the scales should be fairly difficult to remove and careful handling of the fish patient should not result in scale loss. The scales of teleost patients are imbedded within the dermal layer. Consequently, if scale loss is noted, then ulceration and subsequent compromise of the integument is automatically present, as scale loss represents a

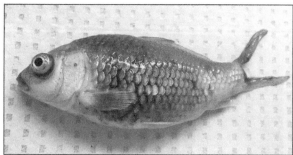

Figure 3.23 Hemorrhagic skin lesions associated with septicemia due to *Aeromonas* sp.

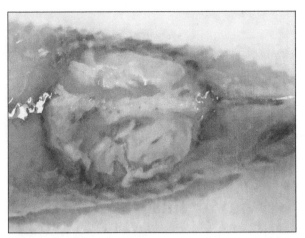

Figure 3.24 Ulcerative skin lesion associated with *Aeromonas* sp.

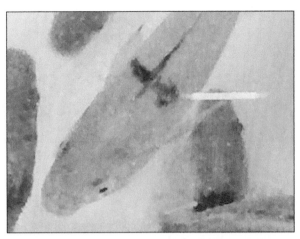

Figure 3.26 Temporary focal hyperpigmentation of skin immediately after placement of invasive fish tag in the musculature of a tilapia.

lesion that extends down to the level of the dermis. Severe edema of the skin or severe coelomic distension can cause the scales to stand out, resulting in a condition that is referred to as "pine-coning" or lepidorthosis (**Figure 3.25**).

Excessive mucous production leading to diffuse or focal discoloration of the skin that appears pale gray/blue or white/yellow may be secondary to poor environmental conditions, ectoparasites, certain viral diseases or irritation due to toxins. Generalized darkening or lightening of the pigment of the skin is often seen as a nonspecific sign of disease in teleost patients. Generalized hyperemia of the skin can be seen in association with bacteremia, viremia or as a response to dermal irritants such as poor water quality or toxins. The chromophores of teleosts are under neuroendocrine control and therefore damage

to the nerves can cause a focal discoloration. This has been documented in cases after intramuscular injection with an irritating substance, insertion of tags into the musculature, or in cases of parasitic infection such as *Myxobolus cerebralis*, which causes "black tail syndrome" in salmonids due to damage to the spinal cord and lower brain stem (**Figure 3.26**). Color changes secondary to certain anesthetics (e.g., metomidate) or severe stress are additional causes of this neuroendocrine effect.

Ectoparasites of the skin may be able to be grossly detected as in the case of leeches, isopods, copepods (e.g., anchor worms) and branchiurans (e.g., fish lice), or may present as small focal white or dark discolorations on the surface of the skin. Several viral diseases such as lymphocystis virus and *Cyprinid herpesvirus 1* (i.e., "carp pox") can cause proliferative growths on the surface of the skin as well. Lymphocystis virus presents as pinpoint coalescing white growths on the surface of the skin, whereas *Cyprinid herpesvirus 1* causes benign pink/white multifocal to coalescing plaques on the surface of the body. Fungal and water mold (e.g., oomycetes) infections often present as cottony growths on the surface of the skin that are best visualized while the patient is still in the water (**Figure 3.27**). As part of the general examination of any fish patient, a skin scrape should be collected and the mucous layer examined by microscopy.

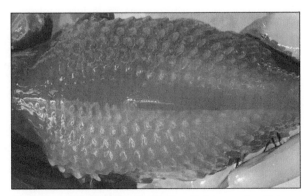

Figure 3.25 Lepidorthosis (i.e., "pine-coning") in fish due to coelomic distension.

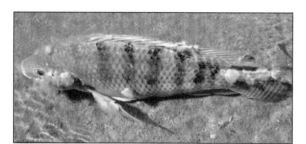

Figure 3.27 Oomycete infestation of skin of a tilapia.

Fins

The fins should be examined for completeness and for any evidence of ulceration, erythema, fraying or parasites. It is also not uncommon to detect bends or previous fractures of individual fin rays, which are palpable as nodular firm callouses. If fin lesions are present, a small fin biopsy can be taken for further investigation as a wet mount under the microscope or for processing for histopathology.

Heart rate

In general, the cardiac activity in fish is monitored by counting the opercular movement over time. However, heart rates in fish can be quantified using a variety of methods including cardiac ultrasonography, Doppler flow or electrocardiography. Of these methods, cardiac monitoring via a Doppler probe is the most commonly used. In general, the probe can be placed into the opercular slit and directed caudoventrally or placed near the heart along the ventrum at the base of the gills (**Figure 3.28**).[26]

Coelom

Fish commonly present with coelomic distension resulting from bacterial, viral, fungal or parasitic infections; metabolic disturbance (e.g., renal/liver failure); neoplasia; polycystic kidney disease in cyprinids; obesity; or egg retention (**Figures 3.29** and **3.30**). It should also be noted that mild to moderate coelomic distension may be a normal clinical finding in an adult gravid female fish that is getting ready to spawn. The coelomic cavity of each patient should be assessed for gross evidence of distension or excessive concavity, which may indicate emaciation. The coelom of each fish patient should also be gently palpated as part of the routine examination.

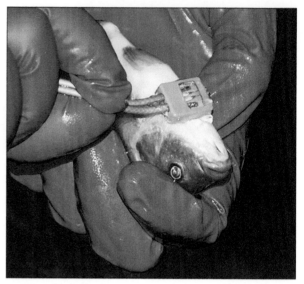

Figure 3.28 Doppler probe placement near the heart along the ventrum.

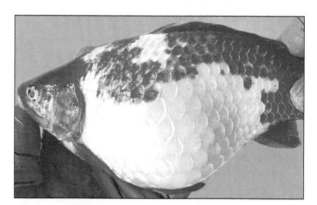

Figure 3.29 Lateral view of goldfish with asymmetric coelomic distension due to polycystic kidney disease.

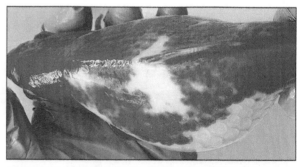

Figure 3.30 Dorsal view of same goldfish in Figure 3.29 with asymmetric coelomic distension due to polycystic kidney disease.

Abnormalities that may be detected on palpation include coelomic masses, organomegaly or coelomic fluid. If large quantities of coelomic fluid are present, a fluid wave may be appreciated on percussion of the coelom, and ballottement may be used to reveal a mass within the fluid-filled cavity.

Vent

The vent should be examined for any signs of erythema, ulceration, protrusion, presence of endoparasites (e.g., *Camallanus* sp.) or prolapse of the gastrointestinal or reproductive organs. Under anesthesia it is also quite common for fish to defecate and the feces can be examined to ensure that they are of normal coloration and consistency for the species. A sample of the feces can also be used to make a direct smear or fecal flotation to examine for parasites or parasite eggs.[27] Light abdominal pressure can often elicit a fecal sample; if the fish does not defecate, a rubber catheter can be inserted into the vent to perform a cloacal flush for obtaining a sample of feces for analysis.

EXTERNAL BIOPSIES

Collection and evaluation of tissue wet mounts is an integral part of the fish clinical workup.[2] External and internal parasites, many of which have distinct motility patterns, are best and most quickly diagnosed in this way. External wet mounts, or external tissue squash preps of small pieces of skin, gills or fin, can be sampled for microscopic evaluation. External wet mounts are a basic and relatively simple diagnostic test that can be used both ante- and postmortem.[28]

Skin scrapes and fin and gill biopsies are easy to obtain and highly informative techniques in clinical examination of fish. Sample collection typically requires minimal equipment and poses low risk to both patient and diagnostician when performed on anesthetized animals. On some occasions (e.g., severely unresponsive patient), the clinician could decide to work with an unanesthetized animal; however, proper handling of the patient is absolutely necessary since the manipulation and collection of samples can cause discomfort in the patient. Experienced clinicians can sample quickly and with

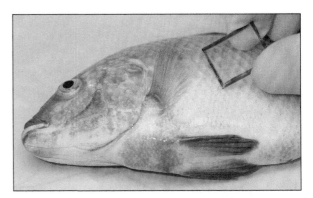

Figure 3.31 Skin biopsy (i.e., scrape) using a coverslip.

minimal distress to an unsedated animal, either by holding the fish in the folds of a net and exposing each area to be sampled one at a time, or with the assistance of an experienced handler. Additionally, the diagnostician must be aware that use of some sedatives and anesthetics can result in sedation-related loss of parasite loads.[29]

Powder-free latex or nitrile gloves should be worn to minimize damage to the skin and to avoid procedure-related removal of external parasites or lesions; similar caveats require careful use of a net or other handling materials. Use of a gloved hand or dark material to cover the eyes of the fish will help reduce stress, stimulation and movement. Discolored areas, excess mucus, hemorrhages, ulcers, erosions, masses or parasites should be sampled as described next.

Skin

In order to obtain a good quality sample, the clinician typically uses a coverslip or the back of a scalpel blade to gently scrape any areas that appear abnormal (e.g., discoloration, thickened mucus, ulcers, erosions, masses or obvious parasites) (**Figure 3.31**). In patients without any "abnormal" external areas, other sites to target include portions of the body that are softer or have fewer scales or where water flow is reduced. Particularly informative areas include the ventrum of fish, behind the pectoral or pelvic fins and around the vent. If scraping near the vent or anus of mature males, careful interpretation is needed since fish milt (i.e., sperm) may mimic flagellate movements; however, sperm typically will

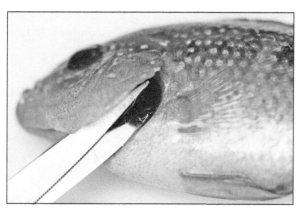

Figure 3.32 Gill biopsy (i.e., clip) excising the tips of several gill filaments.

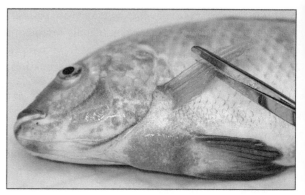

Figure 3.33 Fin biopsy (i.e., clip) excising the tip of the pectoral fin.

not remain motile for more than a minute or two after water activation.

Gills

Gill biopsies are typically collected using scissor blades as a fulcrum and lever, or a pair of forceps to lift the operculum and clip a small section of the gill filaments (**Figure 3.32**). The amount of gill tissue to collect and submit for diagnosis will depend on if the patient is terminal or if the sample is to be collected nonlethally. In the latter, the diagnostician needs to be particularly careful not to cut the gill arch since this structure contains major arterial and venous vessels. As with the skin, the diagnostician should target abnormal areas of the gill. If the fish has been euthanized, the diagnostician can cut a section of the gill arch and examine it microscopically or macroscopically if the sample is too thick for a compound microscope. Additionally, a subsample of the gills, including the gill arch, should be saved in fixative or buffer for histological or molecular diagnosis, respectively. For larger fish, which may appear to bleed more when gills are cut, or for species with fleshier gills, a gill "scrape" can be used to evaluate for parasite or other pathogen load. Gill pathology is often the first sign of poor water quality or external infectious disease. For species that have small gill openings (e.g., seahorses, eels), a catheter or 1 cc syringe with appropriate water can be used to "flush" the gills, with fluid either being suctioned back into the syringe, or the excess fluid allowed to drip into a petri dish or onto a microscope slide for examination.

Fins

Although fin biopsies are not as commonly sampled as gills or skin, in some cases examining a small section from each major fin could be of value. In some fish, hard fin rays and darkly pigmented fins are difficult to evaluate (e.g., normal pigmented cells may be mistaken as a pathologic change) (**Figure 3.33**). For efficacious evaluation of a fin biopsy, the sample should be flattened as much as possible and microscope lighting increased, keeping the condenser closed down for contrast. Changing focus through several different planes will facilitate observation of parasite movement, as will examination along the edges of structures and in the surrounding water.

WET MOUNT EVALUATION

Immediately prior to sample collection, the diagnostician should have prepared slides for biopsy samples by placing one or two small drops of water equidistant on a slide. This will allow for one or two different biopsy samples to be evaluated per slide. A separate coverslip is then placed on each biopsy sample with an adequate amount of water to completely flood the area under the coverslip, and gentle pressure is used to flatten the tissue to allow penetration of light and easier visualization.[28] For external (i.e., skin, gill, and fin) samples, the use of dechlorinated freshwater (not distilled water) for freshwater fish and salt water for marine fish, respectively, is necessary.

During microscopic examination of squash preps/wet mounts, the clinician should use a methodical search pattern (e.g., "mowing the lawn"). Scanning each preparation at 40× (i.e., low power) will help with orientation and identification of areas of interest. Decreasing the condenser aperture or use of phase contrast will help increase contrast and facilitate observation of smaller structures such as protozoan parasites.[30] Most parasites and lesions of interest are visible at 40×–100× magnification. While movement of some parasites, such as the flagellates of the genera *Spironucleus* and *Ichthyobodo*, may be discerned at 100×, specific parasite structures are more apparent at 400×. Individual nonmotile spores of microsporidian parasites are also very small (approximate range 1–5 × 2–8 μm) and are more easily identified at 200×–400×, although their cysts (sporoblastic vesicles) or xenomas may be visible at 40×–100×. Similarly, *Flavobacterium columnare*, the etiologic agent of columnaris disease, is a long, rod-shaped Gram-negative bacteria that can often be found flexing in haystack formations that are more easily observed at 200×–400×.

HEMATOLOGY

Venipuncture

A clinically acceptable blood sample can be readily obtained from most fish species. The most common sampling site to access blood is from the caudal vessels (mixed arterial and venous sample) using a ventral or lateral approach. The site for the ventral approach is along the ventral midline of the caudal peduncle halfway between the tail and anal fin, while the lateral approach is along the lateral midportion of the caudal peduncle along the lateral line of the fish (**Figures 3.34** and **3.35**). For either of these approaches, the needle is inserted under a scale in a cranial direction and advanced at a 45° angle to the vertebral column of the fish. The needle is then withdrawn slightly until blood is obtained. The needle may need to be rotated slightly to allow the beveled edge of the needle better access to the pooled blood supply. Cardiac puncture has been utilized for blood sampling in large fish, but there is a higher risk of death using this technique and it is not recommended for nonlethal sampling. As a last resort, the caudal peduncle can also be severed to obtain a small amount of blood. Though generally not acceptable

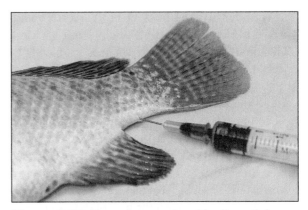

Figure 3.34 **Ventral approach to bleeding a fish.**

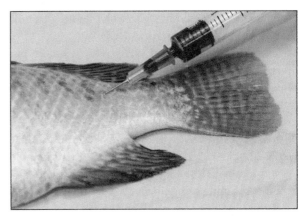

Figure 3.35 **Lateral approach to bleeding a fish.**

for clinical specimens from pet fish, it provides an alternative route for sampling fry and fingerlings as long as the fish are deeply anesthetized or recently euthanized.

In elasmobranchs, venipuncture is body-style specific. Generally, the ventral tail vein is present in all species with tails, and since dorsal recumbency/tonic immobilization is commonly used in elasmobranchs, the tail site is commonly used. Large volumes of blood may be collected safely from this site, although it likely represents a mixed arterial–venous blood sample which needs to be taken into account with blood gas analysis. A lateral tail vein approach, where the needle is passed 90° to the vertebrae and guided carefully just ventral of the vertebral column, may be used in larger species to avoid using longer spinal needles needed to reach the ventral vertebral venus plexus. Most galeomorphs (i.e., sharks) have a dorsal fin sinus present just caudal to the first dorsal fin. The area just caudal to the dorsal fin is often softer and the needle is introduced just off midline at a 45° angle. This sinus can yield small volumes of blood, but packed cell volumes may be lower than blood from the traditional tail vein venipuncture site.[31] This site allows the shark to be in ventral recumbency when collecting blood, which is useful in unsedated but otherwise restrained sharks. Batoid (i.e., rays, skates and sawfishes) body conformation allows for venipuncture in either the wings (i.e., pectoral fins) or the ventral tail. The wing vein method uses a size-appropriate needle to approach the base of the wing next to the body at a 45° angle. The needle is repositioned to fit between cartilage ridges where the ceratotrichia of the wing meet the body. Blood volumes are generally sufficient for most diagnostic needs.

For most biochemical analytes, plasma is preferred over serum, and lithium heparin is recommended for use in most assays and with most fish species.[32,33] Some clinicians have reported hemolysis of blood samples collected in EDTA tubes when fish are anesthetized with tricaine methanesulfonate (MS-222), however, the mechanism for this hemolysis is unknown. Fish blood often clots very quickly so the needle and syringe may need to be heparinized prior to blood collection.

A blood volume collection of 0.5%–1.0% of body weight can be safely taken from most fish. In most cases 1.0 mL can be taken from a 100 g fish and up to 3.0 mL in larger fish, such as production brood stock and adult koi. Most venipuncture in fish can be accomplished using a 1½ inch 21–23 gauge needle on a 1.0 or 3.0 mL syringe. A 1/2 inch 25 gauge needle on a tuberculin (1.0 mL) syringe can be used for small fish. Blood should be used immediately for making blood smears or transferred to a blood tube containing an anticoagulant to minimize clotting. The choice of anticoagulant for preservation of cellular morphology is species-specific with salmonids, cyprinids and sturgeon retaining the best blood cell morphology with heparin, whereas catfish, bass and tilapia blood cells are best preserved in EDTA.[32] Clumped, clotted or hemolyzed blood samples should be discarded.

Hematology

Complete blood counts (CBCs) and biochemical tests can be valuable diagnostic tools in determining the cause of disease in many species. However, normal hematologic parameters, reference interval and interpretation of those values are not available for most fish species. Published hematological data exists for economically important food fish species (e.g., trout, channel catfish, tilapia, striped bass, winter flounder, sturgeon and yellow perch), but these values are not always applicable to pet and ornamental fish.[32–39] Selected hematology and biochemical reference values for a few common ornamental and pet species (i.e., koi, goldfish, pacu and zebrafish) can be found in the literature.[40–44] Environmental conditions such as water quality (temperature, pH, ammonia, nitrite, nitrate, etc.) can significantly affect test results.[45–47] Capture and handling stressors, sampling technique, age, gender, reproductive status, photoperiod, diet, activity level and test methodology are other factors that can affect the results of a CBC and serum or plasma biochemistry results.[40,47]

Interpretation of blood results

Interpretation of blood results in fish is difficult when compared to more common terrestrial species. Nucleated red blood cells and platelets prohibit the use of most automated analyzers used for mammalian blood counts, though two recent studies evaluated the use of in-house blood analyzers for fish.[48,49] Manual evaluation of stained blood smears and the use of a hemocytometer are the most common techniques performed in a clinical setting. Blood smears can be stained with any variation of a Romanowsky stain (Wright/Giemsa/Leishman stains). Natt-Herrick's, Rees-Ecker or modified Dacie's diluents (1:100 or 1:200 dilution of blood to filtered diluent) are commonly utilized for diluting cells for hemocytometer counts of fish species.[50]

Blood cell morphology

Most fish blood cell types appear to have a morphology and function similar to mammalian blood cells (**Figure 3.36**).[50] Erythrocytes are the most numerous blood cell type and are nucleated. Reticulocytes, frequently present in significant numbers in blood smears, are easily recognized by their smaller size and slightly basophilic cytoplasm. Thrombocytes vary in shape depending on their activation state, changing from spiked or oval to round cells as they

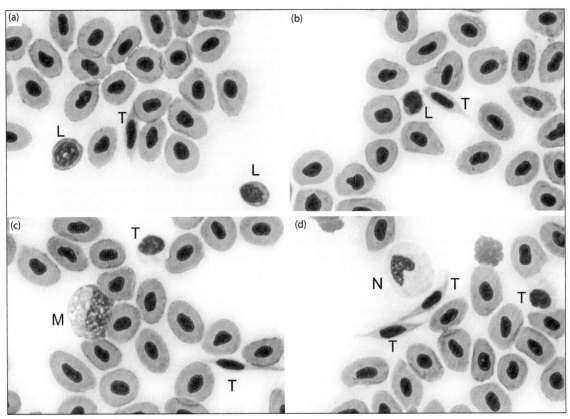

Figure 3.36 Blood cells of a striped bass (*Morone saxatilis*). (a) Lymphocytes (L) and thrombocyte (T). (b) Lymphocyte (L) and thrombocyte (T). (c) Monocyte (M) and thrombocytes (T). (d) Neutrophil (N) and thrombocytes (T). Note that it is possible to see round, oval and spindle-shaped thrombocytes in the same blood smear. (Images courtesy of J. Arnold.)

activate, and may have a segmented or oval nucleus. Lymphocytes can be divided into small or large lymphocytes, though functional differences have not been documented. Neutrophils are one of the largest fish blood cells. The cytoplasm of the neutrophils may have a grainy appearance, and the nucleus is open and usually oval to kidney-bean shaped. Heterophils are similar to neutrophils but with pale eosinophilic to lavender granules in the cytoplasm. Species of fish usually have either neutrophils or heterophils, although some species may have both. Functional differences between fish neutrophils and heterophils have also not been documented. Monocytes are round cells with a deep blue cytoplasm and a round to horseshoe-shaped nucleus. Eosinophils are infrequently observed in fish blood, but are the same size or slightly smaller than neutrophils with distinct eosinophilic granules in the

cytoplasm. Basophils are rarely observed in fish and are similar to mammalian basophils in morphology.

Complete blood count (CBC) abnormalities

The packed cell volume (PCV) can vary within and between species depending on age, gender, activity level, diet, stocking density and water quality. Active species such as tuna have higher normal PCV levels, whereas young fish, elasmobranchs and bottom dwellers have lower normal PCVs.[47] Male fish tend to have higher normal PCVs when compared to female fish of the same age.[40] Obligate air breathers also have higher normal PCVs.[51]

Anemia is typically associated with a PCV less than 20, except in some shark species where a PCV of 20 or less is normal.[47] Anemia in fish has been associated with elevated ammonia and nitrite levels, hypoxia, heavy metal toxicities, poor acclimation to captivity, nutritional disorders including starvation, increased stocking density, use of chlorinated water, stress response, bacterial and viral diseases, inflammatory disease, and parasitism.[47,51–53] A temporary reduction in hemoglobin levels, red blood cell counts and PCV has been observed 24 hours after oral administration of praziquantel at a therapeutic dosage in common carp, *Cyprinus carpio*.[54] An increased PCV (>45) is associated with dehydration in marine fish, hypoxia in marine and freshwater fish, stress, and anesthesia (e.g., MS-222 and benzocaine).[47] The response to hypoxia can be very rapid, and in some cases can occur in less than one hour.[51] Elevated water temperature has also been found to cause an elevated PCV in both goldfish and koi.[40,52]

White blood cell changes occur with many diseases and adverse environmental conditions. A stress leukogram in fish reveals a leukopenia with a lymphopenia and granulocytosis.[47] Elevated white blood cell counts can be found in freshwater fish held at higher water temperatures and those with sepsis.[40,52] A decreased total white count can be found during starvation.[52] Increased lymphocyte counts can be found in normal juvenile fish, husbandry-related disorders and any disease that stimulates the immune system.[47] Lymphopenia is associated with disorders that cause immune suppression such as stress and bacterial sepsis, and has also been found in ciliated protozoan infections.[47,51,52] Inflammation from several causes, including external parasitism, is often accompanied by granulocytosis. Granulocytosis is also seen in sharks with bacterial septicemia and neutrophilia can occur in other fish species with septicemia.[47] Increases in the eosinophil count can sometimes occur with disorders causing inflammation, though eosinophilia due to parasitism is not consistently observed.

Biochemical abnormalities

Muscle damage secondary to capture, anesthesia and excess tissue trauma during sampling can increase creatine kinase (CK) levels, similar to terrestrial species. Alanine aminotransferase (ALT) has been reported to be the most liver-specific enzyme in koi, while a significant elevation in ALT was measured 96 hours after a single oral dose of praziquantel in common carp, *Cyprinus carpio*.[49,54] Lowered blood glucose levels are associated with hepatic disease or injury and sepsis. This is likely due to impairment of the liver's ability to maintain normal glucose levels. Blood glucose is found to be elevated during stress, anesthesia, hypoxia and as an initial response in bacterial septicemia.[52] Serum calcium levels have been observed to be elevated in gravid females, although additional reference interval studies are needed to substantiate this observation.[49] Total protein levels are found to be decreased in males and fish with bacterial septicemia, starvation, chronic stress, renal and hepatic diseases, during spawning, and failure to acclimate to captivity.[52,53] Starvation is also accompanied by a decrease in blood urea nitrogen (BUN).[53] Serum protein levels can be increased in female cyprinids (koi and goldfish) and cyprinids held at higher water temperatures.[40] In one study, rockfish with poor body condition had reduced total protein, albumin, glucose, cholesterol and phosphorus values.[42] Elevated BUN, serum sodium and chloride levels in marine fish can be indicative of gill disease, whereas elevated BUN and decreased sodium and chloride levels have been observed in freshwater fish with gill disease.[40,48,53] Renal disease in marine fish can be accompanied by elevations in magnesium and sulfate levels and an elevation in creatinine.[53] Marine rockfish, *Sebastes* sp., with exophthalmia demonstrated decreased total protein, albumin, sodium, calcium and chloride concentrations when compared to clinically normal fish.[48] The authors suggested this may have been a result of a chronic, low-level malnutrition secondary to the exophthalmia.

Serology

The use of serology for the detection of pathogens and disease conditions in fish is in its infancy; however, a number of ELISA and molecular assays are used in the research setting for the diagnosis and/or confirmation of disease in production (i.e., food) fish, and a few serological assays are available in the research setting for a small number of viral diseases of ornamental pond fish (e.g., koi, carp and goldfish). These include an antibody assay for CyHV-3 (koi herpesvirus, KHV) in koi.[55] The antibody assay for KHV has also been used as a pre-purchase screening test to determine previous exposure to KHV and identify latent carriers. In addition, there are a few research laboratories that have developed serological assays for betanodavirus and ranavirus in fish.[56–58] Unfortunately, very few serological assays have met the standards needed for validation as standard diagnostic methods. However, further development of serological methodology will hopefully advance the use of serology in the future for routine diagnostic purposes.

NECROPSY

If a necropsy is to be performed, fish can be euthanized by a variety of humane methods including immersion, injectable and physical methods (see Chapter 17 on euthanasia). Choice of method will depend on number of fish, size of fish, drug availability, logistics, cost and potential interference with sample analysis, as well as carcass disposition. In addition to the lack of movement, the fish should no longer be responsive to stimuli and have lost the vestibule-ocular reflex (eyes in normal position, parallel to body, regardless of position of the body). The clinician may need to gently press the eye parallel to check this response in fish.[59,60]

Similar to the initial examination of the fish patient, the fish necropsy should be conducted in an organized and thorough manner and follow the same routine each time so that nothing is missed, cross-contamination is avoided, and proper downstream processing of samples and tissues is ensured, which is paramount for microbiological, histological, molecular and microscopic examination. In general, samples collected for bacteriological and fungal recovery are prioritized, with samples collected for virology and molecular diagnosis following, whereas collection of internal tissues for histopathology is generally saved until the end of the necropsy procedure.

MICROBIOLOGICAL SAMPLING

Most of the common bacterial pathogens of fish will grow on nutrient-rich media like blood agar or tryptic soy agar (TSA) supplemented with 5% sheep's blood. If working with brackish or marine water species, it is recommended to also have media supplemented with NaCl or sea salt, since many of the marine organisms, like those in the family *Vibrionaceae*, are halophilic (i.e., salt-loving). There are also a wide range of fish pathogens that are fastidious and need specialized media and growing conditions. For example, the *Flavobacterium* species grow best on Cytophaga agar, whereas Coomassie blue media can be used to rapidly distinguish between *Aeromonas hydrophila* and *A. salmonicida*. Löwenstein-Jensen media or Dorset's egg agar should be used for mycobacterial infections. Some rapid, less fastidious mycobacterial strains will grow on these agars in 4–7 days, whereas other stains may take 30–45 days to grow. In addition, bacterial cultures should be incubated at optimal temperature ranges for the species examined (15°C–18°C for cold-water species, 20°C–22°C for cool-water species, and 25°C–30°C for most warm-water species). Thus, the clinician must communicate with the microbiological laboratory the differential pathogen list generated during the necropsy to better target suspected organisms. For a further discussion of diagnosis of bacterial and fungal pathogens and description of fish pathogens, we refer the reader to other work.[61,62]

External tissue sampling

If skin lesions such as ulcers are present, bacterial culture may be useful. However, careful interpretation is necessary to differentiate primary initiating agents from secondary invaders or water-borne contaminants. In these cases, aseptically remove scales in scaled species at the leading edge of an ulcer to increase probability of culturing primary versus opportunistic agents. Fungal infections can be tentatively diagnosed based on microscopic evaluation and clinical appearance; however, speciation of fungi is difficult even to trained diagnosticians and may require molecular identification or submission to a reference laboratory. In general corn meal agar for oomycetes ("water mold" fungi) and Sabouraud dextrose or potato dextrose agar for fungi is recommended. In general, it is difficult to identify bacterial pathogens during wet mount analysis of external tissues. In some situations, certain pathogens will be included in the differential list due to the frequency in a particular host, tissue or lesion. For example, the particular shape, motility and "haystack" aggregation displayed by *Flavobacterium columnare* allows for a relatively rapid wet mount diagnosis when associated with skin and gill pathology; however, recent findings have demonstrated that other members of the genus and related taxa can display similar pathology and present similar morphology, thus a complete identification of the agent is always recommended.[61-64]

Internal tissue sampling

Following the external examination, at a minimum, the posterior kidney and brain in smaller fish, or the posterior kidney, liver, spleen and brain in larger fish should be sampled for bacteriological analysis. Other internal organs or tissues, the coelomic surface, swim bladder or coelomic fluids may also warrant culture based on clinical signs and/or gross appearance.[61-64]

Kidney culture

In general, the posterior kidney is the main tissue targeted for microbiological analysis. The posterior kidney is easily accessible; its anatomic position is retrocoelomic, decreasing the chance of cross-contamination during the necropsy procedure. The organ filters blood and is part of the mononuclear phagocytic system, thereby increasing chances of detecting organisms during septicemias. There are several different approaches for culture of the kidney. The ventral approach is the most common approach and is preferred if liver and spleen will also be sampled. The lateral approach is particularly useful for larger, deeper bodied fish, whereas the dorsal approach is useful in small to medium-sized fish.[1-3,61-64]

For the ventral approach, the fish should be placed in right lateral recumbency and the exposed lateral body wall disinfected with alcohol. A shallow, ventral incision with a sterile scalpel blade or sharp-pointed scissors should be made caudal to the operculum to serve as an opening for blunt scissors to enter the coelomic cavity and cut out an area of the body wall. This step should avoid penetration of the internal organs and will expose most of the coelomic cavity, visceral organs and swim bladder. From the initial cut, the opening is widened dorsally and caudally, and then from the same point ventrally and caudally, exposing the coelomic cavity. It is important to avoid cutting into any organs, especially the

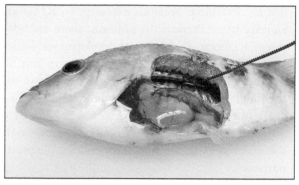

Figure 3.37 **Ventral approach to kidney sampling by opening the coelomic cavity.**

gastrointestinal organs, to prevent contamination of the coelomic cavity. For most teleosts that have a swim bladder, this organ should be deflated and either removed or reflected to one side of the coelomic cavity, and the kidney, which is visible as a red or dark red line or area immediately below the spine, should be exposed. A sterile culture swab or inoculating loop can then be used to sample the tissue (**Figure 3.37**). After cultures have been taken, this opening can be extended cranially, with cuts through or removal of the cleithrum (i.e., crescent-shaped, flat bone caudal to the operculum along the posterior edge of the gill chamber) to expose the anterior section of the coelomic cavity, including the pericardial area and heart.

The lateral approach is similar to the ventral approach except that instead of completely opening a window into the body cavity, scissors or a scalpel blade are used to cut a small slit in the lateral body wall to access the coelomic cavity, allowing for the insertion of a sterile swab or loop into the posterior kidney. In order to correctly conduct this procedure, a good understanding of the anatomy of the species being examined is required (**Figure 3.38**).

For the dorsal approach, the dorsal fin should be removed with scissors to minimize potential contamination, and the dorsal area of the fish wiped with alcohol, in a wide enough region to encompass the area to be cut. Excess alcohol should be allowed to dry or wiped off with sterile gauze prior to incision. A good landmark for the cut in many fish species is the mid-region of the dorsal fin. A sterilized pair of scissors can then be used to cut through

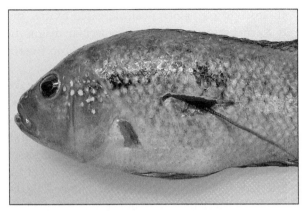

Figure 3.38 Lateral approach to kidney sampling through body incision.

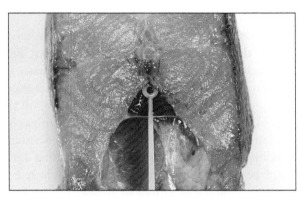

Figure 3.40 Close-up of kidney sampling using dorsal approach shown in Figure 3.39.

skin, muscle, and spinal column to access the kidney (**Figure 3.39**). Typically, blood will be visible leaking from the kidney and surrounding vessels after the cut has been made. A sterile loop can then be inserted directly into the kidney parenchyma and streaked onto the appropriate media (**Figure 3.40**). If the cut is made too deep, contamination from other organs, especially the gastrointestinal tract, will occur. The lateral line may provide an approximate landmark for the cut's ventral most point, along with palpation of the limit of the coelomic cavity.

Brain culture

In order to avoid cross-contamination by opportunistic agents colonizing external tissues, the dorsal midline region of the head slightly behind the eyes for many species should be disinfected with alcohol and then allowed to evaporate. A small, sterile scalpel blade can then be used to cut through the top of the head into the brain case. For larger fish, sterilized bone cutters, an oscillating "stryker" saw or a Dremel tool may be necessary to access the brain. The exposed brain and surrounding cerebrospinal fluid can then be sampled with a sterile inoculating needle or swab, and streaked onto an agar plate or inoculated into a broth media (**Figure 3.41**). Certain bacteria, such as *Streptococcus* sp., are highly neurotropic and can be readily isolated from brain tissue. In suspected streptococcosis, impression smears of brain tissue on a glass slide followed by Gram staining may also be diagnostic.[1-3,61-64]

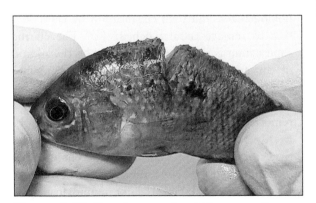

Figure 3.39 Dorsal approach to kidney sampling through incision in dorsum.

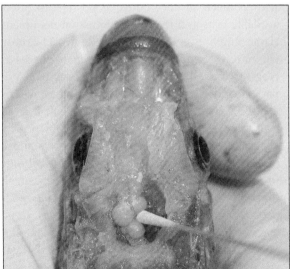

Figure 3.41 Sampling brain after removal of skin and calvarium.

Virology

Historically, the detection of fish viruses has relied upon the observation of cytopathic effects (CPEs) following the inoculation of tissue homogenates on permissive cell lines.[65,66] Although slower than modern molecular techniques, virus isolation is still the "gold standard" diagnostic method as it assures a replicating agent was present in the sample, facilitates additional characterization of the replicating agent and permits challenge studies to be conducted to establish the role of viruses in disease. Viruses from a handful of economically important food fishes have been well studied, including spring viremia of carp virus and koi herpesvirus in common carp *Cyprinus carpio* varieties; viral hemorrhagic septicemia virus (VHSV), infectious hematopoietic necrosis virus (IHNV), and infectious pancreatic necrosis virus in salmon; and channel catfish virus in channel catfish *Ictalurus punctatus*.[65,67] The isolation of these viruses facilitated a better understanding of their *in vitro* behavior (i.e., CPE) within permissive cell lines, virion ultrastructure, nucleic acid type (i.e., RNA or DNA) and phylogenetic affinity, antigenic properties, and *in vivo* behavior to understand pathogenesis including the fulfillment of Koch's/Rivers' postulates verifying that the virus was the causative agent for a given disease.

If a viral etiology is suspected, a diagnostic laboratory familiar with fish viruses should be contacted with as much advance notice as possible to discuss available tests and required submission documents, tissue sampling, and transport strategies. Diagnostic laboratories require time to prepare necessary reagents or cell lines for requested testing. Viral pathogenesis varies considerably among known fish viruses as well as the size and life stage of fish, and thus tissue selection should be reviewed prior to the necropsy.[65-68] Necropsy procedures should be performed by individuals using aseptic technique to minimize bacterial contamination if virus isolation is to be performed. Trained personnel are also needed to note any gross lesions and ensure tissues (e.g., brain, posterior/anterior kidney, spleen, skin, gills, intestinal tract, stomach or others if lesions are observed) are preserved for downstream virus isolation, histology (e.g., 10% neutral buffered formalin or Davidson's fixative), transmission electron microscopy (e.g., glutaraldehyde-based fixative such as Karnovsky's fixative), and molecular diagnostics (e.g., 70%–100% ETOH, RNAlater®, or freezing at −80°C).

During the necropsy, samples should be kept cold on wet ice or cold packs but not frozen, as enveloped viruses can be sensitive to freeze–thaw cycles. Fish <4 cm can be sampled whole after the removal of the yolk sac if present. The entire viscera, which should include the kidney, can be sampled for 4–6 cm fish. The kidney and spleen should be sampled for fish >6 cm, and milt or ovarian fluid can be sampled separately in reproductive individuals. Tissues should be placed in sealed Whirl-Pak® bags and ovarian fluids can be placed in sterile snap cap tubes. Samples can be pooled up to five individuals per bag or tube, and then all samples should be placed within a sealed plastic bag. Ovarian fluid samples should be boxed upright and packed with absorbent material in case of leakage. Samples should be clearly labeled using a label-making printer or neatly handwritten in permanent ink and packed within secondary (e.g., Styrofoam box with cold packs) and tertiary (e.g., labeled cardboard box) containers. Samples should be received by the diagnostic laboratory within 48 hours of collection, and the cold chain (not frozen) must be maintained in transit. If samples are to be delivered by air, it is advisable to ship early in the week to prevent delays resulting in sample delivery on weekends when laboratory staff might not be available to receive them.

Tissue processing for virus isolation begins with suspending the tissues in a dilution medium, followed by homogenization in a Stomacher® or other homogenizer, and then clarification by centrifugation to remove cellular debris.[65,67,68] The clarified supernatant is then decontaminated by the addition of an antibiotic/antimycotic incubation medium and/or filtered through a 450 μm filter. After decontamination, the supernatant is again clarified to remove any final cellular debris and inoculated onto freshly prepared plates or flasks with monolayers that are at least 80% confluent. The choice of cell line and incubation temperature varies by virus.[65,66] Cells should be monitored for cytotoxicity, CPE and contamination on the day after initial inoculation, and afterward for CPE every other day for

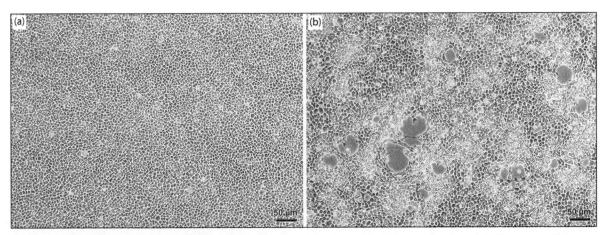

Figure 3.42 Cytopathic effect (CPE) induced by ranavirus (*Frog virus 3*) growing in epithelioma papulosum cyprini cells. (a) Uninfected normal cells. (b) CPE evident by the presence of rounded, refractile cells, and the formation of plaques. (Images courtesy of N. Stilwell.)

at least 14 days. The progression, intensity and type of CPE varies by virus type. Commonly observed CPEs include pyknosis, cytoplasmic vacuolation, cell rounding, formation of syncytia and formation of plaques (**Figure 3.42**). Many well-characterized viruses produce stereotypical CPE; however, testing should be undertaken to corroborate the identity of the viral isolate by its nucleic acid (endpoint and quantitative PCR) or antigenic (plaque reduction serum neutralization assay, fluorescent antibody test, immunoblot) properties.[66] Transmission electron microscopy can also provide useful information about virion ultrastructure; however, some hosts may carry more than one viral species with nearly identical ultrastructural features (e.g., rhabdoviruses VHSV and IHNV in salmon). If CPE is not observed by day 14 post-inoculation, a blind passage should be performed and monitored for an additional 14 days before recording the sample as negative.

Culture-independent diagnostics

Less effort has been devoted and fewer tools have been developed to characterize viruses impacting finfishes from non-food fish aquaculture sectors (i.e., ornamental and tropical species) or wild stocks. In many cases, definitive proof that an epizootic was due to a viral etiology through the fulfillment of the Koch's/Rivers' postulates cannot be accomplished because a permissive cell line is not available or the agent is fastidious and refractory to cell culture. In

these cases, a viral diagnosis is often reached based on a combination of the case history and clinical signs, rule-out of other causes, molecular genetic characterization, histopathologic lesions, and visualization of virus particles within lesions by transmission electron microscopy. For example, blue spot disease has been described in wild northern pike (*Esox lucius*) during spawning aggregations and is believed to be caused by esocid herpesvirus 1 (EsHV1).[69] Although the virus has not been cultured *in vitro*, disease episodes invariably present with the same gross, microscopic and ultrastructural lesions (**Figure 3.43a to d**). A consensus primer set designed against the DNA polymerase of large DNA viruses was used to generate sequence-confirming EsHV1 as a novel alloherpesvirus.[70] Megalocytiviruses within the family *Iridoviridae* are another group of viruses that have proven difficult to cultivate despite numerous opportunities from epizootics in both freshwater and marine fishes reared for food or ornamental use. However, these iridoviruses induce pathognomonic microscopic lesions, with infected cells displaying cytomegaly and stereotypical amphophilic cytoplasmic inclusions within the kidney, spleen and other tissues (**Figure 3.44a to c**).[71] Ultrastructural examination of affected enlarged cells invariably reveals large hexagonal polygonal virus particles often arranged in paracrystalline arrays (**Figure 3.44d and e**).[71] Megalocytivirus detection and genetic characterization can be accomplished using the

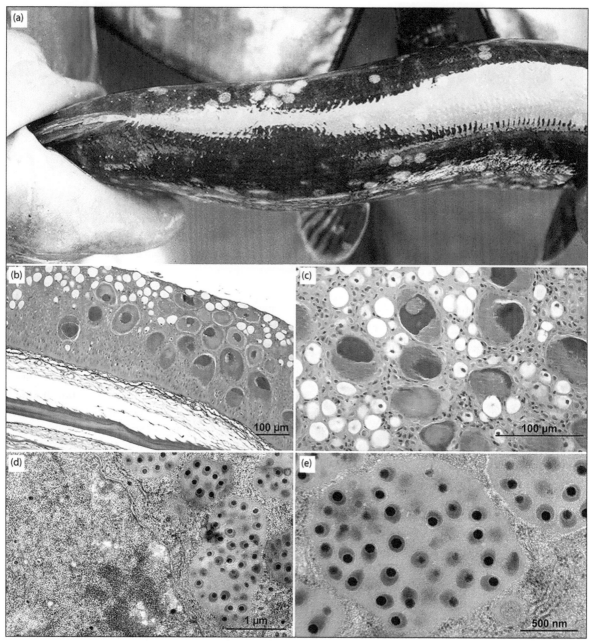

Figure 3.43 (a) Northern pike (*Esox lucius*) displaying bluish-white circular plaques on the dorsal skin characteristic of blue spot disease. (b) Histopathology of affected skin reveals megalocytic epidermal cells displaying karyomegaly. H&E stain. (c) Higher magnification shows cytoplasm containing an abundance of coarse eosinophilic granules and enlarged nuclei containing a homogeneous, flocculent to fine granular, basophilic nucleoplasm with internal membranous structures. H&E stain. (d) Transmission electron photomicrograph of megalocytic epidermal cell displaying the boundary between the nucleus and the cytoplasm. (e) Transmission electron photomicrograph of cytoplasmic vacuoles showing mature virus particles with a hexagonal nucleocapsid with an electron-dense core surrounded by a uniformly staining ellipsoidal tegument layer and a transparent envelope. ([a] Image courtesy of S. Marcquenski. [e] Images from Freitas, J.T. et al., Diseases of *Aquatic Organisms* 2016;122:1–11. With permission.)

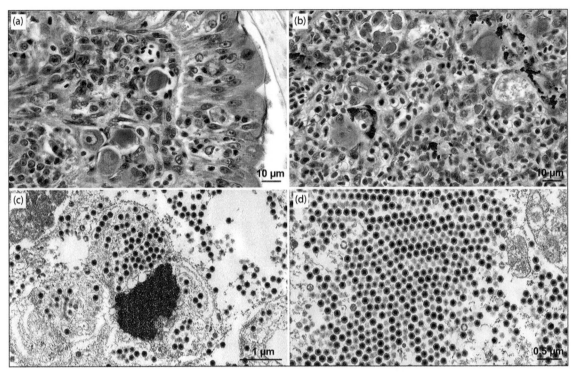

Figure 3.44 (a) Histopathology of liver of threespine stickleback (*Gasterosteus aculeatus*) displaying an irregular focus of coagulative necrosis. H&E stain. (b) Necrotic hepatocytes demonstrating hypereosinophilic cytoplasm, pyknosis, and some karyorrhexis. H&E stain. (c) Transmission electron photomicrograph of splenic parenchyma illustrating numerous virus-infected cells. (d) Transmission electron photomicrograph showing abundant cytoplasmic hexagonal nucleocapsids that are consistent with an iridovirus. (From Waltzek, T.B. et al., *Diseases of Aquatic Organisms* 2012;98:41–56. Images courtesy G. Marty and by permission of Diseases of Aquatic Organisms.)

aforementioned consensus primers that target large DNA viruses.[70,71]

For nearly three decades, amplification of viral nucleic acid by PCR followed by Sanger sequencing (first-generation sequencing) has proven invaluable for the detection and characterization of novel viruses including fish viruses. The strength of PCR is its rapid ability to detect viruses even in low abundance from a range of sample types (cell culture pellets or supernatants, fresh tissue, frozen tissue, and formalin-fixed tissues). However, PCR is a targeted approach requiring previous sequence knowledge to design primers for amplification. This has proven challenging given sequence data for fish viruses within public databases is sparse, with sequences from whole families of RNA viruses lacking altogether (e.g., *Astroviridae*, *Filoviridae*, *Bornaviridae*). One reasonable approach to this problem has been

the use of degenerate primers designed to conserve genomic sequences of well-described vertebrate DNA viruses for the detection of divergent fish DNA viruses.[70] However, the high genetic divergence of known fish DNA viruses to other vertebrate DNA viruses suggests this approach will have limited success in the detection of novel fish RNA given their markedly higher rates of evolution.

The advent of recent viral enrichment strategies paired with high-throughput second-generation sequencing technologies provides several advantages over PCR and Sanger sequencing approaches including: (1) no prior knowledge of the sequence is required for priming, (2) full viral genomes can be recovered given the sheer number of sequence reads generated, and (3) multiple viruses can be discovered in the same sample.[73,74] These techniques have recently led to the discovery of the first fish bunyaviruses,[74] hepadnaviruses,[75] poxviruses,[76] papillomaviruses and polyomaviruses.[77] There is little doubt that second-generation sequencing technologies will greatly expand the known fish viruses in the near future; however, the challenge will be to establish the role of these viruses in disease.

INTERNAL ORGAN EVALUATION

After microbiological sampling, the internal organs should be examined grossly and microscopically as wet mount preparations. The stomach should be examined for the presence of food, hemorrhages, ulcers, granulomas and parasites (i.e., both metazoan and protozoan). For larger fish species or those with more fibrous stomachs, the inner mucosal lining of the stomach should be scraped and examined microscopically. It should be remembered that some species, for example, cyprinids, pipefishes, and parrotfishes, lack a true stomach. The intestinal tract and pyloric cecae should also be checked for the presence of food or fluid, hemorrhages, ulcers, and parasites (especially nematodes and flagellates). The liver should be checked for color, uniformity, fatty consistency, parasites, pigmented macrophage aggregates and granulomas (**Figure 3.45a**). The gallbladder, which is located near or surrounded by the liver, should contain a yellowish to greenish fluid that is normally clear. The size of the gallbladder may vary and can be relatively large in fish that are anorexic or have not eaten for a while. The spleen should be examined for color, size, uniformity, pigmented macrophage aggregates and granulomas (**Figure 3.45b**). The swim bladder should be examined for thickening, hemorrhages, necrosis, fungi and parasites. The swim bladder in some species (e.g., gar, tarpon, arapaima and some catfishes) are highly modified and may contain specialized respiratory tissues. The kidney in some species of fish has anterior and posterior portions that are separate, while some are connected and others are merged (**Figure 3.45c** and **d**). Both the anterior and posterior portions of the kidney should be checked for uniformity, granulomas and parasites. The gonads of fish should be checked for gender, maturity, size, granulomas or hardened structures, which in females is sometimes indicative of degenerating eggs or past "egg-binding" episodes (**Figure 3.45e** and **f**).

Wet mounts of the anterior and posterior kidney, liver, spleen, swim bladder, stomach/spiral valve, intestine (both anterior and posterior portions)/spiral colon, and gonad should be examined for most species (**Figure 3.45g**). In some cases, a wet mount of the brain may be useful, such as in the detection of myxosporidean parasites in the brain of yellow perch (*Perca flavescens*). In larger fish, scrapes of the mucosa of the gastrointestinal organs may be easier and can help rule out some parasitic infestations. Impression smears of the kidney, liver, spleen or brain (and possibly other suspect organs) may be useful after staining. Blotting tissues of excess blood is helpful before making impression smears. Inter- and intraspecies differences can be significant, so familiarity with normal anatomy and normal appearance of wet mounts of these various organs in some common domestic species can help as a starting point. Some good models include salmonids, catfish, tilapia, koi, goldfish, platys and guppies.

Granulomas in wet mounts of fish tissues are a relatively common finding and indicate the presence of an irritating or foreign pathogen or material that has incited a chronic inflammatory response. These granulomas typically appear as "rocklike" masses, often tan to brown in color and are often surrounded by a clear zone consisting microscopically of epithelioid macrophages (**Figure 3.45h**). Granulomas are commonly associated with certain bacterial, fungal and parasitic infections, although these infections may occur without these characteristic lesions. Bacteria that often cause granuloma formation include *Mycobacterium* sp., *Nocardia* sp. and *Francisella* spp. The oomycete causative agent of epizootic ulcerative syndrome, *Aphanomyces invadans*, can cause granuloma formation in the muscle of freshwater and marine fishes. Infection with *Cryptobia iubilans*, a flagellate parasite of several species of cichlids, often results in granuloma formation in the stomach, anterior intestine and associated tissues. Parasitic granulomas can also be seen as a chronic inflammatory response to encysted larval nematodes, larval cestodes, digenean metacercarial or amoebic infections. Granulomas in gonadal tissue may be the result of a bacterial infection like

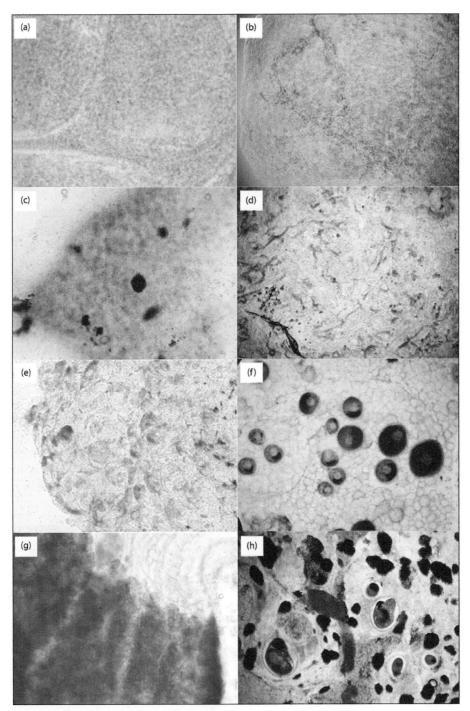

Figure 3.45 Tissue squashes of internal organs. (a) Normal liver of tilapia (*Oreochromis* sp.). (b) Normal spleen of bristlenose catfish (*Ancistrus cirrhosis*). (c) Normal anterior kidney of freshwater angelfish (*Pterophyllum scalare*). (d) Normal posterior kidney of gourami (*Trichopodus* sp.). (e) Normal testis of tilapia (*Oreochromis* sp.). (f) Normal ovary of tilapia (*Oreochromis* sp.). (g) Normal stomach of neon tetra (*Paracheirodon innesi*). (h) Granulomas in liver of tilapia (*Oreochromis* sp.) infected with *Francisella* spp.

Mycobacterium sp. or the result of chronic reabsorption of unlaid eggs in female fish. Scales, spines and plant material can cause foreign-body granulomas as well. Care should be taken to not confuse pigmented macrophage aggregates (PMAs), immune cell aggregates commonly found in anterior and posterior kidney, spleen, and liver of fish, or developing oocytes with granulomas.

Small samples (approximately 0.5–1 cm³) of internal organs, as well as specific lesions, should be preserved in 10% neutral buffered formalin or Davidson's fixative for histology. Organs that should be saved for histopathology include gill, gastrointestinal tract, anterior and posterior kidney, liver, gallbladder, spleen, swim bladder (including rete if present), gonad, heart, brain, skin, muscle, eye, opercula, and pseudobranch. In some instances, sections of spinal cord or neurocranium may also be useful. Tissue samples for electron microscopy should also be saved in an appropriate aldehyde-based fixative such as Karnovsky's fixative.

DIAGNOSTIC IMAGING

Survey radiography

Radiography remains perhaps the most useful non-invasive diagnostic technique in veterinary medicine due to its ease of use, lower cost compared to other diagnostics, amount of valuable information provided and quick implementation. It should be part of all examinations of fish whenever possible.[78–81] Fish less than 6 cm can be radiographed effectively with digital radiography, and multiple exposures allow large fish to be fully evaluated. Radiographs should also be part of every necropsy, as the swim bladder and skeletal system are most effectively evaluated with radiography.

Digital radiography has become the predominant modality and currently exists in two forms. CR refers to "computer radiography," which utilizes a portable cassette and digital processor that reads the cassette after exposure. This process mimics traditional film radiography and replaces the chemical development process with a digital scan. CR plates should be completely sealed in waterproof plastic bags (e.g., Ziploc®) for protection. DR refers to "direct radiography" in which the plate is connected to a computer, without the need for plate processing, for rapid image

procurement. These systems are much more portable and can have better resolution than some CR systems, however, the cord connection between the computer and plate can be a source of water exposure even with the use of protective bags. Wireless DR plates remove the risk that a cord connection causes with water. Although the costs of DR units are decreasing, they cost significantly more than that of CR unit systems.

The standard principles of radiography in companion animal medicine hold true to fish when anatomy allows both lateral and dorso-ventral views. Flatfish and syngnathid anatomy usually reduces the number of views to one. The "standing lateral" view bears unique mention. The patient is placed in ventral recumbency with the beam directed laterally through the body. This view allows evaluation of the swim bladder in its natural orientation, which can help rule in or out a fluid line (**Figure 3.46a** and **b**). A laterally recumbent fish with fluid in the swim bladder can be more difficult to diagnose as the radiolucency of the entire swim bladder is decreased.

Due to improved technology, teleosts and elasmobranchs only need to be out of the physical and physiological support of water for usually seconds to minutes for most radiographic diagnostics. Only MRI remains elusive as a common imaging modality because of the time required to produce effective scans. Super saturating the anesthetic water with

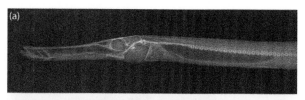
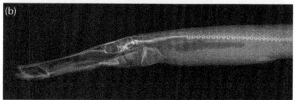

Figure 3.46 Radiograph of trumpetfish (*Aulostomus maculatus*). (a) Lateral view of normal fish. (b) Lateral view with fluid in the swim bladder. Note the decreased radiolucency of the swim bladder and bubble-like appearance of the gas opacity. A standing lateral radiograph would have demonstrated a fluid line.

oxygen prior to diagnostics will benefit the patient. It is recommended (S. Boylan, personal observation) that 115%–150% oxygen saturation (11–15 ppm dissolved oxygen depending on salinity and temperature) be achieved when possible for several minutes before conducting fluoroscopy or CT scans greater than 1 minute. Transported fish have experienced >200% oxygen saturation for more than 10 hours without injury or mortality.

Fish should be removed from their anesthetic bath and tilted with the head down to drain residual water before placing the patient on the cassette. If a contrast agent was given, the fish's oral cavity or vent, depending on the type of contrast study, should be inspected for regurgitated/defecated contrast media. Elasmobranchs are commonly evaluated with contrast studies and are prone to regurgitation. When the patient requires some positional stabilization on a cassette, masking tape provides a radiolucent material that can help stabilize a patient without removing scales or mucous. Various foam pads adapted from companion animal medicine can be used as well.

Radiographic literature on normal fish anatomy is not common.[81–83] As with many exotics, the age, gender, diet and reproductive status may vastly change radiographic anatomy. Hyperostosis, for example, is a normal, age-related change in certain marine teleost skeletons that may be construed as pathologic if the clinician is unfamiliar with Carangidae or certain eel species (**Figure 3.47**).[84] Swim bladder shapes may also change during aging as fish develop "drumming" adult behaviors. During reproduction, ovaries may encompass >25% of the coelomic cavity compared to nonreproductive periods where gonadal tissue is microscopic. Therefore, it is strongly recommended that radiographs of normal members of the species be taken for comparison. Necropsies provide excellent opportunities to generate databases of "normal" anatomy.

Contrast radiography

Contrast radiography is commonly conducted in fish medicine when foreign bodies or changes in appetite occur.[85] If a thorough physical exam, history, survey radiographs, and blood work rule out inappetence from infection/inflammation or

an obvious foreign body, contrast radiography is recommended to find radiolucent foreign bodies, gastrointestinal ruptures, gastrointestinal gas or torsions (**Figure 3.48**). Barium compounds are easy to use and abundant in small animal clinical practices, although regurgitated barium sulfate can adhere to gills, thereby compromising ventilatory capacity in the short term and potentially provoking a long-term inflammatory response. Iodinated liquids, like MD-Gastroview® (37% organically bound iodine), are safer for gastrointestinal ulcers and are less likely to bind to internal obstructions or ulcerated mucosa that can occur with the more viscous barium solutions. Less viscous, iodinated compounds are preferred for rectal administration, as they travel farther in the gastrointestinal system and possess less risk for impaction. The amount of contrast material to use varies on the case. Typically, enough contrast agent is added to fully, but not excessively, distend the stomach. Most carnivorous fish have larger, single-chamber stomachs and/or pyloric ceca compared to filter-feeding species. Cyprinids, an example of

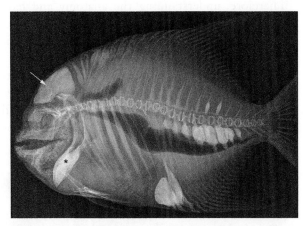

Figure 3.47 Atlantic spadefish (*Chaetodipterus faber*) with hyperostosis and normal adult swim bladder morphology. The swim bladder bifurcates cranially near the Weberian apparatus and progresses dorsal into the expaxial musculature. The caudal aspect of the swim bladder also bifurcates into two branches that extend to the ventral caudal peduncle. The supraoccipital bone (arrow) and cleithrum (*) are radiolucent in juveniles, but are clearly evident in radiography of adults.

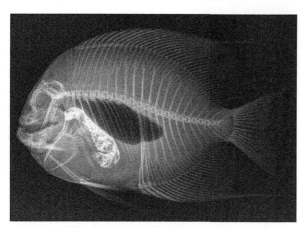

Figure 3.48 Gray angelfish (*Pomacanthus arcuatus*) with Gastroview® contrast agent highlighting an ingested scrub pad used to remove algae in an aquarium. Angelfish are prone to picking and ingesting silicone sealants and other foreign substances that are often radiolucent on survey radiograph.

herbivorous fishes, lack a true stomach and therefore take far less contrast agent. Contrast studies can also be used to delineate gas in the swim bladder versus the gastrointestinal tract (**Figure 3.49**). Therefore, understanding the anatomy and having radiographs of normal individuals will greatly increase the interpretation and diagnostic benefit of contrast radiographic studies.

Ideally, contrast studies should start with lateral, dorsal-ventral and standing lateral survey radiographs without contrast in the sedated patient. Contrast can then be given orally and/or aborally (i.e., via the vent). Most mammalian contrast studies usually require repeat radiographs, which are taken every 15 minutes to every hour for several hours. Fish cannot remain anesthetized for that period of time or experience multiple capture and anesthetic episodes. Given this reduction in the number of contrast images available over the study's design, giving contrast in both the stomach (via feeding needle or red rubber catheter) and the vent (via IV catheter) at the same time is recommended to gain the most from each radiograph (**Figure 3.50**). Catheterization of the bladder for urethrocystography can also be very informative.[86]

SPECIFIC CONDITIONS DIAGNOSED WITH INTERVENTIONAL RADIOGRAPHY/ COMPUTER TOMOGRAPHY

Swim bladder evaluation

Radiography's most common application in fish is evaluation of the teleost swim bladder.[81,82] The two anatomical styles of swim bladder morphology and physiology are physostomous and physoclistous. Physostomous fish possess a patent pneumatic duct connecting the gastrointestinal tract to the swim bladder. These fish often gulp air at the surface to inflate their swim bladder and possess a gas mixture similar to the atmosphere. Physostomous fish are considered "more primitive" in the evolutionary scheme, and the vast majority of these species are freshwater. Cyprinids (koi and goldfish) are the most

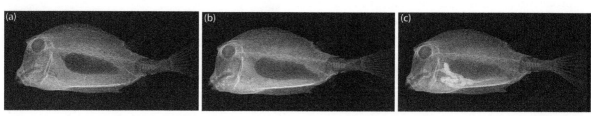

Figure 3.49 Radiographs of a scrawled cowfish (*Acanthostracion quadricornis*). (a) Routine survey radiograph acquired upon acquisition by public aquarium. (b) The same cowfish several years later presenting with abnormal buoyancy. There is an increased gas opacity at the caudal pole of the swim bladder. (c) Standing lateral view of same cowfish with abnormal buoyancy. A contrast radiograph taken 1 hour after 3 mls of oral and 1.5 mls of rectally administered Gastroview® contrast were given confirmed the gas opacity was swim bladder in origin. Interventional radiography allowed a guided swim bladder aspiration that is difficult in cowfishes and boxfishes due to a calcified dermal skeleton.

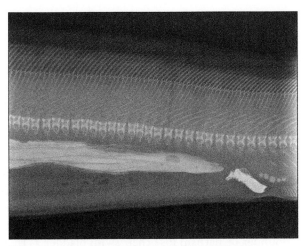

Figure 3.50 Green moray eel (*Gymnothorax funebris*) contrast study. Barium sulfate was given orally and rectally to evaluate the gastrointestinal system due to inappetance. Stomach rugae are clearly visible as contrast material passes through the stomach. Multiple enteroliths are demonstrated adjacent to a rectum infusion of contrast material. Note that the rectally delivered barium sulfate did not disseminate as effectively as the orally administered barium. A liquid iodinated compound would have been better suited for this application.

common physostomous species seen by the companion veterinary practitioner, whereas catfish and baitfish comprise the majority of production-type physostomous fishes. Cyprinids have a bilobed swim bladder with a narrow isthmus between the lobes where the posterior kidney is typically located.[87] Because a connection between the oral cavity and swim bladder exists, opportunistic infections related to poor water quality occur commonly when opportunistic pathogenic bacteria (e.g., aeromonads or atypical mycobacteria) consumed during normal feeding enter the physostomous duct and cause an infection in the lumen of the swim bladder. Fish with infectious aerocystitis (i.e., inflammation of the swim bladder) typically present with abnormal buoyancy, lethargy and a fluid line in the standing lateral radiograph. Interventional radiography is facilitated by placing a radiopaque marker (i.e., coin, needle) where the clinician believes they can make a percutaneous aspiration of swim bladder fluid for cytology and culture. This radiographic-assisted procedure

may prevent an accidental laceration of the posterior kidney or liver, which could result in death.

Certain "fancy" goldfish have been bred for unusual body conformations and thus suffer unusual swim bladder and skeletal abnormalities similar to chondrodystrophic dog breeds. Because each fish is unique in swim bladder anatomy, the best diagnostic imaging occurs when "normal" radiographs have been taken of the individual prior to presentation of a complaint of abnormal buoyancy.

Physoclistous fish use a vascular plexus of blood vessels, or rete, to control the gas volume of the swim bladder. Although most of these fish secrete or absorb oxygen as their primary gas for volume control, nitrogen or a mix of gases are used in a species-specific pattern.[88] Nearly all marine species are physoclistous and therefore suffer catastrophic decompression when brought up from depth rapidly. During ascent, the swim bladder expands as the exterior pressure decreases, and internal organs may prolapse through the mouth or vent when there is no room in the coelom. Benthic species (*Serranidae*/grouper, *Centropristis species*/sea bass, *Lutjanus campechanus*/red snapper) are more prone to catastrophic decompression and suffer mortality hours to weeks after collection.[89–91] "Venting" is a controversial technique practiced by anglers, but veterinarians participating in deep water (>10 m) fish collection should use oxygen saturation, careful swim bladder aspiration and recompression devices to treat these fish.

The clinician needs to be careful not to overinterpret swim bladder radiographs unless they have a strong grasp of normal for the species, gender, age, and so on. The first inclination of most veterinarians is to aspirate what they believe is excessive gas in the swim bladder, which often makes a fish negatively buoyant. The majority of negatively buoyant teleosts die due to contact dermatitis. A floating fish can be maintained in an isolation bin in its original tank indefinitely with supportive care. Isolation bins are appropriately sized containers (e.g., Tupperware®) with holes drilled into the sides for water movement, and flotation foam (i.e., Styrofoam) attached around the edges to keep the bin positively buoyant. These isolation bins separate the fish from tank mate aggression and create a simple, temporary hospitalization environment without the need for a separate system. A lid may be necessary to prevent the patient from jumping out of the isolation bin and back into the main tank population.

Iatrogenic aerocystitis can also occur with repeated swim bladder aspiration. Pathogenic bacteria and fungi can be introduced into a swim bladder, which is not an organ that heals well from infection or inflammation. Clinicians should be prepared to collect all their samples and remove or add gas as needed in as few aspirations as possible. For physostomous fish, sterile "gas" is easily accessible by aspirating the gas from crystalloid fluid bags. This gas composition, however, will not be the enriched oxygen mix common in physoclistous fish. Pure oxygen can be obtained by aspirating gas from balloons filled with medical-grade oxygen and injected into the swim bladder.

Another feature unique to fish is the relationship between the swim bladder and orientation. The teleost swim bladder confers buoyancy but not orientation. Many fish with abnormal buoyancy have normal swim bladder volumes. The positive "belly-up" buoyancy that is a common complaint in sick fish is the same orientation as a healthy fish that is anesthetized. To illustrate the point, the clinician should observe a healthy fish undergoing sedation. As a fish enters a deeper anesthetic state, the fish loses its orientation control and "rolls" into dorsal recumbency with the majority of fish being positively buoyant when anesthetized. Upon recovery from anesthesia, the fish returns to normal buoyancy control and orientation. Many belly-up fish are suffering from vestibular/CNS disease that is preventing normal orientation and not a true swim bladder issue. Treating these cases with antibiotics and anti-inflammatories should be considered first before any swim bladder–invasive procedures are conducted. Identifying the cause of abnormal flotation between true swim bladder disease and vestibular disease is one of the benefits of radiography. The previously mentioned "fancy" goldfish often have irregular, bilobed swim bladders. Some fancy goldfish with hypertrophied wens may have altered buoyancy as they age due to the wen's increasing size. The fish veterinarian should carefully evaluate

the fish, which includes radiographs, but should first address reducing the size of the wen with surgery/cryosurgery (see Chapter 18) and recover the fish for observation before attempting swim bladder aspiration. The abnormal buoyancy may be due solely to the wen, which is readily corrected, though many clinicians' first instinct is to look at the "abnormal" swim bladder and begin aspiration, which usually compromises animal health.

Last, not all fish have swim bladders. The elasmobranchs do not have swim bladders and maintain their neutral buoyancy through a mixture of urea and a fatty liver. Many benthic fish (e.g., flounder or flatfish) lose their swim bladder as they mature from free-swimming fry to benthic adults. Certain pelagic fish like *Echeneis* (i.e., remoras), *Coryphaenids* (i.e., mahi-mahi), and *Rachycentron canadum* (i.e., cobia) also have no swim bladders as adults (**Figure 3.51**).

Subcutaneous emphysema and seahorse brood pouch inflation

Although atypical mycobacteria and *Vibrio* are the most common infectious diseases in syngnathids, subcutaneous emphysema is the most common noninfectious disease of seahorses. Clinical signs almost always include gas accumulation in the distal tail in both male and female seahorses (*Hippocampus erectus* are commonly affected in captivity). Buoyancy control is lost and affected animals fail to feed and die from inappetence and immune suppression sequelae. Treatment with antibiotics (ceftazidime) and carbonic anhydrase inhibitors (acetazolamide immersion or injections) provide temporary relief in less than half of the cases. Aspiration of the gas bubbles also provides temporary relief. Histopathology usually finds sterile, subcutaneous tissue with expanded spaces and little to no inflammation. While the cause may be multifactorial, gas supersaturation is likely the major etiology. A tensiometer/saturometer can be used to determine gas saturation pressure in water. Filtration puts water and its dissolved gases under pressure, and many tanks have constant gas saturation pressures of 15–20 mmHg greater than ambient. In tanks with individuals exhibiting clinical signs, gas saturation pressures are often 25–35 mmHg greater than ambient. Deeper tanks provide a gas saturation refuge

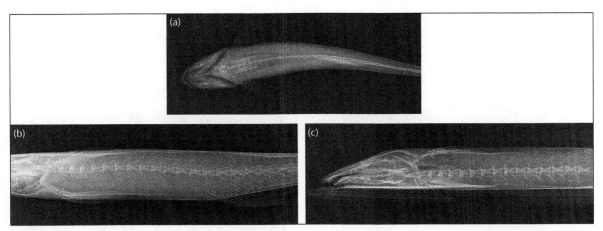

Figure 3.51 Radiographs of a remora/sharksucker (*Echeneis* sp.). (a) Ventral-dorsal view of a normal remora. (b) Lateral view of a remora for evaluation of suspected spinal trauma. (c) Standing lateral, dorsal recumbent view of a normal remora (attachment head organ facing ventrally). Note that no swim bladder is present in any view.

to benthic seahorses because gas saturation is more clinically relevant near the surface. Leaky gaskets, failing pipe joints and cracked pipes allow air to be mixed with water under pressure in a Venturi effect. "Salt creep" on pipes and filters are an indication of leaks that could be the source of air introduction. The water becomes supersaturated, often with nitrogen gas, which creates decompression illness, or the "bends," in highly susceptible species like seahorses. Until saturation is corrected, these cases are chronic and difficult to resolve.

Radiographs are useful to determine if gas emphysema is restricted to just the tail tip or more widespread. Male seahorses possess a rete in their brood pouch that helps them oxygenate the eggs they gestate, and as a result makes males more susceptible to the effects of gas saturation. While both female and male seahorses suffer tail emphysema bubbles, males can concurrently suffer subcutaneous brood pouch emphysema. These cases are invariably fatal, but they should be differentiated from brood pouch gas accumulation. Single-gender tanks (all male) or tanks with unpaired males may experience a phenomenon where adult males inflate their brood pouch without eggs present. These males are positively buoyant and unable to feed. They can be treated symptomatically by "burping" the brood pouch gas with a catheter or similar soft-ended aspirating device. Usually it takes a change in gender population structure for these males

to stop this behavior. Radiographs of males with brood pouch gas accumulation show a solid radiolucent pocket of gas, compared to individuals with subcutaneous brood pouch emphysema that has numerous small gas bubbles present (**Figure 3.52**). It is often helpful to first burp the brood pouch before taking a lateral radiograph to look for subcutaneous emphysema.

Exophthalmia

Gas exophthalmia is common in teleosts with causes including trauma, septicemia, gas supersaturation, and catastrophic decompression syndrome (**Figure 3.53**). Radiographs, fluoroscopy and CT can help aspiration treatments by guiding needle placement and confirming complete gas removal. Injections of intra-ocular isotonic fluids may help consolidate multiple gas pockets into single gas pockets, which are easier to aspirate. Diagnostic imaging can determine gas location and efficacy of therapies, which may include aspiration, hyperbaric oxygen, psuedobranchectomy, antibiotics and anti-inflammatories (**Figure 3.54**).

Spinal trauma

Trauma to the spine is also common in captive fish due to collisions with tank walls or other stationary objects. While difficult to diagnose on gross necropsy, spinal trauma is quickly diagnosed on survey radiographs. Spinal fracture due to tank wall trauma is a common cause of mortality in public

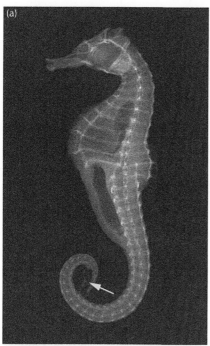

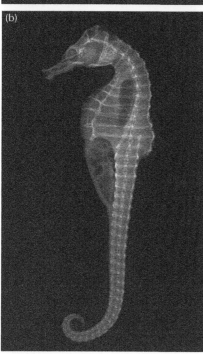

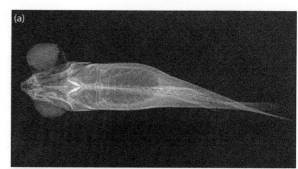

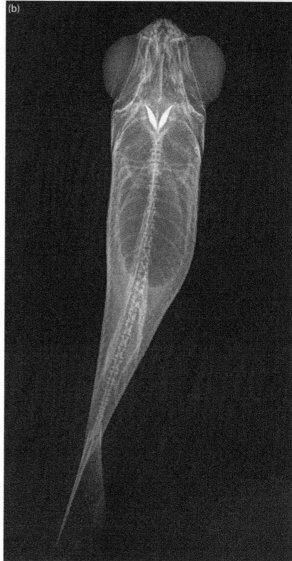

Figure 3.52 Radiograph of a lined seahorse (*Hippocampus erectus*). (a) Male lined seahorse with brood pouch inflation and subcutaneous emphysema (arrow) at tip of tail. (b) Male lined seahorse with "burped" brood pouch revealing subcutaneous emphysema, which carries a far worse prognosis than the animal in **Figure 3.52a**.

Figure 3.53 Radiographs of a black-barred soldierfish (*Myripristis jacobus*). (a) Dorso-ventral view of fish with exophthalmia related to trauma. (b) Dorso-ventral view of eye after aspiration of gas and pseudobranchectomy.

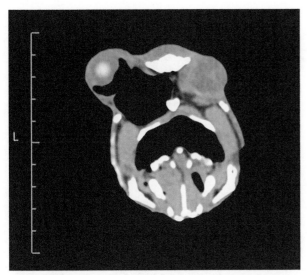

Figure 3.54 Computed tomography (CT) scan of a black sea bass (*Centropristis striata*) head with severe gas exophthalmia in the left eye.

aquaria (**Figure 3.55**). Radiographs commonly find spinal abnormalities that are clinically insignificant (**Figure 3.56**). Among koi hobbyists, spinal fracture can occur due to lightning strikes, avoidance behavior from predators, or impact trauma during breeding season jumping.[92,93]

Endoscopy

Endoscopy is often divided into rigid or flexible endoscopy, with the former having a significant role in fish medicine. Many rigid endoscopic systems are fully portable for site visits and fieldwork.[94] When endoscopy is combined with radiology and/or ultrasound, the diagnostic evaluation of the internal anatomy can equal exploratory surgery with far less risk.[95] The most obvious use of rigid endoscopy is evaluation and/or biopsy of the internal organs through smaller incisions compared to exploratory surgery. Rigid endoscopes are also extremely useful

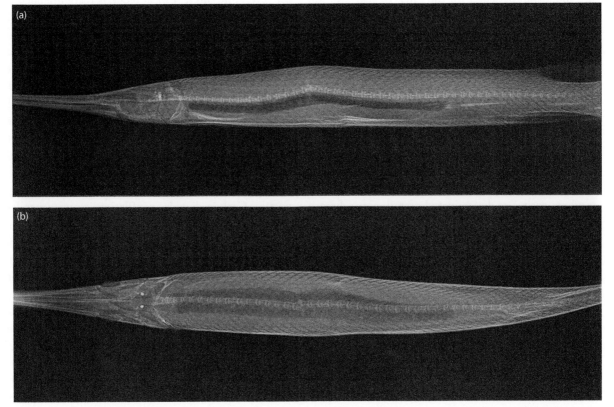

Figure 3.55 Radiographs of a longnose gar (*Lepisosteus osseus*). (a) Lateral view of gar with a spinal fracture caused by hitting tank wall. (b) Dorsal view of same gar with spinal fracture.

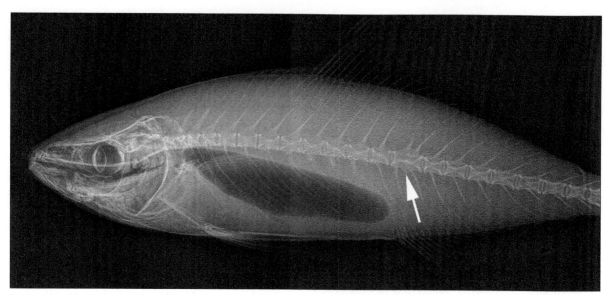

Figure 3.56 Radiograph of rainbow runner (*Elagatis binpinnulata*) acquired postmortem. The spinal abnormality of fused vertebrae (arrow) was either congenital or the result of trauma, and an incidental finding on necropsy.

in evaluating macroscopic gill health and detecting metazoan parasites on the gills. In fish <10 kg, rigid endoscopes can evaluate the oral and upper gastrointestinal systems in the same way that flexible endoscopy works in terrestrial animals. Foreign bodies in the stomach can also be removed safely with endoscopic tools. In larger fish, reproductive and caudal gastrointestinal structures may be evaluated through the vent.

Coelioscopy

Visual evaluation of the internal anatomy is often helpful in complicated cases where hepatic lipidosis, egg binding, ascites or disseminated granulomous disease may be quickly identified. Coelioscopy may be used to identify the gender of young fish when secondary sexual characteristics are absent and small gonad size prevents ultrasonographic identification.[96] Juvenile koi or sturgeon brood stock are often endoscopically sexed without complication.[97–99] Rigid endoscopes have also been used to sterilize male sturgeon while keeping their testicular endocrine function intact by ligating the vas deferens.[100] Preparation for the portal of entry is the same as with surgery. The fish is anesthetized in dorsal recumbency with a fish anesthesia delivery system (see Chapter 17 on anesthesia). Scales are removed only where necessary, and a topical

disinfectant, commonly Betadine, is applied to the area for several minutes. A local block is recommended to reduce pain and bleeding (e.g., buffered lidocaine with epinephrine, 1:1 sodium bicarbonate to epinephrine) and a stab incision is made at the appropriate location with a scalpel blade. Most gender identification surgical approaches start at ventral midline or slightly off midline, cranial to the vent. Incisions are kept small to reduce insufflation gas/fluid loss, reduce coelomic contamination, reduce skin damage/inflammation and reduce the number of sutures necessary to close the wound. Biopsies can be taken for wet mount preparations, cytology, culture, histology or molecular diagnostics. Carbon dioxide insufflation is recommended over atmospheric air, which can create prolonged positive buoyancy if not removed. The nitrogen in atmospheric air can take days to weeks to resolve, whereas residual carbon dioxide can be usually absorbed within 24 hours. A radiograph is recommended post-surgery to evaluate the presence of coelomic gas that should be aspirated prior to recovery. If fluids are chosen for insufflation, those fluids should be isotonic to the species. Standard mammalian cystalloids are appropriate for most freshwater teleosts (e.g., Normosol, LRS). Marine teleost interstitial fluids contain more sodium and chloride than their freshwater counterparts, thus specific marine teleost crystalloid fluids have been developed.[101] Elasmobranchs require a specific electrolyte solution that accounts for their urea concentration.[102] One to three simple interrupted sutures typically close the portal of entry, which may not need any further intervention. Complications during endoscopy may require limited use of systemic antibiotics, analgesics or adjunct wound therapy such as cold laser therapy (see Chapter 18).

Coelioscopy with endoscopic biopsy is a less invasive alternative to exploratory surgery. After imaging (i.e., ultrasound, CT, radiographs, MRI) has found internal anomalies, the next step for diagnosis may be a percutaneous aspiration (with or without ultrasound guidance) or rigid endoscopy biopsy. The approach is the same as mentioned with gonad visualization except the incision site may vary depending on the desired tissue for biopsy. The liver and spleen are the most commonly biopsied organs for culture, histology or molecular diagnostics. Posterior kidney biopsies are more difficult but possible to sample depending on anatomy. Many cyprinid species have the posterior kidney located at the isthmus of the anterior and posterior swim bladder, which is an ideal location for biopsy. Compared to percutaneous aspirations, endoscopic biopsies are often more informative. Bleeding can also be immediately assessed and addressed in organs at high risk for hemorrhage like the spleen, liver and posterior kidney. In fish >3 kg, rigid endoscopes can evaluate the swim bladder lumen when imaging suggests an issue. A lateral approach between ribs is recommended. Incisions for swim bladder endoscopy generally heal uneventfully if hemorrhage and contamination are minimal as the lateral body wall supports the swim bladder until it heals.

Gill evaluation

Unique to fish medicine is the use of a rigid endoscope to completely evaluate the gills without the need for biopsy. In addition, the spiracles or gill slits of most elasmobranchs make standard gill biopsy difficult to impossible. Endoscopy allows full evaluation of each gill arch compared to gill biopsy's small sample and potential risk of hemorrhage (**Figure 3.57a**). Gill biopsies may miss organisms or gill pathology that can be readily diagnosed with endoscopy (**Figure 3.57b**). Fish are lightly anesthetized with the animal kept fully submerged to avoid air pockets that interfere with visualization. Oxygen supplementation is recommended since opercular movements will be reduced or absent. Oxygen saturation should be 115%–150% prior to induction and throughout the examination and recovery. The rigid endoscope is introduced through the opercular opening, gill slit or spiracle, and the gill is evaluated from the arch base to the tips of the primary lamellae. Gill biopsies usually sample only the gill tips to avoid excessive hemorrhage (**Figure 3.57c**). Many infectious agents concentrate at the base of the gill arch where blood is abundant, and the drag of water is less, thus gill biopsies are not sensitive for most gill parasites until the infection is overwhelming. For example, the monogenean *Erpocotyle tiburonis* appears to prefer the last gill slit of bonnethead sharks (*Sphyrna tiburo*) due to reduced drag.[103] This gill slit is the most difficult to biopsy with scissors, but it is easily and safely examined with rigid endoscopy. Saprolegnia infections appear to be more pathogenic in certain fishes like the robust redhorse (*Moxostoma robustum*), where it attacks the base of the gill arch causing mortality without any evidence of the infection in the skin or gill tips (S. Boylan, personal observation). The magnification of rigid endoscopes is sufficient to find the majority of large protozoa and metazoans (i.e., monogeneans, leeches, copepods, fungi) (**Figure 3.57d**).

Gastric examination

Foreign bodies are common in pet fish. Certain marine ornamentals (angelfish, Bermuda chubs) often ingest silicone sealant or cleaning pad fragments, both of which are usually radiolucent and require contrast radiography or endoscopy for diagnosis (**Figure 3.58**). Rigid endoscopes often have tools (baskets, forceps) that may facilitate removal of these foreign bodies through the mouth and avoid surgery. Survey radiographs of trout often find gravel in their stomach, and a quick gastric endoscopic evaluation can determine if the stones are causing inflammation (**Figure 3.59**). Similarly, several grouper species suffer gastric ulceration as they age, which can be quickly diagnosed with noninvasive gastric endoscopy (J. Dill, personal communication).

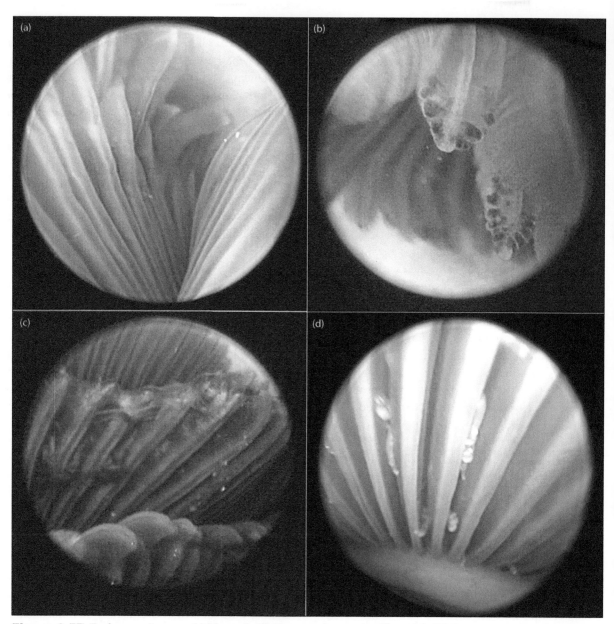

Figure 3.57 Endoscopy images. (a) Normal gill filaments in a striped burrfish (*Chilomycterus schoepfi*). The pallor is due to lighting and not anemia. Endoscopy can often demonstrate red blood cells migrating though the gill capillaries. (b) Telangiectasia in the gills of a black sea bass (*Centropristis striata*). These focal aneurysms of the capillaries are often common after stressful events, such as increased cardiovascular activity, traumatic captures or suboptimal water quality. (c) Tips of gill filaments in a lookdown (*Selene vomer*) where a gill biopsy was recently acquired (upper) compared to normal filaments (lower). (d) Gills of a scamp (*Mycteroperca phenax*) with monogenean infestation. Note that the monogeneans are present at the base of the gill filaments where a gill biopsy would not detect their presence.

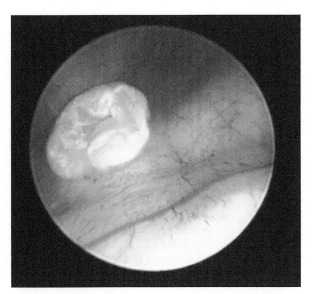

Figure 3.58 Endoscopy of the stomach of a striped burrfish (*Chilomycterus schoepfi*) with contrast (Gastroview®) present as part of an examination looking for a foreign body.

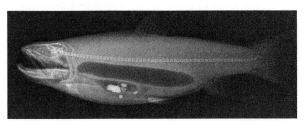

Figure 3.59 Young male brook trout (*Salvelinus fontinalis*) with gravel in an air-inflated esophagus and stomach. Gravel in the stomach is a common occurrence in this species and may be used to aid mechanical digestion.

REFERENCES

1. Stoskopf, M. Clinical examination and procedures. In: *Fish Medicine*. M. Stoskopf, ed. WB Saunders, Philadelphia, 1993; pp. 62–79.
2. Yanong, R.P.E. *Seminars in Avian and Exotic Pet Medicine* 2003;12(2):89–105.
3. Noga, E.J. *Fish Disease: Diagnosis and Treatment*, 2nd ed. Wiley-Blackwell, Ames, Iowa, 2010.
4. Tucker, C.S. Water analysis. In: *Fish Medicine*. M. Stoskopf, ed. WB Saunders, Philadelphia, 1993; pp. 166–198.
5. Klinger, R.E. and Floyd, R.F. *Submission of fish for diagnostic evaluation*, 2013.
6. Floyd, R.F. Behavioral diagnosis. In: *Tropical Fish Medicine, Vet Clinics of North America (Sm Animal Practice)*. M. Stoskopf, ed. 1988;18(2):303–314.
7. Crosby, T.C., Hill, J.E., Watson, C.A., Yanong, R.P. and Strange, R. Effects of tricaine methanesulfonate, Hypno, metomidate, quinaldine, and salt on plasma cortisol levels following acute stress in threespot gourami Trichogaster trichopterus. *Journal of Aquatic Animal Health* 2006;18(1):58–63.
8. King, W., Hooper, B., Hillsgrove, S., Benton, C. and Berlinsky, D.L. The use of clove oil, metomidate, tricaine methanesulphonate and 2-phenoxyethanol for inducing anaesthesia and their effect on the cortisol stress response in black sea bass (*Centropristis striata* L.). *Aquaculture Research* 2005;36(14):1442–1449.
9. Martin, I., Bengt, F. and Robert, S. The efficacy of metomidate, clove oil, Aqui-STM and Benzoak as anaesthetics in Atlantic salmon (*Salmo salar* L.) smolts, and their potential stress-reducing capacity. *Aquaculture* 2003;221:549–566.
10. Thomas, P. and Robertson, L. Plasma cortisol and glucose stress responses of red drum (*Sciaenops ocellatus*) to handling and shallow water stressors and anesthesia with MS-222, quinaldine sulfate and metomidate. *Aquaculture* 1991;96(1):69–86.
11. Strange, R.J. and Schreck, C.B. Anesthetic and handling stress on survival and cortisol concentration in yearling chinook salmon (*Oncorhynchus tshawytscha*). *Journal of the Fisheries Board of Canada* 1978;35(3):345–349.
12. Small, B.C. and Chatakondi, N. Routine measures of stress are reduced in mature channel catfish during and after AQUI-S anesthesia and recovery. *North American Journal of Aquaculture* 2005;67(1):72–78.
13. Lowry, T. and Smith, S.A. Aquatic zoonoses associated with food, bait, ornamental, and tropical fish. *JAVMA* 2007;231(6):876–880.
14. Noble, C., Jones, H.A., Damsgård, B., Flood, M.J., Midling, KØ, Roque, A., Sæther, B.S. and Cottee, S.Y. Injuries and deformities in fish: Their potential impacts upon aquacultural production and welfare. *Fish Physiology and Biochemistry* 2012;38:61–83.
15. Barton, M. *Bond's Biology of Fishes*, 3rd ed. Thomson, Belmont, CA, 2007; pp. 395–396.
16. Hargis Jr., W.J. Disorders of the eye in finfish. *Annual Review of Fish Diseases* 1991;95–117.
17. Williams, C.R. and Whitaker, B.R. The evaluation and treatment of common ocular disorders in teleosts. *Seminars in Avian and Exotic Pet Medicine* 1997; 6(3):160–169.
18. Smartt, J. *Goldfish Varieties and Genetics: Handbook for Breeders*. Fish News Books (Blackwell Science), Iowa State University Press, Ames, IA, 2008.
19. Koppang, E. and Bjerkas, E. The eye. In: *Systemic Pathology of Fish: A Text and Atlas of Normal Tissue Responses in Teleosts, and Their Responses in Disease*, 2nd ed. H.W. Ferguson, ed. Scotian Press, London, 2006; pp. 260–263.

20. Whitaker, B.R. Ocular disorders. In: *BSAVA Manual of Ornamental Fish*. W.H. Wildgoose, ed. British Small Animal Veterinary Association, Gloucester, 2001; p. 151.

21. Evans, D.H., Piermarini, P.M. and Choe, K.P. The multifunctional fish gill: Dominant site of gas exchange, osmoregulation, acid-base regulation, and excretion of nitrogenous waste. *Physiological Reviews* 2005; 85;(1):97–177.

22. Lewis, Jr., W.M. and Morris, D.P. Toxicity of nitrite to fish: A review. *Transactions of the American Fisheries Society* 1986;115(2):183–195.

23. Bengtsson, B.E. Vertebral damage in fish induced by pollutants. In: *Sublethal Effects of Toxic Chemicals on Aquatic Animals*. J.H. Koeman and J.A. Strik, eds. Elsevier, Amsterdam, 1975; pp. 23–30.

24. Anderson, P.A., Huber, D.R. and Berzins, I.K. Correlations of capture, transport, and nutrition with spinal deformities in sandtiger sharks, *Carcharias taurus*, in public aquaria. *Journal of Zoo and Wildlife Medicine* 2012;43(4):750–758.

25. Tate, E.E., Anderson, P.A., Huber, D.R. and Berzins, I.K. Correlations of swimming patterns with spinal deformities in the sand tiger shark, *Carcharias taurus*. *International Journal of Comparative Psychology* 2013;26(1):75–82.

26. Neiffer, D.L. and Stamper, M.A. Fish sedation, anesthesia, analgesia, and euthanasia: Considerations, methods, and types of drugs. *Institute for Laboratory Animal Research Journal* 2009;50(4):343–360.

27. Smith, S.A. Parasites of fish. In: *Veterinary Clinical Parasitology*, 8th ed. A. Zajac, ed. Blackwell Publishing, Ames, IA, 2012; pp. 305–323.

28. Smith, S.A. Non-lethal clinical techniques used in the diagnosis of fish diseases. *Journal of the American Veterinary Medicine Association* 2002;220:1203–1206.

29. Callahan, H.C. and Noga, E.J. Tricaine dramatically reduces the ability to diagnose protozoan ectoparasite (*Ichthyobodo necator*) infections. *Journal of Fish Diseases* 2002;25:433–437.

30. Woo, P.T.K. *Fish Diseases and Disorders, Vol. 1: Protozoan and Metazoan Infections*. 2nd ed. CABI, 2006.

31. Mylniczenko, N.D., Curtis, E.W., Wilborn, R.E. and Young, F.A. Differences in hematocrit of blood samples obtained from two venipuncture sites in sharks. *AJVR* 2006;67(11):1861–1864.

32. Hrubec, T.C. and Smith, S.A. Differences between plasma and serum samples for evaluation of blood chemistry values in rainbow trout, channel catfish, hybrid tilapias and hybrid striped bass. *Journal of Aquatic Animal Health* 1999;11:116–122.

33. Dye, V.A., Hrubec, T.C., Dunn, J.L. and Smith, S.A. Hematology and serum chemistry values for winter flounder (*Pleuronectes americanus*). *International Journal of Recirculating Aquaculture* 2001;2:37–50.

34. Hrubec, T.C., Smith, S.A., Robertson, J.L., Feldman, B., Veit, H.P., Libey, G. and Tinker, M.K. Comparison of hematological reference intervals between culture system and type of hybrid striped bass. *American Journal of Veterinary Research* 1996;57:618–623.

35. Hrubec, T.C., Smith, S.A., Robertson, J.L., Feldman, B., Veit, H.P., Libey, G. and Tinker, M.K. Blood biochemical reference intervals for sunshine bass (*Morone chrysops* × *Morone saxatilis*) in three culture systems. *American Journal of Veterinary Research* 1996;57:624–627.

36. Hrubec, T.C., Cardinale, J. and Smith, S.A. Hematology and plasma chemistry reference intervals for cultured tilapia (*Oreochromis* hybrid). *Veterinary Clinical Hematology* 2000;29:7–12.

37. Hrubec, T.C. and Smith, S.A. Hematology and blood chemistry reference intervals for yellow perch (*Perca flavescens*) raised in recirculation systems. *International Journal of Recirculating Aquaculture* 2004;5:29–42.

38. Knowles, S., Hrubec, T.C., Smith, S.A. and Bakal, R.S. Hematology and plasma chemistry reference intervals for cultured shortnose sturgeon (*Acipenser brevirostrum*). *Veterinary Clinical Pathology* 2006;35(4):434–440.

39. Tavares-Dias, M. and de Moraes F, R. Leukocyte and thrombocyte reference values for channel catfish (*Ictalurus punctatus*), with an assessment of morphologic, cytochemical, and ultrastructural features. *Veterinary Clinical Pathology* 2007;36:49–54.

40. Groff, J.M. and Zinkl, J.G. Hematology and clinical chemistry of cyprinid fish. *Veterinary Clinics of North America: Exotic Animal Practice* 1999;2(5):741–776.

41. Murtha, J.M., Qi, W. and Keller, E.T. Hematologic and serum biochemical values for zebrafish (*Danio rerio*). *Comparative Medicine* 2003;5:37–41.

42. Tripathi, N.K., Latimer, K.S. and Burnley, V.V. Hematologic reference intervals for koi (*Cyprinus carpio*), including blood cell morphology, cytochemistry, and ultrastructure. *Veterinary Clinical Pathology* 2004;33(2):74–83.

43. Tocidlowski, M.E., Lewbart, G.A. and Stoskopf, M.K. Hematologic study of red pacu (*Colossoma brachypomum*). *Veterinary Clinical Pathology* 1997;26(3):119–125.

44. Sakamoto, K., Lewbart, G.A. and Smith, T.M. Blood chemistry values of juvenile red pacu (Piaractus brachypomus). *Veterinary Clinical Pathology* 2001;30(2):50–52.

45. Hrubec, T.C., Robertson, J.L. and Smith, S.A. Effects of temperature on haematologic and biochemical profiles of sunshine bass (*Morone chrysops* × *Morone saxatilis*). *American Journal of Veterinary Research* 1997; 58:126–130.

46. Hrubec, T.C., Robertson, J.L. and Smith, S.A. Effects of ammonia and nitrate concentration on hematologic and serum biochemical profiles of hybrid striped bass (*Morone chrysops* × *Morone saxatilis*). *American Journal of Veterinary Research* 1997;58:131–134.

47. Clauss, T.M., Dove, A.D.M. and Arnold, J.E. Hematologic disorders of fish. *Veterinary Clinics of North America: Exotic Animal Practice* 2008;11(3): 445–462.

48. Harrenstien, L.A., Tornquist, S.J., Miller-Morgan, T.J., Fodness, B.G. and Clifford, K.E. Evaluation of

a point-of-care blood analyzer and determination of reference ranges for blood parameters in rockfish. *Journal of the American Veterinary Medical Association* 2005;226(2):255–265.

49. Palmeiro, B.S., Rosenthal, K.L., Lewbart, G.A. and Shofer, F.S. Plasma biochemical reference intervals for koi. *Journal of the American Veterinary Association* 2007;230(5):708–712.

50. Hrubec, T.C. and Smith, S.A. Hematology of fish. In: *Schalm's Veterinary Hematology*, 6th ed. D.J. Weiss and K.J. Wardrop, eds. Wiley-Blackwell, Ames, 2010; pp. 995–1004.

51. Stoskopf, M. Clinical pathology of freshwater tropical fishes. In: *Fish Medicine*. M. Stoskopf, ed. WB Saunders, Philadelphia, 1993; pp. 543–545.

52. Stoskopf, M. Clinical pathology of carp, goldfish, and koi. In: *Fish Medicine*. M. Stoskopf, ed. WB Saunders, Philadelphia, 1993; pp. 450–453.

53. Stoskopf, M. Clinical pathology of marine tropical fishes. In: *Fish Medicine*. M. Stoskopf, ed. WB Saunders, Philadelphia, 1993; pp. 614–617.

54. Sudova, E., Piackova, V., Kroupova, H., Pijacek, M. and Svobodova, Z. The effect of praziquantel applied *per os* on selected haematological and biochemical indices in common carp (*Cyprinus carpio* L.). *Fish Physiology and Biochemistry* 2009;(35):599–605.

55. University of California, Davis. KHV ELISA. https://www.vetmed.ucdavis.edu/hospital/support-services/lab-services/clinical-laboratory-services/koi-herpes-virus-khv.

56. Munday, B.L., Kwang, J. and Moody, N. Betanodavirus infections of teleost fish: A review. *Journal of Fish Diseases* 2002;25:127–142.

57. Weber, E.S., Waltzek, T.B., Young, D.A., Twitchell, E.L., Gates, A.E., Vagelli, A., Risatti, G.R. and Frasca, Jr., S. Systemic iridovirus infection in the Banggai cardinalfish (*Pterapogon kauderni* Koumans 1933). *Journal of Veterinary Diagnostic Investigations* 2009;21:306–320.

58. Whittington, R.J., Becker, J.A. and Dennis, M.M. Iridovirus infections in finfish—Critical review with emphasis on ranaviruses. *Journal of Fish Diseases* 2010; 33(2):95–122.

59. Kestin, S.C., can de Vis, J.W. and Robb, D.H.F. Protocol for assessing brain function in fish and the effectiveness of methods used to stun and kill them. *Veterinary Record* 2002;150:302–307.

60. Kasumyan, A.O. Vestibular system and sense of equilibrium in fish. *Journal of Ichthyology* 2004;44(Suppl. 2):S224–S268.

61. Buller, N.B. *Bacteria and Fungi from Fish and Other Aquatic Animals: A Practical Identification Manual*. 2nd ed. CABI, 2014.

62. American Fisheries Society Fish Health Section. Blue Book, https://units.fisheries.org/fhs/.

63. Loch, T.P. and Faisal, M. Emerging flavobacterial infections in fish. *Journal of Advanced Research* 2015;6(3):283–300.

64. Loch, T.P., Fujimoto, M., Woodiga, S.A., Walker, E.D., Marsh, T.L. and Faisal, M. Diversity of fish-associated flavobacteria of Michigan. *Journal of Aquatic Animal Health* 2013;3:149–164.

65. Wolf, K. *Fish Viruses and Fish Viral Diseases*. Cornell University Press, Ithaca, NY, 1988.

66. Peters, K. Cell culture of fish cell lines. In: *National Wild Fish Health Survey: Laboratory Procedures Manual*. N. Heil, ed. U.S. Fish and Wildlife Service, Warm Springs, GA, 2009; pp. 10-1–10-16.

67. Plumb, J.A. and Hanson, L.A. Principles of health maintenance. In: *Health Maintenance and Principal Microbial Diseases of Cultured Fishes*, 3rd ed. Wiley-Blackwell, Oxford, 2010.

68. LaPatra, S.E. General procedures for virology. In: *Suggested Procedures for the Detection and Identification of Certain Finfish and Shellfish Pathogens, Blue Book*, 5th ed. Fish Health Section, American Fisheries Society, Bethesda, MD, 2003.

69. Freitas, J.T., Subramaniam, K., Kelley, K.L., Marcquenski, S., Groff, J. and Waltzek, T.B. Genetic characterization of esocid herpesvirus 1 (EsHV1). *Diseases of Aquatic Organisms* 2016;122:1–11.

70. Hanson, L.A., Rudis, M.R., Vasquez-Lee, M. and Montgomery, R.D. A broadly applicable method to characterize large DNA viruses and adenoviruses based on the DNA polymerase gene. *Virology Journal* 2006;3:28.

71. Waltzek, T.B., Marty, G.D., Alfaro, M.E., Bennett, W.R., Garver, K.A., Haulena, M., Weber 3rd, E.S. and Hedrick, R.P. Systemic iridovirus from three-spine stickleback *Gasterosteus aculeatus* represents a new megalocytivirus species (family Iridoviridae). *Diseases of Aquatic Organisms* 2012;98:41–56.

72. Hall, R.J., Wang, J., Todd, A.K. et al. Evaluation of rapid and simple techniques for the enrichment of viruses prior to metagenomic virus discovery. *Journal of Virological Methods* 2014;195:194–204.

73. Datta, S., Budhauliya, R., Das, B., Chatterjee, S., Vanlalhmuaka, and Veer, V. Next-generation sequencing in clinical virology: Discovery of new viruses. *World Journal of Virology* 2015;4:265–276.

74. Waltzek, T.B., Batts, W.N., Winton, J.R. et al. Genomic Characterization of the first fish bunya-viruses through next generation sequencing. *39th Eastern Fish Health Workshop*, April 28–May 2, 2014, Shepherdstown, West Virgina.

75. Hahn, C.M., Iwanowicz, L.R., Cornman, R.S., Conway, C.M., Winton, J.R. and Blazer, V.S. Characterization of a novel hepadnavirus in the white sucker (*Catostomus commersonii*) from the Great Lakes region of the United States. *Journal of Virology* 2015; 89:11801–11811.

76. Gjessing, M.C., Yutin, N., Tengs, T., et al. Salmon gill poxvirus, the deepest representative of the Chordo-poxvirinae. *Journal of Virology* 2015;89:9348–9367.

77. Lopez-Bueno, A., Mavian, C., Labella, A.M., Castro, D., Borrego, J.J., Alcami, A. and Alejo, A. Concurrence

of iridovirus, polyomavirus and a unique member of a new group of fish papillomaviruses in lymphocystis disease affected gilthead seabream. *Journal of Virology* 2016;90:8768–8779.

78. Stetter, M. Diagnostic imaging and endoscopy. *BSAVA Manual of Ornamental Fish* 2001;8:103.

79. Tyson, R., Love, N.E., Lewbart, G. and Bakal, R. Techniques in advanced imaging of fish. *Proceedings American Association of Zoo Veterinarians* 1999;1999: 201–202.

80. Gumpenberger, M., Hochwartner, O. and Loupal, G. Diagnostic imaging of a renal adenoma in a red oscar (*Astronotus ocellatus* Cuvier, 1829). *Veterinary Radiology & Ultrasound* 2004;45(2):139–142.

81. Love, N.E. and Lewbart, G.A. Pet fish radiography: Technique and case history reports. *Veterinary Radiology & Ultrasound* 1997;38(1):24–29.

82. Beregi, A., Szekely, C.S., Békési, L., Szabó, J., Molnár, V. and Molnár, K. Radiodiagnostic examination of the swimbladder of some fish species. *Acta Veterinaria Hungarica* 2001;49(1):87–98.

83. Smith, S.A. and Smith, B.J. Xeroradiographic and radiographic anatomy of the channel catfish, Ictalurus punctatus. *Veterinary Radiology & Ultrasound* 1994;35(5):384–390.

84. Smith-Vaniz, W.F., Kaufman, L.S. and Glowacki, J. Species-specific patterns of hyperostosis in marine teleost fishes. *Marine Biology* 1995;121(4):573–580.

85. Lewbart, G.A., Stone, E.A. and Love, N.E. Pneumocystectomy in a Midas cichlid. *Journal of the American Veterinary Medical Association* 1995;207(3): 319–321.

86. Macrì, F., Passantino, A., Pugliese, M., DiPietro, S., Zaccone, D., Giorgianni, P., Bonfiglio, R. and Marino, F. Retrograde positive contrast urethrocystography of the fish urogenital system. *The Scientific World Journal* 2014;2014:1–4.

87. Britt, T., Weisse, C., Weber, E.S., Matzkin, Z. and Klide, A. Use of pneumocystoplasty for overinflation of the swim bladder in a goldfish. *Journal of the American Veterinary Medical Association* 2002;221(5):690–3.

88. Wittenberg, J.B. The secretion of inert gas into the swim-bladder of fish. *The Journal of General Physiology* 1958;41(4):783–804.

89. Rummer, J.L. and Bennett, W.A. Physiological effects of swim bladder overexpansion and catastrophic decompression on red snapper. *Transactions of the American Fisheries Society* 2005;134(6): 1457–1470.

90. Brown, I., Sumpton, W., McLennan, M. et al. An improved technique for estimating short-term survival of released line-caught fish, and an application comparing barotrauma-relief methods in red emperor (*Lutjanus sebae* Cuvier 1816). *Journal of Experimental Marine Biology and Ecology* 2010;385(1):1–7.

91. Rogers, B.L., Lowe, C.G., Fernandez-Juricic, E. and Frank, L.R. Utilizing magnetic resonance imaging (MRI) to assess the effects of angling-induced barotrauma on rockfish (Sebastes). *Canadian Journal of Fisheries and Aquatic Sciences* 2008;65(7):1245–1249.

92. Bakal, R.S., Love, N.E., Lewbart, G.A. and Berry, C.R. Imaging a spinal fracture in a kohaku koi (Cyprinus carpio): Techniques and case history report. *Veterinary Radiology & Ultrasound* 1998;39(4):318–321.

93. Barlow, A.M. 'Broken backs' in koi carp (*Cyprinus carpio*) following lightning strike. *Veterinary Record* 1993;133(20):503.

94. Divers, S.J., Boone, S.S., Hoover, J.J., Boysen, K.A., Killgore, K.J., Murphy, C.E., George, S.G. and Camus, A.C. Field endoscopy for identifying gender, reproductive stage and gonadal anomalies in free-ranging sturgeon (Scaphirhynchus) from the lower Mississippi River. *Journal of Applied Ichthyology* 2009;25(s2):68–74.

95. Boone, S.S., Hernandez-Divers, S.J., Radlinsky, M.G., Latimer, K.S. and Shelton, J.L. Comparison between coelioscopy and coeliotomy for liver biopsy in channel catfish. *Journal of the American Veterinary Medical Association* 2008;233(6):960–967.

96. Swenson, E.A., Rosenberger, A.E. and Howell, P.J. Validation of endoscopy for determination of maturity in small salmonids and sex of mature individuals. *Transactions of the American Fisheries Society* 2007;136(4):994–998.

97. Matsche, M.A., Bakal, R.S. and Rosemary, K.M. Use of laparoscopy to determine sex and reproductive status of shortnose sturgeon (*Acipenser brevirostrum*) and Atlantic sturgeon (*Acipenser oxyrinchus oxyrinchus*). *Journal of Applied Ichthyology* 2011;27(2):627–636.

98. Falahatkar, B., Gilani, M.H.T., Falahatkar, S. and Abbasalizadeh, A. Laparoscopy, a minimally-invasive technique for sex identification in cultured great sturgeon *Huso huso*. *Aquaculture* 2011;321(3):273–279.

99. Trested, D.G., Goforth, R., Kirk, J.P. and Isely, J.J. Survival of shovelnose sturgeon after abdominally invasive endoscopic evaluation. *North American Journal of Fisheries Management* 2010;30(1):121–125.

100. Hernandez-Divers, S.J., Bakal, R.S., Hickson, B.H., Rawlings, C.A., Wilson, H.G., Radlinsky, M., Hernandez-Divers, S.M. and Dover, S.R. Endoscopic sex determination and gonadal manipulation in Gulf of Mexico sturgeon (*Acipenser oxyrinchus desotoi*). *Journal of Zoo and Wildlife Medicine* 2004;35(4):459–470.

101. Boylan, S.M., Camus, A., Gaskins, J., Oliverio, J., Parks, M., Davis, A. and Cassel, J. Spondylosis in a green moray eel, *Gymnothorax funebris* (Ranzani 1839), with swim bladder hyperinflation. *Journal of Fish Diseases* 2016. doi: 10.1111/jfd.12563.

102. Stamper, M.A. Immobilization of elasmobranchs. In: *The Elasmobranch Husbandry Manual*. M. Smith, D. Warmolts, D. Thoney and R. Hueter, eds. Ohio Biological Survey, Columbus, OH, 2004; p. 293.

103. Bullard, S.A., Frasca Jr, S. and Benz, G.W. Gill lesions associated with *Erpocotyle tiburonis* (Monogenea: Hexabothriidae) on wild and aquarium-held bonnethead sharks (*Sphyrna tiburo*). *Journal of Parasitology* 2001;87(5):972–977.

CHAPTER 4

OCULAR DISORDERS

STEPHEN A. SMITH

EXOPHTHALMIA

Overview: A nonspecific, unilateral or bilateral condition of the eye, commonly called "pop-eye," in which the globe of the eye extends outside its normal limits.

Etiology: Numerous etiologies have been reported to cause exophthalmia including infectious (e.g., viral: infectious pancreatic necrosis [IPN], infectious hematopoietic necrosis [IHN] or viral hemorrhagic septicemia [VHS]; or bacterial: *Aeromonas* sp., *Flavobacterium* sp., *Vibrio* sp., *Edwardsiella ictaluri*, *Renibacterium salmoninarum* or *Mycobacterium* sp.), parasitic, neoplasia, and noninfectious (e.g., gas supersaturation), or as a sequela to impaired renal function or increased abdominal pressure from the accumulation of fluids in the coelomic cavity (**Figures 4.1** and **4.2**).[1-7] Fluid or gas accumulation in the retrobulbar tissues can also cause protrusion of the eye.[1,6]

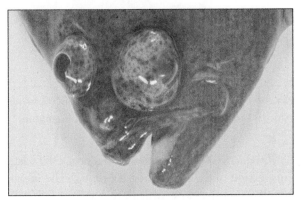

Figure 4.2 Exophthalmia caused by *Mycobacterium* sp. infection associated with the eye of a summer flounder (*Paralichthys dentatus*).

Route of transmission: Depends on specific etiology.

Host range: All freshwater, brackish and marine species are probably susceptible to the various causes of exophthalmia.

Clinical presentation: The globe of the eye expands laterally or circumferentially outside its normal size, or protrusion of the globe outside the normal recesses of the orbit (**Figure 4.3**). The enlarged globe of the eye is predisposed to a variety of infectious diseases or trauma.

Pathology: Anything that expands the posterior segment of the globe (e.g., infectious etiologies, parasites, tumors, increased coelomic pressure) may produce a lateral movement of the globe. Both supersaturation of the water and swim bladder inflammation can cause gas bubbles in the vascular and choroidal gland, resulting in exophthalmos.[6]

Differential diagnosis: This condition should not be confused with telescoping eyes found in a number of goldfish varieties or "bubble eye" goldfish, which have infraorbital lymph-filled sacs of adnexal (i.e., not ocular) origin.

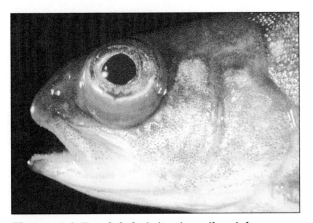

Figure 4.1 Exophthalmia in a juvenile rainbow trout (*Oncorhynchus mykiss*) caused by a systemic bacterial disease.

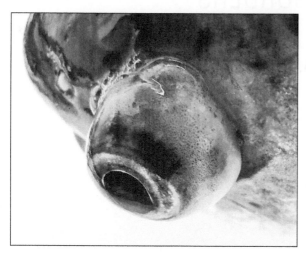

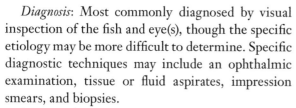

Figure 4.3 Exophthalmia in a rainbow trout (*O. mykiss*) due to supersaturation of gases in the water column.

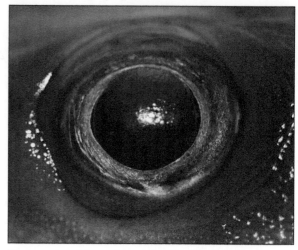

Figure 4.4 Normal eye of cobia (*Rachycentron canadum*).

Diagnosis: Most commonly diagnosed by visual inspection of the fish and eye(s), though the specific etiology may be more difficult to determine. Specific diagnostic techniques may include an ophthalmic examination, tissue or fluid aspirates, impression smears, and biopsies.

Management/control: Depending on the cause of the exophthalmia, this may include correcting environmental conditions (i.e., reducing supersaturated gas concentrations in the water), topical or systemic antibiotics to treat localized ophthalmic or systemic infections, aspiration of excess gases from the globe, or enucleation.

ENOPHTHALMOS

Overview: A condition where the eye decreases in volume and appears retracted or "sunken" into the skull.[8] Though this condition is not specific for any particular infectious disease, enophthalmos may occur with several viral diseases (e.g., koi sleepy disease and koi herpes virus), or bacterial or parasitic (e.g., *Myxobolus* sp.) infections.[1,9] Noninfectious causes may include traumatic injury, social aggression (e.g., "eye snapping"), emaciation and developmental defects. No matter the cause, chronic enophthalmos may result in anophthalmos, where the globe is completely lost and covered by regenerated dermal layers (**Figures 4.4** and **4.5**).[6]

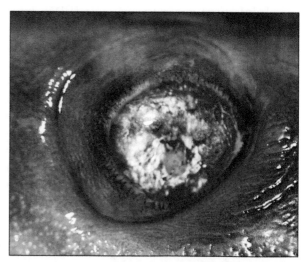

Figure 4.5 Enophthalmos as a result of previous trauma in a cobia (*R. canadum*).

CLOUDY EYE

Overview: A condition where the eye appears to be cloudy or have material in the anterior chamber that makes it appear cloudy.

Etiology: Most commonly the condition is due to a local or systemic infection but may also be due to rapid changes in water quality (i.e., ammonia, nitrites, pH, salinity or osmolality) (**Figure 4.6**). Several protozoan parasites such as *Ichthyophthirius multifiliis*, *Cryptocaryon irritans*, and *Tetrahymena corlissi* have been known to directly infest the epithelium of the cornea, causing

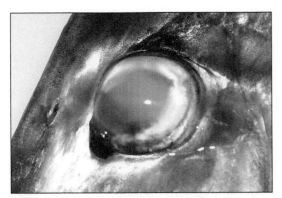

Figure 4.6 Cloudy eye in a lookdown (*Selene vomer*). (Image courtesy of S. Boylan.)

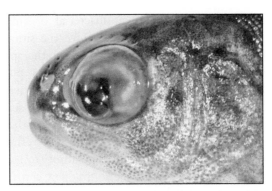

Figure 4.7 Ulcerative keratitis with rupture of the globe in a rainbow trout (*O. mykiss*).

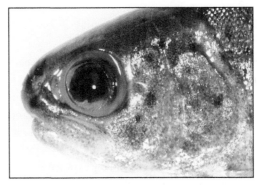

Figure 4.8 Ulcerative keratitis with aphakia in a rainbow trout (*O. mykiss*).

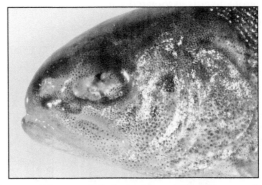

Figure 4.9 Enophthalmos as a result of progressive ulcerative keratitis in a rainbow trout (*O. mykiss*).

it to become cloudy. Occasionally monogeneans (e.g., *Neobenedenia* sp.), turbellarians, and copepods (e.g., *Lernaea* spp. and *Argulus* spp.) may directly parasitize the cornea and surrounding tissues of the eye.[4] Lymphocystis, a generally benign viral disease, has also been reported to affect the cornea and retrobulbar tissues of the eye.[10] Larval digenetic trematodes (e.g., *Austrodiplostomum* spp.) can invade the anterior and posterior chambers of the eye.[11] Dietary deficiencies, such as vitamin A, thiamin or riboflavin, may also contribute to the development of cloudy eye in fish.[6]

Route of transmission: Depends on specific etiology.

Host range: All fish species are presumably susceptible to the various conditions that cause cloudy eye.

Clinical presentation: The condition may be due to corneal edema, corneal opacity or material in the aqueous humor of the eye, all of which may cause the cloudy eye appearance and compromise vision.

Pathology: Both ulcerative keratitis and non-ulcerative keratitis can result in corneal edema and a cloudy appearance to the eye. Superficial abrasions of the eye can rapidly result in corneal ulcerations, which left unchecked can lead to rupture of the globe and subsequent enophthalmos (**Figures 4.7** through **4.9**).[6] Non-ulcerative keratitis can result in edema of the cornea, accumulation of cellular infiltrates and fibroplasia in the anterior chamber, giving the eye a cloudy appearance.[6]

Differential diagnosis: The most common differential would be cataracts. Cloudy eye or corneal edema should not be confused with corneal opacification that commonly occurs postmortem, especially with fish that are chilled.

Diagnosis: Most commonly diagnosed by visual inspection of the eye, though the etiology may be more difficult to identify. The diagnosis should include examination of the water parameters and various systemic diseases.

Management/control: Providing optimal water quality and adequate nutrition is essential. For infectious conditions an antibacterial or antifungal agent may be needed to resolve the situation. Administration of a topical ophthalmic therapeutic for ulcerative keratitis is accomplished by placing the therapeutic on the eye of an out-of-water sedated fish for approximately one minute before placing a layer of n-butyl cyanoacrylate or other ophthalmic adhesive over the ulcerative lesion.[3] In freshwater fish, increasing the environmental salinity to 1–2 ppt (g/L) will reduce the osmotic gradient across the cornea and may help resolve corneal edema. Periodic monitoring for parasitic and bacterial diseases will help reduce the incidence of these etiologies.

UVEITIS

Overview: Uveitis is inflammation of the uvea, which includes the iris, choroidal gland, ciliary body, and associated blood vessels of the eye. As in mammals, anterior uveitis (e.g., anterior chamber and iris) is most commonly diagnosed in fish. This may be caused by a primary infection (i.e., bacterial, viral or fungal) of the eye, the secondary extension of another systemic disease, or a noninfectious (i.e., neoplastic) problem. This condition is often described as a panophthalmitis (**Figure 4.10**). In addition, a granulomatous uveitis associated with vaccination has been reported in Atlantic salmon.[12]

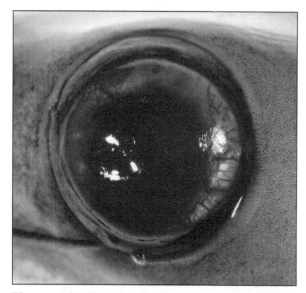

Figure 4.10 Panophthalmitis in a pangasius catfish (*Pangasianodon hypophthalmus*).

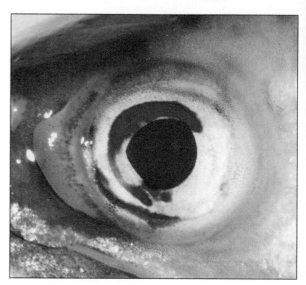

Figure 4.11 Hyphema in the eye of a rainbow trout (*O. mykiss*) infected with enteric redmouth disease (i.e., *Yersinia ruckeri*).

HYPHEMA

Overview: A condition where there is blood in the anterior chamber of the eye. This is usually the result of direct trauma, uveitis, panophthalmitis, or an infectious systemic disease such as with enteric redmouth disease, a bacterial infection of the kidney of salmonids caused by *Yersinia ruckeri*, which often has secondary consequences of hyphema (**Figure 4.11**).

CATARACTS

Overview: A condition of the eye in which the lens becomes cloudy or opaque, resulting in impaired vision or complete blindness.

Etiology: Numerous etiologies have been reported to cause unilateral or bilateral cataracts in both wild and captive fish, including nutritional, infectious, intralenticular parasites, trauma, excess ultraviolet light, changes in water temperature and hereditary factors.[5,13–15] In addition, poor water quality can cause osmotic changes in the lens.[6]

Route of transmission: Depends on the specific etiology.

Host range: All fish species are probably susceptible to cataracts depending on the etiology. Both a nutritional deficiency of vitamin A (hypovitaminosis A) and feeding salmon diets containing a high proportion of animal viscera (e.g., offals) can result in the formation of cataracts (see Chapter 16). A number of freshwater species of fish, such as salmonids and various pan fish (i.e., sunfishes, yellow perch, crappie, croaker, minnows) may serve as the second intermediate (i.e., metacercaria) host for a number of digenetic trematode species (e.g., *Diplostomum* spp.), which have a predisposition to encyst as a metacercarial stage in the lens of the eye.

Clinical presentation: Gradual increasing cloudiness and opacity of the lens of the eye (**Figures 4.12** through **4.14**). Behavioral alterations may include a lack of response to predators or shadows/movement.

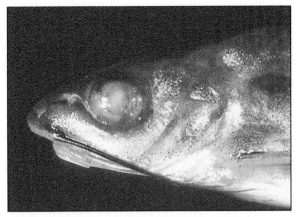

Figure 4.14 Cataracts in a channel catfish (*Ictalurus punctatus*) due to trematode infection of the lens. (Image courtesy of A. Camus.)

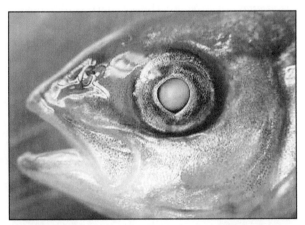

Figure 4.12 Cataracts in the eye of a wild kingfish (*Scomberomorus cavalla*). (Image courtesy of B. Diggles.)

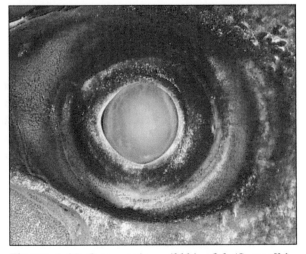

Figure 4.13 Cataracts in a wild kingfish (*S. cavalla*). (Image courtesy of B. Diggles.)

In addition, the fish may lose weight due to the inability to feed or compete for food.

Pathology: The histologic changes seen in cataracts of fish include hydropic swelling of the lens fibers, lysis of fibers, epithelial hyperplasia and intralenticular migration of surface epithelium.[5]

Differential diagnosis: Need to distinguish cataracts from corneal edema or corneal opacity, which cause cloudy eye. Cataracts should also not be confused with lens opacification that normally occurs postmortem.

Diagnosis: Most commonly diagnosed by visual inspection of the eye along with behavior suggesting decreased vision in one or both eyes.

Management/control: Control of cataracts in fish is dependent on the specific etiology with optimal nutrition and diets with adequate vitamin A meeting the nutritional deficiencies, and elimination of the first intermediate host (e.g., snail) of the larval digenetic trematode species preventing the parasitic causes. Several surgical procedures have been used in ornamental or display species to either phacoemulsify and remove the lens from the eye or remove/replace the entire eye for cosmetic reasons.

GAS BUBBLE DISEASE

Overview: A noninfectious condition associated with the supersaturation of dissolved gases, most commonly nitrogen or oxygen, in the water column causing bubbles to form in the eyes and other tissues of the fish.

Etiology: Numerous etiologies are known to cause supersaturation of gases within the water column including leaks in pumps, valves or pipe connections; overaeration of water; sudden extreme temperature gradients; heavy algal blooms; use of spring or well water that has not been sufficiently degassed; and being in close proximity to plunge pools of dams or waterfalls where increased levels of dissolved gases may occur in the water column.[16–18]

Route of transmission: Not applicable.

Host range: The condition has been reported in numerous farmed, aquarium, and wild fish species, though syngnathids (i.e., seahorses and pipefishes) in captivity appear to be more sensitive to increased gas saturation conditions.

Clinical presentation: Clinical signs and mortality vary with species, age, and degree and duration of gas supersaturation. Fish can be affected by acutely or chronically increased levels of gas saturation that manifest in a variety of clinical signs including air bubbles in the anterior chamber of the eye, air emboli in the capillaries of the gills and tissues, and dermal bulla in the skin and fins (**Figures 4.15** through **4.17**).

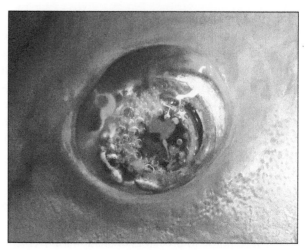

Figure 4.16 Gas supersaturation in red snapper (*Lutjanus campechanus*). (Image courtesy of S. Boylan.)

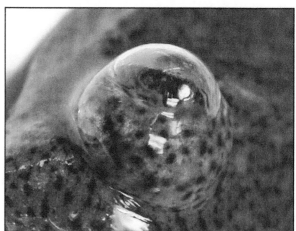

Figure 4.17 Gas supersaturation in a summer flounder (*P. dentatus*) resulting in a large air bubble in the eye. (Image courtesy of S. Boylan.)

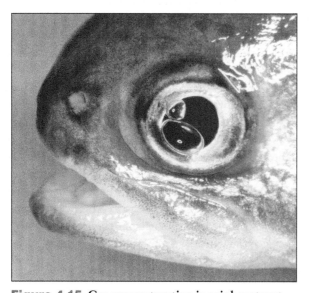

Figure 4.15 Gas supersaturation in rainbow trout (*O. mykiss*) resulting in air bubbles in the anterior chamber of the eye.

Pathology: Retrobulbar gas bubbles can push the globe forward causing exophthalmos, which can result in keratitis, uveitis, panophthalmitis, and cataract formation. Supersaturation of the water can cause emboli to accumulate in the anterior chamber, vasculature, and adnexal structures of the eye.[18]

Differential diagnosis: Though the condition is fairly straightforward to diagnose, the cause can often be difficult to determine.

Diagnosis: Most commonly diagnosed by visual inspection of the eyes, gills and skin for the presence of gas bubbles in the anterior chamber of the globe of the eye (or in the lamellae of the gill or under the epithelium of the skin).

Management/control: Depending on the length of time and the severity of the pathology, the lesions may regress once the cause and/or elevated gas levels are removed. Peribulbar injection of a carbonic anhydrase inhibitor (6 mg/kg acetazolamide) may help resolve gas bubbles within the choroidal gland and anterior chamber.[6] Regular monitoring of water for dissolved gas levels is accomplished with a saturometer that measures differences in total dissolved gas between the atmosphere and water. It must be remembered that even though it might take saturation levels of 104%–110% for overt clinical signs to appear depending on the species involved, levels above 100% even without clinical signs can be chronically stressful to fish.

NEOPLASIA

Overview: Various types of neoplasia have been reported from a number of different species of fish, most commonly in older captive fish.[19,20]

Etiology: Most occur spontaneously, but there are a few reported to be caused by genetic mutations, environmental factors and the *Oncorhynchus mason* virus (i.e., *Herpesvirus salmonis* type 2).[6,21] Some of the eye tumors reported in the literature include melanosarcomas, fibrosarcomas, adenocarcinomas, retinoblastomas, neuronal embryonal tumors, glioneuromas and epitheliomas.[1,6,19–21]

Route of transmission: Not applicable, unless a viral etiology is involved where water or direct contact would be the route of transmission.

Host range: Presumably all fish species are susceptible to neoplasia, though older fish have a higher incidence.

Clinical presentation: Neoplastic conditions of the eye usually present as exophthalmia and/or blindness.

Pathology: Most present as a space-occupying lesion of the various tissues of the eye. As the tumor enlarges, the retrobulbar tissues or globe increase in size, causing exophthalmia.

Differential diagnosis: This condition needs to be differentiated from other causes of exophthalmia including infections, parasites and supersaturation.

Diagnosis: Determination of neoplastic conditions of the eye are primarily diagnosed by enucleation of the globe or at necropsy by histopathology.

Management/control: Control of water quality parameters and avoidance of environmental contaminants. Management of ocular neoplasia in captive fish is either by surgical removal of the tumor or entire eye, or humane euthanasia.

REFERENCES

1. Dukes, T.W. Opthalmic pathology of fishes. In: *The Pathology of Fishes*. W.W. Ribelin and G. Migaki, eds. University of Wisconsin Press, Madison, WI, 1975; pp. 383–398.
2. Hargis, W.J. Disorders of the eye in finfish. *Annual Review Fish Diseases* 1991;1:95–117.
3. Williams, C.R. and Whitaker, B.R. The evaluation and treatment of common ocular disorders in teleosts. *Seminars in Avian and Exotic Pet Medicine* 1997;6(3):160–169.
4. Whitaker, B.R. Ocular disorders. In: *BSAVA Manual of Ornamental Fish*. British Small Animal Veterinary Association, 2001; pp. 147–154.
5. Jurk, I. Ophthalmic disease of fish. *Veterinary clinics Exotic Animal* 2002;5:243–260.
6. Williams, D.L. The fish eye. In: *Ophthalmology of Exotic Pets*. D.L. Williams, ed. Blackwell, Hoboken, NJ, 2012; pp. 211–227.
7. Williams, D.L. and Brancker, W.M. Gross, microscopic and ultrastructural pathology of ocular abnormalities in farmed halibut. *International Journal of Aquaculture and Fishery Sciences* 2018;4(1):1–5.
8. McElwain, A., Ray, C., Su, B., Shang, M., Fobes, M.C., Duncan, P., Thresher, R., Dunham, R.A. and Bullard, S.A. Osteological and histopathological details of unilateral microphthalmia and anophthalmia in juvenile common carp (*Cyprinus carpio*). *Aquaculture* 2013;400–401:135–141.
9. Noor, E.L., Deen, A.I.E. and Zaki, M.S. Eye affection syndrome wild and cultured fish. *Life Science Journal* 2013;10(1):643–650.
10. Dukes, T.W. and Lawler, A.R. The ocular lesions of naturally occurring lymphocystis in fish. *Canadian Journal of Comparative Medicine* 1975;39:406–410.
11. Rosser, T.G., Baumgartner, W.A., Alberson, N.R., Woodyard, E.T., Reichley, S.R., Wise, D.J., Pote, L.M. and Griffin, M.J. *Austrodiplostomum* sp., *Bolbophorus* sp. (Digenea: Diplostomidae), and *Clinostomum* marginatum (Digenea: Clinostomidae) metacercariae in inland silverside *Menidia beryllina* from catfish aquaculture ponds, with notes on the infectivity of *Austrodiplostomum* sp. cercariae in channel catfish *Ictalurus punctatus*. *Parasitology Research* 2016;115:4365–4378.

12. Koppang, E.O., Haugarvoll, E., Hordvik, I., Poppe, T.T. and Bjerkas, I. Granulomatous uveitis associated with vaccination in the Atlantic salmon. *Veterinary Pathology* 2004;41:122–130.

13. Hughes, S.G. Nutritional eye diseases in salmonids: A review. *The Progressive Fish-Culturist* 1985;47: 81–85.

14. Kincaid, H.L. and Calkins, G.T. Rapid classification of nuclear cataracts in lake trout. *The Progressive Fish-Culturist* 1991;53:120–124.

15. Midtlying, P.J., Ahrend, M., Bjerkas, E., Waagbo, R. and Wall, T. Current research on cataracts in fish. *Bulletin of the European Association of Fish Pathologists* 1999;19(6):299–301.

16. Rucker, R.R. Gas-bubble disease in salmonids: A critical review. Technical Paper 58. U.S. Department of the Interior, Fish and Wildlife Service, Washington, DC, 1972.

17. Weitkamp, D.E. and Katz, M. A review of dissolved gas supersaturation literature. *Transactions of the American Fisheries Society* 1980;109:659–702.

18. Smiley, J.E., Okihiro, M.S., Drawbridge, M.A. and Kaufmann, R.S. Pathology of ocular lesions associated with gas supersaturation in white seabass. *Journal of Aquatic Animal Health* 2012;24:1–10.

19. Kagan, R.A., Pinkerton, M.E. and Kinsel, M.J. Neuronal embryonal tumors in fish. *Veterinary Pathology* 2010;47(3):553–559.

20. Mandrioli, L., Sirri, R., Gustinelli, A., Quaglio, F., Sarli, G. and Chiocchetti, R. Ocular glioneuroma with medulloepitheliomatous differentiation in a goldfish (*Carassius auratus*). *Journal of Veterinary Diagnostic Investigation* 2014;26(1):167–172.

21. Kimura, T., Yoshimizu, M. and Tanaka, M. Studies on a new virus (OMV) from oncorhynchus mason-II. *Fish Pathology* 1981;15(3–4):149–153.

CHAPTER 5

SKIN AND FIN DISEASES

PEDRO A. SMITH, DIANE G. ELLIOTT, DAVID W. BRUNO AND
STEPHEN A. SMITH

FURUNCULOSIS

Overview: Furunculosis is caused by an infection with *Aeromonas salmonicida* subspecies *salmonicida*, which can cause a bacterial septicemia in salmonids. The term *furunculosis* stems from the boil-like lesions on the skin and in the musculature of infected fish.[1,2] Even though the disease is named after the raised liquefactive muscle lesions, development of "furuncles" are the exception rather than the rule and generally only occur in older fish suffering from a chronic infection. The distribution is practically worldwide, but absent from salmonid aquaculture in Australia, New Zealand and Chile.

Etiology: Typical *Aeromonas salmonicida* subspecies *salmonicida* is a Gram-negative, nonmotile, facultative, anaerobic rod. An atypical strain of *A. salmonicida* has been isolated from a wide range of cultivated and wild fish species including cyprinids, marine flatfish, and non-salmonids as well as salmonids, inhabiting freshwater, brackish water and marine environments.[3]

Route of transmission: Evidence suggests that fin surfaces were the site of infection for *A. salmonicida* in Atlantic salmon parr that resulted in erosion and lesions.[4] However, skin and fin lesions are not considered a regular feature of seawater epidemics of furunculosis. It was noted that bacterial transmission from fish to fish may start from microcolonies in the gill capillaries of the lamellae with embolic spread and subsequent bacterial colonization of tissues.[5] Transmission may also occur from the release of bacteria from ulcers and transfer from fish to fish by ingestion of *A. salmonicida* and subsequent transfer across the intestinal wall.[6] In addition, the sea louse, *Lepeophtheirus salmonis*, has been shown to experimentally transfer *A. salmonicida* subsp. *salmonicida* via parasitism; however, their role as a mechanical or biological vector has not been determined.[7] *A. salmonicida* can also persist in the immediate surroundings of farms, as its hydrophobic nature supports association with organic waste and fish feed.

Host range: Furunculosis has been recorded in both farmed and wild salmonids including Atlantic salmon (*Salmo salar*), Pacific salmon spp. (*Onchorhynchus gorbuscha*, *O. kisutch*, *O. mykiss*, *O. nerka*, *O. rhodurus*), brown trout (*S. trutta*), Arctic char (*Salvelinus alpinus*), Japanese char (*Salvelinus leucomaenis*), brook trout (*Salvelinus fontinalis*), pollan (*Coregonus pollan*) and lake trout (*Salvelinus namaycush*). In addition, furunculosis has been reported in non-salmonid species such as turbot (*Scophthalmus maximus*), cuckoo wrasse (*Labrus bimaculatus*), goldsinny wrasse (*Ctenolabrus rupestris*), Atlantic cod (*Gadus morhua*) and coalfish (*Polachius virens*).[8–11]

Clinical presentation: Acute and chronic furunculosis can occur and is contingent on water temperature, age of the fish and pathogenicity of the organism. Outbreaks are prompted by stressors including sudden changes in water temperature, handling, crowding and poor water quality. Occurrences of acute furunculosis result in rapid fish death with few or no prior signs of disease, and hence pathological changes are infrequent. For chronic infections the fish show lethargy, inappetence, pale gills and darkening of the skin, although such clinical signs are also reported for other bacterial septicemias. Ventral hemorrhage may be seen near the base of the pectoral, pelvic and anal fins in addition to exophthalmia. Liquefactive, hemorrhagic "boil" lesions occur in the superficial muscle, and raised, fluctuating lesions that may rupture can be seen on the skin surface (**Figure 5.1**). Although such furuncles are characteristic, they are not always present in diseased fish and are not regarded as a diagnostic characteristic.[5] Gross pathology includes ascites, splenomegaly,

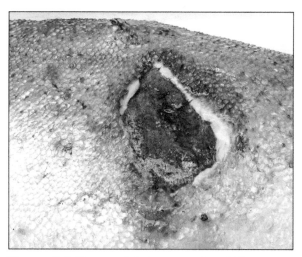

Figure 5.1 Ruptured *Aeromonas salmonicida* furuncle on flank of Atlantic salmon (*Salmo salar*).

subcapsular hemorrhage involving the liver and pyloric ceca. The intestine is devoid of food and often contains exudates of blood, mucus and cellular debris. A carrier state may become established in surviving fish after an infection.

Differential diagnosis: Tissue sections stained with hematoxylin and eosin highlight colonies of bacteria in the heart, kidney, muscle, pancreas and spleen. Motile *Aeromonas* species (e.g., *A. hydrophila*) have been implicated as the causative agents of various fish septicaemias.[12] Other bacterial infections should also be considered as part of a differential diagnosis including those attributed to *Vibrio* spp. infections.

Diagnosis: Sophisticated techniques are available including molecular methods, but primary isolation of the pathogen and hence confirmation are readily achieved from the kidney and other organs using media such as tryptic soy agar (TSA) or brain heart infusion agar (BHIA) incubated at 22°C.[2,13] Most strains of *A. salmonicida* are nonmotile, aerobic, and oxidase-positive and produce a distinct water-soluble brown pigment on media containing tryptone. Diagnosis is based upon gross and histopathological lesions and isolation of the causative agent.

Management/control: The development of oil-based adjuvant vaccines has helped to control furunculosis in farmed salmon with intraperitoneal (IP) immunization providing excellent protection.[14] Currently furunculosis is not considered a major problem in wild or farmed salmon in Norway or the United Kingdom, however in other countries such as Denmark sea-reared rainbow trout can develop furunculosis during the summer.[15] Successful antibiotic treatments may be challenging given the existence of multi-drug resistant isolates or genomic plasticity of the pAsa4 plasmid.[16,17] The use of probiotics to control or limit infection *by A. salmonicida* has shown inconsistent results.[18,19]

AEROMONAS

Overview: An opportunistic bacterial skin and fin disease of all freshwater and occasionally marine fishes.

Etiological agent: The disease, a condition often called "motile aeromonad septicemia," is caused by motile aeromonads of the *Aeromonas hydrophila* complex: *A. hydrophila, A. sobria* and *A. veronii*.[20–22]

Route of transmission: The bacteria is universally distributed in freshwater and sediments, as well as the intestinal tract of fish.[21] The pathogen is readily transmitted horizontally through the water and by direct contact.

Host range: Wild and cultured freshwater fish worldwide are susceptible to *Aeromonas hydrophila* infection, with cultured fish being particularly vulnerable.[21] In addition, *A. hydrophila* has caused disease in amphibians, reptiles, cattle and humans throughout the world.[22,23]

Clinical presentation: The most recognizable clinical signs of disease are hemorrhagic fin and tail erosions, cutaneous hemorrhage and skin ulcerations.

Pathology of disease: A number of virulence factors have been shown to be involved with the pathogenicity of the organism.[24] Acute infections may result in a generalized septicemia with few clinical signs or the fish may exhibit non-specific signs of erythema of the skin, exophthalmia and accumulation of coelomic fluid.[20] Skin infections result in dermal ulceration with focal hemorrhage and inflammation with the underlying musculature eventually becoming necrotic (**Figures 5.2** and **5.3**).[20,25]

Differential diagnosis: Skin and fin lesions caused by other infectious agents such as bacteria (e.g., *A. salmonicida, Flavobacterium columnaris, Renibacterium salmoninarum, Edwardsiella* spp., *Mycobacterium* spp., *Pseudomonas* spp., *Vibrio* spp.) and protozoan

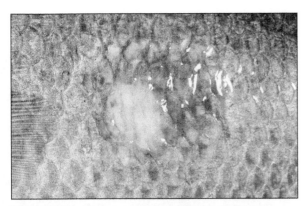

Figure 5.2 *Aeromonas hydrophila* **skin lesion on redbreast sunfish (*Lepomis auritus*).**

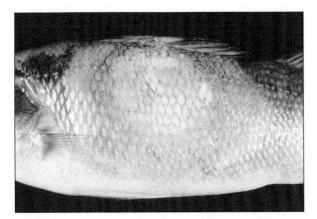

Figure 5.3 *Aeromonas hydrophila* **infection in a cultured yellow perch (*Perca flavescens*).**

ectoparasites must be differentiated from *A. hydrophila* infections. As an opportunistic pathogen, *A. hydrophila* may also exist as a co-infection with other pathogens.

Diagnosis: The motile, Gram-negative bacilli can be isolated on a number of bacteriologic media and can be identified by standard biochemical tests, direct or indirect fluorescent antibody techniques, ELISA, or polymerase chain reaction (PCR) assay.[20-22]

Management/control: As *A. hydrophila* is a ubiquitous organism in both the fish and environment, control is primarily focused on good management practices of reducing stress in the fish by supplying optimal water quality, avoiding overcrowding, proper handling, providing good nutrition, and preventing parasitic or fungal infections. The use of antibiotics, various chemicals and vaccinations have been used with limited success.

EDWARDSIELLOSIS

Overview: Several species of *Edwardsiella*, in addition to *E. ictaluri*, are pathogenic to finfish. Agents of edwardsiellosis previously classified as *E. tarda* affect a wide range of fish taxa including teleosts as well as elasmobranchs in tropical and temperate freshwater and marine environments worldwide.[26,27]

Etiology: *Edwardsiella tarda*, *E. piscicida* and *E. anguillarum* are Gram-negative, motile, short rod bacteria. Following the establishment of the genus *Edwardsiella* in the family Enterobacteriaceae, fish pathogenic *Edwardsiella* other than *E. ictaluri* were considered to be representatives of the species *E. tarda*. Based on recent studies showing phenotypic/ genetic differences and differences in pathology between *E. tarda* isolates from fish and those from humans (including the type strain), it has been proposed that most fish isolates historically classified as *E. tarda* be reclassified into two new taxa: *E. piscicida* and *E. anguillarum*.[28-30] Pathogenicity of these *Edwardsiella* species depends in part on the fish species exposed. For example, *E. piscicida* is more virulent to channel catfish and is involved in more mortality events in this species than is *E. tarda*, whereas *E. anguillarum* is nonpathogenic to channel catfish.[31,33] In comparison, both *E. anguillarum* and *E. piscicida* are pathogenic for eels (*Anguilla* spp.).[28,29]

Route of transmission: Bacteria historically identified as *E. tarda* commonly reside in the intestine of fish and other aquatic animals, can survive for prolonged periods in freshwater and seawater as well as sediment and fouling material on nets, and thrive in organically rich environments.[26] These bacteria are transmitted horizontally from infected animal feces or contaminated mud or water, and likely infect fish by entry through the gills, body surface or gastrointestinal tract. Transmission may be enhanced at water temperatures between 20°C and 30°C.[26] Other factors including integumental injury or coinfection with certain viruses (e.g., aquabirnavirus), bacteria (e.g., *Vibrio harveyi* or *Aeromonas hydrophila*), or ciliated protists (e.g., *Trichodina* sp.) may also augment transmission.[26]

Host range: Edwardsiellosis of fish commonly occurs in warm water species; however, it also has been reported in cold water fishes such as salmonids, turbot (*Scophthalmus maximus*), European eel (*Anguilla anguilla*) and whitefish (*Coregonus lavaretus*).[26,27] Edwardsiellosis is mainly a disease of cultured fish and outbreaks can result in significant mortality.[26] The impact of edwardsiellosis in wild fish is largely unknown, but epizootics have been reported in species such as striped bass (*Morone saxatilis*) and largemouth bass (*Micropterus salmoides*).[34,35]

Clinical presentation: Edwardsiellosis is commonly described as a systemic disease, but mild infections in channel catfish (*Ictalurus punctatus*) have been reported to manifest as small cutaneous lesions located on the posterior-lateral surfaces of the body. External lesions including petechial hemorrhages and ulcers may also occur on the mouth, isthmus, operculum and abdomen. As the disease progresses in channel catfish and certain other fish, deep ulcers and abscesses develop within the skeletal musculature (**Figures 5.4** and **5.5**). The abscesses are often visible from the fish surface as convex, depigmented swollen areas and are filled with malodourous gas and necrotic tissue remnants. External clinical signs observed in various species include exophthalmos and swelling around the eyes, eye opacity, ecchymosis and congestion of the skin and bases of the fins, increased mucus production, fin erosion, abdominal swelling associated with ascites, and swelling and hemorrhage around the vent with occasional rectal prolapse (**Figure 5.6**). In some fish species, reddening of the head associated with subcutaneous hemorrhages has given rise to the name "red-head disease." Fish with edwardsiellosis may also show

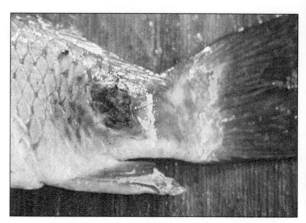

Figure 5.5 Ulcer on caudal peduncle associated with edwardsiellosis in a common carp (*Cyprinus carpio*). (Image courtesy of A. Goodwin, with permission from the collection of J. Plumb.)

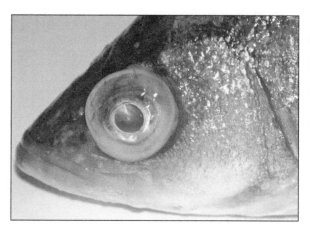

Figure 5.6 Exophthalmos and partial eye opacity associated with edwardsiellosis in a largemouth bass (*Micropterus salmoides*). (Image courtesy of A. Goodwin.)

loss of equilibrium and either lie on their sides at the bottom of a tank, or float on the surface due to swim bladder hyperinflation.

Differential diagnosis: Skin lesions caused by other bacterial pathogens such as *Aeromonas hydrophila*, *Pseudomonas anguilliseptica*, *Vibrio anguillarum* and *Mycobacterium* spp. may appear similar to those caused by edwardsiellosis.

Diagnosis: Identification of the causative bacterium is usually accomplished by isolation on standard media such as brain-heart infusion agar (BHIA) or tryptic soy agar (TSA) at 26°C–30°C for 24–48 h

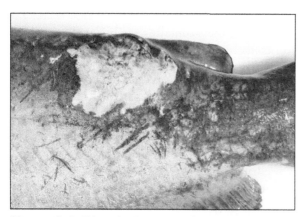

Figure 5.4 *Edwardsiella tarda* infection in a channel catfish (*Ictalurus punctatus*).

with inoculum from internal organs or muscle lesions of infected fish. Isolation success may be improved by a two-step enrichment procedure, with initial inoculation of thioglycollate broth followed by subculture on BHIA.[36] A selective and differential medium, *Edwardsiella tarda* (ET) media enables recovery of the agent of piscine edwardsiellosis from mixed cultures.[37,38] Colonies of piscine *Edwardsiella* phenotypically identified as *E. tarda* show black centers indicative of H_2S production after 24–48 h incubation on ET medium for 24–48 h.

Presumptive diagnosis is based on demonstration that a bacterial isolate is cytochrome oxidase-negative and ferments glucose with both acid and gas production. The triple sugar iron (TSI) reaction is alkaline (slant) and acid (butt), with gas and H_2S production. Most isolates of *E. tarda*, *E. piscicida* and *E. anguillarum* are motile, although some *E. anguillarum* isolates are reported to be non-motile. Assays such as fluorescent antibody tests (FATs) and slide agglutination procedures can be used to rapidly discriminate the causative agents of *Edwardsiella septicemia* from *Edwardsiella ictaluri*. However, because no phenotypic trait has been identified that reliably distinguishes among the species *E. tarda*, *E. piscicida* and *E. anguillarum*, genomic characterization is necessary to specifically identify isolates cultured from fish. Real-time quantitative polymerase chain reaction (qPCR) assays have been developed for each of these *Edwardsiella* species for rapid identification, differentiation and confirmation of isolates from fish tissues or pond water.[32]

Management/control: Edwardsiellosis is commonly treated by oral administration of antibiotics.[26] Nevertheless, antibiotic resistance has been demonstrated in *Edwardsiella* strains isolated from aquaculture facilities, particularly in Southeast Asia.[26] Experimental vaccine formulations have shown promise for prevention of edwardsiellosis but none are commercially licensed.[26,27,39] Other strategies such as administration of immunostimulants or other dietary supplements have also been suggested for increasing resistance of cultured fish to edwardsiellosis.[26] The agents of *Edwardsiella* septicemia are not obligate pathogens and may be widely distributed in the environment and in aquatic animals, so the prevention of entry into or elimination from aquaculture facilities are not considered to be reasonable management options for most facilities. Strict sanitation, provision of optimal water quality and reduction of organic material in aquaculture facilities are recommended to reduce the probability of outbreaks of edwardsiellosis.[26]

ENTERIC SEPTICEMIA OF CATFISH

Overview: Enteric septicemia of catfish (ESC), also known as enteric septicemia or "hole-in-the-head" disease, is one of the most economically significant diseases in the channel catfish aquaculture industry in the United States.[40] Enteric septicemia of catfish is also becoming an increasingly important disease in the cultured catfish industry in Southeast Asia. In addition, ESC has been reported from fishes in Australia, and from diseased and apparently healthy fishes in Europe and the Caribbean.[41-44] The bacterium has narrower host and geographic ranges than the closely related bacterial species historically classified as *E. tarda*.

Etiology: *Edwardsiella ictaluri* is the etiological agent of ESC and is a Gram-negative short rod belonging to the Enterobacteriaceae family. Although *E. ictaluri* is strictly considered a fish microbe, identification of viable bacteria of this species from rectal swabs of fish-eating birds in the United States has raised the possibility that they could serve as vectors.[45]

Route of transmission: Horizontal transmission of *E. ictaluri* from infected fish occurs primarily through the water or via cannibalization of infected fish. Principal routes of entry into catfish include the nares and gastrointestinal tract, and through the gills or abraded skin.[40] The bacterium that enters through the nares may migrate into the olfactory nerve and then into the brain meninges followed by migration into the skull and skin, resulting in the characteristic hole-in-the-head lesion.[46] Fish that survive ESC outbreaks may become long-term carriers.[26] Transmission of the pathogen from spawning adults to progeny has been postulated, but evidence is lacking.[26,27] Infected fish, including clinically diseased or dead fish as well as asymptomatic carriers, are regarded as the primary reservoirs for *E. ictaluri*. Although initial research suggested *E. ictaluri* is an obligate fish pathogen, more recent molecular evidence suggests that the bacterium can persist within the pond environment or disease vectors.[27] Acute outbreaks of ESC in channel catfish are common from late spring to early summer and in autumn when water temperatures are between 18°C and 28°C, but low-level mortality may occur outside this range.[26] Poor water quality, high fish-rearing density, poor nutrition, the presence of other pathogens or parasites, and inadequate sanitation may exacerbate disease.[26]

Host range: *Edwardsiella ictaluri* was first isolated from diseased channel catfish (*Ictalurus punctatus*) in the United States, and infections were originally believed to be restricted to catfish species in the family Ictaluridae.[47] However, natural infections have since been reported in other catfish families including Ariidae, Bagridae, Clariidae, Pangasiidae, Plotosidae and Siluridae, and in non-catfish families including Anguillidae, Cichlidae, Cyprinidae, Moronidae, Plecoglossidae, Salmonidae and Sternopygidae.[26,27,41,48] Infections are most frequent in cultured fish, including food fish, ornamental species, and zebrafish maintained for research (*Danio rerio*). Nevertheless, some isolations of the bacterium have been reported from symptomatic or asymptomatic wild fish such as diseased ayu (*Plecoglossus altivelis*) in Japan, symptomatic tadpole madtom (*Noturus gyrinus*) in the United States, and asymptomatic tandan catfish (*Tandanus tropicanus*) in Australia.[41,49,50] Nearly all isolations of *E. ictaluri* have been made from freshwater fish, but a bacterium characterized as similar to *E. ictaluri* on the basis of biochemical reactions was cultured from diseased sea bass (*Dicentrarchus labrax*) from a marine aquaculture facility in Spain.[42]

Clinical presentation: Disease caused by *Edwardsiella ictaluri* in susceptible species is usually described as an acute septicemia, although infection associated with hole-in-the-head lesions may represent a more chronic, localized encephalitis.[26] External signs of ESC in channel catfish can include hemorrhages (petechiae or ecchymoses) around the mouth and isthmus, on lateral and ventral areas of the body, and at the bases of the fins (**Figure 5.7**). The characteristic hole-in-the-head lesion may initially appear as a swelling on the dorsum of the head (i.e., between or posterior to the eyes) and develops into ulceration

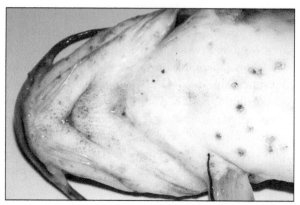

Figure 5.7 Hemorrhagic lesions on the ventral jaw surface (i.e., "chin rash") of a channel catfish (*Ictalurus punctatus*) infected with *Edwardsiella ictaluri*. (Image courtesy of A. Goodwin.)

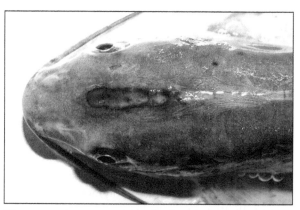

Figure 5.8 Channel catfish (*Ictalurus punctatus*) infected with *Edwardsiella ictaluri* showing characteristic "hole-in-the-head" lesion overlying the frontal bones of the skull. (Image courtesy of A. Goodwin.)

of the fontanelle of the frontal bones of the skull, exposing the brain (**Figure 5.8**). Other external signs of ESC can include exophthalmos, pale gills and abdominal swelling associated with ascites. Small, raised hemorrhagic skin lesions that progress to depigmented or red shallow ulcers can also occur (**Figure 5.9**). Behavioral signs can include sudden decrease in feeding, listlessness, hanging at the water surface in a "head-up, tail-down" posture, and rapid swimming in circles or spirals with erratic swimming bursts. External signs of disease may be absent in channel catfish longer than 15 cm. Catfish overwintering with *E. ictaluri* may exhibit small white

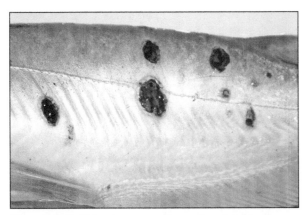

Figure 5.9 Skin ulcers on a channel catfish (*Ictalurus punctatus*) infected with *Edwardsiella ictaluri*. (Image courtesy of A. Goodwin.)

skin ulcerations that are believed to represent healing lesions in disease survivors. Observations of noncatfish species infected with *E. ictaluri* often describe external signs such as hemorrhages, exophthalmos and ascites common to many bacterial septicemias.

Differential diagnosis: In young channel catfish, clinical signs associated with ESC can be similar to those caused by channel catfish virus disease (CCVD). Disease caused by *E. ictaluri* is differentiated from other *Edwardsiella* spp. on the basis of clinical signs; isolation of the bacterium in culture; and identification by biochemical, immunological or molecular testing.

Diagnosis: Diagnosis of *E. ictaluri* infection is usually based on observation of characteristic clinical signs and identification of the causative agent. Primary isolation of *E. ictaluri* is made by inoculating material from the anterior kidney or head lesion/brain onto trypticase soy agar (TSA), McConkey agar, blood agar, or *Edwardsiella* isolation medium (EIM), which is incubated for 2–4 days at 30°C–35°C.[51] The causative agent is a short Gramnegative, cytochrome oxidase-negative rod that produces no indole in tryptone broth. Bacterial colonies appear after 24–48 h incubation at 25°C and growth is sparse at 37°C. The bacterium is nonmotile or weakly motile and does not produce H_2S. Assays such as slide agglutination, microtiter agglutination, and fluorescent antibody tests and enzyme immunoassays (EIAs) are used for confirmatory diagnosis. Both conventional PCR and real-time qPCR assays

have been developed for confirmation of *E. ictaluri* infections in fish.[52,53]

Management/control: Oral antibiotic chemotherapy has been used to control disease caused by *E. ictaluri*, but plasmid-mediated resistance to these antibiotics has been reported.[27] Optimization of husbandry practices is important for reducing impacts of *E. ictaluri* infections. Recommendations include minimization of stressors, prevention of overcrowding, maintenance of high water quality, adherence to strict sanitation, prompt removal of dead fish and provision of high quality diets while avoiding overfeeding.[26,27] Some dietary supplements and immunostimulants have been reported to have beneficial effects in enhancing resistance of channel catfish to ESC.[26]

An attenuated live *E. ictaluri* vaccine (AQUAVAC-ESC®, Merck) commercially licensed in the United States for prevention of ESC in channel catfish is the only licensed ESC vaccine.[40] To conform to industry practices, the vaccine is delivered by immersion to catfish at 7–10 days of age post-hatch when the fish are transported from the hatchery to nursery ponds. However, vaccine efficacy may be limited by delivery to fry when the immune system is not fully functional. An experimental strategy for vaccination of catfish via a single oral dose of live attenuated *E. ictaluri* vaccine mixed with feed has shown promise for improving protection of channel catfish against ESC at the fingerling stage when the immune system is fully developed, but an oral ESC vaccine has not yet been licensed.[54]

PISCIRICKETTSIOSIS

Overview: This is an acute, subacute or chronic systemic bacterial disease affecting a variety of teleost species farmed in brackish and seawater in different locations of the world. The disease is endemic in salmonids cultured along the shores of southern Chile.

Etiology: Piscirickettsiosis is caused by *Piscirickettsia salmonis*, a Gram-negative, non-motile, pleomorphic, facultative intracellular bacterium that multiplies in macrophages and several other cell types of the host.[55]

Route of transmission: This pathogen is shed by infected fish and transmitted to other fish hosts through the water or by direct contact. Survival time of *P. salmonis* in freshwater is short, and transmission through the water in that environment is limited. The role of vertical transmission has not been fully elucidated. It has been reported that salmonid ova can carry the bacterium; however, piscirickettsiosis prevalence in young fish (i.e., fry, parr and pre-smolt stages) is absent or negligible.

Host range: Salmonid fishes are the typical hosts including coho salmon (*Oncorhynchus kisutch*), rainbow trout (*O. mykiss*), Atlantic salmon (*Salmo salar*), Chinook salmon (*O. tshawytscha*) and masou salmon (*O. masou*). Sporadically, *P. salmonis* has caused disease in farmed European seabass (*Dicentrarchus labrax*) from various areas of the Mediterranean Sea and in hatchery-reared white seabass (*Atractoscion nobilis*) from southern California. In addition, *P. salmonis* has caused mortalities in experimentally infected zebrafish (*Danio rerio*) and has been detected in seawater-cultured lumpfish (*Cyclopterus lumpus*) having a clinical disease similar to piscirickettsiosis in salmonids.

Clinical presentation: Clinical signs are nonspecific, and include lethargy, anorexia, skin darkening in the dorsal area of the fish, respiratory distress, coelomic swelling and abnormal swimming. Skin abnormalities are not always present, but in some cases are the only gross lesions shown by fish infected with piscirickettsiosis. Areas with raised scales are usually observed, as well as small nodules that progress to shallow ulcerations (**Figure 5.10**).[56] Petechial and ecchymotic zones of the skin can

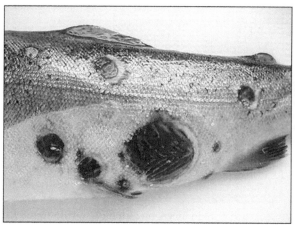

Figure 5.11 Coho salmon (*Oncorhynchus kisutch*) with piscirickettsiosis exhibiting several large, deep ulcers. (Image courtesy of P. Bustos.)

occur either accompanying the lesions already mentioned or by themselves. In some field outbreaks, diseased fish show skin ulcers that are extensive and deep (**Figure 5.11**). It has been experimentally demonstrated that *P. salmonis* can enter through the skin in salmonid fish. Skin sites exposed to *P. salmonis* show progressive bacterial penetration, inflammation and necrosis.[57,58] Integument lesions in nonsalmonid species affected with piscirickettsiosis are rare, and when they occur are usually mild. The septicemic infection causes anemia, reflected by gill paleness and dyspnea, and ascites. Vascular and perivascular necrosis is common, and the internal organs can be eventually affected showing inflammation, hemorrhage, degeneration and necrosis.[55,56] Internal lesions are nonspecific, but some fish may show mottled livers with white to yellowish, circular foci that appear solid or as ring-shaped formations that are indicative of the presence of this disease.[56]

Differential diagnosis: A variety of septicemic infections of fish can share some clinical and/or pathological features with piscirickettsiosis, but due to its closer similarity, francisellosis is probably the most important disease to be considered in a differential diagnosis. Other infectious diseases (e.g., bacterial, parasitic or mycotic) can cause granulomas or nodular abscesses in the liver and require investigation to differentiate these from piscirickettsiosis.

Diagnosis: Diagnosis is based on the identification of the bacteria in fish having clinical and

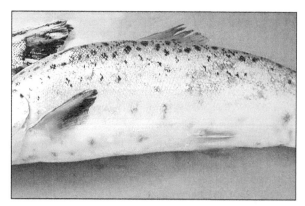

Figure 5.10 Atlantic salmon (*Salmo salar*) with piscirickettsiosis showing raised scales and hemorrhagic shallow ulcerative lesions. (Image courtesy of P. Bustos.)

pathological manifestations of the disease. A presumptive diagnosis is obtained by the observation of organisms morphologically and tinctorially compatible with *P. salmonis* in tissue smears or imprints stained with Gram, Giemsa, Giménez, Pinkerton's method or toluidine blue. Histopathology is helpful to support the diagnosis. Bacterial isolation provides a definitive diagnosis, but this may be difficult as it requires the use of enriched axenic media or fish cell cultures. Identification of the bacterium is carried out using specific antibodies with immunological methods such as immunofluorescence, or more currently, with a variety of PCR tests.[56]

Management/control: Good husbandry practices, which include the use of an optimal aquatic environment (i.e., water quality and quantity), the proper fish biomass and measures to minimize fish stress, are important to decrease the risk of outbreaks of piscirickettsiosis and/or their severity. Biosecurity measures such as the implementation of disinfection procedures, sanitary barriers, frequent mortality removal, appropriate fallowing periods and procedures to avoid moving infected fish are recommended to prevent or control the disease. Epidemiological analyses have shown that greater distances between sea sites lessen the dissemination risk between infected and noninfected fish. Several vaccines are available that have been used extensively in the Chilean salmonid culture, but their efficacy under field conditions has not been optimal. Antibiotics are also frequently used to treat the disease, but consequentially bacterial resistance has been reported.

VIBRIOSIS

Overview: Diseases caused by *Vibrio* spp. affect a wide range of wild and farmed fish species around the world, and occur mostly in marine and brackish water environments, although disease has also been reported in freshwater environments.[59,60] Most outbreaks are associated with relatively warm water temperatures (>15°C), and therefore occur mainly in the summer in temperate climates.[60,61] However, cold-water vibriosis and winter ulcer caused by *Aliivibrio* (~*Vibrio*) *salmonicida* and *Moritella viscosa* (~*Vibrio viscosus*), respectively, rarely occur above 10°C–11°C.[60]

Etiology: Several *Vibrio* species and closely related bacteria cause finfish diseases. The etiologic agents of "classical" vibriosis are *Vibrio* (*Listonella*) *anguillarum* and *V. ordalii*.

Route of transmission: Fish pathogenic vibrios are horizontally transmitted and under appropriate conditions rapidly invade host tissues. *Aliivibrio* (~*Vibrio*) *salmonicida* can be detected in the bloodstream of immersion-challenged fish in as few as 2 h after exposure and can colonize the intestine creating a carrier state.[62] *Vibrio anguillarum* can enter the fish host following oral uptake of contaminated feed or water, and can also enter through the skin, particularly in areas of injury.[61] The bacterium may colonize the skin and posterior intestine with subsequent tissue invasion. It has been suggested that the gill is a portal of entry for *Moritella viscosa* (~*Vibrio viscosus*).[63]

Host range: *Vibrio anguillarum* affects more than 50 diverse saltwater and freshwater fish species worldwide.[61] *Vibrio ordalii* has been recorded primarily in salmonid species in the Pacific Northwest of the United States and Canada, Japan, Australia, New Zealand and Chile, although it has been recorded in non-salmonids such as ayu (*Plecoglossus altivelis*) and rockfish (*Sebastes schlegeli*) in Japan and gilthead seabream in Turkey.[64–67] *Aliivibrio* (~*Vibrio*) *salmonicida* is the causative agent of cold-water vibriosis (i.e., Hitra disease), which principally affects Atlantic salmon (*Salmo salar*), with occasional cases reported in rainbow trout (*Oncorhynchus mykiss*) and Atlantic cod (*Gadus morhua*).[60] Cold-water vibriosis has been described in Norway, Scotland, Iceland, the Faroe Islands, the United States and Canada.[59,60] Winter ulcer mainly affects sea-farmed Atlantic salmon and, to a lesser extent, sea-farmed rainbow trout, with outbreaks restricted to Norway and Iceland.[60] Among other *Vibrio* species that have been most frequently reported as finfish pathogens are *V. harveyi*, which infects a diverse variety of marine species; *V. alginolyticus*, which affects diverse species in warmer waters; *V. splendidus*, which has been implicated in mortality of a variety of marine fish species in Europe and New Zealand; and *V. vulnificus*, which most commonly causes disease in farmed European eels (*Anguilla anguilla*).[60,68] As with *V. anguillarum*, these *Vibrio* spp. are ubiquitous members of the marine microbiota, with a few strains considered as fish pathogens.[60] Among these species, only *V. vulnificus* causes human disease, but the biotypes causing human illness are generally different from those causing fish disease.[59] In addition to the species mentioned, other *Vibrio* spp. and related bacteria have been implicated in isolated disease outbreaks in finfish.[60]

Clinical presentation: *Vibrio* spp. generally cause disseminated systemic infections.[60] External macroscopic signs are considered nonspecific and may include lethargy and weight loss, dark swollen skin lesions that may develop into bleeding ulcers and abscesses, hemorrhages at the bases or other areas of the fins and on the body (especially on lateral and ventral surfaces, at the vent, and around and in the mouth), hemorrhages of the gills, eye opacity, ulceration and exophthalmos, and abdominal distension associated with ascites (**Figures 5.12** through **5.14**). Winter ulcer initially presents as small, raised skin lesions that progress to rounded or oval ulcers that expose underlying muscle, and are characterized by a white demarcation zone separating the lesion from normal tissue.[63] Fish affected by winter ulcer may exhibit lesions for long periods of time and may recover with increasing water temperature.

Differential diagnosis: Skin and fin lesions associated with bacteremia and viremia caused by pathogens such as *Aeromonas salmonicida* and other *Aeromonas* spp. and viral hemorrhagic septicemia virus (VHSV) should be excluded. For suspected cases of winter

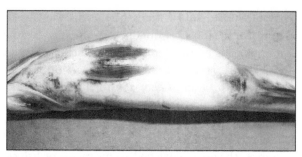

Figure 5.13 Hemorrhagic lesions on the ventral surface and vent of European seabass (*Dicentrarchus labrax*) infected with *Vibrio* (*Listonella*) *anguillarum* serotype O1. (Image courtesy of A. Manfrin.)

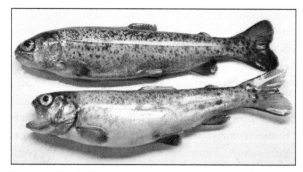

Figure 5.14 Hemorrhages on the head and fin bases of a rainbow trout (*Oncorhynchus mykiss*) infected with *Vibrio anguillarum* (lower) compared to uninfected fish (upper). (Image courtesy of D. Powell.)

ulcer, lesions caused by atypical *Aeromonas salmonicida* infection should also be excluded.

Diagnosis: Preliminary diagnosis of vibriosis is made by detection of curved, motile, Gram-negative rods in the kidney, spleen or blood samples from marine, estuarine or anadromous fish. Culture at 15°C–25°C on standard media such as brain-heart infusion agar (BHIA), tryptic soy agar (TSA) or thiosulfate-citrate-bile salts-sucrose (TCBS) agar may require addition of 0.5%–3.5% NaCl for growth of vibrios.[59,65,68] Most vibrios can be cultured on marine 2216E agar (Difco) after incubation for 2–7 days.[59,63] Confirmatory diagnosis is often made via biochemical or serological testing, and molecular tests have also been developed for identification of some specific agents of vibriosis.[61,65,68,69]

Management/control: Antibiotics have been used to treat outbreaks of vibriosis, but development of

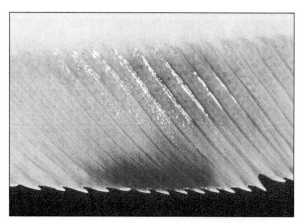

Figure 5.12 Hemorrhage on ventral surface of fin due to vibriosis in a southern flounder (*Paralichthys lethostigma*).

antibiotic resistance of *Vibrio* spp. in aquaculture has been reported.[59,65,70] Commercial vaccines developed for protection against some of the most common agents of vibriosis are mostly inactivated whole-cell preparations delivered by immersion or intraperitoneal (IP) injection, and are often included in multivalent vaccine formulations.[60] Vaccination against *V. anguillarum*, *V. ordalii* and *Aliivibrio* (~*Vibrio*) *salmonicida* has been reported to result in high levels of protection, particularly for fish vaccinated by IP injection, whereas levels of protection are generally lower for fish vaccinated against *Moritella viscosa*. Stressors such as poor water quality or fish handling may contribute to induction of disease, thus improvements in fish husbandry to decrease stress have also been used to reduce impacts of vibriosis in cultured fish populations.

FLAVOBACTERIOSIS

Flavobacteriosis refers to several fish diseases caused by different bacterial species belonging to the genus *Flavobacterium* (formerly *Flexibacter*). This genus consists of Gram-negative, long, slender, non-esporulated microorganisms that have yellow-orange endopigments and display a slow gliding motility on a solid surface. The two most conspicuous species in terms of their global importance as pathogens affecting the skin and fins of fish are *Flavobacterium psychrophilum* and *Flavobacterium columnare*, formerly named *Flexibacter psychrophilus* and *Flexibacter columnaris*, respectively. Both species are ubiquitous freshwater organisms affecting a wide variety of fish species in the wild and in captivity, both in aquaculture and aquariums. Depending on the bacterial species and other factors, flavobacteriosis can affect fish externally, systemically or both. In the former presentation, these bacteria cause disturbances mainly in skin, fins and gills, while in the latter these organisms produce pathological damage in internal organs originating important mortality rates in the diseased fish populations. Another important species of this genus is *F. branchiophilum* that is the etiological agent of bacterial gill disease, a widespread pathological condition of fish in freshwater environments. But since this bacterium specifically affects the respiratory tissue and not skin nor fins, it will not be described further in this section (see "Bacterial Gill Disease" section in Chapter 6).

FLAVOBACTERIOSIS CAUSED BY *FLAVOBACTERIUM PSYCHROPHILUM*

This bacterial species causes two different pathological conditions in fish, bacterial cold-water disease (BCWD) and rainbow trout fry syndrome (RTFS). Although both diseases were first reported affecting rainbow trout, they were initially found at very different times and locations, e.g., BCWD was first observed in the United States in the early 1940s, whereas RTFS was initially recognized in Europe at the late 1980s.[71,72] In most cases of BCWD, the hosts exhibit skin and/or fin lesions, whereas fish with RTFS usually undergo an acute condition and die without showing external manifestations except skin darkening.[72,73]

BACTERIAL COLD-WATER DISEASE

Overview: Bacterial cold-water disease, or "cold water disease" or "peduncle disease," is a systemic disease that affects fry and sometimes juveniles of several teleost species, but typically salmonids, either cultured or in the wild in cold or temperate freshwater (i.e., below 16°C, mainly 5°C–10°C), usually causing only external lesions.

Etiology: This disease is caused by *F. psychrophilum*, a Gram-negative, long slender bacterium.

Route of transmission: Infections are horizontally transmitted through contaminated water. The reservoirs of *F. psychrophilum* include pathogen-carrier fish, bacteria-shedding diseased and dead fish, and water supplies.[74] This bacterium can remain viable for at least 300 days in freshwater.[75] Although there are conflicting results, there is evidence that vertical transmission may also occur since the bacterium has been isolated from milt, ovarian fluid, egg surface and intraovum of sexually mature salmonid fish.[76–81]

Host range: All salmonid species are affected, but coho salmon are particularly susceptible.[82] Although most of the BCWD outbreaks have historically been associated with salmonids, this disease has been described as affecting many non-salmonid teleost, including ayu (*Plecoglossus altivelis*), common carp

(*Cyprinus carpio*), crucian carp (*Carassius carassius*), European eel (*Anguilla anguilla*), pale chub (*Zacco platypus*), perch (*Perca fluviatilis*), roach (*Rutilus rutilus*) and tench (*Tinca tinca*).[83–87] In addition, *F. psychrophilum* has been detected but without clinical signs in Japanese eel (*Anguilla japonica*), fork-tongue goby (*Chaenogobius urotaenia*), Japanese dace (*Trybolodon hakonensis*) and Lake goby (*Rhinogobius brunneus*).[88,89] Finally, *F. psychrophilum* has been isolated from sea lampreys (*Petromyzon marinus*) collected in Lake Ontario, showing skin and fin lesions, which expands the potential susceptible and/or carrier hosts of this pathogen to not only a variety of teleost fish species but to other physiologically and evolutionarily distant vertebrate aquatic animals.[90]

Clinical presentation: First clinical signs are usually fin tip fraying and a rough appearance of the skin. As the infection continues, necrosis develops at the sites of bacterial colonization, often noted on the dorsal and adipose fins. Ulcers and other external lesions can occur in the skin of any area of the body, with a predilection for the caudal peduncle and caudal fin regions.[74] In most cases, the adipose fin and the integument covering the dorsal area of the peduncle become necrotic revealing the underlying musculature (see Chapter 7, **Figure 7.13**). In latter stages of disease, tissue and muscle degeneration progresses to such an extent that the skeletal processes of the caudal fins are fully exposed, yet remain attached to the vertebral column.[80] Along with the external pathology, systemic bacterial infections and extensive internal pathology can also be present in many fish. In the disease form that is more acute, the external lesions are less prevalent, and systemic infections and internal pathology predominate.[74] Several forms of spinal deformations can occur as sequelae in fish that survive after a BCWD outbreak.[76]

Differential diagnosis: Skin and/or fin lesions caused by other infectious agents, including bacteria, fungi and ectoparasites, or primary by mechanical damage (i.e., trauma) of different sorts can be similar to BCWD. In salmonids in freshwater, differential diagnosis should include classical conditions such as Bacterial kidney disease (BKD), furunculosis and columnaris disease, and, in the case of rainbow trout, the emerging pathologies known as red-mark syndrome, warm-water strawberry disease, rush and strawberry disease.[91]

Diagnosis: The observation of characteristic bacteria in Gram-stained preparations and confirmation of *F. psychrophilum* as the causative agent from moribund specimens through primary culture followed by identification through biochemical, serological or genotypic assays is required for diagnosis.[74] Cytophaga agar and other microbiological media with oligonutrients such as Hsu-Shotts and TYE (tryptone yeast extract) are used for laboratory growth of this bacterium.[80]

Management/control: Preventive measures to diminish the risk of having the disease or to decrease its incidence, severity and/or transmissibility are advisable. In wild fish living in freshwater the avoidance of the pathogen is not possible, but in captive cultured fish the use of pathogen-free well or spring water, or the filtering and disinfection with ultraviolet irradiation or ozonation of the inlet water are helpful to eliminate this infection source.[80] Adopting general biosecurity procedures such as facility cleaning and disinfection, and the use of fallowing and quarantine periods are important to control this disease. Once an outbreak has occurred, it is important to promptly remove dead fish to minimize *F. psychrophilum* in the water column.[92]

Although egg disinfection with iodophors (e.g., 100 mg L-1 of active iodine for 10 minutes) or other disinfectants, eliminates most but not all the viable *F. psychrophilum* located at the chorion surfaces, this is recommended to reduce the transmission rate of this bacterium to the progeny. Early administration of chemotherapeutics is more efficient than late treatments to control this infection, and therefore regular surveillance is advisable. However, resistance of *F. psychrophilum* to antimicrobials has been reported and drug sensitivity tests should be carried out before treatment.[93] Vaccines in general have not shown consistent protection and accordingly are not commercially available in many countries.[94]

FLAVOBACTERIOSIS CAUSED BY *FLAVOBACTERIUM COLUMNARE*

Overview: "Columnaris" or "columnaris disease" is an acute to chronic disease that affects many different fish species that live in temperate or warm freshwater ($\geq 15°C$). In its typical form, fish suffer extensive skin, fin and gill damage, with or without

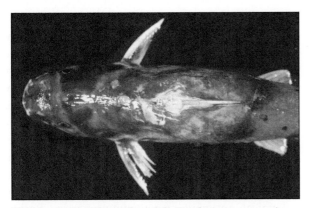

Figure 5.15 Channel catfish (*Ictalurus punctatus*) with classic "saddleback" presentation and yellow pigmentation of *Flavobacterium columnare*.

progression to a systemic invasion that can lead to death on many occasions. Disease designation follows the described characteristic "column-like" bacterial aggregations in wet mount observations of skin and gill lesion samples.[95] Due to the conspicuous yellowish saddle-like shape areas in the skin surrounding the dorsal fin and extending laterally, this morbid condition has also been called "saddleback disease" (**Figure 5.15**). In addition, given that the caudal peduncle tissues of rainbow trout are usually compromised some authors refer to this malady as "peduncle disease" and, finally, in tropical fish it has been named "cotton wool disease" due to the lesion aspect of secondary infections by fungi.[96,97]

Etiology: The causative agent of columnaris disease is the Gram-negative *Flavobacterium columnare*.[98]

Route of transmission: This bacterium is transmitted horizontally from infected to naïve fish by direct and indirect contact or through contaminated water. Although *F. columnare* has been found in reproductive fluids of salmonid fish the occurrence of vertical transmission has not been documented.[81] This opportunistic fish pathogen appears to be ubiquitous and worldwide distributed in freshwater aquatic environments.[97] This organism naturally occurs in a planktonic, free-living state where it can survive for long periods, even in the absence of nutrients.[99] Several water-quality factors affect its survival. However, under certain conditions, this bacterium can remain viable for months or even years outside its hosts in freshwater.[100,101] Besides its planktonic style of life, this bacterium can develop protective biofilms that probably help to preserve it both in and outside its hosts.[102] Fish are the reservoir hosts and they shed *F. columnare* into the medium primarily from diseased individuals but also from carrier fish.

Host range: Columnaris disease affects a wide range of wild and farmed freshwater fish species. Diadromous species, such as salmonids and eels, while spending their life in freshwater, as well as many tropical freshwater aquarium fishes and warm-water food fish species, can also acquire this disease.[97] It has been hypothesized that all freshwater fish species are susceptible to columnaris under environmental conditions favorable to the bacterium and stressful to the fish.[103]

Clinical presentation: Pathological changes are usually confined to gills, skin and fins, but in some cases oral mucosa can be compromised. Systemic infections and internal lesions are uncommon and normally occur after the external tissues have been breached. Disease can be acute, subacute or chronic, depending on the conditions of the outbreak, the fish species and the virulence of the strain involved.[104–106] Mortality rates can be extremely high with 60%– 90% mortality being common.[104] Early clinical signs are usually characterized by the appearance of pale spots in the skin surrounded by hyperemic reddish-tinge areas.[103] Lesions on the gills and fins extend generally from the distal end to the base, and the tissues are necrotic and eroded.[103] Lesions are covered with a yellowish white mucoid exudate consisting largely of swarms of *F. columnare* (**Figure 5.16**).[99]

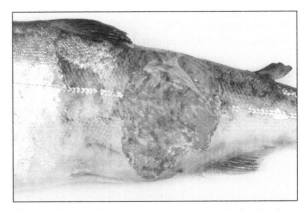

Figure 5.16 *Flavobacterium columnare* infection in coho salmon (*Oncorhynchus kisutch*) with deep ulcer covered by a yellowish white mucoid exudate. (Image courtesy of M. Godoy.)

In the classical presentation, skin lesions begin around the dorsal fin and then increase in size and result in a gray to white lesion that is bilaterally symmetrical.[104] Peduncle skin is also often compromised showing superficial necrosis or ulcers that occur alone or concurrently with the saddle-shape lesions. Secondary infections occur with other bacteria and/or mycotic agents.[107] In warm-water ornamental fish, *F. columnare* is one of the primary causes that facilitate the conspicuous secondary fungal infections termed "cotton wool disease" or "mouth fungus."[96] Although these are the typical presentations of this disease, in some cases fish infected with *F. columnare* may die without any clinical or gross pathological changes.[104]

Differential diagnosis: Columnaris disease should be differentiated from a wide spectrum of other pathological entities that also produce skin, fin and/or gill lesions including infectious and noninfectious conditions. Similar external pathology can be initiated by different infectious agents acting as the primary cause or as secondary contaminants. Some cause pathology in the external tissues, which then can invade internal organs, whereas others show the reverse infection route. Differential diagnosis depends on the host species affected. For example, in cyprinids spring viremia of carp and carp erythrodermatitis should be ruled out, whereas in salmonids bacterial kidney disease should be taken into consideration. Flavobacteriosis caused by *F. psychrophilum* can be confused with columnaris disease and requires differentiation. Mechanical damage can be the primary etiology of external lesions, which become secondarily infected with fungi or bacteria resembling in some cases columnaris disease gross pathology. Fin erosions are common in cultured fish and they may be resolved just by adjusting the fish biomass to the appropriate level.[107] Contaminated lesions of fish that have survived attacks of predators, although normally distinctive, can also be confused with columnaris disease. Finally, there are fish with idiopathic disorders such as the ulcerative dermal necrosis of wild salmonids that may also exhibit external pathology resembling columnaris disease.

Diagnosis: Clinical history, clinical signs and gross pathology consistent with columnaris disease are crucial for preliminary diagnosis. In addition, the observation of long, slender Gram-negative bacteria and the typical "haystack" aggregations in Gram-stained or wet mount preparations from the affected tissues, respectively, is important for a presumptive diagnosis. Gliding motility is not always evident but can be observed on the underside of the cover glass of wet mounts.[104] Identification of the causative agent is required to confirm diagnosis. This bacterium is isolated on low-nutrient agar media, such as Cytophaga, Shieh, Hsu-Shotts or TYES, and identified by typical morphology of its colonies and biochemical, antigenic or genomic properties. Besides isolation, this pathogen can be detected directly from infected tissues using serology as well as conventional and real-time PCR methods.[97,104]

Management/control: Whenever possible prevention is the best approach to control this disease. Decreasing fish biomass density, organic load, and ammonia and nitrite levels are important to diminish the risk of developing columnaris disease. Although not widely available, the use of fish genetically selected for higher resistance to this infection will probably be an important measure to control this disease. Vaccines can elicit immunoprotection against *F. columnare*, and although not always effective, they can sometimes be used as a preventive tool. During the early stages of infection, fish can be treated with antimicrobial baths, whereas in advanced cases therapeutic drugs should be delivered orally by medicated food.

BACTERIAL KIDNEY DISEASE

Overview: Bacterial kidney disease (BKD) is a chronic bacterial disease that occurs in most regions of the world where members of the family Salmonidae are present.[108] Natural disease outbreaks are restricted to salmonid species.[109] Infections commonly manifest as a systemic disease involving hematopoietic kidney tissues and other internal organs, but skin lesions may also be observed in disseminated disease or as localized infections. For example "spawning rash" is a transient infection that has been reported primarily in adult rainbow trout (*Oncorhynchus mykiss*) and other salmonids during the spawning season.[110,111]

Etiology: The causative agent of BKD and salmonid spawning rash is *Renibacterium salmoninarum*, which is a facultative intracellular, Gram-positive, non-motile, non-spore-forming, short rod or diplobacillus.[112,113]

Route of transmission: The bacterium is shed into water by infected fish, and can be transmitted horizontally in freshwater or seawater via the fecal-oral route or by entry into sites of injury to the skin, fins, or eyes.[114] The bacterium is also transmitted vertically in association with the eggs, with some bacteria carried intra-ovum within the yolk.[115] Survival of *R. salmoninarum* in the environment appears limited (≤21 days), but the bacterium can persist for extended periods as subclinical infections in salmonid populations.[114] Although *R. salmoninarum* has been detected in non-salmonid fishes inhabiting the same waters as salmonids, it is unknown whether these species can serve as reservoirs for the pathogen.[116]

Host range: All salmonids are considered susceptible to BKD, and significant economic losses have been reported in cultured Pacific salmon (*Oncorhynchus* spp.) and Atlantic salmon (*Salmo salar*).[117] Clinical BKD has also been recorded in wild salmonids, including populations with no history of supplementation (i.e., wild stocking) with hatchery-reared fish, but disease impacts on free-ranging populations are difficult to assess.[114]

Clinical presentation: Infections generally progress slowly, and clinical disease is uncommon in fish younger than 6–12 months of age.[118] Fish with systemic *R. salmoninarum* may show no external clinical signs, or may present with one or more of the following: lethargy and loss of balance; darkened or mottled skin coloration; abdominal distension produced by ascites; gill pallor associated with anemia; exophthalmos; hemorrhages at the bases of fins and around the vent; superficial vesicles or bullae filled with clear, bloody or turbid fluid; shallow skin ulcers; and abscesses or cystic cavities that extend into the skeletal muscle (**Figure 5.17**).[112] Spawning rash appears as a pustulous dermatitis that may cover large areas of skin with numerous small vesicles or hemorrhagic nodules visible in the epidermis.[112]

Differential diagnosis: Skin lesions associated with pathogens such as *Mycobacterium* spp., *Nocardia* spp., *Carnobacterium maltaromaticum* and *Ichthyophonus* spp. should be excluded.

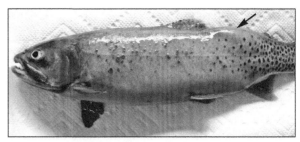

Figure 5.17 Skin lesions including vesicles, shallow ulcers, and an abscess (arrow) associated with systemic BKD in an adult hatchery-reared cutthroat trout (*Oncorhynchus clarkii*). (Image courtesy of J. Drennan.)

Diagnosis: Clinical signs of BKD or spawning rash are not pathognomonic; thus presumptive diagnosis is usually based on microscopic observation of intracellular and extracellular bacteria in stained smears or imprints from infected tissues (**Figure 5.18**). Smears are most frequently made from internal organs such as kidney or spleen. Rapid confirmatory diagnosis is achieved by direct or indirect fluorescent antibody staining of bacteria in smears, other immunological methods (i.e., ELISA), molecular methods (i.e., PCR), or biochemical testing of cultured organisms.[114,119] A number of media formulations have been developed for *R. salmoninarum* culture,

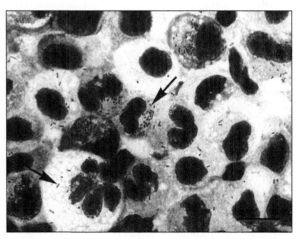

Figure 5.18 *Renibacterium salmoninarum* bacterial cells (arrows) visible within the cytoplasm of phagocytic cells in a Romanowski-stained kidney imprint from a hatchery-reared adult cutthroat trout (*Oncorhynchus clarkii*). Scale bar = 10 μm. (Image courtesy of J. Drennan.)

but the bacterium has an absolute requirement for cysteine, and several weeks can be required for the appearance of visible colonies at optimal incubation temperatures of 15°C–18°C.[113,114]

Management/control: Renibacterium salmoninarum–associated spawning rash may be restricted to skin lesions and may spontaneously resolve after spawning. Systemic BKD is among the more difficult fish diseases to control. Management strategies have included chemotherapy; vaccination; interruption of vertical transmission; and improvements in hygiene, husbandry and biosecurity practices.[109,114,120] Chemotherapeutants have been applied with partial success, but do not completely eliminate the pathogen. A commercial vaccine, containing live cells of a nonpathogenic environmental *Arthrobacter* species, has been licensed for sale in several countries. This vaccine provides significant protection against BKD in juvenile Atlantic salmon but little or no protection of juvenile Pacific salmon.[116] In areas of endemic *R. salmoninarum*, a strategy that has been successfully used for reducing the impact of vertical transmission consists of screening spawning female fish and culling or segregation of eggs from infected females.[121–124] Alleviation of stressful conditions that can exacerbate development of clinical BKD is also important for reducing infections in cultured fish populations.[109] Compartmentalization of BKD management on the basis of fish species and geographic areas, and restriction of movement of fish and eggs from BKD-positive sites, may be an effective strategy for limiting the spread of the disease.[125,126]

MYCOBACTERIOSIS

Overview: Mycobacteriosis occurs in fishes from tropical to subarctic latitudes, and has been reported in wild fish as well as cultured food fish and ornamental species. It has been hypothesized that increased prevalence of mycobacterial infections in some wild fish populations may be linked to environmental stressors such as eutrophication or nutritional stress resulting from a reduced forage base.[127] In cultured fish, disease outbreaks are often related to husbandry factors such as poor water quality, inadequate nutrition, high stocking density or fish handling.[128]

Etiology: A variety of *Mycobacterium* spp. have been named as etiological agents of finfish mycobacteriosis. Historical descriptions have been based on a limited number of characteristics, and some of the archaic mycobacterial species names are now considered synonymous with more completely characterized species.[127] The mycobacterial species most commonly reported as fish pathogens are *M. marinum*, *M. fortuitum* and *M. chelonae*.[129–131] Despite its name, *M. marinum* infects both freshwater and marine fish species in tropical and temperate waters, and is the most widely reported mycobacterial fish pathogen, followed by *M. fortuitum*, which also occurs in both tropical and temperate waters. Infections with *M. chelonae* have been reported primarily from temperate species including salmonids and turbot (*Scophthalmus maximus*).[129] Use of molecular characterization in addition to phenotypic methods has enabled the identification of several additional species of piscine mycobacterial pathogens including *M. abscessus, M. avium, M. gordonae, M. haemophilum, M. montiforense, M. peregrinum/septicum, M. pseudoshottsii, M. shottsii* and *M. salmoniphilum*.[127] Mycobacterial taxonomy is in a state of transition, and it is likely that the full range of mycobacterial species and strains affecting fish is still unknown.[127,131]

Route of transmission: Ingestion of contaminated feed, detritus and water is believed to be a primary mechanism of mycobacterial transmission.[129] The bacterium may also enter through abrasions or other injuries of the integument.[128] Transovarian transmission of mycobacteria has been reported in viviparous fish, but vertical transmission in oviparous species has not yet been demonstrated.[127,131]

Host range: *Mycobacterium* spp. have been associated with disease in more than 165 freshwater, brackish and marine fish species worldwide.[128] All fishes are considered susceptible to mycobacterial infection, but susceptibility to clinical disease varies among species.[127] Non-fish aquatic organisms such as protists, invertebrates and other vertebrates (e.g., frogs, snakes and turtles) can also harbor mycobacteria and may serve as vectors.[127] In addition to causing disease in finfish, aquatic mycobacteria present significant zoonotic concerns, especially for aquarium hobbyists and others who regularly handle fish.[129,132] Human infections caused by aquatic

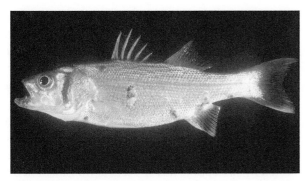

Figure 5.19 Erosion of the lower jaw and preopercle along with shallow hemorrhagic skin lesions associated with a *Mycobacterium marinum* infection in a hybrid striped bass (*Morone saxatilis* × *M. chrysops*). (Image courtesy of A.C. Camus.)

mycobacteria are typically confined to cutaneous lesions of extremities, although deep tissue infections of musculature, tendons and bones have been reported, and systemic infections may rarely occur in immunocompromised individuals.[129,132]

Clinical presentation: Mycobacteriosis in fish is typically a systemic, chronic disease that can remain as a subclinical or slowly progressing infection.[129,133] Affected fish may be lethargic, anorexic and emaciated, and exhibit poor reproductive performance. External lesions are nonspecific and commonly include scale loss and skin ulcers that may appear as shallow ulcerations or as deep hemorrhagic lesions (**Figures 5.19** and **5.20**). Changes in cutaneous pigmentation such as fading or abnormally bright coloration have been observed. Other abnormalities such as unilateral or bilateral exophthalmos, abdominal

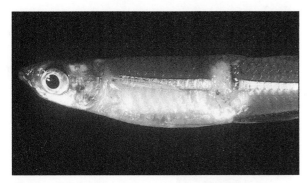

Figure 5.20 Skin ulcer caused by *Mycobacterium marinum* in an inland silverside (*Menidia beryllina*). (Image courtesy of A.C. Camus.)

distension, spinal curvature, or stunting may also occur. Rarely, mycobacteriosis presents as an acute, fulminating disease characterized by rapid morbidity and mortality of fish with few clinical signs.[129]

Differential diagnosis: Skin lesions caused by *Nocardia* spp., *Renibacterium salmoninarum* and *Ichthyophonus* spp. may appear similar to those caused by *Mycobacterium* spp. The genus *Nocardia* stain partially acid-fast but often appear as filamentous, branching rods and also can be distinguished from *Mycobacterium* spp. by biochemical or molecular tests.

Diagnosis: External signs of mycobacteriosis are not pathognomonic, and a presumptive diagnosis can be made by observing the presence of acid-fast bacilli or coccobacilli in affected tissues. Smears of affected tissues can be rapidly stained for detection of acid-fast organisms morphologically consistent with *Mycobacterium* spp.[134] Histopathology is also used to support a diagnosis of mycobacteriosis. Typically, non-branching acid-fast bacteria are present either intracellularly or extracellularly within granulomas, although no acid-fast rods may be visible in sections if few live bacteria are present in tissues, or if tissue decalcification procedures have been applied before staining.[130] Immunohistochemical staining may be useful for detecting mycobacteria in early granulomas.

Mycobacteria can be slow growing and difficult to isolate in culture, and this methodology is not commonly applied for routine diagnosis. A variety of selective media are utilized, and culture at room temperature or the temperature at which suspect infected fish were collected is recommended.[127,131] Identification of mycobacterial species can be time-consuming and costly, and long incubation periods can make interpretation of phenotypic characteristics difficult.[135,136] Therefore, phenotypic characteristics are no longer considered sufficient to differentiate mycobacterial species.[136] Molecular methods such as PCR and gene sequencing are being increasingly used for detection and identification of *Mycobacterium* spp.[135–137] Utilization of quantitative molecular methods is recommended to distinguish mycobacterial DNA detections that represent probable infections from those that likely originate from environmental contaminants.

Management/control: Antimicrobial chemotherapy has occasionally been attempted, especially for treatment of valuable individual fish specimens, but does not eliminate *Mycobacterium* spp. from infected individuals or fish colonies. Additionally, no vaccines are commercially available for the prevention of piscine mycobacteriosis. Fish with mycobacterial infections often have chronic health problems, poor growth and feed conversion rates, and are a source of infection for other fish.[130] Control of mycobacteriosis in fish culture facilities requires destruction of affected stocks and thorough cleaning and disinfection of rearing units, plumbing and equipment. Disinfectants such as ethanol (50%–70%), benzyl-4-chlorophenol-phenylphenol (Lysol®) and sodium chlorite have been shown to rapidly kill *M. marinum* in water, but other disinfectants such as *N*-alkyl dimethyl benzyl ammonium chloride (Roccal®-D, Micronex®) and potassium peroxymonosulfate (Virkon®-S) are ineffective even after prolonged contact times.[138] Sodium hypochlorite (chlorine bleach) may require contact times of 20 minutes or longer at concentrations of 50,000 mg/L to eliminate mycobacteria.[138] Personnel working in facilities where piscine mycobacteriosis may be present should wear appropriate protective clothing and take proper precautions to avoid possible infection.[130] Prevention of mycobacteriosis in fish culture facilities is more cost-effective than treatment. Preventive strategies include stocking with fish from known *Mycobacterium*-free populations, quarantine of new fish isolated from established populations for at least 30–45 days and periodic necropsy of a subsample of fish for mycobacterial examination. Maintenance of fish in optimum water quality and rearing conditions, and regular cleaning of rearing units to reduce biofilms and accumulation of organic material, will help to reduce colonization of mycobacteria and the potential for infection of fish.[130]

LYMPHOCYSTIS

Overview: Lymphocystis is a chronic, or in rare cases subacute, disease affecting many species of teleost fishes in fresh, brackish and marine environments. The disease is generally a self-limiting, benign infection where clinically affected fish have cream to grayish color wart-like masses of the fins and skin.

Etiology: This condition is caused by several types of the lymphocystis disease virus (LDV) that are large iridoviruses belonging to the *Lymphocystivirus* genus.[139–141] The virus induces a pathological hypertrophy of fibroblasts that are mainly located in the dermis of the fish and skin.

Route of transmission: The virus is horizontally transmitted mainly by direct contact, but also through contaminated water and by infected tissues eaten by susceptible hosts. Vertical transmission has not been demonstrated.

Host range: More than 125 different teleost fish species have been reported exhibiting clinical signs of lymphocystis. In general, fish belonging to higher taxonomic orders are susceptible, whereas species of lower orders are less susceptible to this viral infection. Nevertheless, there are exceptions, e.g., salmonids are resistant as expected for fish species of a subfamily belonging to a lower order, whereas smelts, which are phylogenetically related to salmonids, are susceptible to lymphocystis.

Clinical presentation: After a variable incubation period, fish exhibit papilloma-like nodules of varying numbers and size that are frequently located on the fins and skin (**Figures 5.21** and **5.22**). In some cases, gross lesions can also be observed in gills, mouth and occasionally in a variety of internal organs. Generally, the disease is benign and no pathological effects are noticeable in the affected fish except for their unsightliness. Infrequently,

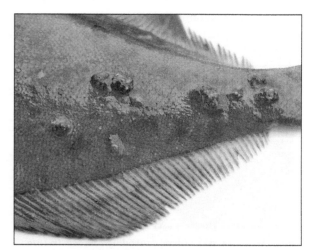

Figure 5.21 Multiple clusters of lymphocystis on the skin of common dab, *Limanda limanda*.

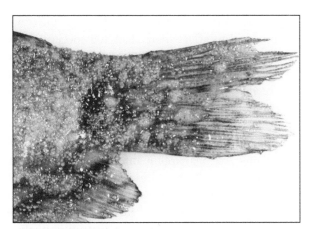

Figure 5.22 Generalized lymphocystis on the skin of gourami, *Trichogaster* sp.

and depending on the severity and location of the lesions, some respiratory and mechanical digestive disturbances can occur and in extremely severe cases the disease can be lethal.

This is generally a self-limiting infection and normally lesions disappear spontaneously ranging from a few weeks to a year. Duration of the clinical signs depends on several factors, water temperature being the most important one. Lower water temperature is associated with longer clinical periods. After remission of clinical signs most fish acquire some degree of immunity and disease reoccurrence is rare, though fish appear to be chronic carriers of the virus.[142]

Differential diagnosis: Besides skin and fin neoplasias, lymphocystis should be differentiated from a variety of external parasitic infestations and from epitheliocystis (*Chlamydiales* spp.).[143] Differential diagnoses should also be made from protozoan infections such as freshwater white spot disease (*Ichthyopthirius multifiliis*), marine white spot disease (*Cryptocaryon irritans*) and *Epystylis* spp., as well as externally encysted digenean trematodes.

Diagnosis: Viral isolation in cell cultures and identification of LDV through different serological and PCR methods is possible, but the primary diagnostic technique is microscopic observation of the tissues with gross pathological appearance using wet mounts and/or histopathology for presumptive and confirmatory diagnosis, respectively.[140,141] Histopathology shows individual cells or clusters of megalocytic fibroblasts surrounded by a distinctive hyaline capsule. These cells exhibit a central, rounded macronucleus and conspicuous basophilic, intracytoplasmatic inclusion bodies in which the LDV replicates.

Management/control: There are currently no vaccines against lymphocystis. Prevention using quarantine and other biosecurity measures to avoid entrance and further dissemination of the virus in naïve fish populations are the most effective methods of disease control. There is no specific treatment against LDV, although when lesions are secondarily contaminated, antibiotics and/or antifungal drugs can be useful in fish recovery. When clinically affected fish are detected, they should be isolated as soon as possible from healthy individuals to avoid disease spread. General good animal husbandry practices and stress minimization are useful to diminish the clinical severity of the disease in individuals and the overall impact of the lymphocystis outbreak in a population.

OOMYCETES

Overview: Oomycetes including *Saprolegnia* spp., *Aphanomyces invadans* and *Achlya* spp. are a ubiquitous group of water molds or pseudofungi. They are widespread and likely endemic to all freshwater ecosystems, and can affect both wild and cultured fish.[144] These pathogens are generally considered agents of secondary infection; despite this, outbreaks can result in major economic losses in farmed animals at all stages of the life cycle.[145] In addition to losses within the aquaculture industry, the decline in natural salmonid populations in many parts of the world has also been attributed to *Saprolegnia* infections.[146] Differences in oomycete pathogenicity is linked with trauma, nutritional status, endocrine changes, temperature and water quality. Temperature appears to play a role in fish susceptibility to saprolegniosis; for example, channel catfish (*Ictalurus punctatus*) become immunocompromised when water temperatures decline and become more susceptible to pathogenic agents.[147] Furthermore, humoral and cellular defensive responses to invading water molds have been observed and may also modulate the gross clinical signs of the resulting infection.[148]

Etiology: The oomycetes form a distinct phylogenetic lineage of eukaryotic organisms that have a life cycle involving sexual and asexual stages that resemble fungi in mycelial growth and mode of nutrition. Within the recognized clades encompassing the taxa *S. diclina* and *S. parasitica*, both act as opportunist and aggressive pathogens of fish and their eggs.[149,150] *Aphanomyces invadans* was originally recognized as the cause of mycotic granulomatosis of ayu (*Plecoglossus altivelis altivelis*) in Japan and as the origin of the seasonal condition epizootic ulcerative syndrome or red spot of striped snakehead (*Channa striata*) and striped mullet (*Mugil cephalus*) from southern Asia and Australia.[151] However, mycotic granulomatosis, epizootic ulcerative syndrome, red spot disease and ulcerative mycosis are all clinically identical and attributed to *A. invadans* infection of stock in fresh and estuarine environments. *Aphanomyces invadans* has an aseptate fungal-like mycelia structure with two typical zoospore forms. The primary zoospore is released at the tip of the sporangium where it forms a spore cluster. This transforms into a free-swimming zoospore that attaches to the skin of the fish where the spore germinates. The hyphae invade the fish skin reaching the skeletal muscle as the target organ and other internal organs.

Route of transmission: Natural infection by *Saprolegnia* spp. are primarily brought about through surface abrasions that breach the normal protective barriers of the skin.[152] It is also possible that the pathogen may gain access to the bloodstream via penetration through the gills or invasion of blood vessels in the superficial lesions. Both *S. parasitica* and *S. australis* can form biofilms with multiple microorganisms, wherein they grow and reproduce. Therefore, natural biofilms may constitute incessant *Saprolegnia* reservoirs in nature and aquaculture.[153] Secondary zoospores of *A. invadans* are transmitted horizontally attaching to the damaged skin of fish and germinating into hyphae. Under adverse conditions the secondary zoospores may also encyst in the environment. The cysts then transform into tertiary generations of zoospores, which plays an important role in the cycle of outbreaks in endemic areas.[154]

Host range: Salmonids (i.e., salmon and trout) and non-salmonids such as tilapia (*Oreochromis* spp.), channel catfish (*Ictalurus punctatus*), carp (*Cyprinus carpio*), eel (*Anguilla anguilla*), perch (*Perca fluviatilis*) and pike (*Esox lucius*) are all susceptible to infection.[155,156]

Aphanomyces invadans shows little host specificity and is reported to affect more than 100 species of wild and cultured finfish, however, carp are known to be naturally resistant to infections with *Aphanomyces invadans*.[157,158]

Clinical presentation: The presence of superficial cotton wool-like tufts, particularly on the integument and gills of host fish or eggs, is generally attributed to *Saprolegnia* infection, and similarly *Achlya* spp. results in a clinical identical scenario.[159] In contrast, *A. invadans* is the etiological agent of an ulcerative mycosis, occurring as necrotizing lesions that typically lead to a mature epithelioid granuloma centered on variable numbers of hyphae. *Saprolegnia*-induced lesions appear gray to white, with circular or crescent-shaped colonies growing by radial extension until adjacent lesions merge (**Figure 5.23**).[160] The vegetative mycelium forms a series of branched, coenocytic filaments creating a whitish cotton, wool- or felt-like mat on the surface of the fish that is largely restricted to the integument and superficial musculature (**Figure 5.24**). However, hyphae can also penetrate the dermal tissues resulting in a diffuse edema and respiratory difficulties.[161] Infection by *A. invadans* can result in scale loss, and red spots on the body surface, head, operculum or caudal peduncle. Large red or gray shallow ulcers, often with a brown necrosis are observed in the later stages. Superficial lesions occur on the flank or dorsum, and are followed by fish losses.[162] An infection by *Saprolegnia* comprises degenerative changes in the muscle mass with consequential diffuse edema. Fish mortality results

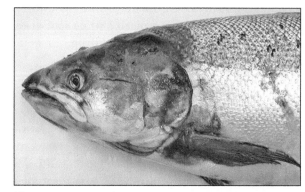

Figure 5.23 Widespread *Saprolegnia*-induced lesions covering the head of an Atlantic salmon (*Salmo salar*).

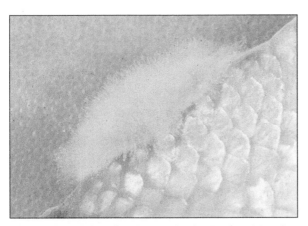

Figure 5.24 Localized fungal infection on skin of a goldfish (*Carassius auratus*).

from progressive destruction of the epidermis by hyphae and impaired osmoregulation. Infection by motile zoospores of *Aphanomyces invadans* can lead to substantial ulceration of the skin, necrosis of muscle with extension to subadjacent structures including the abdominal cavity and cranium, and eventually mortality.[163] Hyphae are associated with the ulcers, infiltrating into myofibers and surrounding connective tissue.[163]

Differential diagnosis: Skin lesions in fish can have diverse etiologies, including infectious agents, toxins, physical causes, predation, and immunological and nutritional deficiencies. However, components in and on the skin have defined roles, and therefore responses to injury or infection largely follow a predetermined response. Careful morphological examination using light microscopy can provide important information that can reveal the pathogenesis of ulcerative syndromes.

Diagnosis: Diagnosis of infection with *Saprolegnia* and *A. invadans* in clinically affected fish can be achieved by histopathology, oomycete isolation or polymerase chain reaction amplification. For diagnostic purposes, the species of *Saprolegnia* responsible for an outbreak may not be practical or necessary, and therefore light microscopy is likely to be the primary diagnostic technique. *Saprolegnia* spp. can be isolated on a low nutrient media such as malt extract agar or Sabouraud agar with incubation at 20°C–22°C and observed for approximately 5 days for newly emerging hyphae tips. The identification

of non-septate hyphae from culture or suspected lesions is used to support a diagnosis. Evidence to distinguish fish lesion isolates from saprophytic isolates using the distinctive cyst coat ornamentation and the determination of esterase isoenzymes is proposed as useful for the screening of potential pathogenic *Saprolegnia*.[164] PCR approaches to examine ribosomal DNA (rDNA) from wide-ranging *Saprolegnia* isolates have been developed with the use of endonuclease *BstUI*. This approach showed identical fingerprints from all strains of *S. parasitica*.[165] *Aphanomyces invadans* is characteristically slow growing in culture, but can be identified to the genus level by inducing sporogenesis and demonstrating typical asexual characteristics.[166] Molecular assays for the detection of *Aphanomyces invadans* have similarly been successful.[167]

Management/control: Both chemical and non-chemical treatments have been used to control saprolegniosis including hydrogen peroxide, sodium chloride, formalin, seawater flushes, potassium permanganate, copper sulfate and ultraviolet irradiation.[168,169] However, some treatments are difficult and there are reservations regarding their efficacy and safety.[170] Eggs infected with oomycetes require the removal of dead or infected eggs at regular intervals, and chemical or therapeutic bath treatments. There is no effective treatment for *A. invadans*–infected fish in the wild or farmed animals. It has been suggested that fish losses could be minimized by adding lime, hydrated lime or salt to the culture water.[166] Currently there are no vaccines available to control oomycetes infection. Overall, the best control for oomycete infections is good management, good water quality, good nutrition and proper handling.

NEOPLASIA

Overview: Several neoplasms (i.e., tumors) that originate from epithelial or mesenchymal cells manifest in the skin and fins of fish. These are some of the more common neoplasia reported in fish, as they are readily observed not only at necropsy but also externally on a live fish.

Etiology: Neoplasia can develop following exposure to certain chemicals, heavy metals, ionizing radiation, chronic inflammation, ultraviolet radiation, pollution and certain viruses, whereas others may be seasonal, of unknown cause or spontaneous in nature.[171-173] A strong correlation between environmental contaminants and induction of skin neoplasia in fishes has been documented.[174,175] Viruses associated with neoplasia development in fish include those in the Herpesviridae, Iridoviridae, Papillomaviridae and Retroviridae families. Within the herpesviruses, the Alloherpesviridae contains the main group of viral etiologies with *Ictalurid herpesvirus* 1 of channel catfish virus, *Cyprinid herpesvirus* 3 (koi herpesvirus) of cyprinids, and the salmonid herpesvirus types 1, 2, 3, 4 and 5 (SalHV 1–5).[176-178] Overall the Alloherpesviridae show a high level of host specificity, the ability to intricately interact with the host defenses and the ability to establish long-term latency.

Route of transmission: Some fish neoplasia can be induced through intraperitoneal injection; however, natural transmission occurs after exposure to pollutants or viruses or spontaneously in some neoplasia.[179] In the case of viral diseases, the virus may be transmitted by diseased fish and/or asymptomatic carriers through the feces, urine and sexual products at spawning. Transmission may also occur from direct contact or through the water, on or in the egg, or through vectors such as rotifers.[180]

Host range: Neoplastic conditions of the skin and fins have been recorded in a wide range of farmed, wild, ornamental and research species, and it is assumed that all fish species are susceptible.

Clinical presentation: Salmon herpesvirus 1 (SalHV-1) is only associated with mild disease in natural outbreaks, and thus is not a major concern in aquaculture, whereas SalHV-5 has only been identified in asymptomatic lake trout, *Salvelinus namaycush*.

Oncorhynchus masou virus

Oncorhynchus masou virus, caused by salmonid herpesvirus type 2 (SalHV-2), is an oncogenic, ulcerative skin condition of masou salmon in Japan. Several other salmonid species are susceptible to SalHV-2 including coho salmon (*O. kisutch*), chum salmon (*O. keta*), sockeye salmon (*O. nerka*) and rainbow trout (*O. mykiss*). Fish show severe exophthalmia and petechial hemorrhage under the lower jaw and along the ventral surface. Epitheliomas occur around the mouth (upper and lower jaw), and to a lesser extent on the caudal fin, operculum and body surface.[181] Infection induces a mandibular epithelial neoplasm, which is characterized as papillomatous.

Epizootic epitheliotropic disease

Epizootic epitheliotropic disease (EED), caused by salmon herpesvirus type 3 (SalHV-3), occurs in lake trout in the Great Lakes region of North America.[178] Epizootic epitheliotropic disease occurs in two forms: an acute form caused by primary virus infection and a chronic form that presents as a papilloma principally of the mouth.

Epidermal papillomatosis

Atlantic salmon papillomatosis, caused by salmon herpesvirus type 4 (SalHV-4), is a benign, epidermal neoplastic condition of the skin and scales of salmon parr, occasionally young adult fish (smolts and grilse) and rainbow trout that have adapted to salt water.[178,182,183] Additional observations of papillomatosis have been reported from rainbow trout reared in freshwater, Atlantic salmon (*Salmo salar*) smolts, cultured eel (*Anguilla japonica*) and koi carp (*Cyprinus carpio*).[184-186] Growths are single or multiple raised plaques with a smooth to nodular texture that is white, brown or pink (**Figure 5.25**). Papillomata vary from a few millimeters to multifaceted growths up to 40 mm where more than half of the body

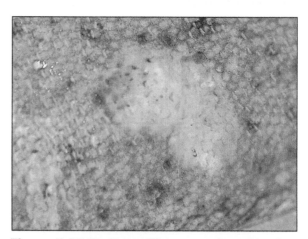

Figure 5.25 Benign papilloma growth on skin of common dab, *Limanda limanda*.

surface may be covered in severely affected fish. The papillomata are generally harmless to the fish, with little dermal involvement, and can spontaneously detach allowing the skin to heal.[187]

Walleye dermal sarcoma

Walleye dermal sarcoma is a seasonal, multifocal cutaneous benign skin neoplasm of adult walleye (*Sander vitreus*) caused by a type C retrovirus.[188] The mesenchymal neoplasm develops from the superficial surface of scales and consists of fibroblast-like cells separated by collagen or osteoid material. The neoplasm is a nonencapsulated nodular mass and the overlaying epidermis is often ulcerated in regressing lesions.[189]

Pigment cell neoplasia

Pigment cell neoplasia is occasionally reported in wild and farmed fishes, with melanomas being the most common type. Melanomas are generally raised, black-pigmented areas and hence visible on the body surface. The neoplasia shows invasion by melanomacrophages in varying degrees of differentiation, with fibrous deposition and metastasis. This is distinctive from an abnormal body coloration reported either as a deficiency or an excess of pigmentation.[190,191] Extensive melanosis and melanoma have occurred in populations of wild coral trout (*Plectropomus leopardus*) where solar ultraviolet B (UVB) radiation was considered the likely cause.[192] In addition, melanosis has been reported in wild populations of smallmouth and largemouth bass, cultured channel catfish and in genetic lines of swordtail × platy crosses and zebrafish (**Figures 5.26** and **5.27**).

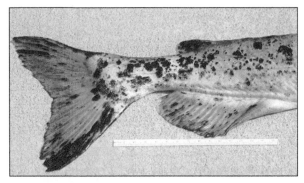

Figure 5.27 Melanosis in a cultured channel catfish (*Ictalurus punctatus*). (Image courtesy of A. Mitchell.)

Chondroma

Chondromas have been reported in Atlantic salmon and neon tetras (*Paracheirodon innesi*) as individual ovoid, white, smooth, firm growths connected to the branchial cartilage and diagnosed as benign cartilaginous neoplastic growth (**Figure 5.28**).[193,194] The growths contain cystic spaces beneath the epidermis with numerous irregular crests of hyaline cartilage beneath the skin. These are surrounded by a loose fibrous matrix of adipose tissue containing strands of immature cartilage.[193,195]

Differential diagnosis: Differential diagnosis of skin neoplasia in fish is generally straightforward with rule outs being infectious hematopoietic necrosis, viral hemorrhagic septicemia, lymphocystis virus, bacterial abscesses and foreign body granulomas. However, most lesions can be clearly differentiated by histology. Viruses are attributed

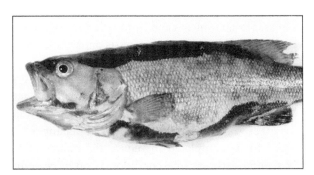

Figure 5.26 Melanosis in a wild smallmouth bass (*Micropterus dolomieu*).

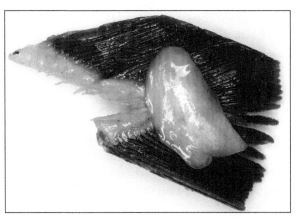

Figure 5.28 Benign chondroma on cartilaginous tissue of gill of rainbow trout (*Oncorhynchus mykiss*).

to most neoplastic conditions of the skin of fish, but no infectious agent has been associated with chondromas and are considered a natural spontaneous occurrence.

Diagnosis: Diagnostic approaches for differentiation of neoplastic lesions in fish are generally gross observation, cytological, histological and ultrastructural examination of the lesions, with topographic localization and histological features used to support a diagnosis of neoplasia. By convention, neoplastic changes are named according to features of differentiation and their degree of malignancy following histological examination, thus descriptions reflect the tissue of origin. As an alternative, specific viral diseases can be diagnosed by virus isolation using cell lines and confirmed by a serum neutralization test using specific antiserum, ELISA, PCR or qPCR, or directly in tissues by immunofluorescence.[177,196–199]

Management/control: Control of skin neoplasia in fish is based on reduction or elimination of the etiology if known, such as reducing exposure to environmental contaminants. Tumor-producing viruses may be controlled by UV, ozone or iodophor treatment of the eggs after fertilization and again at the early eyed stage.[200] The treatment of neoplastic disease in fish is generally not useful, except for valued individuals where surgical intervention may be applicable.

HEAD AND LATERAL LINE SYNDROME

Overview: Head and lateral line erosion (HLLE) or hole-in-the-head (HITH) syndrome is an acute to chronic progressive erosive or ulcerative dermatopathy.

Etiology: Historically, this syndrome has been linked to a number of infectious (i.e., parasitic, viral and bacterial), nutritional and environmental etiologies.[201–204] However, recent evidence suggests that the lesion may be caused by the use of activated carbon in water filtration systems.[205,206] It also may be that this dermatopathy is caused by a combination of different etiologies that show similar lesions.

Route of transmission: Not definitely determined but most likely water exposure.

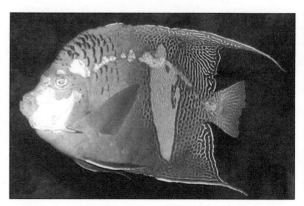

Figure 5.29 Head and lateral line erosion (HLLE) syndrome on face and along lateral line in a captive yellow bar angelfish (*Pomacanthus maculosus*).

Host range: Head and lateral line erosion (HLLE) is most commonly observed in captive marine fishes, while hole-in-the-head (HITH) syndrome (not to be confused with hole-in-the-head of catfish caused by *E. ictaluri*) occurs in freshwater cichlid species (i.e., discus, oscars and angelfish).

Clinical presentation: The syndrome usually starts as focal depigmentation and small erosive skin lesions around the head and/or lateral line of the fish.[205,206] As the disease progresses, the lesions may coalesce and become expansive encompassing the head and entire lateral line (**Figure 5.29**).[206] Though the disease may cause significant disfigurement of the fish, it is rarely fatal.

Differential diagnosis: Skin lesions caused by *Mycobacterium* spp., *Nocardia* spp., *Edwardsiella ictaluri* or other ulcerative conditions may have a similar erosive or "pitting" appearance.

Diagnosis: A presumptive diagnosis is commonly made by noting the species affected and the typical location of erosive lesions in the head and lateral line areas. Stained smears and histopathology of affected tissues often reveal a variety of secondary pathogens such as bacteria, fungi and protozoans.

Management/control: Head and lateral line erosion can generally be reversed by removing all activated carbon and performing large-percentage water changes.[180,200] Greater than 90% water changes may need to be completed to reduce the effects of the activated carbon. The condition is often remedied by moving the affected fish to a new aquarium that has never had fish develop HLLE.

SUNBURN

Overview: Superficial skin lesions along the dorsum of the fish caused by overexposure to ultraviolet rays of the sun.

Etiology: Exposure to long wavelength ultraviolet radiation.[207,208] Fish kept in shallow, unshaded ponds, raceways or tanks can be susceptible to sunburn. Dietary photosensitization, e.g., niacin deficiency, has been shown to render fish susceptible to sunburn.[209,210] There is also the potential for certain chemicals and therapeutics to act as phototoxic agents in fish, e.g., sunburn has been reported in salmonids treated with florfenicol.[211]

Route of transmission: Not applicable.

Host range: Presumably all species of fish are susceptible to sunburn, though white or light-colored fish are especially at risk. The condition has been reported in a variety of salmonids (i.e., trout, salmon and char), paddlefish and koi.[212–214]

Clinical presentation: Reddening, inflammation and epithelial sloughing are generally confined to the dorsal surface of the fish (**Figure 5.30**).[209,212] Mortality, most likely due to osmoregulatory imbalances resulting from the skin lesions, can reach 10%–15% in some affected populations.

Differential diagnosis: Rule outs include bacterial and parasitic infections that cause a superficial dermatopathy.

Diagnosis: Reddened, inflamed skin on the dorsal surface of the fish in the summer. Lesion may appear

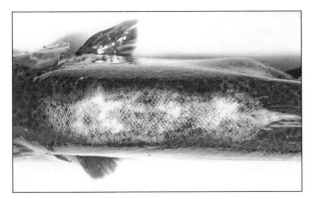

Figure 5.30 Dorsal superficial skin lesion due to sunburn in arctic char (*Salvelinus alpinus*) cultured in shallow raceways.

as a gray patch often located anterior to the dorsal fin.[203,206,207]

Management/control: Providing shade for fish has prevented this condition and even allowed affected fish to return to an apparently normal condition. Anti-inflammatory medicines and vitamin C have been recommended for ornamental species of fish.

PARASITES

There are numerous protozoan and metazoan parasites that can infest the skin and fins of freshwater, brackish and marine fishes. Only a few examples are mentioned here, as there are numerous texts and book chapters devoted to the external and internal parasites of fishes.[215–220]

White spot disease

Overview: A parasitic protozoan disease of the skin, fins and gills of feral and captive freshwater, brackish and marine fishes. This pathogenic disease is commonly called "Ich" or "white spot disease."

Etiology: The parasite of freshwater fish, and sometimes brackish water species, is the ciliate *Ichthyophthirius multifiliis*, and the morphologically and pathologically similar ciliate parasite of marine fishes is *Cryptocaryon irritans*. *Ichthyophthirius multifiliis* has a large horseshoe-shaped macronucleus, whereas *C. irritans* has a large crescent-shaped, lobed macronucleus that is not horseshoe-shaped.[221]

Route of transmission: These holotrichous ciliates invade the skin, fin and gill epithelium of the host causing hyperplasia of the epithelium. Both *I. multifiliis* and *C. irritans* have an obligate fish–associated feeding stage (i.e., trophont) and a reproductive stage (i.e., tomont) in the environment, which ultimately produce free-swimming infective stages (i.e., theronts).[221] The theront penetrates the epithelium and undergoes development into a trophont in a vesicle within the epithelium. When mature, the trophont excysts from the host and differentiates into the tomont, which produces 200–800 tomites. The tomites are released into the environment and become infectious theronts to complete the cycle. The parasite's life cycle and duration of infection in the host are both temperature dependent with the parasite and infection developing more slowly at lower temperatures.[221]

Host range: *Ichthyophthirius multifiliis* appears to parasitize all warm-, cool- and cold-water freshwater fishes, whereas *C. irritans* appears to parasitize marine fishes in waters above temperatures of 19°C.[221]

Clinical presentation: Infestations of *I. multifiliis* or *C. irritans* can often be seen grossly on the skin and fins as the mature trophont stage can range up to 1 mm in size producing the appearance of small, white, raised bumps on the surface of the skin and fins (**Figure 5.31**). Other times the infestation may only appear as small, nonspecific skin lesions where the parasite penetrates through the epithelium of the skin and fins as it enters or exits from the host (**Figure 5.32**). Infected fish will congregate near water intakes, "flash" and rub against the substrate and objects within the environment, have increased opercular rates, and have increased mucus production on the skin and gills.[222] As the infestation progresses, the fish become lethargic and anorexic, and the superficial skin lesions start to ulcerate and become secondarily infected with bacterial and fungal pathogens.[222]

Differential diagnosis: This parasitic disease will need to be differentiated from other conditions causing pale, raised bumps on the skin and fins of fish such as other parasitic (e.g., *Glugea* spp., myxosporideans), viral (e.g., fish pox, lymphocystis) and bacterial (e.g., *Renibacterium salmoninarum*, *Edwardsiella ictaluri*) diseases.

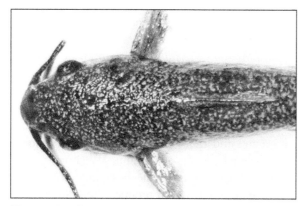

Figure 5.31 Severe infestation of *Ichthyophthirius multifiliis* in a channel catfish (*Ictalurus punctatus*), exhibiting numerous white raised lesions of the skin. (Image courtesy of A. Mitchell.)

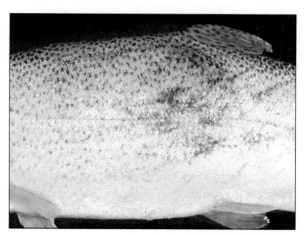

Figure 5.32 *Ichthyophthirius multifiliis* in a rainbow trout (*Oncorhynchus mykiss*) showing shallow erosive skin lesions.

Diagnosis: The diagnosis is made by visual observation of changes in behavior and the appearance of small, raised vesicles or bumps on the skin and fins. The diagnosis is confirmed microscopically by wet mounts of skin or gill biopsies, or by histopathology of affected tissues.

Management/control: Control of these parasites is based on isolation of fish upon arrival and periodic monitoring for infection during the quarantine period. Environmental management of the water with UV treatment or raising the temperature above 30°C for tolerant fish species has been shown to reduce the number of infectious theronts in the water.[221] Immediate removal of infected morbid and dead fish can also help reduce the number of the theronts being released into the water. Treatment is aimed at the free-swimming theront stage and may involve salt or formalin therapy for freshwater fishes, and formalin, copper sulfate or quinine compounds for marine fishes.[221]

Myxosporidiosis

Overview: This is a condition caused by a diverse group of myxosporidean parasites characterized by multicellular spores with polar capsules containing coiled polar filaments.[217,223] The class Myxosporea contains a number of genera including *Henneguya*, *Hoferellus*, *Kudoa*, *Myxobolus*, *Sphaerospora*, *Thelohanellus* and *Unicapsula* that infect a variety of fish tissues.

Etiology: A number of *Myxobolus* species infect the skin and fins of fish including *Myxobolus diversus* in goldfish (*Carassius auratus*), *Myxobolus squamalis* in rainbow trout (*Oncorhynchus mykiss*), *Myxobolus rotundus* in crucian carp (*Carassius carassius*) and *Myxobolus episquamalis* in the flathead gray mullet (*Mugil cephalus*).[217,223]

Route of transmission: These parasites have an obligatory invertebrate oligochaete host for completion of their life cycle.[223] Basically, myxospores are released from the fish host into the environment either by rupture of the cyst or upon death of the host fish. The myxospore is ingested by an oligochaete where the polar filaments are expelled anchoring the parasite to the intestinal epithelium of the oligochaete. The myxospore then releases an amoeboid sporoplasm that penetrates into the intestinal epithelium. The actinospore stage develops within the intestinal epithelium of the oligochaete, which when mature is released to the environment. The actinospore stage is infective to fish, and using a similar process as the myxospore attaches to a suitable host, then a sporoplasm penetrates the epidermis of the fish host. The sporoplasm undergoes a developmental process to form a mature spore completing the life cycle.

Host range: These parasites infect a wide range of freshwater, brackish and marine species of fish, but are especially prevalent in farmed fish populations.

Clinical presentation: Superficial, raised white cysts containing numerous spores can occur on the skin of the head, body and fins of fish (**Figure 5.33**). Generally there is minimal pathology associated

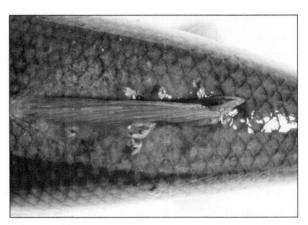

Figure 5.34 Cysts of an unidentified *Myxobolus* sp. on the dorsum of a common carp, *Cyprinus carpio*, showing erosive skin lesions with hemorrhage.

with the cysts, but sometimes the cysts can be associated with focal skin erosion and hemorrhage (**Figure 5.34**). Although the parasites of the skin and fins are generally not a serious problem in the host fish, the disease can reduce the market value of some species of wild and farmed fish.[223]

Differential diagnosis: This parasitic disease needs to be differentiated from other conditions causing raised lesions on the skin and fins of fish such as other parasitic (e.g., *Ichthyophthirius multifiliis*, *Cryptocaryon irritans*, *Glugea* spp.), viral (e.g., fish pox, lymphocystis) and bacterial (e.g., *Renibacterium salmoninarum*, *Edwardsiella ictaluri*) diseases.

Diagnosis: The spores of these parasites can be readily observed in wet mounts of squashed cysts or in histological sections. Morphological characterization of the mature spores can be facilitated by Giemsa, May-Grunwald-Giemsa or silver nitrate staining; however, specific identification is generally not possible.[223] Recently, molecular sequencing using primers for the 18S and internal transcribed spacer (ITS) regions of the rDNA have been used to identify species and to associate the actinospore stages from the oligochaete with the appropriate mature spores in the fish.[223]

Management/control: A number of chemical methods have been tried with only limited success; however, management practices have proven more successful in controlling outbreaks of myxosporideans. The removal of moribund, dead and older age classes of fish reduces the number of infective actinospores released

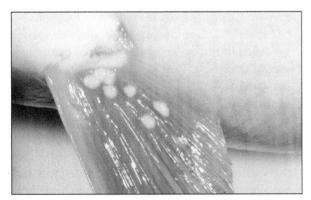

Figure 5.33 Cysts of an unidentified *Myxobolus* sp. on the pectoral fin of a common carp, *Cyprinus carpio*.

into the water.[223] Selecting resistant or non-host species for a particular contaminated site has also proven successful.[223] Alternatively, reducing populations of oligochaetes and other potential intermediate hosts (i.e., bryozoans for *Tetracapsuloides bryosalmonae*) by draining or drying out and liming infected fish ponds interrupts the life cycle of the parasite.[223]

Arthropods (for example, *Lernaea* spp.)

Overview: There are over 2000 species of arthropods (phylum Arthropoda, subphylum Crustacea) parasitic on fish, most of which belong to the class Copepoda.[224] This includes the families Ergasilidae, Lernaeidae, Lernaepodidae, Caligidae and Pennellidae, all of which have species that cause significant pathology in feral and captive fish populations. For instance, *Caligus* spp. and *Lepeophtheirus salmonis* in the family Caligidae are significant pathogens of marine salmonids. In addition, the subphylum Crustacea includes the external parasitic fish lice (subclass Branchiura, for example, *Argulus* spp.) and isopods (order Isopoda).

Etiological agent: Over 100 species of *Lernaea*, commonly called "anchor worms," have been described as external parasites of freshwater fish, especially cyprinids.[224]

Route of transmission: For this arthropod, the holdfast organ and part of the trunk are embedded in host tissue while the remainder of the trunk and elongated abdomen project into the water. At the distal end of the abdomen are usually two egg sacs. The eggs are released into the water and hatch whereupon the larval stages go through three naupliar and five copepodid stages. They then molt into either free-living males or premetamorphosed females. These females are fertilized and then burrow into the fish tissues as they metamorphose into mature females. Larval development is temperature dependent and most outbreaks occur during the warmer summer months when optimal temperatures of 26°C –28°C occur.[224]

Host range: *Lernaea* spp. have a worldwide distribution, with *L. cyprinacea* reported from over 45 species of cyprinids and other fish species.[224]

Clinical presentation: Most adult lernaeids attach to the body surface and become embedded in the superficial layers of the body musculature (**Figure 5.35**). The epithelium around the site of penetration

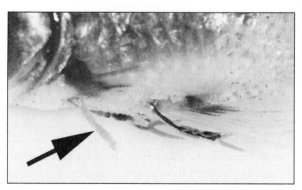

Figure 5.35 One premetamorphosed immature (arrow) and two mature female *Lernaea* sp. with greenish egg sacs on a goldfish (*Carassius auratus*).

becomes hyperplastic with an infiltration of inflammatory cells. There is disruption of the epidermis and dermis, hemorrhage, and muscle necrosis followed by chronic granulomatous fibrosis around the site. The fish may exhibit anorexia, slower growth, and signs of secondary bacterial or fungal infection at the site. Epizootics in cultured fish are often associated with high mortality and even moderate infestations can be severely pathogenic to small fish.[224]

Differential diagnosis: This parasite will need to be distinguished from other arthropods that penetrate or attach themselves to the skin and fins.

Diagnosis: Visual observation of the adult "anchor worm" attached to the body surface of the fish, often with two trailing egg sacs. Specific identification is based on the morphology of the anchors, which consists of two bifurcate dorsal processes and two simple ventral processes.

Management/control: Embedded adult female *Lernaea* are difficult to kill on the host fish, thus control is aimed at breaking the life cycle of the parasite by controlling the larval stages. This may require several treatments over several weeks to kill successive hatches of eggs. In small, confined populations (i.e., ornamental or tropical fish), manual removal of egg cases from females helps reduce the number of larval stages in the environment and number of treatments required. Organophosphate insecticides, particularly trichlorphon, have been used to kill the larval stages, but may be toxic to fish and other invertebrates.[225] Another option is the use of Dimulin® (i.e., diflubenzuron), an insect growth hormone that inhibits chitin formation, to prevent successful molting of the larval stages.[226] Sodium chlorite has also been reportedly used to successfully kill the larval stages.[227] Finally, manual removal of the attached female can be attempted, but usually results in the embedded anchor breaking off in the muscle tissue of the fish. Care should be taken to carefully dissect out the holdfast organ, as leaving the anchor in the tissues can result in a severe granulomatous reaction.

REFERENCES

1. Bernoth, E.M. Furunculosis: The history of the disease and of disease research. In: *Furunculosis: Multidisciplinary Fish Disease Research*. E.M. Bernoth, A.E. Ellis, P.J. Midtlyng, G. Olivier and P. Smith, eds. Academic Press, London, 1997; pp. 1–20.

2. Hiney, M. and Olivier, G. *Furunculosis (Aeromonas salmonicida)*. Fish Disease Group, Department of Microbiology, National University of Ireland, Galway, Galway City, Ireland, 1999; pp. 341–426.

3. Wiklund, T. and Dalsgaard, I. Occurrence and significance of atypical *Aeromonas salmonicida* in non-salmonid and salmonid fish species: A review. *Diseases of Aquatic Organisms* 1988;32(1):49–69.

4. Schneider, R. and Nicholson, B.L. Bacteria associated with fin rot disease in hatchery-reared Atlantic salmon (*Salmo salar*). *Canadian Journal of Fisheries and Aquatic Sciences* 1980;37(10):1505–1513.

5. Bruno, D.W., Munro, A.L. and Needham, E.A. Gill lesions caused by *Aeromonas salmonicida* in sea-reared Atlantic salmon, *Salmo salar* L. *International Council for the Exploration of the Sea Mariculture Committee, CM 1986/F:6*. Thünen-Institut, Braunschweig, Deutschland, 1986.

6. Jutfelt, F., Olsen, R.E., Glette, J., Ringø, E. and Sundell, K. Translocation of viable *Aeromonas salmonicida* across the intestine of rainbow trout, *Oncorhynchus mykiss* (Walbaum). *Journal of Fish Diseases* 2006;29(5):255–262.

7. Novak, C.W., Lewis, D.L., Collicutt, B., Verkaik, K. and Barker, D.E. Investigations on the role of the salmon louse, *Lepeophtheirus salmonis* (Caligidae), as a vector in the transmission of *Aeromonas salmonicida subsp. salmonicida*. *Journal of Fish Diseases* 2016;39(10):1165–1178.

8. Nougayrede, P., Sochon, E. and Vuillaume, A. Isolation of *Aeromonas subspecies salmonicida* in farmed turbot (*Psetta maxima*) in France. *Bulletin of the European Association of Fish Pathologists* 1990;10(5):139–140.

9. Coscelli, G.A., Bermúdez, R., Sancho, A.R., Ruíz, M.V. and Quiroga, M.I. Granulomatous dermatitis in turbot (*Scophthalmus maximus* L.) associated with natural *Aeromonas salmonicida subsp. salmonicida* infection. *Aquaculture* 2014;428–429:111–116.

10. Treasurer, J.W. and Laidler, L.A. *Aeromonas salmonicida* infection in wrasse (Labridae) used as cleaner fish on Atlantic salmon, *Salmo salar* L. farm. *Journal of Fish Diseases* 1994;17(2):155–161.

11. Willumsen, B. *Aeromonas salmonicida subsp. salmonicida* isolated from Atlantic cod and coalfish. *Bulletin of the European Association of Fish Pathologists* 1990;10(3):62–63.

12. Joseph, S.W. and Carnahan, A. The isolation, identification, and systematics of the motile *Aeromonas* species. *Annual Review of Fish Diseases* 1994;4:315–343.

13. Keeling, S.E., Brosnahan, C.L., Johnston, C., Wallis, R., Gudkovs, N. and McDonald, W.L. Development and validation of a real-time PCR assay for the detection of *Aeromonas salmonicida*. *Journal of Fish Diseases* 2013;36(5):495–503.

14. Sommerset, I., Krossøy, B., Biering, E. and Frost, P. Vaccines for fish in aquaculture. *Expert Review of Vaccines* 2005;4(1):89–101.

15. Skall HF, Lorenzen E, Kjær TE, Henriksen NH, Dalsgaard I, Madsen SB, Buchmann K, Krossøy B, and Lorenzen N. Danish sea reared rainbow trout suffer from furunculosis despite vaccination - How can applied research help to solve the problem? In: *Abstracts from DAFINET and ProFish Workshop*, København, Denmark, 2015.

16. Vincent, A.T., Tanaka, K.H., Trudel, M.V., Frenette, M., Derome, N. and Charette, S.J. Draft genome sequences of two *Aeromonas salmonicida subsp. salmonicida* isolates harboring plasmids conferring antibiotic resistance. *FEMS Microbiology Letters* 2015;362(4):1–4.

17. Tanaka, K.H., Vincent, A.T., Trudel, M.V., Paquet, V.E., Frenette, M. and Charette, S.J. The mosaic architecture of *Aeromonas salmonicida subsp. salmonicida* pAsa4 plasmid and its consequences on antibiotic resistance. *PeerJ Preprints* 2016, doi:10.7717/peerj.2595 (accessed 14 May 2017).

18. Smith, P. and Davey, S. Evidence for the competitive exclusion of *Aeromonas salmonicida* from fish with stress inducible furunculosis by a fluorescent pseudomonad. *Journal of Fish Diseases* 1993;16(5):521–524.

19. Gram, L., Løvold, T., Nielsen, J., Melchiorsen, J. and Spanggaard, B. In vitro antagonism of the probiont *Pseudomonas fluorescens* strain AH2 against *Aeromonas salmonicida* does not confer protection of salmon against furunculosis. *Aquaculture* 2001;199(1–2):1–11.

20. Cipriano, R.C., Bullock, G.L. and Pyle, S.W. *Aeromonas hydrophila and motile aeromonad septicemia of fish*. USFWS Fish Disease Leaflet 68, 1984.

21. Aoki, T. Motile aeromonads (*Aeromonas hydrophila*). In: *Fish Diseases and Disorders. Volume 3, Viral, Bacterial and Fungal Infections*. P.T.K. Woo and D.W. Bruno, eds. 1999; pp. 427–453.

22. Janda, J.M. and Abbott, S.L. The genus *Aeromonas*: Taxonomy, pathogenicity, and infection. *Clinical Microbiology Reviews* 2010;23:35–73.

23. Khardori, N. and Fainstein, V. *Aeromonas* and *Plesiomonas* as etiological agents. *Annual Review of Microbiology* 1988;42:395–419.

24. Corral F. del, Shotts E.B. and Brown J. Adherence, haemagglutination and cell surface characteristics of motile aeromonads virulent for fish. *Journal of Fish Diseases* 1990;13:255–268.

25. Huizinga, H.W., Esch, G.W. and Hazen, T.C. Histopathology of red-sore disease (*Aeromonas hydrophila*) in naturally and experimentally infected largemouth bass *Micropterus salmoides* (Lacepede). *Journal of Fish Diseases* 1979;2:263–277.

26. Evans, J.J., Klesius, P.H., Plumb, J.A. and Shoemaker, C.A. *Edwardsiella septicaemia*. In: *Fish Diseases and Disorders. Volume 3, Viral, Bacterial, and Fungal Pathogens*, 2nd ed. P.T.K. Woo and D.W. Bruno, eds. CABI, Cambridge, MA, 2011; pp. 512–569.

27. Griffin, M.J., Greenway, T.E. and Wise, D.J. *Edwardsiella* spp. In: *Fish Viruses and Bacteria: Pathobiology and Protection*. P.T.K. Woo and R.C. Cipriano, eds. CABI, Wallingford, UK, 2017; pp. 190–210.

28. Abayneh, T., Colquhoun, D.J. and Sørum, H. *Edwardsiella piscicida* sp. nov., a novel species pathogenic to fish. *Journal of Applied Microbiology* 2013; 114(3):644–654.

29. Shao, S., Lai, Q., Liu, Q., Wu, H., Xiao, J., Shao, Z., Wang, Q. and Zhang, Y. Phylogenomics characterization of a highly virulent *Edwardsiella* strain ET080813 T encoding two distinct T3SS and three T6SS gene clusters: Propose a novel species as *Edwardsiella anguillarum* sp. nov. *Systematic and Applied Microbiology* 2015;38(1):36–47.

30. Buján, N., Mohammed, H., Balboa, S., Romalde, J.L., Toranzo, A.E., Arias, C.R. and Magariños, B. Genetic studies to re-affiliate *Edwardsiella tarda* fish isolates to *Edwardsiella piscicida* and *Edwardsiella anguillarum* species. *Systematic and Applied Microbiology* 2017, doi:10.1016/j.syapm.2017.09.004 (accessed 11 December 2017).

31. Griffin, M.J., Ware, C., Quiniou, S.M., Steadman, J.M., Gaunt, P.S., Khoo, L.H. and Soto, E. *Edwardsiella piscicida* identified in the southeastern USA by *gyrB* sequence, species-specific and repetitive sequence-mediated PCR. *Diseases of Aquatic Organisms* 2014;108(1):23–25.

32. Reichley, S.R., Ware, C., Greenway, T.E., Wise, D.J. and Griffin, M.J. Real-time polymerase chain reaction assays for the detection and quantification of *Edwardsiella tarda*, *Edwardsiella piscicida*, and *Edwardsiella piscicida*-like species in catfish tissues and pond water. *Journal of Veterinary Diagnostic Investigation* 2015;27(2):130–139.

33. Reichley, S.R., Ware, C., Khoo, L.H., Greenway, T.E., Wise, D.J., Bosworth, B.G., Lawrence, M.L. and Griffin, M.J. Comparative susceptibility of channel catfish, *Ictalurus punctatus*, blue catfish, *Ictalurus furcatus*; and channel (♀) × blue (♂) hybrid catfish to *Edwardsiella piscicida*, *Edwardsiella tarda*, and *Edwardsiella anguillarum*. *Journal of the World Aquaculture Society* 2017, doi:10.1111/jwas.12467 (accessed 11 December 2017).

34. Baya, A.M., Romalde, J.L., Green, D.E., Navarro, R.B., Evans, J., May, E.B. and Toranzo, A.E. Edwardsiellosis in wild striped bass from the Chesapeake Bay. *Journal of Wildlife Diseases* 1997;33(3):517–525.

35. Francis-Floyd, R., Reed, P., Bolon, B., Estes, J. and McKinney, S. An epizootic of *Edwardsiella tarda* in largemouth bass (*Micropterus salmoides*). *Journal of Wildlife Diseases* 1993;29(2):334–336.

36. Amandi, A., Hiu, S.F., Rohovec, J.S. and Fryer, J.L. Isolation and characterization of *Edwardsiella tarda* from fall chinook salmon (*Oncorhynchus tshawytscha*). *Applied and Environmental Microbiology* 1982;43(6):1380–1384.

37. Lindquist, J.A. Medium and procedure for the direct, selective isolation of *Edwardsiella tarda* from environmental water samples. In: *Abstracts of the General Meeting of the American Society Microbiology*. AMS National Meeting, Dallas, Texas, 1991.

38. Castro, N., Toranzo, A.E., Nuñez, S. and Magariños, B. Evaluation of the selective and differential ET medium for detection of *Edwardsiella tarda* in aquaculture systems. *Letters in Applied Microbiology* 2011;53(1):114–119.

39. Park, S.B., Aoki, T. and Jung, T.S. Pathogenesis and strategies for preventing *Edwardsiella tarda* infection in fish. *Veterinary Research* 2012, http://veterinaryresearch.biomedcentral.com/articles/10.1186/1297-9716-43-67 (accessed 11 December 2017).

40. Klesius, P.H. and Pridgeon, J.W. Vaccination against enteric septicemia of catfish. In: *Fish Vaccination*. R. Gudding, A. Lillehaug and Ø. Evensen, eds. John Wiley & Sons, Chichester, UK, 2014; pp. 211–225.

41. Kelly, E., Martin, P.A.J., Gibson-Kueh, S. et al. First detection of *Edwardsiella ictaluri* (Proteobacteria: Enterobacteriaceae) in wild Australian catfish. *Journal of Fish Diseases* 2018;41(1):199–208.

42. Blanch, A.R., Pintó, R.M. and Jofre, J.T. Isolation and characterization of an *Edwardsiella* sp. strain, causative agent of mortalities in sea bass (*Dicentrarchus labrax*). *Aquaculture* 1990;88(3–4):213–222.

43. Popović, N.T., Hacmanjek, M. and Teskeredžić, E. Health status of rudd (*Scardinius erythrophthalmus hesperidicus* H.) in Lake Vrana on the Island of Cres, Croatia. *Journal of Applied Ichthyology* 2001;(1):43–45.

44. Soto, E., Griffin, M., Arauz, M., Riofrio, A., Martinez, A. and Cabrejos, M.E. *Edwardsiella ictaluri* as the causative agent of mortality in cultured Nile tilapia. *Journal of Aquatic Animal Health* 2012;24(2):81–90.

45. Taylor, P.W. Fish-eating birds as potential vectors of *Edwardsiella ictaluri*. *Journal of Aquatic Animal Health* 1992;4(4):240–243.

46. Shotts, E.B., Blazer, V.S. and Waltman, W.D. Pathogenesis of experimental *Edwardsiella ictaluri*

infections in channel catfish (*Ictalurus punctatus*). *Canadian Journal of Fisheries and Aquatic Sciences* 1986;43(1):36–42.

47. Hawke, J.P. A bacterium associated with disease of pond cultured channel catfish. *Journal of the Fisheries Research Board of Canada* 1979;36(12):1508–1512.

48. Hawke, J.P., Kent, M., Rogge, M., Baumgartner, W., Wiles, J., Shelley, J., Savolainen, L.C., Wagner, R., Murray, K. and Peterson, T.S. Edwardsiellosis caused by *Edwardsiella ictaluri* in laboratory populations of zebrafish *Danio rerio*. *Journal of Aquatic Animal Health* 2013;25(3):171–183.

49. Sakai, T., Kamaishi, T., Sano, M., Tensha, K., Arima, T., Iida, Y., Nagai, T., Nakai, T. and Iida, T. Outbreaks of *Edwardsiella ictaluri* infection in ayu *Plecoglossus altivelis* in Japanese rivers. *Fish Pathology* 2008;43(4):152–157.

50. Klesius, P., Lovy, J., Evans, J., Washuta, E. and Arias, C. Isolation of *Edwardsiella ictaluri* from tadpole madtom in a southwestern New Jersey river. *Journal of Aquatic Animal Health* 2003;15(4):295–301.

51. Shotts, E.B. and Waltman, W.D. A medium for the selective isolation of *Edwardsiella ictaluri*. *Journal of Wildlife Diseases* 1990;26(2):214–218.

52. Williams, M.L. and Lawrence, M.L. Verification of *Edwardsiella ictaluri*-specific diagnostic PCR. *Letters in Applied Microbiology* 2010;50(2):153–157.

53. Bilodeau, A.L., Waldbieser, G.C., Terhune, J.S., Wise, D.J. and Wolters, W.R. A real-time polymerase chain reaction assay of the bacterium *Edwarsiella ictaluri* in channel catfish. *Journal of Aquatic Animal Health* 2003;15(1):80–86.

54. Wise, D.J., Greenway, T.E., Byars, T.S., Griffin, M.J. and Khoo, L.H. Oral vaccination of channel catfish against enteric septicemia of catfish using a live attenuated *Edwardsiella ictaluri* isolate. *Journal of Aquatic Animal Health* 2015;27(2):135–143.

55. Bartholomew, J., Arkush, K.D. and Soto, E. Chapter 20: *Piscirickettsia salmonis*. In: *Fish Viruses and Bacteria Pathobiology and Protection*. P.T.K. Woo and C. Rocco, eds. CABI, Wallingford, UK, 2017; pp. 272–285.

56. Branson, E.J. and Nieto Diaz-Munoz, D. Description of new disease condition occurring in farmed coho salmon, *Oncorhynchus kisutch* (Walbaum), in South America. *Journal of Fish Diseases* 1991;14(2):147–156.

57. Smith, P.A., Pizarro, P., Ojeda, P., Contreras, J., Oyanedel, S. and Larenas, J. Routes of entry of *Piscirickettsia salmonis* in rainbow trout *Oncorhynchus mykiss*. *Diseases of Aquatic Organisms* 1999;37(3):165–172.

58. Smith, P.A., Rojas, M.E., Guajardo, A., Contreras, J., Morales, M.A. and Larenas, J. Experimental infection of coho salmon *Oncorhynchus kisutch* by exposure of skin, gills and intestine with *Piscirickettsia salmonis*. *Diseases of Aquatic Organisms* 2004;61(1–2):53–57.

59. Actis, L.A., Tolmasky, M.E. and Crosa, J.H. Vibriosis. In: *Fish Diseases and Disorders. Volume 3, Viral, Bacterial, and Fungal Pathogens*, 2nd ed. P.T. Woo and D.W. Bruno, eds. CABI, Cambridge, Massachusetts, 2011; pp. 570–605.

60. Colquhoun, D.J. and Lillehaug, A. Vaccination against vibriosis. In: *Fish Vaccination*. R. Gudding, A. Lillehaug and Ø. Evensen, eds. John Wiley & Sons, Chichester, UK, 2014; pp. 172–184.

61. Frans, I., Michiels, C.W., Bossier, P., Willems, K.A., Lievens, B. and Rediers, H. *Vibrio anguillarum* as a fish pathogen: Virulence factors, diagnosis and prevention. *Journal of Fish Diseases* 2011;34(9):643–661.

62. Bjelland, A.M., Johansen, R., Brudal, E., Hansen, H., Winther-Larsen, H.C. and Sørum, H. *Vibrio salmonicida* pathogenesis analyzed by experimental challenge of Atlantic salmon (*Salmo salar*). *Microbial Pathogenesis* 2012;52(1):77–84.

63. Løvoll, M., Wiik-Nielsen, C.R., Tunsjø, H.S., Colquhoun, D., Lunder, T., Sørum, H. and Grove, S. Atlantic salmon bath challenge with *Moritella viscosa*—Pathogen invasion and host response. *Fish & Shellfish Immunology* 2009;26(6):877–884.

64. Ruiz, P., Poblete, M., Yáñez, A.J., Irgang, R., Toranzo, A.E. and Avendaño-Herrera, R. Cell-surface properties of *Vibrio ordalii* strains isolated from Atlantic salmon *Salmo salar* in Chilean farms. *Diseases of Aquatic Organisms* 2015;113(1):9–23.

65. Toranzo, A.E., Magariños, B. and Avendaño-Herrera, R. Vibriosis: *Vibrio anguillarum*, *V. ordalii* and *Aliivibrio salmonicida*. In: *Fish Viruses and Bacteria: Pathobiology and Protection*. P.T.K. Woo and R.C. Cipriano, eds. CABI, Wallingford, UK, 2017; pp. 314–333.

66. Muroga, K., Jo, M. and Masumura, K. *Vibrio ordalii* isolated from diseased ayu (*Plecoglossus altivelis*) and rockfish (*Sebastes schlegeli*). *Fish Pathology* 1986;21(4): 239–243.

67. Akayli, T., Timur, G., Albayrak, G. and Aydemir, B. Identification and genotyping of *Vibrio ordalii*: A comparison of different methods. *The Israeli Journal of Aquaculture—Bamidgeh* 2010;62(1):9–18.

68. Haenen, O.L.M., Fouz, B., Amaro, C. et al. Vibriosis in aquaculture: 16th EAFP Conference, Tampere, Finland, 4th September 2013. *Bulletin of the European Association of Fish Pathologists* 2014;34(4):138–147.

69. Chatterjee, S. and Haldar, S. Vibrio related diseases in aquaculture and development of rapid and accurate identification methods. *Journal of Marine Science: Research & Development* 2012;S1:002.

70. Kashulin, A., Seredkina, N. and Sørum, H. Coldwater vibriosis. The current status of knowledge. *Journal of Fish Diseases* 2017;40(1):119–126.

71. Davis, H.S. Care and diseases of trout. *Research Report No. 12. US Department of the Interior. US Government Printing Office*, Washington DC, 1946.

72. Lorenzen, E., Dalsgaard, I., From, J., Hansen, E.M., Horlyck, V., Korsholm, H., Mellergaard, S. and Olesen, N.J. Preliminary investigations of fry mortality syndrome in rainbow trout. *Bulletin of the European Association of Fish Pathologists* 1991;11: 77–79.

73. Bernardet, J.F., Baudin-Laurencin, F. and Tixerant, G. First identification of "*Cytophaga psychrophila*" in France. *Bulletin of European Association of Fish Pathologists* 1988;8:104–105.

74. Starliper, C.E. Bacterial coldwater disease of fishes caused by *Flavobacterium psychrophilum*. *Journal of Advanced Research* 2011;2:97–108.

75. Madetoja, J., Nystedt, S. and Wiklund, T. Survival and virulence of *Flavobacterium psychrophilum* in water microcosms. *FEMS Microbiology Ecology* 2003;43(2): 217–223.

76. Holt, R.A. *Cytophaga psychrophila*, the causative agent of bacterial cold-water disease in salmonid fish. PhD thesis. Oregon State University, Corvallis, OR, 1987.

77. Brown, L.L., Cox, W.T. and Levine, R.P. Evidence that the causal agent of bacterial coldwater disease *Flavobacterium psychrophilum* is transmitted within salmonid eggs. *Diseases of Aquatic Organisms* 1997;29: 213–218.

78. Ekman, E., Borjeson, H. and Johansson, N. *Flavobacterium psychrophilum* in Baltic salmon *Salmo salar* brood fish and their offspring. *Diseases of Aquatic Organisms* 1999;37(3):159–163.

79. Cipriano, R.C. Intraovum infection caused by *Flavobacterium psychrophilum* among eggs from captive Atlantic salmon broodfish. *Journal of Aquatic Animal Health* 2005;17(3):275–283.

80. Cipriano, R.C. and Holt, R.A. *Flavobacterium psychrophilum*, cause of bacterial cold-water disease and rainbow trout fry syndrome. *Fish Disease Leaflet No. 86. United States Department of Interior*. US Geological Service, National Fish Health Research Laboratory, Kearneysville, WV, 2005.

81. Loch, T.P. and Faisal, M. Gamete-associated flavobacteria of the oviparous chinook salmon (*Oncorhynchus tshawytscha*) in lakes Michigan and Huron, North America. *Journal of Microbiology* 2016; 54(7):477–486.

82. Holt, R.A., Rohovec, J.S. and Fryer, J.L. Bacterial cold-water diseases. In: *Bacterial Diseases of Fish*. V. Inglis, R.J. Roberts and N.R. Bromage, eds. Blackwell, Oxford, UK, 1993; pp. 3–22.

83. Iida, Y. and Mizokami, A. Outbreaks of coldwater disease in wild ayu and pale chub. *Fish Pathology* 1996;31:157–164.

84. Lee, K.B. and Heo, G.J. First isolation and identification of *Cytophaga psychrophila* from cultured ayu in Korea. *Fish Pathology* 1998;33:37–38.

85. Nakayama, H., Tanaka, K., Teramura, N. and Hattori, S. Expression of collagenase in *Flavobacterium psychrophilum* isolated from cold-water disease-affected ayu (*Plecoglossus altivelis*). *Bioscience, Biotechnology and Biochemistry* 2015;80:135–144.

86. Lehmann, J., Mock, D., Stuerenberg, F.J. and Bernardet, J.F. First isolation of *Cytophaga psychrophila* from a systemic disease in eel and cyprinids. *Diseases of Aquatic Organisms* 1991;10:217–220.

87. Madetoja, J., Dalsgaard, I. and Wiklund, T. Occurrence of *Flavobacterium psychrophilum* in fish-farming environments. *Diseases of Aquatic Organisms* 2002;52:109–118.

88. Izumi, S., Liu, H., Aranishi, F. and Wakabayashi, H. A novel serotype of *Flavobacterium psychrophilum* detected using antiserum against an isolate from amago, *Oncorhynchus masou rhodurus* Jordan & Gilbert, in Japan. *Journal of Fish Diseases* 2003;26: 677–680.

89. Amita, K., Hoshino, A., Honma, T. and Wakabayashi, H. An investigation on the distribution of *Flavobacterium psychrophilum* in the Umikawa River. *Fish Pathology* 2000;35:193–197.

90. Elsayed, E.E., Eissa, A.E. and Faisal, M. Isolation of *Flavobacterium psychrophilum* from sea lamprey, *Petromyzon marinus* L. with skin lesions in Lake Ontario. *Journal of Fish Diseases* 2006;29(10):629–632.

91. Oidtmann, B., LaPatra, S.E., Verner-Jeffreys, D. et al. Differential characterization of emerging skin diseases of rainbow trout – a standardized approach to capturing disease characteristics and development of case definitions. *Journal of Fish Diseases* 2013;36: 921–937.

92. Madetoja, J., Nyman, P. and Wiklund, T. *Flavobacterium psychrophilum*, invasion into and shedding by rainbow trout *Oncorhynchus mykiss*. *Diseases of Aquatic Organisms* 2000;43(1):27–38.

93. Miranda, C.D., Smith, P., Rojas, R., Contreras-Lynch, S. and Vega, J.M.A. Antimicrobial susceptibility of *Flavobacterium psychrophilum* from Chilean salmon farms and their epidemiological cut-off values using agar dilution and disk diffusion methods. *Frontiers in Microbiology* 2016;7:1880.

94. Gómez, E., Méndez, J., Cascales, D. and Guijarro, J.A. *Flavobacterium psychrophilum* vaccine development: A difficult task. *Microbial Biotechnology* 2014;(5):414–423.

95. Davis, H.S. A new bacterial disease of fresh-water fishes. In: *Bulletin of the Bureau of Fisheries. Volume XXXVIII, Document 924*. US Government Printing Office, Washington DC, 1922; pp. 261–287.

96. Bernardet, J.F. and Bowman, J.P. The genus *Flavobacterium*. In: *The Prokaryotes: A Handbook on the Biology of Bacteria. Volume 7, Proteobacteria: Delta and Epsilon Subclasses. Deeply Rooting Bacteria*. M. Dworkin and S. Falkow, eds. Springer, New York, 2006; pp. 481–531.

97. Declercq, A.M., Haesebrouck, F., Van den Broeck, W., Bossier, P. and Decostere, A. Columnaris disease in fish: A review with emphasis on bacterium-host interactions. *Veterinary Research* 2013;44(1):27.

98. Bernardet, J.F., Segers, P., Vancanneyt, M., Berthe, M., Kersters, K. and Vandamme, P. Cutting a Gordian knot: Emended classification and description of the genus *Flavobacterium*, emended description of the family Flavobacteriaceae, and proposal of *Flavobacterium hydatis* nom. nov. (Basonym, *Cytophaga*

aquatilis Strohl and Tait 1978). *International Journal of Systematic Bacteriology* 1996;46:128–148.

99. Lange, M.D., Farmer, B.D., Declercq, A.M., Peatman, E., Decostere, A. and Beck, B.H. Sickeningly sweet: L-rhamnose stimulates *Flavobacterium columnare* biofilm formation and virulence. *Journal of Fish Diseases* 2017, doi:10.1111/jfd.12629.

100. Kunttu, H. Characterizing the bacterial fish pathogen *Flavobacterium columnare* and same factors affecting its pathogenicity. Academic dissertation, University of Jyväskilä, 2010.

101. Kunttu, H.M.T., Sundberg, L.R., Pulkkinen, K. and Valtonen, E.T. Environment may be the source of *Flavobacterium columnare* outbreaks at fish farms. *Environmental Microbiology Reports* 2012;4:398–402.

102. Cai, W., De La Fuente, L. and Arias, C.R. Biofilm formation by the fish pathogen *Flavobacterium columnare*: Development and parameters affecting surface attachment. *Applied Environmental Microbiology* 2013;79(18):5633–5642.

103. Wakabayashi, H. Columnaris disease. In: *Bacterial Diseases of Fish*. V. Inglis, R.J. Roberts and N.R. Bromage, eds. Blackwell, Oxford, UK, 1993; pp. 23–39.

104. La Frentz, B.R., Goodwin, A.E., Shoemaker, C.A. Columnaris disease. In: *FHS Blue Book: Suggested Procedures for the Detection and Identification of Certain Finfish and Shellfish Pathogens*. American Fisheries Society, Fish Health Section. 2014. http://afs-fhs.org/bluebook/bluebook-index.php.

105. Pacha, R.E. and Ordal, E.J. Myxobacterial diseases of salmonids. In: *A Symposium on Diseases of Fishes and Shellfishes, Volume 5*. S.F. Snieszko, ed. American Fisheries Society special publication, 1970; pp. 243–257.

106. Soto, E., Mauel, M.J., Karsi, A. and Lawrence, M.L. Genetic and virulence characterization of *Flavobacterium columnare* from channel catfish (*Ictalurus punctatus*). *Journal of Applied Microbiology* 2008;104(5):1302–1310.

107. Ferguson, H.W. Chapter 3 Skin. In: *Systemic Pathology of Fish*, 2nd ed. H.W. Ferguson, ed. Scottian Press, London, 2006; p. 69.

108. Wiens, G.D. Bacterial kidney disease (*Renibacterium salmoninarum*). In: *Fish Diseases and Disorders. Volume 3, Viral, Bacterial, and Fungal Pathogens*, 2nd ed. P.T.K. Woo and D.W. Bruno, eds. CABI, Cambridge, MA, 2011; pp. 338–374.

109. Elliott, D.G. *Renibacterium salmoninarum*. In: *Fish Viruses and Bacteria: Pathobiology and Protection*. P.T.K. Woo and R.C. Cipriano, eds. CABI, Wallingford, UK, 2017; pp. 286–297.

110. Ferguson, H.W. Chapter 3 Skin. In: *Systemic Pathology of Fish*, 2nd ed. H.W. Ferguson, ed. Scottian Press, London, 2006; pp. 77–78.

111. American Fisheries Society, Fish Health Section. *FHS Blue Book: Suggested Procedures for the Detection and Identification of Certain Finfish and Shellfish Pathogens*. AFS-FHS, 2016, https://units.fisheries.org/fhs/fish-health-section-blue-book-2016/.

112. Bruno, D.W., Noguera, P.A. and Poppe, T.T. *A Colour Atlas of Salmonid Diseases*, 2nd ed. Springer, London, 2013.

113. Sanders, J.E. and Fryer, J.L. *Renibacterium salmoninarum* gen. nov., sp. nov., the causative agent of bacterial kidney disease in salmonid fishes. *International Journal of Systematic Bacteriology* 1980;30(2):496–502.

114. Pascho, R.J., Elliott, D.G. and Chase, D.M. Comparison of traditional and molecular methods for detection of *Renibacterium salmoninarum*. In: *Molecular Diagnosis of Salmonid Diseases, Volume 3, Reviews: Methods and Technologies in Fish Biology and Fisheries*. C.O. Cunningham, ed. Kluwer Academic Publishers, Dordrecht, The Netherlands, 2002; pp. 157–209.

115. Evelyn, T.P.T., Prosperi-Porta, L. and Ketcheson, J.E. Persistence of the kidney-disease bacterium, *Renibacterium salmoninarum*, in coho salmon, *Oncorhynchus kisutch* (Walbaum), eggs treated during and after water-hardening with povidone-iodine. *Journal of Fish Diseases* 1986;9(5):461–464.

116. Elliott, D.G., Wiens, G.D., Hammell, K.L. and Rhodes, L.D. Vaccination against bacterial kidney disease. In: *Fish Vaccination*. R. Gudding, A. Lillehaug and Ø. Evensen, eds. John Wiley & Sons, Chichester, UK, 2014; pp. 255–272.

117. Evenden, A.J., Grayson, T.H., Gilpin, M.L. and Munn, C.B. *Renibacterium salmoninarum* and bacterial kidney disease: The unfinished jigsaw. *Annual Review of Fish Diseases* 1993;3:87–104.

118. Evelyn, T.P.T. Bacterial kidney disease—BKD. In: *Bacterial Diseases of Fish*. V. Inglis, R.J. Roberts and N.R. Bromage, eds. Halsted Press, New York, 1993; pp. 177–195.

119. OIE. Bacterial kidney disease (*Renibacterium salmoninarum*). In: *Manual of Diagnostic Tests for Aquatic Animals*, 4th ed. World Organisation for Animal Health (Office International des Épizooties), Paris, 2003; pp. 167–184.

120. Elliott, D.G., Pascho, R.J. and Bullock, G.L. Developments in the control of bacterial kidney disease of salmonid fishes. *Diseases of Aquatic Organisms* 1989;6:201–215.

121. Gudmundsdóttir, S., Helgason, S., Sigurjónsdóttir, H., Matthíasdóttir, S., Jónsdóttir, H., Laxdal, B. and Benediktsdóttir, E. Measures applied to control *Renibacterium salmoninarum* infection in Atlantic salmon: A retrospective study of two sea ranches in Iceland. *Aquaculture* 2000;186:193–203.

122. Meyers, T.R., Korn, D., Glass, K., Burton, T., Short, S., Lipson, K. and Starkey, N. Retrospective analysis of antigen prevalences of *Renibacterium salmoninarum* (Rs) detected by enzyme-linked immunosorbent assay in Alaskan Pacific salmon and trout from 1988 to 2000 and management of Rs in hatchery chinook and coho salmon. *Journal of Aquatic Animal Health* 2003;15(2):101–110.

123. Munson, A.D., Elliott, D.G. and Johnson, K. Management of bacterial kidney disease in chinook salmon hatcheries based on broodstock testing by enzyme-linked immunosorbent assay: A multiyear study. *North American Journal of Fisheries Management* 2010;30:940–955.

124. Faisal, M., Schulz, C., Eissa, A., Brenden, T., Winters, A., Whelan, G., Wolgamood, M., Eisch, E. and VanAmberg, J. Epidemiological investigation of *Renibacterium salmoninarum* in three *Oncorhynchus* spp. in Michigan from 2001 to 2010. *Preventive Veterinary Medicine* 2012;107:260–274.

125. Murray, A.G., Munro, L.A., Wallace, I.S., Allan, C.E.T., Peeler, E.J. and Thrush, M.A. Epidemiology of *Renibacterium salmoninarum* in Scotland and the potential for compartmentalised management of salmon and trout farming areas. *Aquaculture* 2012;324–325:1–13.

126. Hall, M., Soje, J., Kilburn, R., Maguire, S. and Murray, A.G. Cost-effectiveness of alternative management policies for bacterial kidney disease in Atlantic salmon aquaculture. *Aquaculture* 2014;434:88–92.

127. Gauthier, D.T. and Rhodes, M.W. Mycobacteriosis in fishes: A review. *The Veterinary Journal* 2009; 180(1):33–47.

128. Lewis, S. and Chinabut, S. Mycobacteriosis and nocardiosis. In: *Fish Diseases and Disorders. Volume 3, Viral, Bacterial, and Fungal Pathogens*, Second Edition. P.T.K. Woo and D.W. Bruno, eds. CABI, Cambridge, MA, 2011; pp. 397–423.

129. Decostere, A., Hermans, K. and Haesebrouck, F. Piscine mycobacteriosis: A literature review covering the agent and the disease it causes in fish and humans. *Veterinary Microbiology* 2004;99(3–4):159–166.

130. Francis-Floyd, R. Mycobacterial infections in fish. *Southern Regional Aquaculture SRAC Publication No. 4706*. Department of Agriculture, SRAC, Stoneville, MS, 2011. http://fisheries.tamu.edu/files/2013/09/SRAC-Publication-No.-4706-Mycobacterial-Infections-of-Fish.pdf.

131. Gauthier, D.T. and Rhodes, M.W. Mycobacterium spp. In: *Fish Viruses and Bacteria: Pathobiology and Protection*. P.T.K. Woo and R.C. Cipriano, eds. CABI, Wallingford, UK, 2017; pp. 245–257.

132. Kušar, D., Zajc, U., Jenčič, V., Ocepek, M., Higgins, J., Žolnir-Dovč, M. and Pate, M. Mycobacteria in aquarium fish: Results of a 3-year survey indicate caution required in handling pet-shop fish. *Journal of Fish Diseases* 2017;40(6):773–784.

133. Austin, B. and Austin, D.A. *Bacterial Fish Pathogens*, 5th ed. Springer, London, 2012.

134. Zhao, D., Yang, X.M., Chen, Q.Y., Zhang, X.S., Gu, C.J. and Che, X.Y. A modified acid-fast staining method for rapid detection of *Mycobacterium tuberculosis*. *Journal of Microbiological Methods* 2012;91(1):128–132.

135. Jacobs, J.W., Stine, C.B., Baya, A.M. and Kent, M.L. A review of mycobacteriosis in marine fish. *Journal of Fish Diseases* 2009;32(2):119–130.

136. Kaattari, I.M., Rhodes, M.W., Kaattari, S.L. and Shotts, E.B. The evolving story of *Mycobacterium tuberculosis* clade members detected in fish. *Journal of Fish Diseases* 2006;29(9):509–520.

137. Zerihun, M.A., Hjortaas, M.J., Falk, K. and Colquhoun, D.J. Immunohistochemical and Taqman real-time PCR detection of mycobacterial infections in fish. *Journal of Fish Diseases* 2011; 34(3):235–246.

138. Mainous, M.E. and Smith, S.A. Efficacy of common disinfectants against *Mycobacterium marinum*. *Journal of Aquatic Animal Health* 2005;17(3):284–288.

139. Kvitt, H., Heinisch, G. and Diamant, A. Detection and phylogeny of Lymphocystivirus in sea bream *Sparus aurata* based on the DNA polymerase gene and major capsid protein sequences. *Aquaculture* 2008;275(1–4):58–63.

140. Borrego, J.J., Valverde, E.J., Labella, A.M. and Castro, D. Lymphocystis disease virus: Its importance in aquaculture. *Reviews in Aquaculture* 2017; 9(2):179–193.

141. Zheng, F., Liu, H., Guo, X. and Wang, B. Isolation and identification of a new isolate of lymphocystis disease virus isolated from black rockfish (*Sebastes schlegelii*) in China. *Aquaculture* 2016; 451:340–344.

142. Lorenzen, K. and Dixon, P.F. Prevalence of antibodies to lymphocystis virus in estuarine flounder *Platichthys flesus*. *Diseases of Aquatic Organisms* 1991;11:99–103.

143. Nylund, S., Steigen, A., Karlsbakk, E., Plarre, H., Andersen, L., Karlsen, M., Watanabe, K. and Nylund, A. Characterization of "Candidatus Syngnamydia salmonis" (Chlamydiales, Simkaniaceae), a bacterium associated with epitheliocystis in Atlantic salmon (*Salmo salar* L.). *Archives of Microbiology* 2015;197:17–25.

144. van West, P. *Saprolegnia parasitica*, an oomycete pathogen with a fishy appetite: New challenges for an old problem. *Mycologist* 2006;20(3):99–104.

145. Bruno, D.W., van West, P. and Beakes, G. Saprolegnia and other oomycetes. In: *Fish Diseases and Disorders. Volume 3: Viral, Bacterial and Fungal Infections*, 2nd ed. P.T.K. Woo and D.W. Bruno, eds. CABI, Cambridge, Massachusetts, 2011; pp. 669–720.

146. van den Berg, A.H., McLaggan, D., Diéguez-Uribeondo, J. and van West, P. The impact of the water moulds *Saprolegnia diclina* and *Saprolegnia parasitica* on natural ecosystems and the aquaculture industry. *Fungal Biology Reviews* 2013;27(2):33–42.

147. Bly, J.E., Lawson, L.A., Szalai, A.J. and Clem, L.W. Environmental factors affecting outbreaks of winter saprolegniosis in channel catfish, *Ictalurus punctatus* (Rafinesque). *Journal of Fish Diseases* 1993;16(6):541–549.

148. Noga, E.J. Water mold infections of freshwater fish: Recent advances. *Annual Review of Fish Diseases* 1993;3:291–304.

149. Lamour, K.H., Win, J. and Kamoun, S. Oomycete genomics: New insights and future directions. *FEMS Microbiology Letters* 2007;274(1):1–8.

150. Thoen, E., Vrålstad, T., Rolén, E., Kristensen, R., Evensen, Ø and Skaar, I. Saprolegnia species in Norwegian salmon hatcheries: Field survey identifies *S. diclina* sub-clade IIIB as the dominating taxon. *Diseases of Aquatic Organisms* 2015;114(3):189–198.

151. Karunasagar, I., Karunasagar, I. and Otta, S.K. Disease problems affecting fish in tropical environments. *Journal of Applied Aquaculture* 2003;13(3–4):231–249.

152. Singhal, R.N., Jeet, S. and Davies, R.W. Experimental transmission of *Saprolegnia* and *Achlya* to fish. *Aquaculture* 1987;64(1):1–7.

153. Ali, S.E., Thoen, E., Vrålstad, T., Kristensen, R., Evensen, Ø and Skaar, I. Development and reproduction of *Saprolegnia* species in biofilms. *Veterinary Microbiology* 2013;163(1–2):133–141.

154. Choudhury, T.G., Singh, S.K., Parhi, J., Barman, D. and Das, B.S. Common fungal diseases of fish: A review. *Environment and Ecology* 2014;32(2):450–456.

155. Bly, J.E., Lawson, L.A., Dale, D.J., Szalai, A.J., Durborow, R.M. and Clem, L.W. Winter saprolegniosis in channel catfish. *Diseases of Aquatic Organisms* 1992;13:155–164.

156. Copland, J.W. and Willoughby, L.G. The pathology of *Saprolegnia* infections of *Anguilla anguilla* L. elvers. *Journal of Fish Diseases* 1982;5(5):421–428.

157. Kamilya, D. and Baruah, A. Epizootic ulcerative syndrome (EUS) in fish: History and current status of understanding. *Reviews in Fish Biology and Fisheries* 2014;24(1):369–380.

158. Yadav, M.K., Pradhan, P.K., Sood, N., Chaudhary, D.K., Verma, D.K., Chauhan, U.K., Punia, P. and Jena, J.K. Innate immune response against an oomycete pathogen *Aphanomyces invadans* in common carp (*Cyprinus carpio*), a fish resistant to epizootic ulcerative syndrome. *Acta Tropica* 2016;155:71–76.

159. Hussein, M.M., Hassan, W.H. and Mahmoud, M.H. Pathogenicity of *Achlya proliferoides* and *Saprolegnia diclina* (Saprolegniaceae) associated with saprolegniosis outbreaks in cultured Nile tilapia (*Oreochromis niloticus*). *World Journal of Fish and Marine Sciences* 2013;5(2):188–193.

160. Hatai, K. and Hoshiai, G. Mass mortality in cultured coho salmon (*Oncorhynchus kisutch*) due to *Saprolegnia parasitica* Coker. *Journal of Wildlife Diseases* 1992;28(4):532–536.

161. Bruno, D.W. and Stamps, D.J. Saprolegniasis of Atlantic salmon, *Salmo salar* L., fry. *Journal of Fish Diseases* 1987;10(6):513–517.

162. Fraser, G.C., Callinan, R.B. and Calder, L.M. Aphanomyces species associated with red spot disease: An ulcerative disease of estuarine fish from eastern Australia. *Journal of Fish Diseases* 1992;15(2):173–181.

163. Boys, C.A., Rowland, S.J., Gabor, M., Gabor, L., Marsh, I.B., Hum, S. and Callinan, R.B. Emergence of epizootic ulcerative syndrome in native fish of the Murray-Darling river system, Australia: Hosts, distribution and possible vectors. *PLOS ONE* 2012;7(4), doi:10.1371/journal.pone.0035568 (accessed 14 May 2017).

164. Beakes, G. and Ford, H. Esterase isoenzyme variation in the genus *Saprolegnia*, with particular reference to the fish-pathogenic *S. diclina-parasitica* complex. *Journal of General Microbiology* 1983;129(8):2605–2619.

165. Molina, F.I., Jong, S.C. and Ma, G. Molecular characterization and identification of *Saprolegnia* by restriction analysis of genes coding for ribosomal RNA. *Antonie van Leeuwenhoek* 1995;68(1):65–74.

166. Lilley, J.H., Callinan, R.B., Chinabut, S., Kanchanakan, S., Macrae, I.H. and Phillips, M.J. *Epizootic ulcerative syndrome (EUS) Technical Handbook*. Aquatic Animal Health Research Institute, Bangkok, 1998.

167. Vandersea, M.W., Litaker, R.W., Yonnish, B. et al. Molecular assays for detecting *Aphanomyces invadans* in ulcerative mycotic fish lesions. *Applied and Environmental Microbiology* 2006;72(2):1551–1557.

168. Waterstrat, P.R. and Marking, L.L. Communications: Clinical evaluation of formalin, hydrogen peroxide, and sodium chloride for the treatment of *Saprolegnia parasitica* on fall chinook salmon eggs. *The Progressive Fish-Culturist* 1995;57(4):287–291.

169. Gieseker, C.M., Serfling, S.G. and Reimschuessel, R. Formalin treatment to reduce mortality associated with *Saprolegnia parasitica* in rainbow trout, *Oncorhynchus mykiss*. *Aquaculture* 2006;253(1–4):120–129.

170. Leal, J.F., Neves, M.G., Santos, E.B. and Esteves, V.I. Use of formalin in intensive aquaculture: Properties, application and effects on fish and water quality. *Reviews in Aquaculture* 2016, doi:10.1111/raq.12160 (accessed 14 May 2017).

171. Anders, K. and Yoshimizu, M. Role of viruses in the induction of skin tumours and tumour-like proliferations of fish. *Diseases of Aquatic Organisms* 1994;19:215–232.

172. Getchell, R.G., Casey, J.W. and Bowser, P.R. Seasonal occurrence of virally induced skin tumors in wild fish. *Journal of Aquatic Animal Health* 1998;10(2):191–201.

173. Coffee, L.L., Casey, J.W. and Bowser, P.R. Pathology of tumors in fish associated with retroviruses: A review. *Veterinary Pathology* 2013;50(3):390–403.

174. Kinae, N., Yamashita, M., Tomita, I., Kimura, I., Ishida, H., Kumai, H. and Nakamura, G. A possible correlation between environmental chemicals and pigment cell neoplasia in fish. *The Science of the Total Environment* 1990;94(1–2):143–153.

175. Hedrick, R.P., Groff, J.M., Okihiro, M.S. and McDowell, T.S. Herpesviruses detected in papillomatous skin growths of koi carp (*Cyprinus carpio*). *Journal of Wildlife Diseases* 1990;26(4):578–581.

176. Hanson, L., Dishon, A. and Kotler, M. Herpesviruses that infect fish. *Viruses* 2011;3(11):2160–2191.

177. Glenney, G.W., Barbash, P.A. and Coll, J.A. A quantitative polymerase chain reaction assay for the detection and quantification of epizootic epitheliotropic disease virus (EEDV; Salmonid Herpesvirus 3). *Journal of Aquatic Animal Health* 2016;28(1): 56–67.

178. Hanson, L., Doszploy, A., van Beurden, S.J., de Oliveira, P.H. and Waltzek, T. Alloherpesviruses of fish. In: *Aquaculture Virology*. F. Kibenge and M. Godoy, eds. Academic Press, London, 2016; pp. 1–32.

179. Mulcahy, M.F. and O'Leary, A. Cell-free transmission of lymphosarcoma in northern pike *Esox lucius* L. *(Pisces; Esocidae) Experientia* 1970;26:891.

180. McAllister, P.E. and Herman, R.L. Epizootic mortality in hatchery-reared lake trout *Salvelinus namaycush* caused by a putative virus possibly of the herpesvirus group. *Diseases of Aquatic Organisms* 1989;6(2): 113–119.

181. Yoshimizu, M. and Kasai, H. Oncogenic viruses and oncorhynchus masou virus. In: *Fish Diseases and Disorders. Volume 3, Viral, Bacterial and Fungal Infections*, 2nd ed. P.T.K. Woo and D.W. Bruno, eds. CABI, Cambridge, Massachusetts, 2011; pp. 276–301.

182. Carlisle, J.C. and Roberts, R.J. An epidermal papilloma of the Atlantic salmon I: Epizootiology, pathology and immunology. *Journal of Wildlife Diseases* 1977;13(3):230–234.

183. Roberts, R.J. and Bullock, A.M. Papillomatosis in marine cultured rainbow trout *Salmo gairdneri* Richardson. *Journal of Fish Diseases* 1979;2(1):75–77.

184. Bylund, G., Valtonen, E.T. and Niemelä, E. Observations on epidermal papillomata in wild and cultured Atlantic salmon *Salmo salar* L. in Finland. *Journal of Fish Diseases* 1980;3(6):525–528.

185. Calle, P.P., McNamara, T. and Kress, Y. Herpesvirus-associated papillomas in koi carp (*Cyprinus carpio*). *Journal of Zoo and Wildlife Medicine* 1999;30(1): 165–169.

186. Yu, J., Kim, D.W. and Park, S.W. Epidermal papilloma on the snout of cultured eel, *Anguilla japonica* (Temminck and Schlegel, 1847) in Korea. *World Journal of Fish and Marine Sciences* 2014;6(1):119–123.

187. Ottensen, O.H., Noga, E.J. and Amin, A. Histopathology of culture-associated skin erosions and papillary hyperplasia of Atlantic halibut, *Hippoglossus hippoglossus* (L.). *Journal of Fish Diseases* 2010;33(6):489–496.

188. Martineau, D., Bowser, P.R., Renshaw, R.R. and Casey, J.W. Molecular characterization of a unique retrovirus associated with a fish tumor. *Journal of Virology* 1992;66(1):596–599.

189. Martineau, D., Bowser, P.R., Wooster, G. and Forney, J.L. Histologic and ultrastructural studies of dermal sarcoma of walleye (Pisces: *Stizostedion vitreum*). *Veterinary Pathology* 1990;27(5):340–346.

190. Jawad, L.A. and Al-Kharusi, L.H. A reported case of abnormal pigmentation in the epaulet grouper

191. *Epinephelus stoliczkae* (Day, 1875) collected from the Sea of Oman. *Anales de Biología* 2013;35:41–44.

191. Muto, N., Takayama, K. and Kai, Y. First record of abnormal body coloration in a rockfish *Sebastes trivittatus* (Scorpaenoidei: Sebastidae). *Ichthyological Research* 2016;63(1):197–199.

192. Sweet, M., Kirkham, N., Bendall, M., Currey, L., Bythell, J. and Heupel, M. Evidence of melanoma in wild marine fish populations. *PLOS ONE* 2012;7(4), doi:10.1371/journal.pone.0041989 (accessed 14 May 2017).

193. Bruno, D.W. and Mitchell, C.G. Branchial chondroma from farmed Atlantic salmon, *Salmo salar* L. *Bulletin of The European Association of Fish Pathologists* 1995;15(3):107–108.

194. Sirri, R., Mandrioli, L., Bacci, B., Morini, M. and Bettini, G. Snout chondroma in a neon tetra *Paracheirodon innesi*. *Fish Pathology* 2010;45(2): 84–87.

195. Mesbah, M., Rezaie, A. and Dezfuly, T. Case report of chondroma in a grass carp (*Ctenopharyngodon idella*). *Veterinary Research Forum* 2016;7(2):173–176.

196. Aso, Y., Wani, J., Klenner, D.A. and Yoshimizu, M. Detection and identification of *Oncorhynchus masou* virus (OMV) disease by polymerase chain reaction (PCR). *Bulletin of Fisheries Sciences, Hokkaido University* 2001;52(2):111–116.

197. Ciulli, S., Pinheiro, A., Volpe, E., Moscato, M., Jung, T.S., Galeotti, M., Stellino, S., Farneti, R. and Prosperi, S. Development and application of a real-time PCR assay for the detection and quantitation of lymphocystis disease virus. *Journal of Virological Methods* 2015;213:164–173.

198. Valverde, E.J., Cano, I., Labella, A., Borrego, J.J. and Castro, D. Application of a new real-time polymerase chain reaction assay for surveillance studies of lymphocystis disease virus in farmed gilthead seabream. *BMC Veterinary Research* 2016;12:71, doi:10.1186/s12917-016-0696-6 (accessed 14 May 2017).

199. Garcia-Rosado, E., Castro, D., Cano, I., Pérez-Prieto, S.I. and Borrego, J.J. Serological techniques for detection of lymphocystis virus in fish. *Aquatic Living Resources* 2002;15(3):179–185.

200. Yoshimizu, M. and Nomura, T. Oncorhynchus masou virus (OMV) epidemiology and its control strategy. *Bulletin of National Research Institute of Aquaculture* 2001;Suppl. 5:11–14.

201. Hemdal, J.F. A reported case of head and lateral line erosion (HLLE), potentially caused by a bacterial infection in a marine angelfish. *Drum and Croaker* 1989;22:2–3.

202. Varner, P. and Lewis, D. Characterization of a virus associated with head and lateral line erosion syndrome in marine angelfish. *Aquatic Animal Health* 1991;3:198–205.

203. Gardner, G.R. and LaRoche, G. Copper induced lesions in estuarine teleosts. *Journal of the Fisheries Research Board of Canada* 1973;30:363–367.

204. Morrison, C.M., O'Neil, D. and Wright, J.R. Jr. Histopathology of "hole-in-the-head" disease in the Nile tilapia, *Oreochromis niloticus*. *Aquaculture* 2007;273:427–433.

205. Hemdal, J. and Odum, R.A. The role of activated lignite carbon in the development of head and lateral line erosion in the ocean surgeon. *North American Journal of Aquaculture* 2011;73(4):489–492.

206. Stamper, M.A., Kittell, M.M., Patel, E.E. and Corwin, A.L. Effects of full-stream carbon filtration on the development of head and lateral line erosion syndrome (HLLES) in ocean surgeon. *Journal of Aquatic Animal Health* 2011;23(3):111–116.

207. Bullock A.M. 1988. Solar ultraviolet radiation: A potential environmental hazard in the cultivation of farmed finfish. In: *Recent Advances in Aquaculture, Volume 3*. J.E. Muir and R.J. Roberts, eds. Croom Helm, Beckenham, Kent, UK, pp. 139–224.

208. Noceda, C., Sierra, S.G. and Martinez, J.L. Histopathology of UV-B irradiated brown trout *Salmo trutta* skin. *Diseases of Aquatic Organisms* 1997;31: 103–108.

209. Bullock, A.M. and Roberts, R.J. Sunburn lesions in salmonid fry: A clinical and histological report. *Journal of Fish Diseases* 1981;4:271–275.

210. DeLong, D.C., Halver, J.E. and Yasutake, W.T. A possible cause of sunburn in fish. The *Progressive Fish-Culturist* 1959;21(3):111–113.

211. Aquaflor. Product bulletin. 2016. Merck Animal Health, http://www.aquaflor-usa.com/pdfs/Aquaflor_ Product_Bulletin_FINAL.pdf.

212. Dunbar, C.E. Sunburn in fingerling rainbow trout. *The Progressive Fish-Culturist* 1959;21:74.

213. Bullock, A.M., Roberts, R.J., Waddington, P. and Bookless, W.D.A. Sunburn lesions in koi carp. *Veterinary Record* 1983;112(23):551.

214. Ramos, K.T., Fries, L.T., Berkhouse, C.S. and Fries, J.N. Apparent sunburn of juvenile paddlefish. *The Progressive Fish-Culturist* 1994;56:214–216.

215. Hoffman, G.L. *Parasites of North American Freshwater Fishes*. Cornell University Press, Ithaca, NY, 1999.

216. Woo, P.T.K. and Buchmann, K. *Fish Parasites: Pathobiology and Protection*. CAB International, London, 2012; p. 383.

217. Lom, J. and Dykova, I. Protozoan parasites of fishes. In: *Developments in Aquaculture and Fisheries Science*, Volume 26. Elsevier Science, Amsterdam, 1992; p. 316.

218. Smith, S.A. and Noga, E.J. General Parasitology of Fish. In: *Fish Medicine*. M.K. Stoskopf, ed. W.B. Saunders, Philadelphia, 1992; pp. 131–148.

219. Longshaw, M. and Feist, S.W. Parasitic diseases. In: *BSAVA Manual of Ornamental Fish*, 2nd edition. W.H. Wildgoose, ed. British Small Animal Veterinary Association, Gloucester, UK, 2001; pp. 167–183.

220. Bruno, D.W., Nowak, B. and Elliott, D.G. Guide to the identification of fish protozoan and metazoan parasites in stained tissue sections. *Diseases of Aquatic Organisms* 2006;70:1–36.

221. Dickerson, H.W. *Ichthyophthirius multifiliis* and *Cryptocaryon irritans* (Phylum Ciliophora). In: *Fish Diseases and Disorders*. Volume 1, Protozoan and Metazoan Infections. P.T.K. Woo, ed. CAB International, Wallingford, UK, 2006; pp. 116–153.

222. Hines, R.S. and Spira, D.T. Ichthyophthiriasis in the mirror carp *Cyprinus carpio* (L.) III. Pathology. *Journal of Fish Biology* 1974;6:189–196.

223. Feist, S.W. and Longshaw, M. Phylum Myxozoa. In: *Fish Diseases and Disorders*. Volume 1, Protozoan and Metazoan Infections. P.T.K. Woo, ed. CAB International, Wallingford, UK, 2006; pp. 230–296.

224. Lester, R.J.G. and Hayward, C.J. Phylum Arthropoda. In: *Fish Diseases and Disorders Volume 1: Protozoan and Metazoan Infections*. P.T.K. Woo, ed. CAB International, Wallingford, UK, 2006; pp. 466–565.

225. Sarig, S. *Disease of Fishes. Book 3, The Prevention and Treatment of Diseases of Warmwater Fishes under Subtropical Conditions, with Special Emphasis on Intensive Fish Farming*. TFH Publications, Neptune City, NJ, 1971; p. 127.

226. Hoffman, G.L. and Lester, R.J.G. Crustacean parasites of fish. *International Journal for Parasitology* 1987;17:1030–1031.

227. Dempster, R.P., Morales, P. and Glennon, F.X. Use of sodium chlorite to combat anchor worm infestation of fish. *The Progressive Fish-Culturist* 1988;50:51–55.

CHAPTER 6

GILL DISEASES

STEPHEN A. SMITH

KOI HERPESVIRUS

Overview: Koi herpesvirus (KHV) disease is a highly contagious viral disease of feral and cultivated carp, especially ornamental varieties (i.e., koi).[1–4]

Etiological agent: The cause of KHV is cyprinid herpesvirus-3 (CyHV-3), an enveloped herpesvirus in the family Alloherpesviridae.[5] This virus has also been known as carp interstitial nephritis and gill necrosis virus.[1]

Route of transmission: All age groups of carp appear to be susceptible to KHV, but younger fish up to 1 year of age appear to be more susceptible to clinical disease.[6,7] Transmission of KHV is horizontal with virus from infected fish shed in the feces, urine, sloughed gill cells and skin mucus.[1] The virus is spread through the water; however, other fish species, invertebrates, piscivorous birds and mammals may also be involved in the transmission of the virus.[1] The virus remains active in water for at least 4 hours at water temperatures of 23°C–25°C.[8]

Host range: Natural infections of KHV have only been reported in common carp (*Cyprinus carpio*), varieties of the species (e.g., koi carp) and some carp × goldfish hybrids.[1,9–11] Other cyprinids such as goldfish (*Carassius auratus*) and grass carp (*Ctenopharyngodon idella*) may harbor the virus but generally do not show clinical signs of disease.[12]

Clinical presentation: Though the clinical signs of KHV are generally nonspecific, one of the most common clinical signs associated with KHV infections in koi are gill lesions including areas of hemorrhage, inflammation, sloughing of gill epithelium and necrosis (**Figure 6.1**). In most cases, accompanying secondary bacterial and parasitic protozoal and monogenean infections may be the most obvious gill pathogen.[2,3,13] Other external signs of KHV may include excessive mucus production,

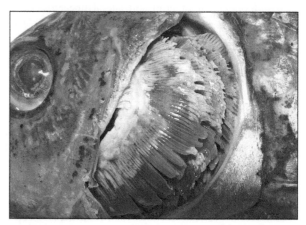

Figure 6.1 Necrotic gill lesions in a koi infected with koi herpesvirus (KHV) disease. (Image courtesy of J. Haugland.)

endophthalmia (i.e., sunken eyes), pale areas to ulcerations of the skin and hemorrhage of the fins. The disease is temperature dependent, occurring between 16°C and 25°C.[2,3,7,8] Morbidity can reach 100% in susceptible populations, whereas mortality is typically 70%–80%, but can be as high as 90%–100%.[3,10]

Pathology of disease: The virus primarily enters fish through the epithelium of the skin and gill tissue.[14] Gill, kidney, spleen, liver and pancreas are the organs in which KHV is most abundant during the course of an overt infection where inflammatory infiltrates and necrosis are evident.[15–17] The loss of osmoregulatory function of the gill, kidney and intestine contribute to the observed mortality.[15] Survivors of KHV are considered chronically infected and have been shown to intermittently shed the virus when temperatures are permissive.[18]

Differential diagnoses: This disease must be differentiated from other viral diseases of carp (e.g., spring viremia of carp), and other bacterial and parasitic infections of the gill.[4,19]

Diagnosis: Cell culture isolation of KHV has been used in the past but is not considered to be as sensitive as current polymerase chain reaction (PCR)–based methods.[3] Immunodiagnostic methods (e.g., ELISA and immunofluorescence tests) have also been used for the diagnosis of KHV.[3]

Management/control: There is no chemotherapeutic treatment for KHV disease and an effective vaccine is currently not available. Thus, avoiding exposure to the virus along with a good biosecurity and quarantine program are probably the best methods for prevention of the disease. Raising the water temperature above the submissive temperatures has been shown to decrease mortalities, but survivors are considered chronic carriers of the virus. Depopulation of the remaining exposed individuals of an infected population should be considered. All systems and equipment exposed to the infection should be sanitized with an appropriate disinfectant.[20]

BACTERIAL GILL DISEASE

Overview: A superficial bacterial disease of the gills of cultured salmonids.

Etiological agent: The infectious agent of bacterial gill disease (BGD) is *Flavobacterium branchiophilium*, a yellow-pigmented, Gram-negative, nonmotile, rod-shaped bacterium.[21,22]

Route of transmission: *Flavobacterium branchiophilium* is highly contagious to salmonids with the bacteria readily adhering to gill tissue.[23] The bacterium is ubiquitous in the water and can persist in the water and sediment. Fish in the water source may also contribute as reservoirs of the bacteria.[23] Bacterial gill disease typically occurs in association with environmental stressors such as overcrowding, overfeeding, low dissolved oxygen, inadequate water flow, elevated ammonia levels, increased organic matter in tanks or raceways, and increased turbidity of water.[23]

Host range: Bacterial gill disease has a broad salmonid host range and worldwide distribution; basically the disease can be found almost everywhere salmonids are intensively culture. In addition to salmonids, *F. branchiophilium* has been reported to cause disease in walleye (*Stizostedion vitreum*), rohu (*Labeo rohita*), catla (*Catla catla*), silver carp (*Hypophthalmichthys molitrix*) *and* common shiners (*Luxilus cornutus*).[22,24–27]

Clinical presentation: Clinical signs of BGD include lethargy, loss of appetite and signs of respiratory distress (e.g., gasping at the surface of the water, orientation facing into the flow of water).[23] The bacteria primarily colonizes the external surface of the gill tissue with gill filaments appearing pale and swollen. The infection is not generally associated with the yellow mucoid exudate typical of columnaris (*F. columnare*) infections in warm-water fish.

Pathology of disease: There may be hyperplasia and hypertrophy of gill epithelium, fusion of lamellae and clubbing of gill filaments.[28] Severe infections may exhibit mucus cell hyperplasia, epithelial cell degeneration and necrosis.[29,30] Body surface lesions are not typical.[23]

Differential diagnosis: Differentials would include diseases causing gill pathology in salmonids and other fish such as columnaris (*F. columnare*), protozoan parasites, monogeneans and fungal infections.

Diagnosis: A presumptive diagnosis can be made from the characteristic behavior demonstrated by the fish, previous facility history and the presence of Gram-negative filamentous rod-shaped bacteria in wet mounts. Histopathology will show epithelial hyperplasia, clubbing and fusion of gill lamellae, and accumulations of long, thin Gram-negative bacteria. A definitive diagnosis is based on isolation of the bacteria on the selective media Cytophaga agar.[31] Serologic and PCR assays have also been developed but are primarily used for research.[32–36]

Management/control: Control is based on good management principles of optimizing water quality and reducing stresses, i.e., reducing overcrowding, not overfeeding, and removal of detritus and uneaten feed from tanks or raceways.

COLUMNARIS

Overview: A localized bacterial infection of the gills, skin and fins or a systemic infection of freshwater fish, especially warm water species.

Etiology: The disease, commonly called "columnaris" or "columnaris disease," is caused by *Flavobacterium columnare*, a Gram-negative, yellow-pigmented bacteria[37–39] (see Chapter 5).

Host range: Columnaris affects a wide range of wild and cultured freshwater fish and it is presumed

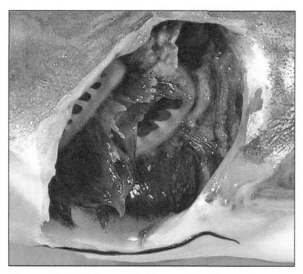

Figure 6.2 Columnaris disease (*Flavobacterium columnare*) showing necrosis of lamellae and yellowish mucoid mass of bacteria on gills of a channel catfish (*Ictalurus punctatus*). (Image courtesy of L. Khoo.)

that all warm- and cool-freshwater species are susceptible, and less commonly are cold water-species susceptible.[39]

Route of transmission: The bacteria are transmitted horizontally through the water or by direct contact. This typically opportunistic fish pathogen appears to be ubiquitous and distributed worldwide in freshwater aquatic environments.[39,40]

Clinical presentation: The lesions are usually confined to the gills, skin (i.e., "saddle-back" presentation) and fins. Lesions on the gills usually extend from the distal tips of the lamellae and progress toward the base, and chronically infected tissues often become necrotic. Gill lesions are usually covered with a yellowish mucoid mass consisting mostly of *F. columnare* colonies (**Figure 6.2**).[39,41]

Pathology: Histopathology shows the epithelium of the lamellae becomes dissociated from the capillary bed due to the edematous accumulation of fluids.[42] The associated blood vessels become congested and there are scattered masses of Gram-negative bacteria throughout the epithelium.[42]

Differential diagnosis: As both *Flavobacterium columnare* and *F. branchiophilium* cause gill pathology, these two related pathogens should be differentiated based presumptively on species affected (i.e., warm-water vs. cold-water fish), and the presence or

absence of yellowish material and necrotic gill tissues. Additional possible etiologies include viral, bacterial and parasitic infections, as well as noninfectious problems such as poor water quality, chemical toxicants and trauma.

Diagnosis: A suggestive history, clinical signs and gross pathology consistent with columnaris are usually sufficient for a preliminary diagnosis. The presence of long slender, flexing bacteria in typical "haystack" aggregations in wet mounts of affected gill tissue or other lesions supports the presumptive diagnosis. Specific identification of the causative agent requires isolation on Cytophaga, Hsu-Shotts or TYES (tryptone yeast extract salts) agar followed by standard biochemical, serological or molecular assays.

Management/control: The best approach to control columnaris is through good management by optimizing water quality and reducing stresses, i.e., reducing fish densities, reducing organic load, and removal of detritus and uneaten feed from tanks or raceways. In addition, there are a number of chemicals (i.e., oxidizing agents and quaternary ammonias) and one approved therapeutic (i.e., Aquaflor) that have been used to treat this disease in captive fish.

Epitheliocystis

Overview: A typically chronic benign infectious disease characterized by cysts in the gill epithelium of wild or farmed fish.

Etiological agent: The causative agents of this disease are Gram-negative intracellular chlamydia-like bacteria that are part of the order Chlamydiales.[43–45] Recent research has shown that other organisms may also produce "epitheliocystis-like" lesions in the gills of fish.[46,47]

Route of transmission: Though not proven, horizontal transmission through the water is the assumed route of transmission. Presumably the cysts rupture and release the infectious agent into the water.

Host range: Disease of freshwater, marine and anadromous fish of more than 20 families (i.e., 90+ species) from both warm- and cold-water environments.[48–50]

Clinical presentation: Clinical signs of overt infections include lethargy, flared opercula, increased gill mucus and increased respiratory rates. Cysts may appear as transparent to white elongated nodules along the gill filaments. Although the gills are the most frequent site of infection, epithelial tissues of the skin, pseudobranch and esophagus may also be affected.[45]

Pathology of disease: Epitheliocystis is characterized by cysts in the branchial epithelia of the host. Cysts may also be found as an incidental finding in individuals without clinical disease. Cysts are hypertrophic host cells (i.e., mucus, chloride and epithelial cells) filled with the chlamydia-like organisms.[45] The host response is generally limited, and there is usually little to no mortality associated with most infections. However, proliferative infections may cause severe mortalities in cultured juvenile fish.[51,52]

Differential diagnosis: This disease must be differentiated from cysts having a viral etiology, or from cysts caused by opisthokonts (e.g., *Dermocystidium* sp.), protozoans (e.g., *Ichthyophthirius multifiliis, Loma* sp.) or bacterial pathogens.

Diagnosis: Squash preparations of gill tissue show a cyst with a thick capsule and homogeneous basophilic granular contents.[45] Although histopathology may be used to provide a definitive diagnosis, no serological methods are available for the specific diagnosis of these infections. Electron microscopy is required for a specific diagnosis where the intracellular forms can be distinguished.[46,53,54]

Management/control: There are a few anecdotal reports of chemotherapeutics being used to treat this disease, but control efforts generally focus on reducing stressful environmental conditions such as decreasing stocking densities, reducing nutrient loads and reducing large salinity changes.[45,47,55]

BRANCHIOMYCOSIS

Overview: A localized to diffuse fungal disease, commonly called "gill rot," of the gill tissue of freshwater fish.[56,57]

Etiological agent: There are primarily two species of *Branchiomyes* that are responsible for this disease and includes *B. sanguinis* and *B. demigrans*. Both species produce branched, non-septate hyphae.

Route of transmission: Fungal spores are released into the water and transmitted horizontally to other fish. Spores adhere to the gill tissue, germinate and

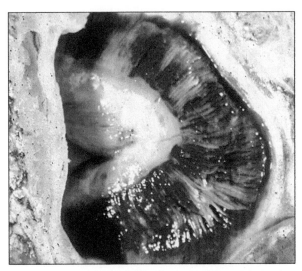

Figure 6.3 Necrotic gill lesions in a cultured hybrid tilapia (*Oreochromis* spp.) infected with *Branchiomyces* sp.

produce hyphae, which penetrate the epithelium and blood vessels of the gill.

Host range: Most species of freshwater fish are susceptible to branchiomycosis, though those cultured in intensive production systems are predisposed to the disease. Outbreaks have been reported in tilapia, carp, channel catfish and eels.[58–61]

Clinical presentation: The fish becomes lethargic, anorexic, and shows signs of respiratory distress (e.g., increased opercular rates, gulping at the water surface). The gills develop areas of paleness (i.e., ischemia), swollen gill filaments, and as the disease progresses, areas of hemorrhage and necrosis (**Figure 6.3**).

Pathology of disease: The disease is characterized by focal areas of infarctive necrosis of the gills. Fungal hyphae develop in lamellar epithelium or penetrate blood vessels causing obstruction, thrombosis and necrosis of gill tissues. In channel catfish, infection of the blood vessels is primarily confined to the gill arches and the base of the primary lamellae.[60] This intravascular hyphal infection occludes the blood vessels presumably decreasing respiratory efficiency of the gill.[60]

Differential diagnosis: Numerous viral, bacterial and parasitic diseases cause similar lesions that are limited to the gill tissue.

Diagnosis: The diagnosis is based on clinical signs, macroscopic and microscopic examination of the gill tissue. The fungus can be cultured on Sabouraud dextrose agar at 25°C–32°C followed by speciation based on morphological or molecular identification.

Management/control: Reducing stress in the fish by decreasing population densities, reducing feeding rates, increasing aeration and increasing water exchanges may lessen the clinical effects of the infection. Removal of morbid and dead fish, and strict sanitation and disinfection procedures are essential for disease control.

SAPROLEGNIA

Overview: An opportunistic, saprophytic infection of the gills of wild and cultured fish caused by one or more genera of water molds of the class Oomycetes (see "Oomycetes" in Chapter 5).

Etiology: There are numerous oomycete fish pathogens including the genera *Saprolegnia*, *Aphanomyces* and *Achlya*.[60,62–64] Several of the *Saprolegnia* spp. are significant pathogens of the gills of fish, with *S. diclina* and *S. parasitica* being the most commonly reported.[65,66]

Route of transmission: Free-swimming zoospores are released into the water from the spore cluster at the tip of the mature zoosporangium.[62,64] The zoospores attach to areas of epithelial abrasion of the gill and skin of a fish where the spore germinates producing hyphae.[62,64]

Host range: As *Saprolegnia* spp. has little host specificity, it is presumed that all freshwater fish, and some brackish water fish, are susceptible to infection.

Clinical presentation: Focal to generalized *Saprolegnia* lesions are easily identified by their superficial whitish cotton- or wool-like tufts of mycelium that are generally restricted to the surface of the gill, fins or skin (**Figure 6.4**). Sometimes the hyphal mass of a *Saprolegnia* infection will have a red, brown or gray appearance due to particles and other debris in the water that become trapped within the mycelial growth.

Pathology: Hyphae of *Saprolegnia* spp. rarely penetrate the deeper tissues of the fish, unlike *Aphanomyces invadans* or the *Branchiomyes* spp. that typically penetrate the deeper tissues of the gill. Infection of the gill tissue causes epithelial hyperplasia, which

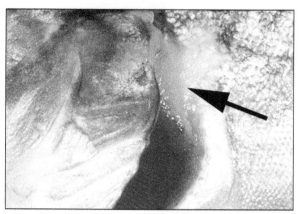

Figure 6.4 **Saprolegniasis (arrow) on gill of cultured rainbow trout (*Oncorhynchus mykiss*).**

results in impaired osmoregulation and respiratory difficulties.[62]

Differential diagnosis: Since most *Saprolegnia* infections are considered secondary infections, it is important to look for the underlying primary cause.

Diagnosis: A presumptive diagnosis of saprolegniasis is made by visual observation of the cotton-like fungal growth on the surface of the gill tissue. The diagnosis may be supported by microscopic examination of wet mounts and observing the branched non-septate hyphae, or by histopathology using a silver stain to highlight the fungal hyphae. *Saprolegnia* spp. can be isolated on a low nutrient media such as malt extract agar or Sabouraud agar, and incubated at 20°C–22°C for 5 days. Specific identification of the oomycete may be achieved by examination of the fine structure of the zoospore and cyst, or by PCR assay, though the speciation of *Saprolegnia* responsible for an outbreak may not be practical or necessary.[62,64,67]

Management/control: Chemicals such as formalin, hydrogen peroxide, sodium chloride, potassium permanganate and iodophores have been used to control the free-swimming infectious zoospores but are generally not effective against the vegetative mycelial growth on the fish.[68–70] Ozone and UV irradiation have also been used to limit the spread of fungal disease.[71] Prevention and control involve good management practices that ensure good water quality, optimal nutrition, external parasite control, avoidance of overcrowding, proper handling and grading of fish, and reducing negative social interactions.[62]

PROLIFERATIVE GILL DISEASE

Overview: Proliferative gill disease (PGD), also called "hamburger gill disease," is a parasitic disease of the gills of channel catfish (*Ictalurus punctatus*).

Etiological agent: Proliferative gill disease is caused by *Henneguya ictaluri*, a myxosporean parasite that has a required oligochaete intermediate host (i.e., *Dero digitate*) in which the infectious actinospore (historically called *Aurantiactinomyxon ictalurid*) develops.[72,73]

Route of transmission: The oligochaete worm releases the actinospore stage into the water where it comes into contact and attaches to the skin of the fish.[73] The sporoplasm from the actinospore penetrates the fish, migrates to the gills and other internal organs as part of its complex developmental life cycle, and finally develops multicellular spores in the gills that are released into the water.[73] The optimal temperature range for the disease is 16°C–25°C.[72]

Host range: Channel catfish (*Ictalurus punctatus*) is the only host species in which *Henneguya ictaluri* can complete its life cycle. Channel catfish hybrids with blue catfish (*I. furcatus*) are partially refractive to the parasite and may not allow the parasite to complete its life cycle.[74]

Clinical presentation: Affected fish demonstrate lethargy, reduced feeding activity, and congregation in shallow areas near incoming water or aerators.[72] The gills appear to be swollen with areas of hemorrhage adjacent to necrotic areas (**Figure 6.5**). Young fish recently stocked into ponds appear to be the most severely affected.

Pathology of disease: There is extensive gill hyperplasia and hypertrophy with focal areas of collagen loss leading to chondrolysis and dyschondroplasia accompanied by an extensive inflammatory response in the acute and subacute stages of the disease.[73,75,76] Other organs (e.g., stomach, heart, liver, kidney and spleen) may harbor the developing parasite, but are not usually associated with inflammation or significant pathology.[73]

Differential diagnosis: The main differentials would be diseases causing gill pathology in channel catfish such as protozoan parasites, monogeneans and branchiomycosis.

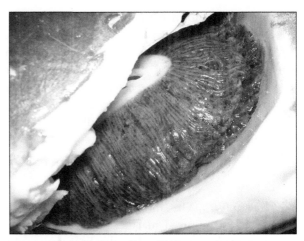

Figure 6.5 Proliferative gill disease (PGD) in a channel catfish (*I. punctatus*) showing swollen gill tissue with areas of hemorrhage adjacent to necrotic areas. (Image courtesy of L. Khoo.)

Diagnosis: A history of recently stocked young fish exhibiting signs of respiratory distress supported by histopathology of gill tissues is sufficient for a diagnosis. Unfortunately, the myxospores of *H. ictalurid* cannot be differentiated microscopically from other *Henneguya* spp. A PCR and quantitative polymerase chain reaction (qPCR) assay have been developed for the detection and specific identification of both *Henneguya ictaluri* and the actinospore stage in tissue and pond water allowing for earlier detection before clinical signs.[77,78]

Management/control: No effective preventive or therapeutic agent currently exist for PGD; however, applying hydrated lime to dry ponds prior to filling with water can significantly reduce the number of *Dero* spp. in the pond.[72] Attempts at biological control by stocking ponds with organisms (i.e., fish and invertebrates) that feed on *Dero* sp. have not been successful. Using qPCR to estimate the number of *Dero* sp. in a pond may help determine which ponds are suitable for stocking young naive fish.[79,80]

AMOEBIC GILL DISEASE

Overview: Amoebic gill disease (AGD) is a parasitic disease of the gills of fish, primarily cultured salmonids.

Etiological agent: The amoeba infecting the gills of saltwater salmonids belong to the genera

Neoparamoeba (formerly *Paramoeba*) with *Neoparamoeba perurans*, *N. pemaquidensis* and *N. branchiphilia* being the primary species causing AGD in the marine environment.[81–84] There are also a number of freshwater amoeba species belonging to the genera *Thecamoeba*, *Protacanthamoeba* and *Acanthamoeba* that cause similar clinical signs and pathology in freshwater cultured salmonids.[85–89]

Route of transmission: The facultative, amphizoic parasites are transmitted horizontally through the water.

Host range: The disease is most commonly observed in cultured marine and freshwater salmonids. A similar disease has also been reported in marine turbot (*Psetta maxima*), sea bass (*Dicentrarchus labrax*) and ballan wrasse (*Labrus bergylta*).[90,91] Infestations of amoeba on the gills of freshwater fish, commonly called "nodular gill disease," have been reported in rainbow trout (*Oncorhynchus mykiss*), coho salmon (*O. kisutch*), Atlantic salmon (*Salmo salar*), arctic char (*Salvelinus alpinus*), sturgeon (*Scaphirhynchus albus*) and tilapia (*Oreochromis aureus* and *O. nilotica*).[85–87,92,93]

Clinical presentation: Fish become lethargic, have an increased respiratory rate and flared operculum, and congregate near the water surface. The gills have increased mucus and show multifocal patches of swollen, pale tissue (**Figures 6.6** and **6.7**). Clinical disease is most commonly observed at temperatures greater than 16°C and salinities above 32%, with other factors such as high stocking densities, smolt size, suspended organic matter and biofouling, and previous gill damage also affecting the onset of disease.[84] Mortality rates typically range from 10% to 20%, but losses as high as 70% have occasionally been reported.

Pathology of disease: There is a prominent epithelial hyperplasia resulting in lamellar fusion with a significant leucocyte infiltration. The parasite can be found most commonly palisading along the surface of the lamellae.[86,87]

Differential diagnosis: Other viral, bacterial, parasitic and fungal diseases that cause increased mucus on the gills and respiratory distress.

Diagnosis: The diagnosis of AGD is made by macroscopic examination of the gills supported by gill smears and histopathology. Conventional PCR and

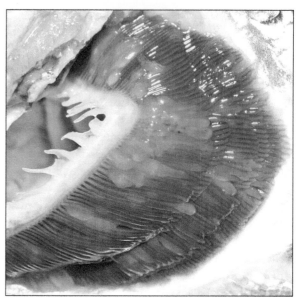

Figure 6.6 Amoebic gill disease in a cultured Atlantic salmon (*Salmo salar*) demonstrating diffuse pale, thickened mucoid patches and swollen gill tissue. (Image courtesy of M. Powell.)

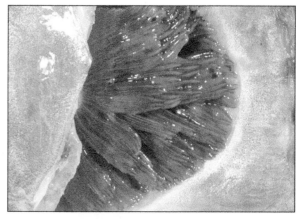

Figure 6.7 Nodular (i.e., amoebic) gill disease in a cultured freshwater rainbow trout (*O. mykiss*) exhibiting increased mucus and multifocal patches of pale, swollen gill tissue.

real-time TaqMan PCR methods can be used to identify the species of amoeba.[94,95]

Management/control: Freshwater baths and hydrogen peroxide are used as treatments for marine infections, while formalin has been used for freshwater amoebic infections.[84]

Glochidiosis

Overview: An obligatory parasitic larval stage of certain freshwater bivalve molluscs that encysts within the epithelium (i.e., gills and skin) of host fish.[96]

Etiological agent: The first larval stage of some freshwater mussels in the families Unionidae and Margaritiferidae.

Route of transmission: Immature glochidia are released by the adult mussel and attach by various mechanisms to the gill tissue of the host fish.[96,97] The glochidia become covered with a layer of epithelial tissue and undergo metamorphosis.

Host range: Numerous freshwater species of fish within the worldwide distribution of unionids (i.e., North America, Europe, China and Southeast Asia). However, most mussel species are host specific in that their glochidia will only complete metamorphosis on one host species or only a few species of fish.[98,99]

Clinical presentation: No clinical signs are usually exhibited by fish with glochidia, though an infestation may alter behavior of infected fish by reducing their activity and subsequent dispersal in the wild.[100] Rarely the pathology associated with a heavy infestation may reduce the ability of gases to diffuse across the epithelium of the gill surface, and result in an infected individual showing signs of respiratory distress (**Figure 6.8**).

Pathology: The presence of the glochidia incites a focal epithelial hyperplasia causing fusion of adjacent secondary gill lamellae.[101,102] There may also be a localized increase in the number of mucus

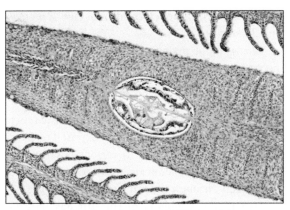

Figure 6.9 Histopathology of gill tissue showing bivalve morphology of glochidia and the resulting intense hyperplasia of the lamellae. H&E stain.

cells and eosinophilic granular cells.[101] Once the mature glochidia drops off the host (i.e., excysts), the gill tissue will repair itself by re-epithelialization of the hyperplastic areas. Some species of glochidia have a relatively short maturation period (i.e., weeks) on the fish host, whereas other species may overwinter on the gills of the fish and excyst in the spring.

Differential diagnosis: The embedded glochidia often grossly resemble encysted digenetic trematode larvae (i.e., metacercaria). Other differentials include cysts of a number of parasitic protozoan species, epitheliocystis or lymphocystis.

Diagnosis: Glochidia are distinguished by their unique thin-shelled bivalve morphology, which can be seen using a dissecting scope or by histopathology (**Figure 6.9**). Specific identification of the glochidia mussel species can be accomplished with molecular techniques.[103–105]

Management/control: This condition is not generally a problem for most wild or captive fishes. Filtration or avoidance of water containing freshwater unionids is a method for preventing an infestation; however, once the infestation occurs, no treatment is available to remove the encysted glochidia.

NEOPLASIA

Overview: Neoplasms of the gill tissues (i.e., gill filaments and gill arch) in fish are rare and either spontaneous lesions or induced following exposure to a

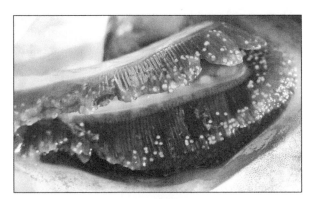

Figure 6.8 Numerous glochidia of the wavy-rayed lampmussel (*Lampsilis fasciola*) encysted in the gills of a smallmouth bass (*Micropterus dolomieu*). (Image courtesy of B. Fisher.)

variety of environmental conditions (see "Neoplasia" in Chapter 5).[106]

Etiology: The majority of gill neoplasia is spontaneous in nature with no known cause though chemical contamination and viral etiologies should always be considered.

Route of transmission: Due to the expansive surface area of the gills that is constantly exposed to the surrounding water, exposure to various environmental agents including chemicals and infectious agents is most likely through the gill tissues.

Host range: Neoplasia of the gill has only been recorded in a few wild and farmed food and ornamental species, and induced by various chemical exposures in several laboratory fishes. However, it is assumed that all fish species are susceptible. Reports of spontaneous neoplasia include branchioblastomas or branchial lamellar neoplasm in wild salmonids, branchial chondroma in a farmed Atlantic salmon (*Salmo salar*), adenoma in a brown trout (*Salmo fario*), branchioblastomas in koi carp (*Cyprinus carpio*), branchioblastomas and lymphosarcoma in sunshine bass (*Morone saxatilis* × *M. chrysops*), osteochondroma in gilthead sea bream (*Sparus aurata*), and osteoblastic osteosarcoma in a barbel (*Barbus barbus plebejus*) (see Chapter 5, **Figure 5.28**).[106–112] Chemically induced neoplasia has been reported in medaka, zebrafish and platyfish × swordtails.[113–115]

Clinical presentation: Most neoplasms of the gill tissue present as soft to firm whitish growths attached to the supporting branchial cartilage. Rarely do they interfere with respiration.

Pathology: Most neoplastic masses are grossly visible and connected to the gill arch. They have the potential to differentiate into cartilage, pillar cells, and other epithelial or mesenchymal elements of the normal gill tissues.[111]

Differential diagnosis: The differential diagnosis should include granulomatous responses to bacterial infections, encysted parasites (i.e., digenetic trematode larvae) or foreign bodies. The differential may also need to distinguish between thyroid tumors and thyroid hyperplasia (i.e., goiter), which commonly occur in the branchial cavity (**Figure 6.10**) (see "Goiter" in Chapter 9).

Diagnosis: The diagnostic approach for neoplastic gill lesions in fish include gross observation,

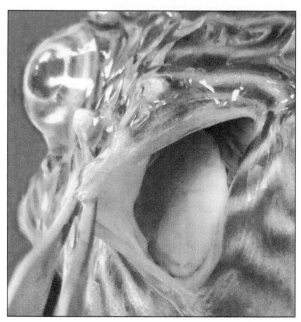

Figure 6.10 Branchial thyroid mass on the gills of a striped burfish (*Chilomycterus schoepfi*). (Image courtesy of S. Boylan.)

cytological, histological and ultrastructural examination, with histology being the primary diagnostic technique.

Management/control: As the cause for most gill neoplasia is not known, control effort should focus on reducing exposure to environmental contaminants or pathogens.

GAS BUBBLE DISEASE

Overview: A condition associated with the super-saturation of dissolved gases, most commonly nitrogen or oxygen, in the water column causing bubbles to form in the capillaries of the gills (see "Gas Bubble Disease" in Chapter 4).

Etiology: Numerous etiologies are known to cause super-saturation of the water including leaks in system plumbing, sudden extreme temperature changes, heavy algal blooms, and use of ground water that has not been sufficiently degassed.[116,117]

Route of transmission: Not applicable.

Host range: The condition has been reported in numerous wild, farmed and aquarium species.

Clinical presentation: Clinical signs may include loss of equilibrium, abnormal buoyancy and aimless

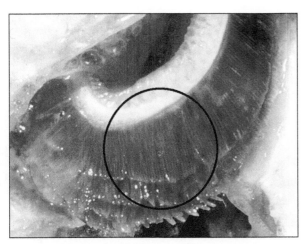

Figure 6.11 Gas bubble disease (i.e., super-saturation) in a cultured rainbow trout (*O. mykiss*) showing pale, ischemic areas (circle) along the gill filaments.

swimming, with spasmodic convulsions just prior to death.[118] Overt gross lesions include air emboli in the capillaries of the gills with or without petechial hemorrhages (**Figure 6.11**). Other tissues (i.e., eyes, skin and fins) may also demonstrate air bubbles.[117,118]

Pathology: Air bubbles in capillaries of the secondary lamellae prevent normal circulation of blood through the gills (**Figure 6.12**). This reduces the efficiency of gas (i.e., oxygen, carbon dioxide) transfer across the gill surface causing hypoxia in the fish.

Differential diagnosis: This problem is not difficult to diagnose, but the underlying cause can often be challenging to determine.

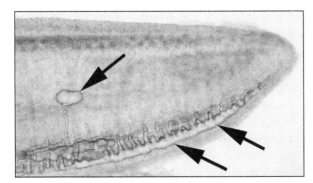

Figure 6.12 Wet mount of gill tissue of a bluegill (*Lepomis* sp.) with gas bubble disease showing elongated air bubbles (arrows) within the vessels of the gill. (Image courtesy of S. Boylan.)

Diagnosis: The condition is most commonly diagnosed by visual inspection of the gills for the presence of gas emboli in the capillaries of the gill lamellae.

Management/control: Lesions generally regress once the elevated gas levels are eliminated. Monitoring culture water for elevated dissolved gas levels with a saturometer helps to avoid the problem before lesions occur.

MISCELLANEOUS PARASITIC PROBLEMS

Besides the previously mentioned parasitic diseases of the gill (i.e., proliferative gill disease, amoebic gill disease and glochidiosis), there are numerous other protozoan and metazoan parasites that may infest the gill tissue of freshwater, brackish and marine fish.[119–124] Though most do not produce readily distinguishable specific gross lesions, many cause substantial histologic lesions and significant clinical signs in the fish.[120,121,124] Though too numerous to list, a few deserve special mention as important parasites of the gill. One of the more common protozoan parasites of freshwater fish is *Ichthyophthirius multifiliis*, or *Cryptocaryon irritans* in marine fishes, both commonly called "Ich" or "white spot disease" (see "White Spot Disease" in Chapter 5). They are holotrich ciliates that invade the epithelium of the host as part of their developmental cycle causing hyperplasia of the epithelium. These parasites are one of the larger protozoans, and individual trophonts (i.e., feeding stage) can sometimes be seen grossly as small, raised white spots on the skin and fins, but are generally not as easily observed on the gills. Another group of important protozoan pathogens of the gills are the trichodinids, which are peritrichous ciliates. These mobile parasites cause irritation to the gills by their feeding activity and movement over the gill surface causing the epithelium to become hyperplastic. *Ichthyobodo* (~*Costia* spp.) *necator* is one of the more pathogenic protozoans that can be found either attached or detached from the gill. This is an extremely small flagellate that uses at least one of its flagella to attach to the epithelial cells and causes hyperplasia of the gill tissue. Several parasitic dinoflagellates (e.g., *Amyloodinium ocellatum*, *Piscinoodinium* spp. and *Oodinium* spp.) are major pathogens of tropical and cultured marine and freshwater species. In the trophont stage, these parasites have rhizoids that penetrate the host cells and allow the parasite to attach to and feed off the epithelial tissues of the gills. In the aquarium trade this condition is commonly called "velvet disease" due to the brownish coloration large numbers of trophonts give the gill tissue.

Some of the more important metazoan parasites of the gills include the parasitic flatworms called monogeneans.[119,122,124] The most common species affecting the gills of fish belong to the families Dactylogyridae and Gyrodactylidae. The monogeneans have a direct life cycle with either a viviparous (i.e., live-bearing) or oviporus (i.e., egg laying) method of reproduction. These parasites have a posterior opisthaptor or attachment organ armed with hooks, clamps or anchors, which allows the monogenean to firmly attach to the epithelial tissues of the gills, while the anterior end of the flatworm has an oral opening for feeding. Both the attachment and feeding activity of the monogenean causes irritation to the gill tissue and results in hyperplasia of the gill epithelium. Several species of Digenea (i.e., digenetic trematodes) also have a larval stage (i.e., metacercaria) that encysts in the epithelial tissue of the fish gill.[124] Fish commonly serve as a secondary intermediate host for these parasites, with molluscs generally serving as the first intermediate host. These parasites usually cause only a localized cartilaginous and epithelial tissue response around the encysted parasite. Larger parasites that may be observed attached to the gill tissue of fish include copepods in the families Ergasilidae and Lernaeopodidae, which contain the species *Ergasilus* and *Salmonicola*, respectively (**Figures 6.13** and **6.14**). More than 100 species of these two genera, commonly called "gill lice," are parasitic on the gills of freshwater or marine species.[124] Only the mature females are parasitic, whereas the juvenile stages (i.e., nauplii and copepodid stages) and mature males are free-living in the water. The mature females have a modified second antennal segment that is used for either piercing or encircling the gill filament or gill arches. The attachment and feeding activity of the copepod causes localized swelling, epithelial hyperplasia,

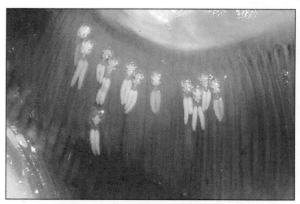

Figure 6.13 Adult female *Ergasilus* sp. with paired egg masses on the gill filaments of a wild-caught northern pike (*Esox lucius*). (Image courtesy of A. Thomsen.)

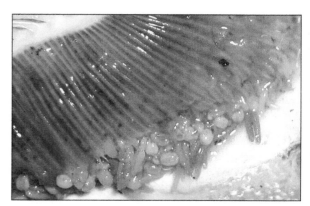

Figure 6.14 Heavy infestation of adult *Salmincola* sp. ("gill lice") attached to the gills of a trout. (Image courtesy of C. Banner.)

hemorrhage with inflammation, occlusion of the filament vessels and atrophy of the tips of the gill filaments.[124]

Typical behavior of fish clinically infected with either protozoan and metazoan parasites include increased opercular rates, sporadic gasping, flashing (i.e., rubbing or scratching against the substrate or objects), lack of shoaling activity, lethargy, hiding and loss of coordination. Diagnosis can be based on direct visual observations or nonlethal gill biopsies and wet mount observations for rapid determination of the presence of a parasitic infestation. A more extensive evaluation may require microscopic evaluation of the tissues to ascertain the species and extent of the infestation.

Most control methods for parasitic infestations of the gills of fish involve the use of chemicals to either kill the parasites on the host or one of its life stages in the water.[119,120,124] Control of digenean infections on the gills of fish is most commonly accomplished through the elimination of the snail intermediate host using molluscicides, environmental manipulation, weed control or molluscophagous fish.[124]

REFERENCES

1. OIE. *Manual of Diagnostic Tests for Aquatic Animals.* http://www.oie.int/standard-setting/aquatic-manual/access-online/ (accessed 22 June 2018).
2. Hedrick, R.P., Gilad, O., Yun, S., Spangenberg, J.V., Marty, G.D., Nordhausen, R.W., Kebus, M.J., Bercovier, H. and Eldar, A. A herpesvirus associated with mass mortality of juvenile and adult koi, a strain of common carp. *Journal of Aquatic Animal Health* 2000;12:44–57.
3. Haenen, O.L.M., Way, K., Bergmann, S.M. and Ariel, E. The emergence of koi herpesvirus and its significance to European aquaculture. *Bulletin of the European Association of Fish Pathologists* 2004;24:293–307.
4. Pokorova, D., Vesely, T., Piackova, V., Reschova, S. and Hulova, J. Current knowledge on koi herpesvirus (KHV): A review. *Veterinary Medicine–Czech* 2005;50:139–147.
5. Waltzek, T.B., Kelley, G.O., Stone, D.M., Way, K., Hanson, L., Fukuda, H., Hirono, I., Aoki, T., Davison, A.J. and Hedrick, R.P. Koi herpesvirus represents a third cyprinid herpesvirus (CyHV-3) in the family *Herpesviridae. Journal of General Virology* 2005;86:1659–1667.
6. Bretzinger, A., Fischer-Scherl, T., Oumouna, M., Hoffmann, R. and Truyen, U. Mass mortalities in koi carp, *Cyprinus carpio*, associated with gill and skin disease. *Bulletin of the European Association of Fish Pathologists* 1999;19:182–185.
7. Sano, M., Ito, T., Kurita, J., Yanai, T., Watanabe, N., Miwa, S. and Iida, T. First detection of koi herpesvirus in cultured common carp *Cyprinus carpio* in Japan. *Fish Pathology* 2004;39:165–167.
8. Perelberg, A., Smirnov, M., Hutoran, M., Diamant, A., Bejerano, Y. and Kotler, M. Epidemiological description of a new viral disease afflicting cultured *Cyprinus carpio* in Israel. *Israeli Journal of Aquaculture* 2003;55:5–12.
9. Hedrick, R.P., Waltzek, T.B. and McDowell, T.S. Susceptibility of koi carp, common carp, goldfish and goldfish x common carp hybrids to cyprinid herpesvirus-2 and herpesvirus-3. *Journal of Aquatic Animal Health* 2006;18:26–34.
10. Bergmann, S.M., Lutze, P., Schutze, H., Fischer, U., Dauber, M., Fichtner, D. and Kempter, J. Goldfish

(*Carassius auratus*) is a susceptible species for koi herpesvirus (KHV) but not for KHV disease. *Bulletin of the European Association of Fish Pathologists* 2010;30:74–84.
11. Bergmann, S.M., Sadowski, J., Kielpinski, M., Bartlomiejczyk, M., Fichtner, D., Riebe, R., Lenk, M. and Kempter, J. Susceptibility of koi × crucian carp and koi × goldfish hybrids to koi herpesvirus (KHV) and the development of KHV disease (KHVD). *Journal of Fish Diseases* 2010;33:267–272.
12. Bergmann, S.M., Schutze, H., Fischer, U., Fichtner, D., Riechardt, M., Meyer, K., Schrudde, D. and Kempter, J. Detection of koi herpes-virus (KHV) genome in apparently healthy fish. *Bulletin of the European Association of Fish Pathologists* 2009;29:145–152.
13. Walster, C.I. Clinical observations of severe mortalities in koi carp, *Cyprinus carpio*, with gill disease. *Fish Veterinary Journal* 1999;3:54–58.
14. Costes, B., Stalin Raj, V., Michel, B., Fournier, G., Thirion, M., Gillet, L., Mast, J., Lieffrig, F., Bremont, M. and Vanderplasschen, A. The major portal of entry of koi herpesvirus in *Cyprinus carpio* is is the skin. *Journal of Virology* 2009;83:2819–2830.
15. Gilad, O., Yun, S., Adkison, M.A., Way, K., Willits, N.H., Bercovier, H. and Hedrick, R.P. Molecular comparison of isolates of an emerging fish pathogen, koi herpesvirus, and the effect of water temperature on mortality of experimentally infected koi. *Journal of General Virology* 2003;84:2661–2667.
16. Dishon, A., Perelberg, A., Bishara-Shieban, J., Ilouze, M., Davidovich, M., Werker, S. and Kotler, M. Detection of carp interstitial nephritis and gill necrosis virus in fish droppings. *Applied and Environmental Microbiology* 2005;71:7285–7291.
17. Pikarsky, E., Ronen, A., Abramowitz, J., Levavi-Sivan, B., Hutoran, M., Shapira, Y., Steinitz, M., Perelberg, A., Soffer, D. and Kotler, M. Pathogenesis of acute viral disease induced in fish by carp interstitial nephritis and gill necrosis virus. *Journal of Virology* 2004;78:9544–9551.
18. St-Hilaire, S., Beevers, N., Way, K., Le Deuff, R.M., Martin, P. and Joiner, C. Reactivation of koi herpesvirus infections in common carp *Cyprinus carpio. Diseases of Aquatic Organisms* 2005;67:15–23.
19. Goodwin, A.E. Differential diagnosis: SVCV vs KHV in koi. *FHS/AFS Newsletter* 2003;31:9–13.
20. Kasai, H., Muto, Y. and Yoshimizu, M. Virucidal effects of ultraviolet, heat treatment and disinfectants against koi herpesvirus (KHV). *Fish Pathology* 2005;40:137–138.
21. Bernardet, J.F., Segers, P., Vancanney, T.M., Berthe, F., Kerstera, K. and Vandamme, P. Cutting the Gordian Knot: Emended classification and description of the Genus *Flavobacterium*, emended description of the Family Flavobacteriaccae, and proposal of *Flavobacterium hydatis* nom. nov. (Basonym, *Cytophaga aquatilis* Strohl and Tait 2978). *International Journal of Systematic Bacteriology* 1996;46(1):128–148.

22. Wakabayashi, H., Huh, G.J. and Kimura, N. *Flavobacterium branchiophila* sp. nov., a causative agent of bacterial gill disease of freshwater fishes. *International Journal of Systematic Bacteriology* 1989;39:213–216.

23. Starliper C.E. Bacterial gill disease. USFW Blue Book, 2012. https://units.fisheries.org/fhs/wp-content/uploads/sites/30/2017/08/1.2.1-BGD_2014.pdf.

24. Nagel, T. Intensive culture of fingerling walleyes on formulated feed. *The Progressive Fish-Culturist* 1976;38(2):90–91.

25. Farkas, J. Filamentous *Flavobacterium* sp. isolated from fish with gill diseases in cold water. *Aquaculture* 1985;44:1–10.

26. Ostland, V.E., Lumsden, J.S., MacPhee, D.D. and Ferguson, H.W. Characteristics of *Flavobacterium branchiophilum*, the cause of salmonid bacterial gill disease in Ontario. *Journal of Aquatic Animal Health* 1994;6:13–26.

27. Swain, P., Mishra, S., Dash, S., Nayak, S.K., Mishra, B.K., Pani, K.C. and Ramakrishna, R. Association of *Flavobacterium branchiophilum* in bacterial gill disease of Indian major carps. *Indian Journal of Animal Science* 2007;77(7):646–649.

28. Speare, D.J., Ferguson, H.W., Beamish, F.W.M., Yager, J.A. and Yamashiro, S. Pathology of bacterial gill disease: Ultrastructure of branchial lesions. *Journal of Fish Diseases* 1991;14:1–20.

29. Speare, D.J., Ferguson, H.W., Beamish, F.W.M., Yager, J.A. and Yamashiro, S. Pathology of bacterial gill disease in rainbow trout: Sequential development of lesions during natural outbreaks of disease. *Journal of Fish Diseases* 14:21–32.

30. Ostland, V.E., Ferguson, H.W., Prescott, J., Stevenson, R.M.W. and Barker, I. K. Bacterial gill disease of salmonids: Relationship between the severity of gill lesions and bacterial recovery. *Diseases of Aquatic Organisms* 1990;9:5–14.

31. Anacker, R.L. and Ordal, E.J. Studies on the myxobacterium *Chondrococcus columnaris*. I. Serological typing. *Journal of Bacteriology* 1959;78:25–32.

32. Huh, G.J. and Wakabayashi, H. Detection of *Flavobacterium* sp., a pathogen of bacterial gill disease, using the indirect fluorescent antibody technique. *Fish Pathology* 1987;12:233–242.

33. MacPhee, D.D., Ostland, V.E., Lumsden, J.S. and Ferguson, H.W. Development of an enzyme-linked immunosorbent assay (ELISA) to estimate the quantity of *Flavobacterium branchiophilum* on the gills of rainbow trout *Oncorhynchus mykiss*. *Diseases of Aquatic Organisms* 1995;21:13–23.

34. Speare, D.J., Markham, R.J.F., Despres, B., Whitman, K. and MacNair, N. Examination of gills from salmonids with bacterial gill disease using monoclonal antibody probes for *Flavobacterium branchiophilum* and *Cytophaga columnaris*. *Journal of Veterinary Diagnostic Investigation* 1995;7:500–505.

35. Toyama, T., Kita-Tsukamoto, K. and Wakabayashi, H. Identification of *Flexibacter maritimus*, *Flavobacterium branchiophilum* and *Cytophaga columnaris* by PCR targeted 16S ribosomal DNA. *Fish Path* 1996;31(1):25–31.

36. Warsen, A.E., Krug, M.J., LaFrentz, S., Stanek, D.R., Loge, F.J. and Call, D.R. Simultaneous discrimination between 15 fish pathogens by using 16S ribosomal DNA PCR and DNA microarrays. *Applied and Environmental Microbiology* 2004;70(7):4216–4221.

37. Bernardet, J.F. and Bowman, J.P. The genus *Flavobacterium*. In: *The Prokaryotes: A Handbook on the Biology of Bacteria. Volume 7, Proteobacteria: Delta and Epsilon Subclasses. Deeply Rooting Bacteria*. M. Dworkin and S. Falkow, eds. Springer, New York, 2006; pp. 481–531.

38. Declercq, A.M., Haesebrouck, F., Van den Broeck, W., Bossier, P. and Decostere, A. Columnaris disease in fish: A review with emphasis on bacterium-host interactions. *Veterinary Research* 2013;44(1):27.

39. Loch, T.P. and Faisal, M. Emerging flavobacterial infections in fish: A review. *Journal of Advanced Research* 2015;6:283–300.

40. Kunttu, H.M.T., Sundberg, L.R., Pulkkinen, K. and Valtonen, E.T. Environment may be the source of *Flavobacterium columnare* outbreaks at fish farms. *Environmental Microbiology Reports* 2012;4:398–402.

41. Wakabayashi, H. Columnaris disease. In: *Bacterial Diseases of Fish*. V. Inglis, R.J. Roberts and N.R. Bromage, eds. Blackwell, Oxford, UK, 1993; pp. 23–39.

42. Pacha, R.E. and Ordal, E.J. Histopathology of experimental columnaris disease in young salmon. *Journal of Comparative Pathology* 1967;77(4):419–423.

43. Paperna, I. and Sabnai, I. Epitheliocystis disease in fishes. In: *Fish Diseases*, W. Ahne, ed. Springer, Berlin, 1980; pp. 228–234.

44. Moulder, J.W. Order II. Chlamydiales (Stortz and Page, 1971). In: *Bergey's Manual of Systematic Bacteriology*, Vol. 1. N. Kreig, ed. Williams & Wilkins, Baltimore, 1984; pp. 729–739.

45. Nowak, B.F. and LaPatra S.E. Epitheliocystis in fish. *Journal of Fish Diseases* 2006;29:573–588.

46. Stride, M.C., Polkinghorne, A. and Nowak, B.F. Chlamydial infections of fish: Diverse pathogens and emerging causes of disease in aquaculture species. *Veterinary Microbiology* 2014;171:258–266.

47. Blandford, M.I., Taylor-Brown, A., Schlacher, T.A., Nowak, B. and Polkinghorne, A. Epitheliocystis in fish: An emerging aquaculture disease with a global impact. *Transboundary and Emerging Diseases* 2018;1–11.

48. Hoffman, G.L., Dunbar, C.E., Wolf, K. and Zwillenberg, L.O. Epitheliocystis, a new infectious disease of the bluegill (*Lepomis macrochirus*). *Antonie van Leeuwenhoek* 1969;35:146–158.

49. Zachary, A. and Paperna, I. Epithelicystis disease in the striped bass *Morone saxatilis* from the Chesapeake Bay. *Canadian Journal of Microbiology* 1977;28:1404–1414.

50. Paperna, I. Epitheliocystis infections in wild and cultured sea bream (*Sparus aura*ta, Sparidae) and grey mullets (*Liza ramada*, Mugilidae). *Aquaculture* 1977;10:169–176.

51. Terence, M., Bradley, T.M., Newcomer, C.E. and Maxwell, K.O. Epitheliocystis associated with massive mortalities of cultured lake trout *Salvelinus namaycush*. *Diseases of Aquatic Organisms* 1988;4:9–17.

52. Crespo, S., Grau, A. and Padros, F. Epitheliocystis disease in the cultured amberjack, *Seriola dumerili* Risso (Carangidae). *Aquaculture* 1990;90:197–207.

53. Wolke, R.E., Wyand, D.S. and Khairallah, L.H. A light and electron microscopic study of epitheliocystis disease in the gills of Connecticut striped bass (*Morone saxatilis*) and white perch (*Morone americanus*). *Journal of Comparative Pathology* 1970;80:559–563.

54. Paperna, I., Sabnai, I. and Castel, M. Ultrastructural study of epitheliocystis organisms from gill epithelium of the fish *Sparus aurata* (L.) and *Liza ramada* (Risso) and their relation to the host cell. *Journal of Fish Diseases* 1978;1:181–189.

55. Goodwin, A.E., Park, E. and Nowak, B.F. Successful treatment of largemouth bass, *Micropterus salmoides* (L.), with epitheliocystis hyperinfection. *Journal of Fish Diseases* 2005;28:623–625.

56. Meyer, F.P. and Robinson, J.A. Branchiomycosis: A new fungal disease of North American fishes. *The Progressive Fish-Culturist* 2011;74–77.

57. Khoo, L. Fungal diseases in fish. *Journal of Exotic Pet Medicine* 2000;9:102–111.

58. Paperna, I. and Smirnova, M. Branchiomyces-like infection in a cultured tilapia (Oreochromis hybrid, Cichlidae). *Diseases of Aquatic Organisms* 1997;31:233–238.

59. Ibrahim, K.S. Isolation and pathological study of branchiomycosis from the commercial pond of common carp (*Cyprinus carpio*) fish in Governorate of Duhok, Iraq. *Iraqi Journal of Veterinary Medicine* 2011;35:1–9.

60. Khoo, L., Leard, A.T., Waterstrat, P.R., Jack, S.W. and Camp, K.L. Branchiomyces infection in farm-reared channel catfish, *Ictalurus punctatus* (Rafinesque). *Journal of Fish Diseases* 1998;21:423–431.

61. Egusa, S. and Ohira, Y. Branchiomycosis of pond-cultured eels. *Fish Pathology* 1972;7:79–83.

62. Bruno D.W. and Wood B.P. *Saprolegnia* and other Oomycetes. P.T.K. Woo, and D.W. Bruno, eds. *Fish Diseases and Disorders*, Vol. 3: *Viral, Bacterial and Fungal Infections*. CABI, Wallingford, Oxon, UK, 1999; pp. 599–659.

63. Gozlan, R.E., Marshall, W.L., Lilje, O., Jessop, C.N., Gleason, F.H. and Andreou, D. Current ecological understanding of fungal-like pathogens of fish: What lies beneath? *Frontiers in Microbiology* 2014;5(62):1–16.

64. Van West, P. *Saprolegnia parasitica*, an oomycete pathogen with a fishy appetite: New challenges for an old problem. *Mycologist* 2006;20:99–104.

65. Hatai, K. and Hoshiai, G. Mass mortality in cultured coho salmon (*Oncorhynchus kisutch*) due to *Saprolegnia parasitica* Coker. *Journal of Wildlife Diseases* 1992;28:532–536.

66. Hussein, M. and Hatai, K. Pathogenicity of *Saprolegnia* species associated with outbreaks of salmonid saprolegniosis in Japan. *Fisheries Science* 2002;68:1067–1072.

67. Earle, G. and Hintz, W. New approaches for controlling *Saprolegnia parasitica*, the causal agent of a devastating fish disease. *Tropical Life Sciences Research* 2014;25:101–109.

68. Gieseker, C.M., Serfling, S.G. and Reimschuessel, R. Formalin treatment to reduce mortality associated with *Saprolegnia parasitica* in rainbow trout, *Oncorhynchus mykiss*. *Aquaculture* 2006;253:120–129.

69. Zaki, M.S., Fawzi, O.M. and El-Jackey, J. Pathological and biochemical studies in *Tilapia nilotica* infected with *Saprolegnia parasitica* and treated with potassium permanganate. *American-Eurasian Journal of Agricultural and Environmental Sciences* 2008;3:677–680.

70. Sudova, E., Machova, J., Svobodova, Z. and Vesely, T. Negative effects of malachite green and possibilities of its replacement in the treatment of fish eggs and fish: A review. *Veterinarni Medicina (Praha)* 2007;52(12):527–539.

71. Fornerisa, G., Bellardib, S., Palmegianoc, G.B., Sarogliad, M., Sicuroa, B., Gascoe, L. and Zoccarato, I. The use of ozone in trout hatchery to reduce saprolegniasis incidence. *Aquaculture* 2003;221:157–166.

72. Durborow R.M., Crosby D.M. and Delomas T. Proliferative gill disease (hamburger gill disease). SRAC Publication No. 475. 2015.

73. Belem, A.M.G. and Pote, L.M. Portals of entry and systemic localization of proliferative gill disease organisms in channel catfish *Ictalurus punctatus*. *Diseases of Aquatic Organisms* 2001;48:37–42.

74. Rosser, T.G. Characterization of myxozoan parasites associated with catfish aquaculture in Mississippi with notes on the development of *Henneguya ictaluri* in susceptible and non-susceptible catfish hosts. PhD dissertation, Mississippi State University, Starkville, Mississippi. 2017.

75. Lovy, J., Goodwin, A.E., Speare, D.J., Wadowska, D.W. and Wright, G.M. Histochemical and ultrastructural analysis of pathology and cell responses in gills of channel catfish affected with proliferative gill disease. *Diseases of Aquatic Organisms* 2011;94:125–134.

76. Wise, D.J., Griffin, M.J., Terhune, J.S., Pote, L.M. and Khoo, L.H. Induction and evaluation of proliferative gill disease in channel catfish fingerlings. *Journal of Aquatic Animal Health* 2008;20:236–244.

77. Whitaker, J.W., Pote, L.M., Khoo, L., Shivaji, R. and Hanson, L. The use of polymerase chain reaction assay to diagnose proliferative gill disease in channel catfish (*Ictalurus punctatus*). *Journal of Veterinary Diagnostic Investigation* 2001;13:394–398.

78. Griffin, M.J., Wise, D.J., Camus, A.C., Mauel, M.J., Greenway, T.E. and Pote, L.M. A real-time polymerase chain reaction assay for the detection of the myxozoan parasite *Henneguya ictaluri* in channel catfish. *Journal of Veterinary Diagnostic Investigation* 2008;20:559–566.

79. Whitaker, J.W., Pote, L.M. and Hanson, L.A. Assay to detect the actinospore and myxospore stages of proliferative gill disease in oligochaetes and pond water. *North American Journal of Aquaculture* 2005;67: 133–137.

80. Griffin, M.J., Pote, L.M., Camus, A.C., Mauel, M.J., Greenway, T.E. and Wise, D.J. Application of a real-time PCR assay for the detection of *Henneguya ictaluri* in commercial channel catfish ponds. *Diseases of Aquatic Organisms* 2009;86:223–233.

81. Kent, M.L., Sawyer, T.K. and Hedrick, R.P. *Paramoeba pemaquidensis* (Sarcomastigophora: Paramoebidae) infestation of the gills of coho salmon, *Oncorhynchus kisutch*, reared in seawater. *Diseases of Aquatic Organisms* 1988;5:163–169.

82. Clark, A. and Nowak, B.F. Field investigations of amoebic gill disease in Atlantic salmon, *Salmo salar* L., in Tasmania. *Journal of Fish Diseases* 1999;22: 1–11.

83. Wong, F.Y.K., Carson, J. and Elliott, N.G. 18S ribosomal DNA-based PCR identification of *Neoparamoeba pemaquidensis*, the agent of amoebic gill disease in sea-farmed salmonids. *Diseases of Aquatic Organisms* 2004;60:65–76.

84. Ruane N.M. and Jones S.R.M. Amoebic gill disease (AGD) of farmed Atlantic salmon (*Salmo salar* L.). Leaflet No. 60, ICES Identification Leaflets for Diseases and Parasites of Fish and Shellfish. 2013.

85. Sawyer, T.K., Hnath, J.G. and Conrad, J.F. *Thecamoeba hoffmani* sp. n. (Amoebida: Thecamoebidae) from gills of fingerling salmonid fish. *Journal of Parasitology* 1974;60:677–682.

86. Wolf, J.C. and Smith, S.A. What's your diagnosis? Mortality and pale thickened gills in rainbow trout. *Laboratory Animals* 2000;29:23–24.

87. Smith, S.A., Hughes, K.P. and Luoma, J. Amoebic gill infestation in pallid sturgeon, *Scaphirhynchus albus*. *Bulletin of the European Association of Fish Pathologists* 2002;22:400–402.

88. Buchmann, K., Nielsen, T., Sigh, J. and Bresciani, J. Amoebic gill infections of rainbow trout in freshwater ponds. *Bulletin of the European Association of Fish Pathologists* 2004;24:87–91.

89. Dyková, I., Kostka, M., Wortberg, F., Nardy, E. and Pecková, H. New data on aetiology of nodular gill disease in rainbow trout, Oncorhynchus mykiss. *Folia Parasitologica* 2010;57(3):157.

90. Munday, B.L., Zilberg, D. and Findlay, V. Gill disease of marine fish caused by infection with *Neoparamoeba pemaquidensis*. *Journal of Fish Diseases* 2001;24: 497–507.

91. Karlsbakk, E., Olsen, A.B., Einen, A.C.B., Mo, T.A., Fiksdal, I.U., Aase, H., Kalgraff, C., Skår, S.A. and Hansen, H. Amoebic gill disease due to *Paramoeba perurans* in ballan wrasse (*Labrus bergylta*). *Aquaculture* 2013;412–413:41–44.

92. Bullock, G., Herman, R., Heinen, J., Noble, A., Weber, A. and Hankins, J. Observations on the occurrence of bacterial gill disease and amoeba gill infestation in rainbow trout cultured in a water recirculation system. *Journal of Aquatic Animal Health* 1994;6:310–317.

93. Speare, D.J. Nodular gill disease (amoebic gill infestation) in arctic char, *Salvelinus alpinus*. *Journal of Comparative Pathology* 1989;121:277–282.

94. Young, N.D., Dyková, I., Nowak, B.F. and Morrison, R.N. Development of a diagnostic PCR to detect *Neoparamoeba perurans*, agent of amoebic gill disease. *Journal of Fish Diseases* 2008;31:285–295.

95. Fringuelli, E., Gordon, A.W., Rodger, H., Welsh, M.D. and Graham, D.A. Detection of *Neoparamoeba perurans* by duplex quantitative Taqman real-time PCR in formalin-fixed, paraffin-embedded Atlantic salmonid gill tissues. *Journal of Fish Diseases* 2012;35:711–724.

96. Kat, P.W. Parasitism and the Unionacea (Bivalvia). *Biological Reviews of the Cambridge Philosophical Society* 1984;59:189–208.

97. Barnhart, M.C., Haag, W.R. and Roston, W.N. Adaptations to host infection and larval parasitism in Unionoida. *Journal of the North American Benthological Society* 2008;27:370–394.

98. Williams, J.D., Warren, M.L., Cummings, K.S., Harris, J.L. and Neves, R.J. Conservation status of freshwater mussels of the United States and Canada. *Fisheries* 1993;18:6–22.

99. Bogan, A.E. Global diversity of freshwater mussels (Mollusca, Bivalvia) in freshwater. *Developments in Hydrobiology: Freshwater Animal Diversity Assessment* 2008;595:149–166.

100. Horky, P., Douda, K., Maciak, M., Zavorka, L. and Slavik, O. Parasite-induced alterations of host behaviour in a riverine fish: The effects of glochidia on host dispersal. *Freshwater Biology* 2014;59:1452–1461.

101. Treasurer, J.W. and Turnbull, T. The pathology and seawater performance of farmed Atlantic salmon infected with glochidia of *Margaritifera margaritifera*. *Journal of Fish Biology* 2000;57:858–866.

102. Howerth, E.W. and Keller, A.E. Experimentally induced glochidiosis in smallmouth bass (*Micropterus dolomieu*). *Veterinary Pathology* 2006;43:1004–1007.

103. Kneeland, S.C. and Rhymer, J.M. A molecular identification key for freshwater mussel glochidia encysted on naturally parasitized fish hosts in Maine, USA. *Journal of Molluscan Studies* 2007;73:279–282.

104. Gerke, N. and Tiedemann, R. A PCR-based molecular identification key to the glochidia of European freshwater mussels (Unionidae). *Conservation Genetics* 2001;2:287–289.

105. Zieritz, A., Gum, B., Kuehn, R. and Geist, J. Identifying freshwater mussels (Unionoida) and parasitic glochidia larvae from host fish gills: A molecular key to the North and Central European species. *Ecology and Evolution* 2012;2:740–750.

106. Groff, J.M. Neoplasia in fishes. *Veterinary Clinics of North America: Exotic Animal Practice* 2004;7:705–756.

107. Bruno, D.W. and Mitchell, C.G. Branchial chondroma from farmed Atlantic salmon, *Salmo salar* L. *Bulletin of the European Association of Fish Pathologists* 1995;15:107–108.

108. Sarkar, H.L. and Dutta-Chaudhuri, R. On the occurrence of adenoma in the gill apparatus of a trout, *Salmo fario. Transactions of the American Microscopical Society* 1964;83:93–96.

109. Knusel, R., Brandes, K., Lechleiter, S. and Schmidt-Posthaus, H. Two independent cases of spontaneously occurring branchioblastomas in koi carp (*Cyprinus carpio*). *Veterinary Pathology* 2007;44:237–239.

110. Nash, G. and Porter, C. Branchial osteochondroma in a gilthead sea bream, *Sparus aurata* L., cultured in the Gulf of Aqaba. *Journal of Fish Diseases* 1985;8:333–336.

111. Thiyagarajah, A., MacMillan, J.R. and Munson, A.D. Neoplasms in cultured sunshine bass. *Journal of Fish Diseases* 2001;24:551–556.

112. Manera, M. and Biavati, S. Branchial osteogenetic neoplasm in a barbel, *Barbus barbus plebejus*. *Diseases of Aquatic Organisms* 1999;37:231–236.

113. Brittelli, M.R., Chen, H.H.C. and Muska, C.F. Induction of branchial (gill) neoplasms in the medaka fish (*Oryzias latipes*) by N-methyl-N9-nitro-N-nitrosoguanidine. *Cancer Research* 1985;45:3209–3214.

114. Spitsbergen, J.M., Tsai, H.W., Reddy, A., Miller, T., Arbogast, D., Hendricks, J.D. and Bailey, G.S. Neoplasia in zebrafish (*Danio rerio*) treated with 7,12-dimethylbenz[a] anthracene by two exposure routes at different developmental stages. *Toxicologic Pathology* 2000;28:705–715.

115. Kimura, I., Ando, M., Kinae, N., Wakamatsu, Y., Ozato, K. and Harshbarger, J.C. MNNG carcinogenesis of the gill in platyfish × swordtail F hybrids and in medaka. *Gann* 1984;43:36.

116. Rucker, R.R. Gas-bubble disease in salmonids: A critical review. Technical Paper 58. U.S. Department of the Interior, Fish and Wildlife Service, Washington DC. 1972.

117. Smiley, J.E., Okihiro, M.S., Drawbridge, M.A. and Kaufmann, R.S. Pathology of ocular lesions associated with gas supersaturation in white seabass. *Journal of Aquatic Animal Health* 2012;24:1–10.

118. Machado, J.P., Garling, D.L., Kevern, N.R., Trapp, A.L. and Bell, T.G. Histopathology and the pathogenesis of embolism (gas bubble disease) in rainbow trout (*Salmo gairdneri*). *Canadian Journal of Fisheries and Aquatic Sciences* 1987;44:1985–1994.

119. Smith, S.A. and Noga, E.J. General parasitology of fish. In: *Fish Medicine*. M.K. Stoskopf, ed. W.B. Saunders, Philadelphia, 1992; pp. 131–148.

120. Lom J. and Dykova I. *Protozoan Parasites of Fishes. Developments in Aquaculture and Fisheries Science*, Volume 26. Elsevier Science, 1992.

121. Bruno, D.W., Nowak, B. and Elliott, D.G. Guide to the identification of fish protozoan and metazoan parasites in stained tissue sections. *Diseases of Aquatic Organisms* 2006;70:1–36.

122. Hoffman, G.L. 1999. *Parasites of North American Freshwater Fishes*. Cornell University Press, Ithaca, NY, 1999.

123. Longshaw, M. and Feist, S.W. Parasitic diseases. In: *BSAVA Manual of Ornamental Fish*, 2nd ed. W.H. Wildgoose, ed. British Small Animal Veterinary Association, Gloucester, UK, 2001; pp. 167–183.

124. Woo P.T.K. ed. *Fish Diseases and Disorders. Volume 1, Protozoan and Metazoan Infections*. CAB International, Wallingford, UK, 2006.

CHAPTER 7

MUSCULOSKELETAL DISEASES

150

JOHN S. LUMSDEN

LIP FIBROMA

Overview: Proliferative masses on the lip(s) of freshwater angelfish (*Pterophyllum scalare*). Reported to occur at an incidence of <1% in three farmed populations in Florida and occasionally in commercial populations of angelfish.[1] The condition generally occurs in older or geriatric individuals, though it may rarely occur in younger fish. To date, this condition has only been reported in captive angelfish.

Etiology: Several clinical features support the involvement of an infectious agent in the etiology of this lesion. More than one fish in the population will generally be affected and often many fish are affected and both C-type and A-type retroviral particles have been identified in fibroblasts of these tumors.[1,2] However, cell-free extracts taken from tumor tissue were not successful in reproducing the lesion, and several subsequent investigations using molecular techniques have not confirmed a viral etiology.

Clinical presentation: Well-circumscribed, proliferative oral masses, often of both the upper and lower arcades, progressively increase in size and may enlarge sufficiently to interfere with feeding (**Figure 7.1**). These expanding lesions can also mechanically ulcerate.

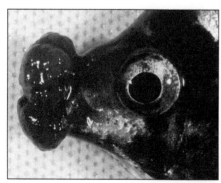

Figure 7.1 Lip fibroma in a freshwater angelfish (*Pterophyllum scalare*). (Image courtesy of S.A. Smith.)

Pathology: The histological description of the tumor is fairly consistent; loose masses of dermal spindle cells resembling fibroblasts overlain by a hyperplastic, often pedunculated, labial epithelium with embedded osseous metaplasia and developing teeth.[2,3] The classification of the type of neoplasm has varied however. The presence of retroviral particles in fibroblasts supports a diagnosis of a fibroma; however, the consistent presence of immature tooth buds in the neoplasm and their arrangement suggests that tooth cells such as odontoblasts are the neoplastic cell type and the remaining cellular changes are metaplastic.[1,2,4] Other terms such as odontoblastoma or odontogenic hamartoma have therefore also been used.[4,5]

Differential diagnosis: Oral neoplasms in fish are not uncommon, particularly in wild demersal (i.e., bottom-dwelling) fish exposed to pollutants. However, no other neoplasms at this site have been described in angelfish.[2] Proliferative masses composed of reactive mesenchymal tissues can also be common in some species of captive fish associated with repetitive trauma.

Diagnosis: A proliferative/hyperplastic oral mass as described in freshwater angelfish should provide a presumptive diagnosis. Confirmation of a diagnosis requires histopathology. Excisional biopsies can be performed if euthanasia is not desired.

Management/control: If affected populations are noted they should be isolated from other angelfish. Affected fish in large commercial breeding populations should be euthanized, as there is potentially a genetic/infectious component. One of the palliative treatments for this condition has been to excise the growth from the oral area; however, the dermal mass often regrows. In addition, removing the mass generally removes the underlying lip structures of the fish and does not improve the ability to feed.

SKELETAL DEFORMITIES, INCLUDING OPERCULAR, JAW AND OTHER

Overview: These conditions have numerous commonalities so they are dealt with initially together. Opercular, jaw and other skeletal deformities are reported to occur together or separately depending on the situation and fish species in question. Identification of separate etiologies and pathogenesis of these complex conditions is difficult. In general, axial and appendicular skeletal deformities can be fairly common, in part, simply due to the large numbers of fish viewed in commercial settings. The clinical impact of these deformities can also be less in buoyant animals, however, and this can allow genetic causes for deformities to accumulate in some settings. These conditions should be considered multifactorial and complex in their pathogenesis with genetic, infectious, nutritional, management, and environmental causes and interactions. In addition, the same lesion in different species may have different causes. Triploidy has been associated with an increased prevalence of malformations.[6]

Opercular complex deformity

The buccal pump, required in most fish for optimal respiration, relies on fully developed opercular bone(s) and an intact branchiostegal membrane. Congenital or acquired loss of bone, epithelial tissue or both lead to reduced respiratory efficiency and predisposes fish to greater clinical impacts of reduced water quality.

Etiology: Multiple examples have been documented and include genetic/familial, congenital but not proven to be genetic (e.g., semiopal culum); congenital, associated with egg incubation temperature; acquired unknown; nutritional, specifically a deficiency of vitamin C; and acquired associated with infectious agents, e.g., bacterial gill disease, sea lice and others.[7-14] Importantly, as with many other acquired lesions in fish, recovery from unilateral opercular anomalies have been reported to occur frequently.[15] This would be particularly true if the anomaly was limited to the branchiostegal membrane; however, fibroplasia following infectious disease with a lack of epithelial regrowth has also

been reported.[13] A pathogenesis whereby unossified fibrous bone is subjected to excessive demand leading to the appearance of osteochondrosis in juvenile fish has been proposed.[11]

Clinical presentation: Opercular complex deformity can be bi- or unilateral, the latter typically more common and can involve both the opercular bone, which can be shortened/reduced or folded, and the branchiostegal membrane.[11] Lack of apposition of the branchiostegal membrane to the epithelium at the terminal edge of the branchial cavity leads to reduced efficiency of the buccal pump and reduced irrigation of the gills. The resulting decreased efficiency in respiration, particularly in fish with bilateral lesions, is significant in reduced oxygen waters and also impacts feed conversion and growth rates.[11,13]

Differential diagnosis: Visual diagnosis is straightforward but identification of cause can be very difficult. These lesions can appear at any time and in most captive populations are expected to be present at low rates. A progressive or sudden increase in prevalence should suggest further diagnostics to rule out infectious causes.

Management/control: Proper control of egg incubation water temperatures and control of infectious diseases may limit the occurrence of some of these conditions. Other factors require a more holistic approach to population health.[11]

Skeletal malformations

A complex skeleton with multiple bones that develop and are ossified at different rates and are affected by a variety of stressors may lead to a complex set of problems that are often grouped together.

Etiology: Multiple causes have been documented.[16,17] Numerous studies have suggested that elevated egg incubation temperatures in Atlantic salmon are associated with vertebral deformities.[18,19] In one study in Atlantic salmon, elevated egg incubation temperature did not increase the incidence of vertebral malformations but did increase opercular, fin and jaw malformations.[9] Both Mendelian and polygenic influences on some deformities have been suggested; however, more comprehensive studies in gilthead sea bream have demonstrated that environmental effects are most important and that

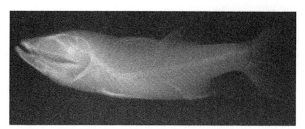

Figure 7.2 Radiograph of hybrid striped bass (*Morone chrysops* × *Morone saxatilis*) with spinal deformity (i.e., lordosis) due to lack of swim bladder development. (Image courtesy of S.A. Smith.)

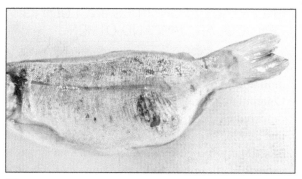

Figure 7.4 Rainbow trout (*Oncorhynchus mykiss*) with "short-tail" and experimental bacterial coldwater disease.

heritability was not significant for lordosis or opercular defects.[20,21] A higher rate of skeletal deformities has also been associated with high-density production.[22,23] Prevention of proper swim bladder inflation during development (e.g., a layer of oil on the surface of the water) is associated with skeletal abnormalities in larval fish, particularly lordosis (**Figure 7.2**).[24] Deficiencies of vitamin C and phosphorus, and an excess of or deficiency of vitamin A are documented.[17] Developmental malformations in yolk sac larvae, including twinning, are quite common and have been attributed to pollutants, metals (e.g., selenium, copper and cadmium), genetics and environmental causes.[16,25]

Clinical presentation: Varied clinical signs but include lordosis, kyphosis, scoliosis, and shortened or fused vertebrae leading to anterior posterior shortening of the body, i.e. "short tail" (**Figures 7.3** and **7.4**).[26] Many of these defects do not appear, or have clinical impact, until later in development, e.g., at or after smoltification.[27] Once again it is

worth noting that substantial healing and remodeling can occur after vertebral damage or fusion has occurred.[28] Delayed development and therefore detection of the true prevalence of these lesions is very challenging, but since the economic impact of many of these lesions can be significant, early detection could reduce some of the impact.[7,17]

Diagnosis: Detection of skeletal deformities is quite straightforward; they may be phenotypically obvious or detected by radiography (**Figure 7.5**).

Management/control: In most intensively reared commercial populations, active monitoring of skeletal anomalies should be practiced early if the scope of the problem justifies the expense.[29] Sorting of affected sea bream in early life stages has reduced the economic impact realized at harvest.[17] At later points in production, however, the expense has already been incurred.

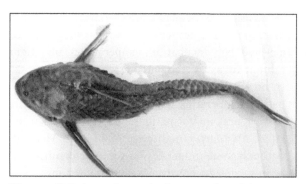

Figure 7.3 Aquarium-raised armored catfish (*Hypostomus* sp.) with skeletal curvature (i.e., scoliosis).

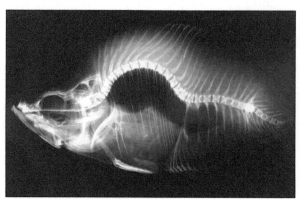

Figure 7.5 Radiograph of a fish with spinal deformity.

Deformed jaw: Kype and grilsing

Jaw deformities were also present in many of the studies referenced earlier describing complex alterations of numerous tissues. The specific condition discussed here is spawning jaw or kype, while "screamer disease" is covered with nutritional issues later. The development of a kype is a secondary sexual characteristic of male salmon (**Figure 7.6**). Some salmon are semelparous and have a single reproductive season before death, whereas others, like the Atlantic salmon, are iterparous and can spawn multiple times after they are sexually mature. Some Atlantic salmon partially lose their kype while some do not. Pre-spawn mature anadromous salmon males (i.e., grilse), distinct from post-spawned males (i.e., kelts), also develop abnormal jaws (i.e., grilsing) but have stopped eating and growing. The histological characteristics of each are distinct.[30]

Etiology: The cause of grilsing is complex, as the factors that influence sexual maturation are complex. Photoperiod, genetics, growth rate and body condition, feeding, and production systems all influence early maturation.[31]

Clinical presentation: Atlantic salmon can undergo early maturation within the first year after smoltification and can be as small as 10 cm total length and represent a major cause of economic loss in commercial production.[32] Affected fish are smaller than conspecifics and have undergone sexual maturation including the characteristic hooked lower jaw. They typically have decreased growth and feed conversion

efficiency, have reduced flesh quality, and experience increased mortality.[32–34]

Diagnosis: Routine production monitoring will detect elevated early sexual maturation. However, the challenge is predicting which groups will experience the greatest degree of maturation and therefore losses.

Management/control: The factors presently receiving the greatest effort as solutions are photoperiod manipulation and genetics.[31]

NUTRITION AND MUSCULOSKELETAL ABNORMALITIES

Overview: The nutritional requirements for many species of fish remain poorly defined, particularly under the demanding conditions of commercial production. Nutritional issues are a common cause of reduced production in species newly under aquaculture production. The implication of specific nutrients in the development of many musculoskeletal deformities is complicated by the multifactorial nature of their pathogenesis, however, the importance of several key nutrients is unquestionable.[16,17,35,36] The specific conditions covered here in greater detail include the effects of retinoic acid (vitamin A) excess and deficiency, ascorbic acid (vitamin C) and phosphorus deficiency on skeletal development, and vitamin E deficiency on muscle function. Other dietary components no doubt influence the development and function of the musculoskeletal system (see Chapter 16).

Vitamin A

Etiology: Retinol (vitamin A) excess and deficiency. Although there are varied effects, particularly dependent on the stage of growth, excess retinol most importantly causes precocious mineralization, whereas a deficiency of vitamin A reduces collagen synthesis and bone formation producing net bone loss.[36]

Clinical presentation: Both an excess and a deficiency may produce scoliosis.[16] Experimentally, excessive retinoic acid is teratogenic with pharyngeal cartilage affected in flounder embryos and vertebral compression/deformities in juveniles.[37,38] Immersion of flounder larvae in retinoic acid receptor agonists resulted in jaw malformations.[39] Other clinical signs of hypervitaminosis A include reduced growth,

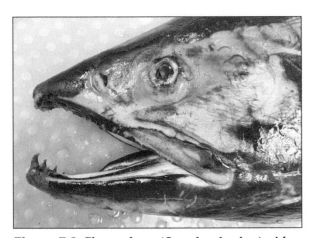

Figure 7.6 Chum salmon (*Oncorhynchus keta*) with kype. (Image courtesy of S. Russell.)

blindness, hemorrhage and anemia, clinical signs also described for retinol deficiency.[36,40]

Vitamin C

Etiology: Ascorbic acid (vitamin C) is required for proper hydroxylation and maturation of collagen, and for osteoblast function and mineralization of bone. Ascorbic acid supplementation is required in commercial diets since fish cannot synthesize this vitamin. Any teleost species would be susceptible; however, species requirements vary widely.

Clinical presentation: Affected fish may have hemorrhages and spinal deformities (e.g., lordosis and scoliosis) with vertebral fractures (e.g., broken back disease). Scorbutic fish may have distorted gill filaments and arches and opercular abnormalities.[41,42] They may also not grow at optimum rates and may have lower survival rates.[12] Higher temperatures worsen the clinical signs of disease because minimum needs are higher.[43,44] Younger fish are also most susceptible, as they experience increased bone growth and turnover.[44]

Pathology: Distortion of cartilage particularly of the gill filaments and in the sclera of the eye is common. Affected cartilage is disorganized, hyperplastic and has increased matrix. Chrondrocyte degeneration and pyknosis was also noted as an early lesion. Fractures were also present in juvenile rainbow trout and channel catfish with vertebra affected prominently.[41,42]

Phosphorus deficiency

Etiology: Phosphorus deficiency can result in reduced growth and skeletal deformities.[45] Phosphorus deficiency has become more important with the need for lower phosphorus in fish diets to reduce environmental impacts. Appropriate phosphorus and calcium levels are both required for normal skeletal growth, and concentrations in bones and tissues are closely interrelated. Sufficient calcium and/or magnesium can be obtained from hard or salt water unlike phosphorus. Single nutrient deficiencies are also relatively uncommon. As a relevant example, "screamer disease" was postulated to involve a lack or imbalance in dietary phosphorus in addition to inadequate vitamin C exacerbated by high water temperatures (>20°C).[46]

Clinical presentation: Softening of bones and distorted vertebral spines were noted in phosphorus deficiency of rainbow trout and in phosphorus-depleted Atlantic salmon, which also had scoliosis.[47,48] The clinical presentation of screamer disease was a characteristic ankyloses of the mandibular articulation, and the most obvious abnormality was a fixed and permanently open (i.e., agape) jaw. Other lesions included spinal shortening, fractured vertebrae, and rarefaction of osseous and cartilaginous tissues resulting in softening/folding, particularly of the opercula and vertebral spines.[46]

Pathology: Consistent lesions in screamer disease included a highly cellular cartilage that was excessive/hyperplastic with a lack of ossification. Where ossification had occurred, osteoclastic activity was prominent.[46]

Differential diagnoses: Fish with phosphorus deficiency are most likely to have bones that are soft and bend, whereas scorbutic fish will have bones that break. There may be more than one concurrent nutritional excess/deficiency, however.

Diagnosis: Histopathology is required, as the nature of the lesions may direct subsequent analyses. Radiology may also be useful. Diagnosis of nutritional deficiencies should include a chemical analysis of feed for phosphorus and calcium and their ratios, as well as vitamin A and vitamin C. Skeletal tissues and muscle should also be analyzed. Tissue concentrations are the most reliable indicator of ascorbate status in fish.[41]

Management/control: Nutritional requirements are species-specific and are also influenced by age/stage of production, water temperature and growth rate/feed conversion rates. Detailed nutritional requirements are available for only a few species. In addition, with increased pressure to incorporate greater amounts of plant protein and to reduce environmental impacts, further research will be needed. Ascorbic acid and many other feed constituents have a limited shelf-life, and stored feed should be renewed regularly.

Nutritional myopathy

Etiology: Nutritional myopathy in teleosts has been clearly demonstrated to occur in some conditions with a deficiency of alpha-tocopherol (vitamin E) or in some instances with dietary lipids that have undergone oxidation. There is little published evidence for a role of selenium as demonstrated in mammals. Oxidized lipid and/or vitamin E deficiency is often associated with lipoid liver disease, sekoke disease in carp and with steatitis.[46,49–51] Fish with these conditions may or may not have a myopathy, and fish with a myopathy may also have lipoid liver disease/steatitis.[49,52,53] In addition, there are numerous reports of fish species suspected of having a nutritional myopathy, but a cause has not been proven.[54]

Clinical presentation: Fish with a myopathy have reduced growth rates and increased mortality. Other clinical signs associated with myopathy, steatitis or lipoid liver disease include anemia, "tail-down" swimming position and darkened color. Seahorses suspected of having a nutritional myopathy had a reduced or absent "snick," the suctioning of prey requiring the nuchal muscles.[54] Affected fish died of numerous secondary infections, whereas supplementation of the diet saw the reversal of clinical signs.[54]

Pathology: There are several characteristic histological features of "bland" nutritional myopathy. These include degeneration of the sarcoplasm with myofiber contraction and necrosis and phagocytosis by macrophages. Thinned remaining fibers may exhibit central rowing of nuclei, and in chronic stages there is marked variation in fiber size. An important feature is the relative lack of inflammatory response and the lack of mineralization (**Figure 7.7**). In addition, muscle groups affected are in some cases bilaterally symmetrical.

Differential diagnoses: Numerous infectious agents may produce a myopathy; however, histopathology, culture, etc. should allow differentiation. There are several reports of idiopathic myopathies, e.g., in walleye *Stizostedion vitreum* and Siamese fighting fish *Betta splendens*. However, the light microscopic lesions differ markedly in character from nutritional myopathy: necrotizing and granulomatous myositis with caseonecrotic cores and mineralization.[16,55]

Diagnosis: As for other nutritional disorders, histopathology, radiology and chemical analysis of feed and tissues may be required.

Management/control: The same as for other nutritional disorders previously discussed. Fish feeds require sufficient antioxidants and must be stored

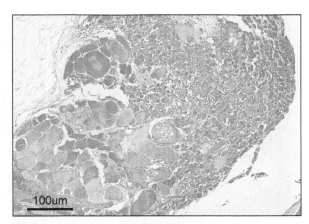

Figure 7.7 Seahorse (*Hippocampus kuda*) with myopathy due to suspected nutritional deficiency. H&E stain. (Image courtesy of V. LePage.)

under cool, dry conditions. Feed should be dated and used in a reasonable time frame. Reversal of these conditions with supplementation or with a new diet is variable.

ELECTROCUTION

Overview: Electrocution is most commonly due to lightning strikes or stray voltage from equipment.[16,56]

Etiology: Electrocution is usually due to a lightning strike of the water or of a building holding fish, or stray voltage from improperly grounded equipment, e.g., pumps or heaters.[16,56,57] Lesions associated with the use of direct current electrofishing can appear identical to the previous situations. Voltage appears to be more lethal in low water hardness (i.e., soft water).

Clinical presentation: Affected fish are usually dark, may have increased respiration and open mouths, but will have reduced swimming ability with flaccidity of the posterior portion of the body. They may appear to have crooked backs with the deviation at or just behind the dorsal fin (**Figure 7.8**). Larger fish are more likely to be affected.

Pathology: Spinal fracture(s) are caused by hypercontraction of myotomes at the site of greatest force (**Figure 7.9**). There will be extensive hemorrhage at the lesion and local myonecrosis (**Figure 7.10**).

Diagnosis: Palpation with crepitus. Radiography can be used but is not usually required. Spinal fracture and hemorrhage at the site is usually sufficient

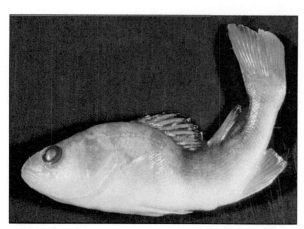

Figure 7.8 Spinal deformity in a yellow perch (*Perca flavescens*) as a result of electroshock in a production system due to stray voltage from an improperly grounded water chiller. (Image courtesy of S.A. Smith.)

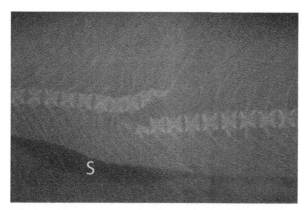

Figure 7.9 Radiograph of rainbow trout (*Oncorhynchus mykiss*) with a complete spinal fracture after electrocution. S, swim bladder. (Image courtesy of R. Moccia.)

for a diagnosis. There may be a history of the weather having recently been stormy.

Management/control: Check electrical equipment for proper grounding. Severely affected fish should be euthanized, as they will not recover.

NONPARASITIC INFECTIOUS MYOSITIS

Overview: There are numerous causes of myositis due to infectious agents where the musculoskeletal system is secondarily affected. Only a few key pathogens that notably and consistently target the musculoskeletal system are covered.

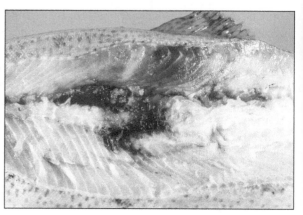

Figure 7.10 The same rainbow trout as **Figure 7.9** with hemorrhage and myonecrosis at site of fracture. (Photo courtesy of R. Moccia.)

Edwardsiella tarda and *E. piscicida*

Edwardsiellosis (i.e., "Edwardsiella septicemia," "red disease" of eels, "emphysematous putrefactive disease" of catfish, "fish gangrene") affects a range of fish species in freshwater and marine environments around the world, and is particularly common in warm water.[58] As for many of the infectious agents, particularly bacteria, lesions in filtering organs are common, however, muscle lesions are often present. *Edwardsiella tarda* is also a zoonotic agent.[59]

Etiology: The majority of this disease is caused by *E. tarda*; however, recently some isolates once considered as *E. tarda* are now classified as *E. piscicida*.[60] They are phenotypically and biochemically indistinguishable and require DNA sequencing techniques to differentiate.

Route of transmission: Horizontal transmission with the bacterium present in water, ponds and in the intestines of fish. Since these bacteria are not obligate pathogens, poor management or stressful conditions are commonly associated with mortality events, which often occur chronically.

Host range: Numerous species including freshwater and marine fishes. Examples include channel catfish (*Ictalurus punctatus*), Japanese eel (*Anguilla japonica*), barramundi (*Lates calcarifer*), olive flounder (*Paralichthys olivaceus*) and red sea bream (*Pagrus major*).[61]

Clinical presentation: Varied but consistent with systemic infection including exopthalmia; ascites; erosions of the skin; and pale, inflamed gill tissue.

Expansive lesions are often present in muscle, which are characteristically foul smelling on release of the liquid content and often surrounded by zones of hemorrhage.

Pathology: The majority of descriptions have histocytes as the dominant cell type and granulomatous inflammation as the dominant reaction in most tissues, often progressing to abscessation.[58] *Edwardsiella tarda* causes abscesses filled with cells enlarged with bacteria, necrotic debris and gas in the muscle of channel catfish.[62] In red sea bream, liquefied abscesses were noted in muscle adjacent to the kidney.[63]

Differential diagnosis: *Aeromonas hydrophila* and *Vibrio anguillarum*, both of which can affect muscle, or other systemic bacterial infections.

Diagnosis: Culture on trypticase soya agar (TSA) or other media followed by biochemical characterization. Enzyme immunoassay has been used.[64] Loop-mediated isothermal amplification and various polymerase chain reaction (PCR) assays are now also available.[65] Differentiation of *E. piscicida* from *E. tarda* requires more advanced PCR techniques and multilocus sequence analysis.[60]

Management/control: Numerous reports describe efficacious experimental vaccines.[61] Good management practices will limit the impact of this disease.

Renibacterium salmoninarum

Bacterial kidney disease (BKD) caused by *Renibacterium salmoninarum* is one of the most important infectious diseases that significantly affects muscle. The detrimental impact in *Oncorhynchus* salmon species has been so great, particularly in Chinook salmon, that this species is no longer farmed to a great extent in British Columbia and only in smaller-sized, low-density operations.

Etiology: *Renibacterium salmoninarum* is a Gram-positive diplobacillus that belongs to the Micrococcus-Arthrobacter sub-group of the actinomycetes.[66] Isolates from different hosts or regions have proved quite homogenous by most typing methods; however, multilocus variable-number tandem-repeat genotyping may be more promising.[67]

Route of transmission: Both horizontal and vertical transmission are documented for this organism.[68,69]

Host range: Salmonids including salmon and trout. The disease was first described in Atlantic salmon as

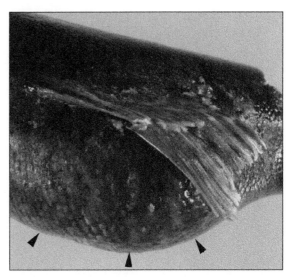

Figure 7.11 Speckled trout (*Salvelinus fontinalis*) with lateral expansion of musculature (arrowheads) due to infection with *R. salmoninarum*. (Image courtesy of H. Ferguson.)

"Dee disease" and subsequently in numerous other salmonids.[67] Chinook and Atlantic salmon sustain the greatest economic impact.

Clinical presentation: The kidney and other internal organs are targeted initially with skeletal muscle impacted largely by extension from the kidney once the infection has progressed. The chronic nature of the disease, however, means that muscle lesions may be the first clinical signs noticed in well-grown fish. The lesions may extend to and distort the dermis and the profile of the fish (**Figure 7.11**). Large lesions often have cavernous bullae that may contain fluid (**Figure 7.12**).

Pathology: Extensive sheets of enlarged macrophages with a smaller number of neutrophils. Cells often contain large numbers of bacteria that stain poorly with H&E unless present in overwhelming numbers. Gram stain will pinpoint the characteristic diplobacilli in cells and in tissue/fluid.

Differential diagnosis: Bacterial diseases such as *Aeromonas salmonicida* subsp. *salmonicida* or furunculosis, nephrocalcinosis, or *Carnobacterium piscicola*.

Diagnosis: Immunofluorescence of kidney tissue is often used for regulatory screening, whereas the aquaculture industry often uses an ELISA on homogenized kidney tissue.[70,71] The advantages of the ELISA are greater sensitivity and rapid results

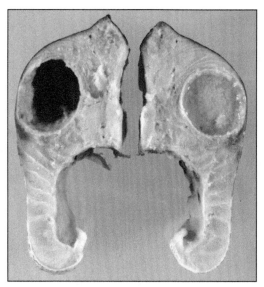

Figure 7.12 Salmon with suspect *R. salmoninarum* cavitation lesion of muscle. (Image courtesy of H. Ferguson.)

that are quantitative facilitating decisions in broodstock management. PCR assays are also used as is histopathology. Culture is slow, requiring weeks and specialized media, and is not widely used.

Management/control: Antimicrobials are generally ineffective. Targeted use of erythromycin in broodstock before spawning and ELISA screening to eliminate heavily infected fish can reduce the burden in fry. Good husbandry practices including site fallowing and maintaining appropriate stocking densities can reduce losses due to BKD. A vaccine with variable efficacy is available.[72]

Ichthyophoniasis

Similar to *R. salmoninarum*, filtering organs are primarily impacted by ichthyophoniasis. However, muscle is often infected as well, and these lesions can have significant economic impact.

Etiology: Ichthyophoniasis is caused by *Ichthyophonus hoferi*, a protistan parasite whose taxonomic classification is unclear.

Route of transmission: Ingestion of infected fish is proposed to be the most important mode of spread to piscivorous fish.[73] The route of infection in wild planktivorous fish is unclear.[74] Experimentally, intraperitoneal injection of isolated parasites or repeated feedings resulted in the highest infection rates.[74] There is no evidence for vertical transmission. Incorporation of infected marine fish in the food stream has been implicated as the source in most cultured settings.

Host range: Wild marine fish and anadromous fish worldwide are most commonly affected; however, there are examples of infection in cultured marine fish and in wild freshwater fish.[75]

Clinical presentation: There are usually minimal or no clinical signs. though affected fish may be emaciated. Infected rainbow trout have decreased swimming performance.[76] Gross lesions in herring are termed "sandpaper skin" and represent either raised inflammatory lesions or pigmented ulcers. Rainbow trout may have petechial hemorrhages and similar lesions as herring.[77] The lesions in these fish are most intense over the caudal third of the body.

Pathology: The muscle lesions are histiocyte-rich, multifocal to coalescing foci (granulomas or granulomatous inflammation) in tissues including muscle. Unencapsulated schizonts may be single or multiple and will be typically surrounded by inflammation. The roughly spherical schizonts range in size from 50 to 250 μm and are periodic acid-Schiff (PAS)–positive.

Differential diagnosis: Other invasive fungi and *Dermocystidium* spp. need to be ruled out.

Diagnosis: Culture is considered to be the most sensitive detection technique, particularly in low-intensity infections. PCR and qPCR, histology and squash preparations of tissues are also used alone or in combination with culture.[78,79]

Management/control: No chemotherapeutants are available. Avoidance of feeding unsterilized fish offal to cultured fish and elimination of heavily infected individuals is recommended.

Flavobacterium psychrophilum

Etiology: *Flavobacterium psychrophilum* is the causative agent of bacterial coldwater disease (BCWD) and rainbow trout fry syndrome (RTFS). Some presentations of BCWD are characterized by a necrotizing myositis and others with a cephalic osteochondritis.[80,81] *Flavobacterium psychrophilum* also commonly targets the vertebral cartilage and bone.[16] Fin or tail rot is also a common presentation as well (**Figure 7.13**). It should be noted that to date sub-groups (i.e., genotypes or other) of isolates have not been associated with distinct clinical presentations.[82]

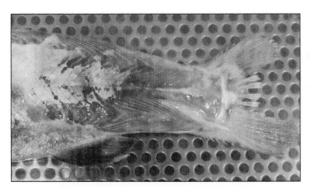

Figure 7.13 Rainbow trout (*Oncorhynchus mykiss*) with bacterial coldwater disease (BCWD) due to *F. psychrophilum*.

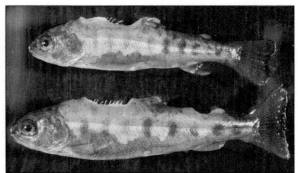

Figure 7.14 Juvenile rainbow trout (*Oncorhynchus mykiss*) with bacterial coldwater disease (BCWD) ulcerative lesions along dorsal surface of fish. (Image courtesy of S.A. Smith.)

Route of transmission: The bacteria is predominantly transmitted horizontally and in large numbers from dead fish and those with ulcerative lesions. Disease is most common at ~12°C and below. Both cephalic osteochondritis and retinal scleritis and necrotic myositis result from systemic spread with localization to the cartilage/bone or muscle. The disease may also be transmitted vertically.[83]

Host range: Commercially most important in salmonids in freshwater worldwide, but numerous other species are also affected.[84] *Oncorhynchus* sp. are particularly susceptible with rainbow trout aquaculture affected most severely. The impact of vertical transmission on host immunity (i.e., tolerance) or on disease is poorly understood but is potentially very important.[83]

Clinical presentation: There are several clinical presentations of BCWD; however, the two of concern here are cephalic osteochondritis and necrotic myositis.[85] Apart from mortality, rainbow trout with cephalic osteochondritis have exophthalmos and intraocular hemorrhage, whereas those with necrotic myositis have large muscular lesions filled with bloody fluid that can markedly expand the overlying dermis and may eventually ulcerate.[81] Young rainbow trout may have ulcerative lesions of the dorsal fin and caudal peduncle (**Figure 7.14**). Fish that survive BCWD outbreaks will often have a spinal deformity.

Pathology: The cartilage of the branchial arches and cranium are the primary targets in cephalic osteochondritis with lysis, pyogranulomatous inflammation and often some degree of fibrosis if the fish survives.[81] Similar lesions are noted when *F. psychrophilum* affects the vertebrae, and the inflammatory response often extends to the spinal cord. Large bullae in the muscle filled with hemorrhage and necrotic debris with large numbers of filamentous organisms characterize necrotic myositis. Similar lesions were reproduced in experimental infections.[80]

Differential diagnosis: *Aeromonas salmonicida*, BKD, whirling disease, and any septicemic disease (in smaller fish with RTFS). PCR can readily discriminate *F. psychrophilum* from the numerous other yellow-pigmented, Gram-negative species that cause disease in salmonids.[86]

Diagnosis: Culture of the organism on Cytophaga or similar agar is straightforward; however, incubation should be at 15°C and growth can be slow. The organism in cartilage and bone is poorly or not visible using most histologic stains. Immunohistochemistry demonstrates the filamentous organisms well in these situations.[81]

Management/control: Antimicrobial treatment, though *F. psychrophilum* is inherently resistant to sulfa combinations.[87] Commercial vaccines exist, however they are not widely available. Important management strategies include a reduction in stocking density and careful monitoring of inappetence followed by rapid treatment.[85] Culturing fish at or above 15°C will profoundly limit the disease; however, this is rarely possible. Resistant strains of fish have been developed, as the heritability of disease resistance is moderate.[88]

Motile aeromonads and *Aeromonas salmonicida* subsp. *salmonicida*

The motile aeromonads are a complex of organisms that cause systemic fish disease with muscle often involved; the same applies to *Aeromonas salmonicida* subsp. *salmonicida*.

Etiology: *Aeromonas salmonicida* subsp. *salmonicida* (hereafter simply *A. salmonicida*) is the cause of furunculosis, a disease that produces "furuncles" or necrotizing muscle lesions in the muscle of salmonids and other cold-water species (**Figure 7.15**). Motile aeromonads, hereafter referred to as *A. hydrophila* for simplicity, cause muscle lesions as part of systemic disease, and most severely and commonly in warmer water species.

Route of transmission: Transmission is horizontal for both organisms. Although fish can be affected year-round, *A. hydrophila* septicemia is most common in the spring with rising water temperatures.

Host range:

- *A. salmonicida*—Classically a disease of salmonids, with charr (*Salvelinus alpinus*) and brook trout (*Salvelinus fontinalis*) particularly susceptible and most likely to present with necrotizing muscle lesions. Other salmonids will develop muscle involvement more commonly in chronic infections. Furunculosis has had a large economic impact in Atlantic salmon aquaculture. Atypical strains of *A. salmonicida* (e.g., subsp. *achromogenes*) can infect a broad range of non-salmonid fish including goldfish and carp.[89]

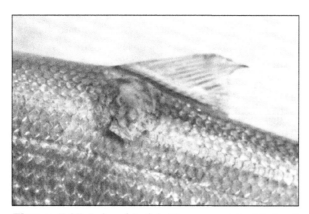

Figure 7.15 Lake whitefish (*Coregonus sp.*) with focal necrotizing myositis caused by *A. salmonicida* subsp. *salmonicida*. (Image courtesy of H. Ferguson.)

- *A. hydrophila*—Has greatest impact in warmer freshwater groups of fish, e.g., channel catfish, carp and tilapia, but can also infect brackish and saltwater fish less commonly.

Clinical presentation: Typical for many systemic bacterial diseases; however, the muscle lesions, when present, can be the initial reason that an abnormality is noticed. The muscle lesions can be very large, occur anywhere on the body, and may even penetrate and extend to the abdominal cavity.

- *A. salmonicida*—The term "furuncle" is a misnomer as fish do not have hair follicles, inflammation of which is termed "furunculosis." The term is widespread and historical and so continues to be used. Furuncles are not consistently present in fish infected with *A. salmonicida* but tend to be more commonly present in fish that are chronically infected or in fish that are relatively resistant to infection, e.g., rainbow trout. Since muscle lesions are an expression of systemic spread with localization in the secondary vasculature network beneath the dermis, susceptible species like brook trout may have furuncles along with other systemic lesions. The lesions are expansive with ulceration through the dermis occurring as the disease progresses.
- *A. hydrophila*—Chronic infection with motile aeromonads will often be limited to the dermis and musculature with hemorrhage and ulceration of the epidermis/dermis occurring initially with spread to muscle.[90]

Pathology:

- *A. salmonicida*—Early muscle lesions with *A. salmonicida* are commonly localized near the secondary vasculature between the deep dermis and musculature. Macrophages predominate, but neutrophils are also present, and there are often numerous Gram-negative bacteria. Liquefactive lesions expand as myonecrosis becomes extensive and are filled with fluid, fibrin, inflammatory cells, cellular debris, hemorrhage and bacteria (**Figure 7.16**).[91]

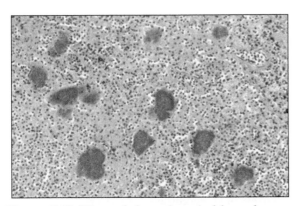

Figure 7.16 Histopathology of a typical furuncle caused by *A. salmonicida* subsp. *salmonicida* that includes hemorrhage, necrotic debris and bacterial microcolonies. H&E stain. (Image courtesy of H. Ferguson.)

A. hydrophila—Red-sore disease in striped bass (*Morone saxatilis*) and its hybrids, largemouth bass (*Micropterus salmoides*) and other species is initially centered on the epidermis and dermis with hemorrhage, inflammation, waterlogging (i.e., movement of water into tissues that lack an overlying epidermis)/edema that then progresses to ulceration with extensive necrosis of muscle in chronic lesions (**Figure 7.17**). The muscle lesions have been described as lacking inflammatory cells; however, the lack is likely due in part to lysis of cells from waterlogging of tissues.[90]

Differential diagnosis: Numerous bacteria including *Vibrio* spp., *F. psychrophilum*, *Streptococcus* spp. and *Pseudomonas* spp.

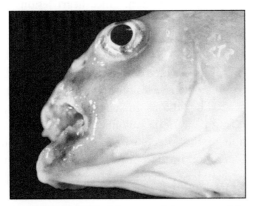

Figure 7.17 Cichlid with necrotizing stomatitis caused by motile *Aeromonas* septicemia. (Image courtesy of H. Ferguson.)

Diagnosis: Culture and biochemical characterization are most important, but other diagnostic and molecular assays have also been developed.[89]

A. salmonicida—Culture from lesions or kidney tissue using TSA or brain heart infusion agar (BHIA) often produces a brown pigment in the media; however, this is not a constant finding.

A. hydrophila—Culture using TSA or BHIA media, however, numerous concurrent bacteria will grow. To facilitate preferential growth of motile aeromonads in primary culture Rimler-Shotts (RS agar) or SGAP-10C can be used.[92,93] Speciation of the *A. hydrophila* complex can be challenging and molecular tools should provide greater clarity.

Management/control:

A. salmonicida—Elimination/reduction of *A. salmonicida* in eggs is best achieved by treatment with iodine compounds. However, efficacy can be limited by organic matter, soft acidic water and high numbers of organisms.[89] Salmonid stocks that carry *A. salmonicida* without clinical signs may be "stress-tested" by injection of prednisolone.[94] Resistant strains of brook and brown trout have been developed over several decades, but resistance to *A. salmonicida* in Atlantic salmon has only moderate heritability.[95,96] The significant impact of furunculosis on Atlantic salmon aquaculture has led to numerous other strategies to blunt its impact. Vaccination using killed-bacterins with oil adjuvant and intraperitoneal injection have been very effective in reducing the commercial impact of furunculosis in Atlantic salmon aquaculture.[97] They are typically a multivalent preparation combined with *Vibrio anguillarum/ordalli/salmonicida*. There can be side effects, however, primarily due to the adjuvant, including peritonitis and reduced growth rates. However, recent shifts to smaller injection volumes may limit this deleterious impact.[98] Antimicrobial resistance has been demonstrated to both oxytetracycline and oxolinic acid.[99]

A. hydrophila—Heterogeneity of isolates and antigenic diversity is a barrier to effective control beyond the typical good management practices. Experimental killed and live attenuated vaccines may play a role in the future.[100,101] Infection is precipitated by stress and poor management in many situations and so reduced impact can be achieved by improved management.

Heart and skeletal muscle disease, and pancreas disease/sleeping disease

These diseases are grouped together because of the similarity of the lesion produced in red muscle fibers of salmonids. Red "slow" muscle is normally found as a wedge under the lateral line and is important for locomotion. Compared to the other major type of muscle (i.e., white), red muscle is more highly vascularized with greater numbers of mitochondria. This type of muscle fibers may also be seen associated with opercula or with some fins.[16]

Etiology: Heart and skeletal muscle disease (HSMI) is associated with piscine reovirus (PRV). The term "associated" is appropriate, as growth of the virus on cell lines has proved problematic and is therefore due to a lack of repeatable fulfillment of Koch's postulates.[102,103] However no on-farm case of HSMI is known to have occurred without the presence of PRV, and there is a strong epidemiological relationship between the histological lesions and presence of the virus.[104] Pancreas disease (PD) and the closely similar sleeping disease (SD) are caused by salmonid alphavirus (SAV).[105] There are six subtypes of the virus; however, viral determinants of disease variability remain to be determined.

Route of transmission: Fish injected with tissue homogenates containing PRV can horizontally transmit the virus; however, development of characteristic lesions is variable.[102,103,106] Pancreas disease and SD are transmitted horizontally.[105]

Host range: Salmonids, most importantly Atlantic salmon for HSMI and PD, and rainbow trout for SD. Heart and skeletal muscle disease is present in Norway, Scotland, Chile and more recently in British Columbia, Canada, and is presently considered the

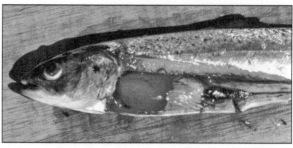

Figure 7.18 Atlantic salmon (*Salmo salar*) "pinhead" with marked cachexia due to pancreas disease. (Image courtesy of H. Ferguson.)

third most important disease of Atlantic salmon in Norway.[104,107]

Clinical presentation: The course of clinical disease of HSMI and PD/SD can be quite prolonged and vary by phase. Importantly, this affects the choice of diagnostic test. HSMI is typically characterized by low mortality (<20%) but very high morbidity. Abnormal swimming and anorexia can also be present, but runting is not described.[104] Pancreas disease will present with a decrease in appetite in the acute phase with mortality in the chronic phase and runting of a proportion of affected fish during recovery (**Figure 7.18**). Sleeping disease will have low mortality until the subacute to chronic phases when appetite decreases and mortalities increase. It is in the recovery phase when lethargy/sluggish swimming/"sleeping behavior" is most commonly present.[105] In rainbow trout "sleeping" or fish lying on their sides or on the bottom of the tank/raceway can be present at any stage of production. Since heart lesions can be present in all three diseases, there may be ascites and other lesions associated with heart failure.

Pathology: In fish affected by HSMI, skeletal lesions are restricted to the red muscle.[106] Fish with PD or SD may have lesions in both the red and white muscle. The lesions include hyaline degeneration and fragmentation, myofiber swelling, and infiltration of the affected myofibers by macrophages. Regeneration is often present, characterized by central rowing of sarcolemma nuclei and basophilia. The degree of inflammation varies but is most prominent in the red muscle in fish with HSMI or SD. There may be a limited degree of fibrosis in fish with severe lesions.

Differential diagnosis: Cardiomyopathy syndrome must be differentiated: There are no pancreatic lesions and muscle lesions are not restricted to the red fibers and are limited in severity.[108,109] Fish with HSMI also have no pancreatic lesions. Nutritional myopathy is also a differential given that there can be a limited inflammatory response, particularly in fish with PD.

Diagnosis: Careful attention to the range of lesions present and sampling over time is required if only histopathology is used to make a diagnosis. The viral etiologies can be detected by qPCR and immunohistochemistry (IHC), but virus isolation is not typically performed for routine diagnosis. The viruses are either difficult (SAV) or extremely difficult to grow (PRV) and CPE is often not present.

Management/control: General best management practices for infectious disease are applied to reduce the impact of these diseases. Reduction of the clinical impact is most critical and review of movement practices of viremic fish and of stress is needed. Control of sea lice may also be important, as they have been hypothesized to play a role in transmission of SAV.[110] Effective commercial vaccines for pancreas disease are now available.

PARASITIC INFECTIOUS MYOSITIS

Overview: Numerous species of protozoan and metazoan parasites infect the musculoskeletal system of fish as larval stages or adults. They may parasitize only a single type of fish or may be nonspecific in their infectivity. Some cause significant pathology and/or death of the host fish, whereas others cause minimal harm to the host.

Kudoa thyrsites

Although *Kudoa* species can cause space occupying cyst lesions and myositis, antemortem clinical signs are not typical.[111] The primary economic impact in many species, including Atlantic salmon, is after harvest due to myoliquefaction or "soft flesh" of the tissues.

Etiology: Dozens of species of parasites affect a range of fish species.[111] *Kudoa thyrsites* alone affects numerous species of fish, and this parasite will be the focus of much of the information to follow.

There is evidence that *K. thyrsites* itself is a complex assemblage of distinct geographic subpopulations.[111] Morphological classification needs to be supplemented by further DNA analysis to clarify phylogeny.

Route of transmission: Myxosporeans do not demonstrate direct transmission and require additional host(s), however, these are often not known.[111]

Host range: Each *Kudoa* species has a distinct host range. *Kudoa thyrsites* infects multiple species of fish and has a global distribution.[112]

Clinical presentation: Cysts of varying size may be present and can be macroscopically visible either with or without dissection of the muscle depending on the species of *Kudoa* and the species of fish affected. There are few antemortem clinical signs documented. Since *K. thyrsites* can be present in the hearts of *Oncorhynchus* spp. and in other tissues, further investigation may reveal a greater antemortem impact.

Pathology: *Kudoa thyrsites* does not cause macroscopic cyst formation, however many other species do.[111] As a generalization, no host reaction is present when the parasite is within intact myofibers. Fiber degeneration and release of myxospores stimulates a strong response dominated by macrophages.[111]

Differential diagnosis: Other myxosporeans or infectious agents affecting muscle. Lesions are multifocal and only inflammation may be noted in a given section, particularly in light infections. Lesions that have only nonsporulated stages cannot be differentiated using light microscopy.

Diagnosis: Gross examination and light microscopy can be used. However, rapid assays are required to detect affected fish after harvest and before sale since post mortem myoliquefaction ("soft flesh" or "milky flesh") is the most important economic impact (**Figure 7.19**).[111] A quantitative 18S rDNA PCR for *K. thyrsites* was found to perform acceptably compared with histology to predict flesh quality.[113]

Management/control: There are no vaccines or chemotherapeutants for *Kudoa* spp. The economic impact of *K. thyrsites* in Atlantic salmon in the British Columbia aquaculture industry is managed by classification of sites based on historical incidence. Movement of smolts from low-risk to higher-risk sites sequentially can reduce the impact, and there is recent evidence for acquired resistance.[114]

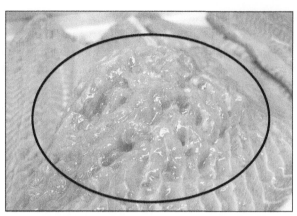

Figure 7.19 Atlantic salmon (*Salmo salar*) fillet with myolysis (circle) due to *Kudoa thyrsites*. Myolysis occurs after euthanasia and processing. (Image courtesy of D. Morrison.)

Myxobolus cerebralis

Whirling disease, caused by *Myxobolus cerebralis*, is an important disease that has significant clinical impact on wild trout in infected freshwater bodies. The parasite originated in Europe but is now present in North America, Asia, Africa and Oceania.[115]

Etiology: *Myxobolus cerebralis* is a myxozoan parasite with myxospores and actinospores.

Route of transmission: Due to the importance of the disease and the attention that this parasite has received as opposed to other myxosporeans, the life cycle of *M. cerebralis* is well understood. Myxospores are released from dying fish into the environment and ingested by *Tubifex tubifex*, an aquatic oligochaete worm. Sexual reproduction occurs in *T. tubifex*, and actinospores actively seek salmonids and attach to and penetrate the epidermis.

Host range: Many *Oncorhynchus*, *Salmo* and *Salvelinus* species can be infected; however, rainbow trout, cutthroat trout and sockeye salmon are most commonly affected. Mountain whitefish (*Prosopium williamsoni*) are also susceptible.[115] Susceptibility decreases with increasing age as cartilage becomes ossified.[116]

Clinical presentation: The clinical signs typically described for whirling disease are not exclusive to this disease but should place it as a potential consideration, particularly in areas where the parasite is endemic. Juvenile salmonids that are less than a year of age that exhibit whirling behavior, have a blackened tail, or have skeletal deformities, including a shortened operculum or nose, indented cranium, or scoliosis, should be suspect.

Pathology: The lesions produced by infection can vary with the fish affected; susceptible species have more severe lesions centered on the cranium and central nervous system, whereas more resistant species, e.g. brown trout (*Salmo trutta*), have less severe lesions that are more common in the ribs and vertebrae.[117] In rainbow trout the most important lesions are necrosis of cranial cartilage associated with trophozoites and/or spores with, often extensive, histocytic inflammation of adjacent tissues. Older fish may have spores present in bone with little or no inflammation. Cranium, vertebrae, ribs, fin rays and branchial arches can all be affected.

Differential diagnosis: Similar clinical signs can be caused by numerous infectious agents that can infect cranial tissues. *Flavobacterium psychrophilum* can cause whirling behavior and spinal deformities. Several other myxosporea can infect the brain and spinal cord of rainbow trout, and are morphologically similar, confusing the diagnostic process. However, *M. neurotropas* produces no inflammation.[119] *Myxobolus kisutchi*, *M. neurobius*, *M. arcticus* and others have also been identified in the central nervous tissue of salmonids.[120]

Diagnosis: Histology and PCR are confirmatory methods for diagnosis that often follow a presumptive diagnosis based on clinical signs and/or a pepsin-trypsin digest of cranial tissues. Histology and PCR will detect the presence of both presporogonic and sporogonic stages.[115,118]

Management/control: Avoidance of infection is the most effective strategy. The lack of management strategies for wild stocks apart from restrictions on fish movement has seen whirling disease spread to many U.S. states. Aquaculture operations can effectively prevent disease by keeping fry in concrete raceways or other artificial systems, and preventing exposure of susceptible ages of fish to *T. tubifex*. Ultraviolet irradiation of incoming hatchery water can also be effective.[121]

Glugea

Glugea is one genus of many microsporean (i.e., microsporidean) parasites that affect fish. Microsporeans are strictly intracellular parasites.

Classification of microsporidea is based on spore morphology, fish species and host affected, although molecular analysis is modifying this somewhat.[122]

Etiology: The genus *Glugea* infects many species of fish and many tissue sites since connective tissue cells are targeted.[122]

Route of transmission: Direct transmission by ejection of the infectious sporoplasm via the polar tube from the spore into host cells. Ingestion of spores with initial infection of intestinal cells and then spreading to other organs has also been documented. There is a simple life cycle including merogony and sporogony that both take place in the host cell cytoplasm.

Host range: A broad range of fish species in both freshwater and marine environments is affected. A single species of *Glugea* can also infect more than one species of fish. Notable species include *Glugea hertwegi* in smelt (*Osmerus mordax*), *G. anomala* in sticklebacks (*Gasterosteus aculeatus*), *G. plecoglossi* in ayu (*Plecoglossus altivelis*) and *G. stephani* in English sole (*Parophrys vetulus*).

Clinical presentation: White to black cyst-like structures, often multiple, that displace normal tissue and protrude from the dermis (**Figure 7.20**).

Pathology: Massive hypertrophy of infected cells yield a xenoma that can result in marked atrophy of surrounding tissue. A xenoma may contain meronts, sporonts and mature spores, often with the latter centrally located. Depending on the stage of development, xenomas may be surrounded by a dystrophic parasite-induced wall including remnants of atrophied adjacent cells and host fibroblasts. On dissolution of the xenoma, a more notable host response

includes more intense fibroplasia and large numbers of histocytes ingesting spores.

Differential diagnosis: Other microsporeans including *Heterosporis* spp. and *Pleistophora* spp. that affect muscle and histiozoic myxosporeans.

Diagnosis: Histology can be used to identify microsporidia to the generic level, but definitive classification requires electron microscopy to determine spore morophology. PCR diagnosis is becoming more common as is sequencing of small subunit ribosomal rRNA genes.

Management/control: Avoidance of infection is the best practice. The impact of microsporeans on most cultured fish is limited. A number of chemotherapeutants, including fumagillin and albendazole, are effective experimentally, but none are approved for use in food fish.[123]

Pleistophora hyphessobryconis

Pleistophora hyphessobryconis is a microsporidean parasite that causes widespread myositis that has considerable clinical impact in susceptible fish.

Etiology: *Pleistophora hyphessobryconis* is the cause of "neon tetra disease" in the neon tetra (*Paracheirodon innesi*) and other tropical fishes.

Route of transmission: Natural transmission of microsporeans is direct. Experimental infection by ingestion of spores produced reproduction of disease.[123] Autoinfection, spread from a myocyte to adjacent myocytes, is possible. Infection of 8-day-old neon tetras has also been documented, raising the likelihood of vertical transmission.[124]

Host range: This agent demonstrates fairly broad host specificity, and numerous fish species apart from the neon tetra have been demonstrated to be infected with *P. hyphessobryconis* of which the majority are tropical aquarium fish.[124] Distinct but morphologically similar microsporeans are potentially responsible for some of these, as identity is often made on limited morphological characterization. More recently zebrafish (*Danio rerio*) have been identified to be naturally and experimentally infected.[124]

Clinical presentation: There are often no clinical signs apart from mortality. Closer examination of a portion of affected fish will typically reveal areas of depigmentation/pallor in the epidermis that overlay

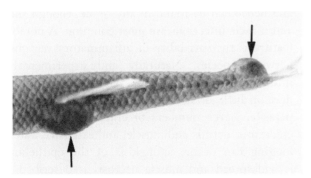

Figure 7.20 Cyst-like masses (arrows) of *Glugea* sp. that protrude from the dermis. (Image courtesy of H. Ferguson.)

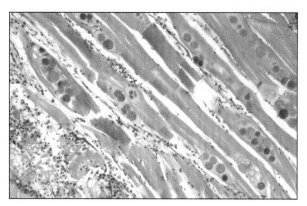

Figure 7.21 *Pliestophora* sp. infection of muscle in a neon tetra (*Paracheirodon innesi*). H&E stain. (Image courtesy of H. Ferguson.)

areas of swollen and edematous muscle. Spinal curvature has also been reported.[124]

Pathology: Myocytes are expanded by numerous sporophorus vesicles that contain developing stages and mature spores. Disruption of myomeres and loss of sarcoplasm are usually present, and vesicles may completely occupy myomeres. There may be no inflammation present or it may be extensive (**Figure 7.21**). Myolysis/myonecrosis is accompanied by inflammation, and the response is histocytic with cells that contain numerous phagocytosed spores.[124,125] Cellular hypertrophy does not occur.[122]

Differential diagnosis: Morphologically similar microsporeans, particularly those in the genus *Ovipleistophora* and *Heterosporis* should be included in the differential.

Diagnosis: Histopathology is the primary diagnostic technique used in most cases followed by electron microscopy for species confirmation. Spores are Gram-positive.[125] Classification of *Pleistophora* species, based on ultrastructure and small submit rRNA gene sequences, is ongoing.[124]

Management/control: Avoidance of infection is the main control method. Purchase of fish from commercial suppliers, including aquarium stores, should be cautious. Fish can be subclinically infected for at least a year and routine quarantine procedures may not be sufficient to detect mild infections even when fish are sacrificed and examined histologically.[124]

Tetrahymena

Tetrahymena spp. are mostly saprozoic protozoa; however, fish infections are increasingly described. They are small pyriform holotrichous ciliophorans that can act as histophagus parasites of fish, invertebrates and amphibians.[126]

Etiology: *Tetrahymena corlissi* is the most important species that causes disease in freshwater fish.[127] *Uronema* spp. and *Miamiensis* spp. cause a similar disease (i.e., scuticociliatosis) in marine species of fish.[128,129]

Route of transmission: Invasion from the environment is most common, as *Tetrahymena* are usually free-living. However, horizontal transmission from infected fish is a significant source of infection for tank mates.

Host range: A common cause of disease in freshwater aquarium fish, either in commercial culture or aquaria, and many fish are susceptible. Notable species include guppies (*Poecilia reticulata*), angelfish (*Pterophyllum scalare*), platy (*Xiphophorus maculates*) and neon tetras, golden perch (*Macquaria ambiqua*), goldfish (*Carassius auratus*), and koi (*Cyprinus carpio koi*).[130–132] Food fish like Atlantic salmon, hybrid striped bass, and yellow perch can also be infected.[133]

Clinical presentation: Lesions may be raised, and pale or depigmented. They can occur anywhere on the body. Depigmentation of the dermis can be present when necrosis of dermal cells, including the pigment cells, occurs and when the dermis is waterlogged. Fish may also die without visible lesions.

Pathology: These ciliates can be highly invasive, particularly in susceptible species like the guppy and hence can be found in any tissue, though skin and muscle infections are most common. A notable feature is the variability in inflammatory response between species. Naturally and experimentally infected guppies, which experience high mortality, develop little or no inflammatory response to the parasite. Large numbers of ciliates can penetrate epidermis, dermis and muscle, and extensive waterlogging can occur. Spongiosis of the epithelium is widespread and muscle necrosis is described.[134] Erythrocytes, and likely other cells/cell content, have been noted inside the parasite.[134] In contrast, koi and goldfish, which are more resistant to infection, generate an inflammatory response that is dominated by histocytes.[132] Atlantic salmon had dermal depigmentation and erosion with spongiosis, and an infiltrate of macrophages, lymphocytes and plasma cells. Local muscle necrosis was extensive with loss of striation and granular degeneration of myofibers.[133]

Differential diagnosis: The most important primary differential diagnosis would be other invasive ciliates. Similar gross lesions could be present with columnaris.

Diagnosis: Histopathology is the gold standard for diagnosis. Wet mounts of dermal lesions would also reveal ciliates. *Tetrahymena* are easily cultured and are used as vectors and for development of vaccines for other diseases. Hence molecular assays are readily available but they are not used diagnostically.[135]

Management/control: Treatment of golden perch with dimetridazole resulted in a cessation of mortality and healing of ulcers in affected fish in several days.[131] There is a lack of chemotherapeutants for food fish. Niclosamide, albendazole and chloroquine all had some efficacy on *in vitro* survival of the parasite and oral niclosamide reduced mortality in the guppy.[136] Experimental infections in the guppy revealed that infection was worse when poor environmental conditions (e.g., high ammonia and low water temperature) were present.[130]

Digenetic trematodes

A large group of metazoan parasites that commonly infect fish as either an intermediate or final (i.e., definitive) host.[137,138] They may cause mortality, but in most cases the primary economic impact is downgrading of flesh quality/appearance. Affected flesh may appear unappealing but is completely safe to eat if thoroughly cooked. There are a few digeneans that are zoonotic.

Etiology: Yellow grub or *Clinostomum* sp., blackspot or *Neascus* sp. and the tissue fluke *Bolbophorus damnificus* are examples specifically dealt with here. Blackspot can be caused by more than one genus and species of Neodiplostomidae (i.e., neascus stage) including *Posthodiplostomum citicola*, *Uvulifer ambloplitis* and others.

Route of transmission: The life cycle of digeneans is complex and indirect. Fish can be intermediate or final hosts. Often the metacercaria is the "quiescent"

life stage in the second intermediate host (i.e., fish) with completion of the life cycle in piscivorous birds. The encysted metacercaria is often the stage encountered in fish health investigations.

Host range: Clinostomids infect a broad range of fish and consist of numerous species of parasite. *Clinostomum marginatum* is important in North America, while *C. complanatum* is important outside North America. The taxonomy of Clinostomids is currently in flux.[139] Encysted *Neascus* spp. cause blackspot in a large number of fish species worldwide. *Bolbophorus damnificus* affects the channel catfish (*I. punctatus*) and is highly pathogenic in juvenile fish.

Clinical presentation: Clinostomid metacercaria are very large and yellow in color, and therefore easily noted externally under or in the skin (**Figure 7.22**). Blackspots are small and unsightly, and in fish valued for their appearance (e.g., koi) can have an economic impact (**Figure 7.23**). Blackspot infections in very high numbers have rarely been associated with mortality depending on the fish species and site of infection.[137] Both the yellow grub and blackspot

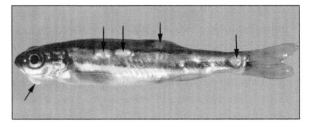

Figure 7.22 Encysted larval digeneans (arrows) in a baitfish. (Image courtesy of H. Ferguson.)

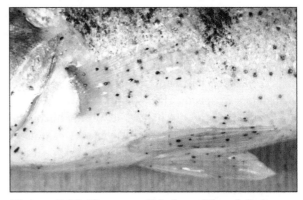

Figure 7.23 Numerous "blackspot" larval digeneans in the fins and skin of a yellow perch (*Perca flavescens*). (Image courtesy of H. Ferguson.)

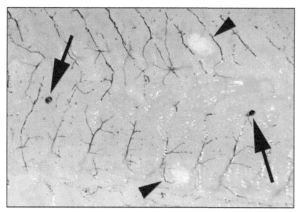

Figure 7.24 Yellow grub (arrowhead) and blackspot (arrow) parasites in the muscle of a blue gill (*Lepomis macrochirus*). (Image courtesy of S.A. Smith.)

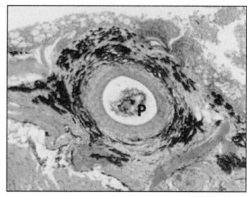

Figure 7.25 Histopathology of "blackspot" larval digenean in a pumpkinseed (*Lepomis gibbosus*). Note that the black pigmentation is due to the host's melanomacrophage response surrounding the parasite (P). H&E stain. (Image courtesy of S.A. Smith.)

metacercarial stages are often readily noticeable in the muscle (**Figure 7.24**). There are few characteristic gross clinical signs for *B. damnificus*. Parasitism with *B. damnificus* may also increase mortality in juvenile channel catfish due to *E. ictaluri*.[140] In most situations, small numbers of any of these parasites have little impact on fish health.

Pathology: Digeneans demonstrate some degree of host and tissue specificity. Encapsulated metacercaria is the most common presentation; however, not all metacercaria are encapsulated. The capsule (i.e., cyst or connective tissue capsule) is composed of both host-derived and parasite-derived proteins. The host response, the peripheral portion of the capsule, is typically composed of fibrosis of varying exuberance with melanomacrophages and lymphocytes most commonly present. The characteristic blackspot is produced when the host response includes a preponderance of melanomacrophages, and even though the parasite may be killed by the host response the spot of black pigment will often remain (**Figure 7.25**).

Differential diagnosis: There are a large number of digenean species that infect fish, and identification of larvae can be challenging if only histological sections are available. Adult digeneans can also be difficult to differentiate from cestodes in sections. Whole specimens and consulting a relevant taxonomic key may be required.

Diagnosis: Histopathology is often the primary technique; however, speciation of larvae is often poor using histology alone. For speciation, whole specimens

should be removed from the fish and examined with a dissecting scope.[137] There is also an increasing bank of DNA nucleotide sequences for digeneans, particularly those that are a concern for fish health that may reveal life history, and taxonomy and assist in diagnosis.[139]

Management/control: Interruption of the life cycle is presently the only practical course of action. Reduction in intensity of infection is often the goal rather than elimination of the parasite. Raising freshwater fish in tanks or raceways will help reduce or eliminate the snail host, but this is not practical in many aquaculture operations where fish are cultured in earthen ponds. Several control strategies in combination may have some impact (e.g., molluscivorous fish, molluscicides such as copper sulfate, netting over pens and scaring birds). Praziquantel in the water or orally is effective but may not be approved for use in food fish.[138]

REFERENCES

1. Francis-Floyd, R., Bolon, B., Fraser, W. and Reed, P. Lip fibromas associated with retrovirus-like particles in angel fish. *Journal of the American Veterinary Medical Association* 1993;202(3):427–429.
2. Martineau, D. and Ferguson, H.W. Neoplasia. In: *Systemic Pathology of Fish*, 2nd ed. 2006; pp. 313–334.
3. Coffee, L.L., Casey, J.W. and Bowser, P.R. Pathology of tumors in fish associated with retroviruses: A review. *Veterinary Pathology* 2013;50:390–403.
4. Harshbarger, J.C. Neoplasia and developmental anomalies. In: *BSAVA Manual of Ornamental Fish*, 2nd ed. 2001; pp. 219–224.

5. Groff, J.M. Neoplasia in fishes. *Veterinary Clinics Exotic Animal Practice* 2004; 7:705–756.

6. Madsen, L., Arnberg, J. and Dalsgaard, I. Spinal deformities in triploid all-female rainbow trout (*Oncorhynchus mykiss*). *Bulletin European Association of Fish Pathology* 2000;20:206–208.

7. Afonso, J.M., Montero, D., Robaina, L., Astorga, N., Izquierdo, M.S. and Gines, R. Association of a lordosis-scoliosis-kyphosis deformity in gilthead seabream (*Sparus aurata*) with family structure. *Fish Physiology and Biochemistry* 2000;22:159–163.

8. Handwerker, T.S. and Tave, D. Semiopperculum: A nonheritable deformity in Mozambique tilapia. *Journal of Aquatic Animal Health* 1994;6:85–88.

9. Ornsrud, R., Gil, L. and Waagbo, R. Teratogenicity of elevated egg incubation temperature and egg vitamin A status in Atlantic salmon, *Salmo salar* L. *Journal of Fish Diseases* 2004;27:213–223.

10. Kazlauskiene, N., Leliuna, E. and Kesminas, V. Peculiarities of opercular malformations of salmon (*Salmo salar* L.) juveniles reared in the Peimena salmon hatchery. *Acta Zoologica Lutuanica* 2006;16:312–316.

11. Koumoundouros, G., Oran, G., Divanach, P., Stefanakis, S. and Kentouri, M. The opercular complex deformity in intensive sea bream (*Sparus aurata* L.) larviculture. Moment of apparition and description. *Aquaculture* 1997;156:165–177.

12. Soliman, A.K., Jauncey, K. and Roberts, R.H. The effect of varying forms of dietary ascorbic acid on the nutrition of juvenile tilapias (*Oreochromis niloticus*). *Aquaculture* 1986;52:1–10.

13. Speare, D. and Ferguson, H.W. Gills and pseudobranchs. In: *Systemic Pathology of Fish*, 2nd ed. 2006; pp. 25–62.

14. Frasca, S., Kirsipuu, V.L., Russell, S., Bullard, S.A. and Benz, G.W. Opercular lesion in wild black drum, *Pogonias cromis* (Linnaeus, 1766), associated with attachment of the sea louse *Sciaenophilus tenuis* (Copepoda: Siphonostomatoida: Caligidae). *Acta Ichthyologica et Piscatoria* 2004;34:115–127.

15. Beraldo, P. and Canavese, B. Recovery of opercular anomalies in gilthead sea bream, *Sparus aurata* L.: Morphological and morphometric analysis. *Journal of Fish Diseases* 2011;34:21–30.

16. Turnbull J. Musculoskeletal system. In: *Systemic Pathology of Fish*, 2nd ed. 2006; pp. 289–311.

17. Boglione C., Costa C. Skeletal deformities and juvenile quality. In: *Sparidae: Biology and Aquaculture of Gilthead Seabream and Other Species*, 1st ed. 2011; pp. 233–294.

18. Baeverfjord, G., Lein, I., Asgard, T., Rye, M., Storset, A. and Siikavoupi, S.I. Vertebral deformities induced by high temperatures during embryogenesis in Atlantic salmon (*Salmo salar*). Toward predictable quality. *Abstracts at Aquaculture Europe 99, EAS special publication* 1999;27:6–7.

19. Wargelius, A., Fhelldal, P.G. and Hansen, T. Heat shock during early somitogenesis induces caudal vertebral column defects in Atlantic salmon (*Salmo salar*). *Developmental Genes and Evolution* 2005;215:350–357.

20. Mair, G.C. Caudal deformity syndrome (CDS): An autosomal recessive lethal mutation in the tilapia, *Oreochromis niloticus* (L.). *Journal of Fish Diseases* 1992;15:71–75.

21. Castro, J., Pino-Querido, A., Hermida, M. and Martinez, P. Heritability of skeleton abnormalities (lordosis, lack of operculum) in gilthead seabream (*Sparus aurata*) supported by microsatellite family data. *Aquaculture* 2008;279:18–22.

22. Koumoudouros, G., Divanach, P. and Kentouri, M. The effect of rearing conditions on the development of saddleback syndrome and caudal fin deformities in *Dentex dentex* (L.). *Aquaculture* 2001;200:285–304.

23. Russo, T., Scardi, M., Boglione, C. and Cataudella, S. Rearing morphologies and morphological quality in aquaculture: An application of the self-organizing map to the study of skeletal anomalies and meristic counts in gilthead seabream (*Sparus aurata* L.1758). *Aquaculture* 2010;315:69–77.

24. Chatain, B. Abnormal swimbladder development and lordosis in sea bass (*Dicentrarchus labrax*) and sea bream (*Sparus auratus*). *Aquaculture* 1994;119:371–379.

25. Jezierska, B., Lugowska, K. and Witeska, M. The effects of heavy metals on embryonic development of fish (a review). *Fish Physiology and Biochemistry* 2009;35:625–640.

26. Gil-Martens, L., Obach, A., Ritchie, G. and Witten, P.E. Analysis of a short tail type in farmed Atlantic salmon (*Salmo salar* Linnaeus., 1758). *Fish Veterinary Journal* 2005;8:71–79.

27. Witten, P.E., Gil-Martens, L., Hall, B.K., Huysseune, A. and Obach, A. Compressed vertebrae in Atlantic salmon (*Salmo salar*): Evidence for metaplastic chondrogenesis as a skeletogenic response late in ontogeny. *Diseases of Aquatic Organisms* 2005;64:237–246.

28. Witten, P.E., Obach, A., Huysseune, A. and Baeverfjord, G. Vertebrae fusion in Atlantic salmon (*Salmo salar*): Development, aggravation and pathways of containment. *Aquaculture* 2006;258:164–172.

29. Boglione, C., Pulcini, D., Scardi, M., Palamara, E., Russo, T. and Cataudella, S. Skeletal anomaly monitoring in rainbow trout (*Onchorhynchus mykiss*, Walbaum 1792) reared under different conditions. *PLOS ONE* 2014;9:e96983. doi: 10.1371/journal.pone.0096983.

30. Witten, P.E. and Hall, B.K. Seasonal changes in the lower jaw skeleton in male Atlantic salmon (*Salmo salar* L.): Remodeling and regression of the kype after spawning. *Journal of Anatomy* 2003;203:435–450.

31. Good, C. and Davison, J. A review of factors influencing maturation of Atlantic salmon, *Salmo salar*, with focus on water recirculation aquaculture system environments. *Journal of the World Aquaculture Society* 2016;47:605–632.

32. McClure, C.A., Hammell, K.L., Moore, M., Dohoo, I.R. and Burnley, H. Risk factors for early sexual maturation in Atlantic salmon in seawater farms in New

Brunswick and Nova Scotia, Canada. *Aquaculture* 2007;272:370–379.

33. Aksnes, A., Gjerde, B. and Roald, S.O. Biological, chemical and organoleptic changes during maturation of farmed Atlantic salmon, *Salmo salar*. *Aquaculture* 1986;53:7–20.

34. St-Hilaire, S., Ribble, C., Whitaker, D.J. and Kent, M. Prevalence of *Kudoa thyrsites* in sexually mature and immature pen-reared Atlantic salmon (*Salmo salar*) in British Columbia, Canada. *Aquaculture* 1998;162:69–77.

35. Cahu, C., Infante, J.Z. and Takeuchi, T. Nutritional components affecting skeletal development in fish larvae. *Aquaculture* 2003;227:254–258.

36. Lall, S.P. Disorders of nutrition and metabolism. *Fish Diseases and Disorders* 2010;2:202–237.

37. Suzuki, T., Oohara, I. and Kurokawa, T. Retinoic acid given in late embryonic stage depresses Sonic hedgehog and *Hoxd-4* expression in the pharyngeal area and induces skeletal malformation in flounder (*Paralichthys olivaceus*) embryos. *Development, Growth and Differentiation* 1999;41:143–152.

38. Takeuchi, T., Dedi, J., Haga, Y., Seikai, T. and Watanabe, T. Effect of vitamin A compounds on bone deformity in larval Japanese flounder (*Paralichthys olivaceus*). *Aquaculture* 1998;169:155–165.

39. Haga, Y., Suzuki, T., Kagechika, H. and Takeuchi, T. A retinoic acid receptor-selective agonist causes jaw deformity in the Japanese flounder *Paralichthys olivaceus*. *Aquaculture* 2003;221:381–392.

40. Hermann, K. Teratogenic effects of retinoic acid and related substances on the early development of the zebrafish (*Brachydanio rerio*) as assessed by a novel scoring system. *Toxicology in Vitro* 1995;9:267–283.

41. Dabrowski, K., El-Fiky, N., Kock, G., Frigg, M. and Wieser, W. Requirement and utilization of ascorbic acid and ascorbic sulfate in juvenile rainbow trout. *Aquaculture* 1990;91:317–337.

42. Lim, C. and Lovell, R.T. Pathology of the vitamin C deficiency syndrome in channel catfish (*Ictalurus punctatus*). *Journal of Nutrition* 1978;108:1137–1146.

43. Labrie, L., Komar, C., Terhune, J., Camus, A. and Wise, D. Effect of sublethal exposure to the trematode *Bolbophorus* spp. on the severity of enteric septicemia of catfish in channel catfish fingerlings. *Journal of Aquatic Animal Health* 2004;16:231–237.

44. Sato, M., Kondo, K. and Yoshinaka, P. Effect of water temperature on the skeletal deformity in ascorbic acid deficient trout. *Bulletin of the Japanese Society for Scientific Fisheries* 1983;49:443–446.

45. Sigiura, S.H., Hardy, R.W. and Roberts, R.J. The pathology of phosphorus deficiency in fish—A review. *Journal of Fish Diseases* 2004;27:255–265.

46. Roberts, R.J., Hardy, R.W. and Sugiura, S.H. Screamer disease in Atlantic salmon, *Salmo salar* L., in Chile. *Journal of Fish Diseases* 2001;24:543–549.

47. Shearer, K.D. and Hardy, R.W. Phosphorus deficiency in rainbow trout (*Salmo gairdneri*) fed a diet containing deboned fillet scrap. *The Progressive Fish Culturist* 1987;49:192–197.

48. Baeverfjord, G., Asgard, T. and Shearer, K.D. Development and detection of phosphorus deficiency in Atlantic salmon, *Salmo salar* L. parr and post smolts. *Aquaculture Nutrition* 1998;4:1–11.

49. Bell, J.G., McEvoy, J., Tocher, D.R. and Sargent, J.R. Depletion of α-tochopherol and astaxanthin in Atlantic salmon (*Salmo salar*) affects autoxidative defense and fatty acid metabolism. *The Journal of Nutrition* 2000;130:1800–1808.

50. Smith, C.E. The prevention of liver lipoid degeneration (ceroidosis) and microcytic anaemia in rainbow trout *Salmo gairdneri* Richardson fed rancid diets: A preliminary report. *Journal of Fish Diseases* 1979;2:429–437.

51. Cowey, C.B., Degener, E., Tacon, A.G.J. and Youngson, A. The effect of vitamin E and oxidized fish oil on the nutrition of rainbow trout (*Salmo gairdneri*) grown at natural, varying water temperatures. *British Journal of Nutrition* 1984;51:443–451.

52. Yokote, M. Sekoke disease, spontaneous diabetes in carp. *Bulletin of the Freshwater Fisheries Research Laboratory* 1970;20:39–72.

53. Roberts, R.J., Richards, R.H. and Bullock, A.M. Pansteatitis in rainbow trout *Salmo gairdneri* Richardson: A clinical and histopathological study. *Journal of Fish Diseases* 1979;2:85–92.

54. LePage, V., Young, J., Dutton, C.J. et al. Diseases of captive yellow seahorse *Hippocampus kuda* Bleeker, pot-bellied seahorse *Hippocampus abdominalis* Lesson and weedy seadragon *Phyllopteryx taeniolatus* (Lacepede). *Journal of Fish Diseases* 2015;38:439–450.

55. Holloway, H.L. and Smith, C.E. A myopathy in North Dakota walleye, *Stizostedion vitreum* (Mitchell). *Journal of Fish Diseases* 1982;5:527–530.

56. Roberts, R.J. Miscellaneous non-infectious disease. In: *Fish Pathology*, 4th ed. 2012; pp. 425–438.

57. Pasnik, D.J., Smith, S.A. and Wolf, J.C. Accidental electroshock of fish in a recirculation facility. *The Veterinary Record* 2003;153:562–564.

58. Evans, J., Klesius, J., Plumb, P.H. and Shoemaker, C.A. Edwardsiella septicaemias. *Diseases and Disorders of Fish* 2011;3:512–569.

59. Hirai, Y., Asahata-Tago, S., Ainoda, Y., Fujita, T. and Kikuchi, K. *Edwardsiella tarda* bacteremia. A rare but fatal water- and foodborne infection: Review of the literature and clinical cases from a single centre. *Canadian Journal of Infectious Disease and Medical Microbiology* 2015;26:313–318.

60. Griffin, M.J., Quiniou, S.M., Cody, T., Tabuchi, M., Ware, C., Cipriano, R.C., Mauel, M.J. and Soto, E. Comparative analysis of *Edwardsiella* isolates from fish in the eastern United States identifies two distinct genetic taxa amongst organisms phenotypically classified as *E. tarda*. *Veterinary Microbiology* 2013;165:358–372.

61. Park, S.B., Aoki, T. and Jung, T.S. Pathogenesis of and strategies for preventing *Edwardsiella tarda* infection in fish. *Veterinary Research* 2012;43:67.

62. Darwish, A., Plumb, J.A. and Newton, J.C. Histopathology and pathogenesis of experimental infection with *Edwardsiella tarda* in channel catfish. *Journal of Aquatic Animal Health* 2000;12:255–266.

63. Miyazaki, T. and Kaige, N. Comparative histopathology of edwardsiellosis in fishes. *Fish Pathology* 1985;20:219–227.

64. Rogers, W.A. Serological detection of two species of *Edwardsiella* infecting catfish. *Developments in Biological Standardization* 1981;49:169–172.

65. Savan, R., Igarashi, A., Matsuoka, S. and Sakai, M. Sensitive and rapid detection of edwardsiellosis in fish by a loop-mediated isothermal amplification method. *Applied and Environmental Microbiology* 2004; 70:621–624.

66. Wiens, G.D., Rockey, D.D., Wu, Z. et al. Genome sequence of the fish pathogen *Renibacterium salmoninarum* suggests reductive evolution away from an environmental Arthobacter ancestor. *Journal of Bacteriology* 2008;190:6970–6982.

67. Matejusova, I., Bain, N., Colquhoun, D.J. et al. Multilocus variable-number tandem-repeat genotyping of *Renibacterium salmoninarum*, a bacterium causing bacterial kidney disease in salmonid fish. *BMC Microbiology* 2013;13:285.

68. Evelyn, T.P.T., Prosperi-Porta, L. and Ketcheson, J.E. Experimental intra-ovum infection of salmonid eggs with *Renibacterium salmoninarum* and vertical transmission of the pathogen with such eggs despite their treatment with erythromycin. *Diseases of Aquatic Organisms* 1986;1:197–202.

69. McKibben, C.L. and Pascho, R.J. Shedding of *Renibacterium salmoninarum* by infected Chinook salmon *Oncorhynchus tschawytscha*. *Diseases of Aquatic Organisms* 1999;38:75–79.

70. American Fisheries Society, Fish Health Section. *FHS Blue Book: Suggested Procedures for the Detection and Identification of Certain Finfish and Shellfish Pathogens.* AFS-FHS, Bethesda, MD, 2012.

71. BKD White Paper: Evaluation of Bacterial Kidney Disease (BKD) impacts on the Canadian salmon aquaculture industry. Fisheries and Oceans Canada. 2010.

72. Elliott, D.G., Wiens, G.D., Hammell, K.L. and Rhodes, L.D. Vaccination against bacterial kidney disease. In: *Fish Vaccination.* R. Gudding, A. Lillehaug and O. Evensen, eds. 2014; pp. 255–272.

73. Kocan, R., Hershberger, P., Mehl, T., Elder, N., Bradley, M., Wildermuth, D. and Stick, K. Pathogenicity of *Ichthyophonus hoferi* for laboratory-reared Pacific herring (*Clupea pallasi*) and its early appearance in wild Puget Sound herring. *Diseases of Aquatic Organisms* 1999;35:23–29.

74. Hershberger, P.K., Hart, L.M., MacKenzie, A.H., Yanney, M.L., Conway, C.M. and Elliot, D.G. Infecting Pacific herring with *Ichthyophonus* sp. in the laboratory. *Journal of Aquatic Animal Health* 2015;27:217–221.

75. Gavryuseva, T.V. First report of *Ichthyophonus hoferi* infection in young coho salmon *Oncorhynchus kisutch*

(Walbaum) at a fish hatchery in Kamchatka. *Russian Journal of Marine Biology* 2007;33:43–48.

76. Kocan, R., LaPatra, S., Gregg, J., Winton, J. and Hershberger, P. *Ichthyophonus*-induced cardiac damage: A mechanism for reduced swimming stamina in rainbow trout. *Journal of Fish Diseases* 2006;29:521–527.

77. Hershberger PK. Ichthyophonus disease (Ichthyophoniasis). American Fisheries Society, Fish Health Section. 2014.

78. Hamazaki, T., Kahler, E., Borba, B.M. and Burton, T. PCR testing can be as accurate as culture for diagnosis of *Ichthyophonus hoferi* in Yukon River Chinook salmon *Oncorhynchus tshawytscha*. *Diseases of Aquatic Organisms* 2013;105:21–25.

79. Kocan, R.M., Gregg, J.L. and Hershberger, P.K. Diagnostic methodology is critical for accurately determining the prevalence of *Ichthyophonus* infections in wild fish populations. *Journal of Parasitology* 2011;97:344–348.

80. Lumsden, J.S., Ostland, V.E. and Ferguson, H.W. Necrotic myositis in cage cultured rainbow trout *Oncorhynchus mykiss* (Walbaum), caused by *Flexibacter psychrophilum*. *Journal of Fish Diseases* 1996;19:113–119.

81. Ostland, V.E., McGrogan, D.G. and Ferguson, H.W. Cephalic osteochondritis and necrotic scleritis in intensively reared salmonids associated with *Flexibacter psychrophilus*. *Journal of Fish Diseases* 1997;20:443–451.

82. Hesami, S., Allen, K.J., Metcalf, D., Ostland, V.E., ManInnes, J.I. and Lumsden, J.S. Phenotypic and genotypic analysis of *Flavobacterium psychrophilum* isolates from Ontario salmonids with coldwater disease. *Canadian Journal of Microbiology* 2008;54:619–629.

83. Ekman, E., Akerman, G., Balk, L. and Norrgren, L. Nanoinjection as a tool to mimic vertical transmission of *Flavobacterium psychrophilum* in rainbow trout *Oncorhynchus mykiss*. *Diseases of Aquatic Organisms* 2003;55:93–99.

84. Nematollahi, A., Decostere, A., Pasmans, F. and Haesebrouck, F. *Flavobacterium psychrophilum* infections in salmonid fish. *Journal of Fish Diseases* 2003;26:563–574.

85. Lumsden, J.S., Young, K., MacInnes, J.I., Russell, S. and Hesami, S. Management approaches for coldwater disease caused by *Flavobacterium psychrophilum*. *Proceedings of the Canadian Freshwater Aquaculture Symposium, AAC Special Publication* 2004;11:111–117.

86. Loch, T.P. and Faisal, M. Emerging flavobacterial infections in fish: A review. *Journal of Advanced Research* 2015;6:283–300.

87. Hesami, S., Parkman, J., MacInnes, J.I., Gray, J.T., Gyles, C.L. and Lumsden, J.S. Antimicrobial susceptibility of *Flavobacterium psychrophilum* isolates from Ontario. *Journal of Aquatic Animal Health* 2010;22:39–49.

88. Silverstein, J.T., Vallejo, R.L., Palti, Y., Leeds, T.D., Rexroad, C.E., Welch, T.J., Wiens, G.D. and Ducrocq, V. Rainbow trout resistance to bacterial cold-water disease is moderately heritable and is not adversely correlated with growth. *Journal of Animal Science* 2009;87:860–867.

89. Cipriano, R.C. and Austin, B. Furunculosis and other aeromonad diseases. *Fish Diseases and Disorders* 2011;3:424–483.

90. Huizinga, H.W., Esch, G.W. and Hazen, T.C. Histopathology of red-sore disease (*Aeromonas hydrophila*) in naturally and experimentally infected largemouth bass *Micropterus salmoides* (Lacepede). *Journal of Fish Diseases* 1979;2:263–277.

91. Roberts, J.R. The bacteriology of teleosts. In: *Fish Pathology*, 2nd ed. 1989; pp. 289–320.

92. Schotts, E.B. and Rimler, R. Medium for isolation of *Aeromonas hydrophila*. *Journal of Applied Microbiology* 1973;26:550–553.

93. Huguet, J. and Ribas, F. SGAP-10C agar for the isolation and quantification of *Aeromonas* from water. *Journal of Applied Bacteriology* 1991;70:81–88.

94. Cipriano, R.C., Ford, L.A., Smith, D.R., Schachte, J.H. and Petrie, C.J. Differences in detection of *Aeromonas salmonicida* in covertly infected salmonid fishes by the stress-inducible furunculosis test and culture-based assays. *Journal of Aquatic Animal Health* 1997;9:108–113.

95. Ehlinger, N.F. Selective breeding of trout for resistance to furunculosis. *New York Fish and Game Journal* 1977;24:25–36.

96. Bailey, J.K., Olivier, G. and Friars, G.W. Inheritance of furunculosis resistance in Atlantic salmon. *Bulletin of the Aquaculture Association of Canada* 1993;4:90–92.

97. Lillehaug, A., Lunder, T. and Poppe, T.T. Field testing of adjuvanted furunculosis vaccines in Atlantic salmon, *Salmo salar* L. *Journal of Fish Diseases* 1992;15:485–496.

98. Mydtlyng, P.J. and Lillihaug, A. Growth of Atlantic salmon *Salmo salar* after intraperitoneal administration of vaccines containing adjuvants. *Diseases of Aquatic Organisms* 1998;32:91–97.

99. Inglis, V., Frerichs, G.N., Millar, S.D. and Richards, R.H. Antibiotic-resistance of *Aeromonas salmonicida* isolated from Atlantic salmon, *Salmo salar* L, in Scotland. *Journal of Fish Diseases* 1991;14:353–358.

100. Anbarasu, K., Thangakrishnan, K., Arun, B.V. and Chandran, M.R. Assessment of immune response in freshwater catfish (*Mystus vittatus* Bloch) to different bacterins of *Aeromonas hydrophila*. *Indian Journal of Experimental Biology* 1998;36:990–995.

101. Liu, Y.J. and Bi, Z.X. Potential use of a transposon Tn916-generated mutant of *Aeromonas hydrophila* J-1 defective in some exoproducts as a live attenuated vaccine. *Preventive Veterinary Medicine* 2007;78:79–84.

102. Garver, K.A., Johnson, S.C., Polinski, M.P., Bradshaw, J.C., Marty, G.D., Snyman, H.N., Morrison, D.B. and Richard, J. Piscine orthoreovirus from Western North America is transmissible to Atlantic salmon and sockeye salmon but fails to cause heart and skeletal muscle inflammation. *PLOS ONE* 2016;11:e0146229, Pmid:26730591.

103. Kongtorp, R. and Taksdal, T. Studies with experimental transmission of heart and skeletal muscle inflammation in Atlantic salmon, *Salmo salar* L. *Journal of Fish Diseases* 2009;32:253–262.

104. Di Cicco E, Ferguson HW, Schulze AD, Kaukinen KH, Li S, Vanderstichel R, Wessel O, Rimstad E, Gardner IA, Hammell KL, and Miller KM. Heart and skeletal muscle inflammation (HSMI) disease diagnosed on a British Columbia salmon farm through a longitudinal farm study. *PLOS ONE* 2017; doi.org/10.1371/journal.pone.0171471.

105. Graham, D.A. and McLoughlin, M.F. Salmonid alphaviruses. *Fish Disease and Disorders* 2011;3:245–275.

106. Kongtorp, R.T., Kjerstad, A., Taksdal, T., Guttvik, A. and Falk, K. Heart and skeletal muscle inflammation in Atlantic salmon, *Salmo salar* L.: A new infectious disease. *Journal of Fish Diseases* 2004;27:351–358.

107. Marine Harvest, A.S.A. *Marine Harvest Annual Report to US Securities and Exchange Commission*. Commission File Number: 001-36275. 2015.

108. Ferguson, H.W., Roberts, R.J., Richards, R.H., Collins, R.O. and Rice, D.A. Severe degenerative cardiomyopathy associated with pancreas disease in Atlantic salmon, *Salmo salar* L. *Journal of Fish Diseases* 1986;20:95–98.

109. Ferguson, H.W., Poppe, T. and Speare, D.J. Cardiomyopathy in farmed Norwegian salmon. *Diseases of Aquatic Organisms* 1990;8:225–231.

110. Karlsen, M., Hodneland, K., Endresen, C. and Nylund, A. Genetic stability within the Norwegian sub-type of salmonid alphavirus (family *Togaviridae*). *Archives of Virology* 2005;151:861–874.

111. Moran, J.D.W., Whitaker, D.J. and Kent, M.L. A review of the myxosporean genus *Kudoa* Maglitsch, 1947, and its impact on the international aquaculture industry and commercial fisheries. *Aquaculture* 1999;172:163–196.

112. Whipps, C.M. and Kent, M.L. Phylogeography of the cosmopolitan marine parasite *Kudoa thyrsites* (Myxozoa: Myxosporea). *Journal of Eukaryotic Microbiology* 2006;53:364–373.

113. Funk, V.A., Raap, M., Sojonky, K., Jones, S., Robinson, J., Fallkenberg, C. and Miller, K.M. Development and validation of an RNA- and DNA-based quantitative PCR assay for determination of *Kudoa thyrsites* infection levels in Atlantic salmon *Salmo salar*. *Diseases of Aquatic Organisms* 2007;75:239–249.

114. Jones, S.R.M., Cho, S., Nguyen, J. and Mahony, A. Acquired resistance to *Kudoa thyrsites* in Atlantic salmon *Salmo salar* following recovery from a primary infection of the parasite. *Aquaculture* 2016;451:457–462.

115. MacConnell, E., Bartholomew, J. Whirling disease of salmonids. In: *FHS Blue Book: Suggested Procedures for the Detection and Identification of Certain Finfish and Shellfish Pathogens*. AFS-FHS: Bethesda, Maryland. 2010.

116. Ryce, E.K.N., Zale, A.V., MacConnell, E. and Nelson, M. Effects of fish age versus size on the development of whirling disease in rainbow trout. *Diseases of Aquatic Organisms* 2005;63:69–76.

117. Hedrick, R.P., McDowell, T.S., Gay, M., Marty, G.D., Georgiadis, M.P. and MacConnell, E. Comparative susceptibility of rainbow trout *Onchorhynchus mykiss*

and brown trout *Salmo trutta* to *Myxobolus cerebralis*, the cause of salmonid whirling disease. *Diseases of Aquatic Organisms* 1999;37:173–183.

118. Kelley, G.O., Zagmutt-Vergara, J., Leutenegger, M., Myklebust, K.A., Adkison, M.A., McDowell, T.S., Marty, G.D., Kahler, A.L., Bush, A.L., Gardner, I.A. and Hedrick, R.P. Evaluation of five diagnostic methods for the detection and quantification of *Myxobolus cerebralis*. *Journal of Veterinary Diagnostic Investigation* 2004;16:202–211.

119. Hogge, C.I., Campbell, M.R. and Johnson, K.A. A new species of myxozoan (Myxosporea) from the brain and spinal cord of rainbow trout (*Onchorhynchus mykiss*) from Idaho. *Journal of Parasitology* 2008;94:218–222.

120. Hallett, SL and JL Bartholomew. *Myxobolus cerebralis* and *Ceratomyxa shasta*. In: *Fish Parasites: Pathology and Protection*, P.T.K. Woo and K. Buchmann, eds. CABI International, Wallingford, Oxfordshire, UK, 2012; pp. 131–162.

121. Hedrick, R.P., McDowell, T.S., Marty, G.D., Mukkatira, K., Antonio, D.B., Andree, K.B., Bukhari, Z. and Clancy, T. Ultraviolet irradiation inactivates the waterborne infective stages of *Myxobolus cerebralis*: A treatment for hatchery water supplies. *Diseases of Aquatic Organisms* 2000;42:53–59.

122. Dykova, I. Phylum Microspora. *Fish Diseases and Disorders* 2006;1:205–229.

123. Speare, D.J., Athanassopoulou, F., Daley, J. and Sanchez, J.G. A preliminary investigation of alternatives to fumagillin for the treatment of *Loma salmonae* infection in rainbow trout. *Journal of Comparative Pathology* 1999;121:241–248.

124. Saunders, J.L., Lawrence, C., Nichols, D.K., Brubaker, J.F., Peterson, T.S., Murray, K.N. and Kent, M.L. *Pleistophora hyphessobryconis* (Microsporidea) infecting zebrafish (*Danio rerio*) in research facilities. *Diseases of Aquatic Organisms* 2010;91:47–56.

125. Canning, E.U., Lom, J. and Dykova, I. Description of species infecting fish: *Pleistophora hyphessobryconis* Schaperclaus, 1941. *The Microsporidia of Vertebrates* 1986;101–107.

126. Bruno, D.W., Nowak, B. and Elliott, D.G. Guide to the identification of fish protozoan and metazoan parasites in stained tissue sections. *Diseases of Aquatic Organisms* 2006;70:1–36.

127. Basson, L. and Van As, J. Trichodinidae and other ciliophorans (Phylum Ciliophora). *Fish Disease and Disorders* 2006;1:154–182.

128. Hoffman, G.L., Landolt, M., Camper, J.E., Coats, D.W., Stookey, J.L. and Burek, J.D. A disease of freshwater fishes caused by *Tetrahymena corlissi* Thompson, 1955, and a key for identification of holotrich ciliates

of freshwater fishes. *The Journal of Parasitology* 1975; 61:217–223.

129. Cheung, P.J., Nigrelli, R.F. and Ruggieri, G.D. Studies on the morphology of *Uronema marinum* Dujardin (Ciliatea: Uronematidae) with a description of the histopathology of the infection in marine fishes. *Journal of Fish Diseases* 1980;3:295–303.

130. Jing, S.J., Kitamura, S., Song, J.Y. and Oh, M.J. 2007. *Miamiensis avidus* (Ciliophora: Scuticociliatida) causes systemic infection of olive flounder *Paralichthys olivaceus* and is a senior synonym of *Philasterides dicentrarchi*. *Diseases of Aquatic Organisms* 2007;73:227–234.

131. Leibowitz, M.P., Ariav, R. and Zilberg, D. Environmental and physiological conditions affecting *Tetrahymena* sp. infection in guppies, *Poecilia reticulate* Peters. *Journal of Fish Diseases* 2005;28:539–547.

132. Herbert, B. and Graham, P. Tetrahymenosis, columnaris disease and motile aeromonad septicemia in golden perch, *Macquaria ambigua* (Richardson), from Australia. *Diseases in Asian Aquaculture VI* 2008;179–192.

133. Sharon, G., Pimenta Leibowitz, M., Chettri, J.K., Isakov, N. and Zilberg, D. Comparative study of infection with *Tetrahymena* of different ornamental fish species. *Journal of Comparative Pathology* 2014;150:316–324.

134. Ferguson, H.W., Hicks, B.D., Lynn, D.H., Ostland, V.E. and Bailey, J. Cranial ulceration in Atlantic salmon *Salmo salar* associated with *Tetrahymena* sp. *Diseases of Aquatic Organisms* 1986;2:191–195.

135. Leibowitz, M.P. and Zilberg, D. *Tetrahymena* sp. infection in guppies, *Poecilia reticulata* Peters: Parasite characterization and pathology of infected fish. *Journal of Fish Diseases* 2009;32:845–855.

136. Gaertig, J., Gao, Y., Tishgarten, T., Clark, T.G. and Dickerson, H.W. Surface display of a parasite antigen in the ciliate *Tetrahymena thermophila*. *Nature Biotechnology* 1999;17:462–465.

137. Leibowitz, M.P., Chettir, J.K., Ofir, R. and Zilberg, D. Treatment development for systemic *Tetrahymena* sp. infection in guppies, *Poecilia reticulata* Peters. *Journal of Fish Diseases* 2010;33:473–480.

138. Bullard, S.A. and Overstreet, R.M. Digeneans as enemies of fishes. *Fish Diseases* 2008;817–976.

139. Paperna, I. and Dzikowski, R. Digenea (*Phylum Platyhelminthes*). *Fish Diseases and Disorders* 2006; 1:345–390.

140. Overstreet, R.M., Curran, S.S., Pote, L.M., King, D.T., Blend, C.K. and Grater, W.D. *Bolbophorus damnificus* n. sp. (Digenea: Bolbphoridae) from the channel catfish *Ictalurus punctatus* and American white pelican *Pelecanus erythrorbynchos* in the USA based on life-cycle and molecular data. *Systematic Parasitology* 2002;52:81–96.

CHAPTER 8

COELOMIC DISORDERS

CHRISTINE L. DENSMORE

COELOMIC DISTENSION

Dropsy

Overview: Dropsy is a commonly applied term for coelomic (i.e., abdominal) distention due to ascites, or the effusion and collection of fluid freely throughout the coelomic cavity. It is a nonspecific syndrome and a clinical presentation, as opposed to a defined disease. Dropsy, or ascites, is generally a sign of another ongoing disease process, oftentimes one that is multisystemic and impacting coelomic organs and tissues.

Etiology: Dropsy may be caused by a variety of potential etiological agents, both infectious and noninfectious. Generally, dropsy is associated with infectious disease processes associated with viral, mycotic or bacterial infection. In particular, pathogenic aeromonad, pseudomonad and vibrio bacteria have all been associated with free serous fluid accumulation in the coelomic cavity among various species of fishes.[1] Stressors such as rapid change in water temperature may predispose fish to bacterial diseases associated with dropsy.[2] *Rhabdovirus carpio*, the causative agent of spring viremia of carp (SVC), is another of the more recognized causative agents associated with dropsy among some cyprinids and other fishes.[3] Dropsy associated with SVC has also been more specifically called "infectious dropsy."[4] Parasitism of the coelomic cavity or coelomic organs and infections of mixed etiologies have also been associated with dropsy.[2]

Clinical presentation: Clinically affected fish display coelomic distension of varying degrees of severity (**Figures 8.1** and **8.2**). Severely affected scaled fish may have protrusion of the scales that causes them to stand erect from the body surface, causing lepidorthosis or a "pine cone" appearance (**Figure 8.3**). Although dropsy is not unique to any taxonomic group of fishes, it is especially well recognized among pond cultured and hobbyist cyprinids.

Differential diagnosis: As dropsy is more accurately defined as a clinical presentation of disease rather than a disease entity, the differential diagnoses are numerous, including not only the potential etiologies that lead to free coelomic fluid accumulation but also other various causes of coelomic distension: neoplasia, organomegaly, gastrointestinal obstruction, egg-binding.

Diagnosis: Diagnostic imaging may be useful in determining if coelomic distention is related to fluid accumulation or some other cause. If free coelomic fluid is suspected or observed, coeliocentesis and evaluation of the coelomic fluid through cytology and microbial (i.e., bacterial, viral and fungal) culture may often be diagnostically useful.

Management/control: Treatment and control options depend upon the underlying etiology.

Cichlid bloat, Malawi bloat

Overview: Generally considered a disease syndrome similar to dropsy, affecting specifically Malawi cichlids, a popular group of ornamental fish among aquarium hobbyists.

Etiology: Causative agents are varied and underlying infectious diseases, parasitism, and nutritional imbalances have been associated with cichlid bloat.[5,6] Among potential bacterial etiologies, both clostridiosis (*Clostridium difficile*) and francisellosis (*Francisella noatunensis subsp. orientalis*) have been reported in association with Malawi bloat.[6,7]

Clinical presentation: Clinically affected fish may display coelomic distension characterized internally by ascites, hemorrhage into the coelomic cavity, organomegaly and granulomatous inflammation of organs particularly the digestive tract.[5,7] Additional signs may include anorexia, dyspnea, lethargic behavior and mortality.

Differential diagnosis: Like dropsy, Cichlid or Malawi bloat is a clinical syndrome rather than a

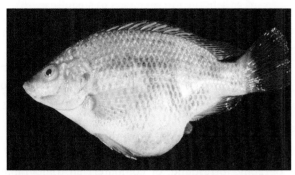

Figure 8.1 Severe coelomic distention in a female tilapia (*Oreochromis* sp.) due to cystic ovaries. (Image courtesy of S.A. Smith.)

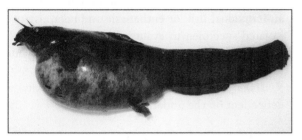

Figure 8.2 Severe coelomic distention in a female madtom (*Noturus* sp.) due to cystic ovaries. (Image courtesy of S. Boylan.)

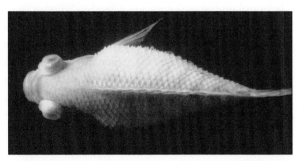

Figure 8.3 Lepidorthosis (i.e., "pine-cone" appearance) in tilapia (*Oreochromis* sp.) due to coelomic distension. (Image courtesy of S.A. Smith.)

specific disease. Differential diagnoses include the potential etiologies described for dropsy, as well as other various causes of coelomic distension that can impact Malawi cichlids, including neoplasia, organomegaly and gastrointestinal obstruction.

Diagnosis: Diagnostic imaging may be helpful in determining if coelomic distension is related to fluid accumulation or some other cause. If free coelomic fluid is suspected or observed, coeliocentesis and evaluation of the coelomic fluid through cytology and microbial culture may often be diagnostically useful.

Management/control: Treatment and control options vary and depend upon determination of the underlying etiology.

Salmonid water belly

Overview: Water belly occurs among salt water pen-reared salmonid fish, including Atlantic salmon (*Salmo salar*), Chinook salmon (*Oncorhynchus tshawytscha*) and rainbow trout (*Oncorhynchus mykiss*). This condition is idiopathic and presents as marked coelomic distension related largely to the accumulation of seawater in the stomach (**Figure 8.4**). Although it may clinically resemble dropsy, the fluid accumulation occurs within the gastrointestinal tract and not free within the coelomic cavity.

Etiology: The etiology has not been determined, although it is associated with dietary changes such as intensive feeding regimes and food composition, particularly related to fat and carbohydrates.[8]

Clinical presentation: Water belly has been reported to occur in sea-reared salmon and trout in both the Pacific Northwest (United States and Canada) and Europe.[9] Fish show severe distension of the coelomic cavity and mortality may also result. On necropsy, the stomach is fluid (seawater) filled, with stomach contents accounting for up to 40% of whole body weight.[10] Development of this condition is likely to

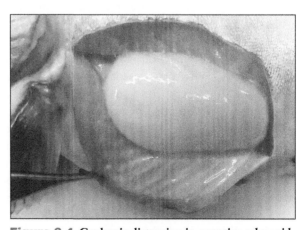

Figure 8.4 Coelomic distension in a captive salmonid due to "water belly," an idiopathic condition where there is an accumulation of sea water in the stomach. (Image courtesy S. Boylan.)

be chronic and as a result the stomach may be thin-walled and the liver may be atrophied.

Differential diagnosis: Differentials include ascites (i.e., dropsy), organomegaly, neoplasia and gastrointestinal obstruction.

Diagnosis: Gross external observation of marked coelomic distension coupled with the signalment (e.g., farmed salmonid) may provide a presumptive diagnosis. Verification that the coelomic distension is related solely to an enlarged seawater-filled stomach may be documented on necropsy.

Management/control: In some instances, dietary changes such as reduction of the feeding rate have been reported to improve this condition among affected fish.[11]

Miscellaneous etiologies (noneffusive)

Overview: In addition to the accumulation of free fluid within the coelomic cavity, many other factors affecting the size of coelomic organs or contents of the coelomic cavity may potentially result in apparent gross distension of the fish. Coelomic distension is a clinical sign of disease related to one or more coelomic organs or tissues, and further diagnosis is usually required to identify the true underlying etiology and appropriate management options.

Etiology: Distension of the coelomic cavity that is not related to effusion and/or accumulation of free fluid may be attributable to various underlying causes such as organomegaly, overinflation of the swim bladder, egg retention in ripe females, parasitism, and neoplasia associated with coelomic tissues or organs.

Clinical presentation: Grossly apparent distention of the body cavity may present to varying degrees. In subtle cases, comparing the body profile of an individual fish to another presumably normal specimen of the same species and life stage may help to identify any distension and whether it is general or localized. For laterally compressed fish, observing them from above in dorso-ventral orientation is most likely helpful. In more severe cases, protrusion of scales (i.e., lepidorthosis) over the lateral body walls may be evident, as seen in severe cases of dropsy. Coelomic distension may be generalized or restricted to a specific quadrant or region of the body cavity. Depending on the etiology and severity,

other nonspecific clinical signs may present, such as anorexia, lethargy, ataxia or abnormal swimming behavior, and hyperpigmentation.

Differential diagnosis: Dropsy and peritonitis should also be considered in the differential diagnosis list along with the potential underlying etiologies previously mentioned.

Diagnosis: Identification of the underlying cause is potentially aided by imaging techniques such as radiography, ultrasound, or computerized tomography, if available. Coeliocentesis to check for and evaluate coelomic fluid content may help rule out dropsy and its potential infectious etiologies. Exploratory surgery or laparoscopy for a nonlethal diagnosis of an individual fish, or euthanasia and necropsy of an isolated specimen to evaluate disease within multiple individuals or a population of fish may provide a more definitive diagnosis.

Management/control: Management options are dependent on the underlying etiology.

COELOMIC INFLAMMATION

Steatitis

Overview: Also known as "yellow fat disease," steatitis is an inflammatory condition affecting adipose tissue. Usually, steatitis is described affecting coelomic adipose stores that are associated with the mesentery and sometimes associated with pancreatic tissue among fishes. Still, the condition has been reported to affect other fat stores in fish as well, such as pericardial adipose tissue, fins or skin.[12] The condition is most frequently reported in cultured fish in association with unsuitable diets, but may also occur in wild fish.

Etiology: Steatitis is generally nutritional in origin and commonly associated with lipid peroxidation. It occurs in fish fed rancid feed or other feed items with unsuitable lipid components in the diet. For example, steatitis has been reported to occur among hatchery fish that were fed liver as a starter feed.[13]

Clinical presentation: Clinical signs may vary, but inflammation of the visceral adipose tissue may present grossly as discolored (cream to yellow) masses in the coelomic cavity where fat stores are normally found (**Figure 8.5**). Histologically, steatitis may appear as granulomatous inflammation with lymphocytic, eosinophilic granular and giant

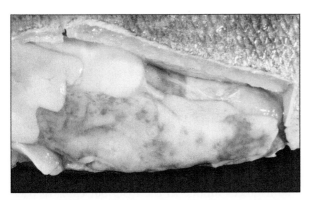

Figure 8.5 Steatitis in a cultured yellow perch (*Perca flavescens*). (Image courtesy of S.A. Smith.)

cells, as well as fibrosis. Inflammation may produce adhesions that involve coelomic organs. Additional clinical signs not involving the coelomic cavity may occur if the steatitis involves other body tissues. Fin loss and ulcerative skin lesions have been described in an atypical case in channel catfish.[12] In addition, muscle involvement and necrosis has been reported in conjunction with steatitis. Lethargy, hyperpigmentation and increased mortality in a population of farmed Atlantic bluefin tuna (*Thunnus thynnus*) has also been associated with steatitis.[14]

Differential diagnosis: Differentials include infectious or noninfectious peritonitis, liver lipidosis, multisystemic diseases associated with granulomatous inflammation (e.g., mycobacteriosis and norcardiosis), and pancreatitis.

Diagnosis: Diagnosis is based on gross and histological findings and ruling out potential differential causes. Identification of the underlying (i.e., nutritional) etiology and a positive response to correction of the dietary anomaly is confirmatory.

Management/control: Management is dependent on identifying and correcting the underlying nutritional etiology. An appropriate change of feed is often corrective for the population of fish.

Infectious peritonitis

Overview: Infectious peritonitis is a generalized inflammation of the peritoneal lining of the coelomic cavity caused by an infectious agent. It is often associated with multisystemic diseases, accompanied by infection and inflammation of coelomic organs. Numerous etiological agents are possible.

Etiology: There are multiple microbial agents associated with peritonitis in fish. The majority of reports of peritonitis in fish describe bacterial etiologies, and the list of potential causative agents is extensive. *Streptococcus* spp. (Gram-positive cocci) has produced multisystemic disease in fish species including tilapia.[15] Mycobacteriosis in fish (*Mycobacterium* spp., acid-fast positive short bacilli) often involves multiple coelomic organs and can be associated with peritonitis as well.[16] *Vagococcus salmoninarum* (Gram-positive bacillus) has been associated with an infectious peritonitis among Atlantic salmon (*Salmo salar*), rainbow trout (*Oncorhynchus mykiss*) and brown trout (*Salmo trutta*).[17] Aeromonad and pseudomonad bacteria are causative agents of various multisystemic and hemorrhagic diseases among fish species and are also associated with peritonitis. For example, *Pseudomonas fluorescens*, the agent of a hemorrhagic septicemia among tropical aquarium fish, marine fish, and pond fish, is often associated with fibrinous peritonitis.[18] Besides bacterial agents, the rickettsial pathogen *Piscirickettsia salmonis* has also been shown to produce peritonitis lesions in association with multisystemic disease among cultured salmonid fish.[19] Systemic diseases caused by fungal pathogens may also include peritonitis. Examples include phaeohyphomycosis (*Veronaea botryosa*) in cultured sturgeon, and granulomatous peritonitis caused by *Fusarium solani* in a desert pupfish (*Cyprinodon macularius*) and in a pink-tailed triggerfish (*Melichhthys vidua*).[20,21]

Traumatic injury may also be an underlying cause of peritonitis, and it may be resultant from predation, fighting or various fishing activity. For instance, retained fish hooks penetrating through the gastrointestinal tract may produce an infectious peritonitis associated with secondary bacterial infection in species that are fished commercially or recreationally.[22] Venting, the process of inserting a hollow needle through the abdominal wall to release gasses from barotraumatized fish, can also lead to an infectious peritonitis.[23] Spawning stress has also been identified as a precursor to bacterial peritonitis among fish.[24]

Clinical presentation: Clinical signs will vary with the etiological agent and species affected but generally include nonspecific indicators of disease such as anorexia and lethargy as well as increased mortality in the population. Coelomic distension may be noted with serous to serosanguinous exudate. Inflammatory change is also generally evident on necropsy, appearing as focal to diffuse discolored lesions or hemorrhage along the peritoneum and affecting coelomic organs. Various causative agents such as *Mycobacterium* spp. or intracoelomic protozoans may also produce a granulomatous inflammatory response apparent as nodules on coelomic organs.[16,25] A pseudomembrane covering coelomic organs may also form in association with inflammatory change, as is noted in a case of peritonitis associated with pasteurellosis among farmed Atlantic salmon.[26] Intracoelomic adhesions may also be present (**Figure 8.6**).

Differential diagnosis: Infectious peritonitis may be associated with a variety of microbial agents of infectious disease among fishes, including bacteria, rickettsia, fungi and fungal-like organisms, and protozoans. Intracoelomic parasitism by helminths, such as larval cestodes, may also produce similar lesions. Noninfectious causes of peritonitis such as aseptic vaccine reactions in the peritoneum, and other causes of ascites and abdominal distension can also be differentials.

Diagnosis: Diagnosis is likely to be based on microbial culture or molecular-based detection of the causative organism. Peritoneal effusion may be a readily available source of diagnostic material for cytology and microbial culture, obtained either by coeliocentesis in a live fish or necropsy in a recently

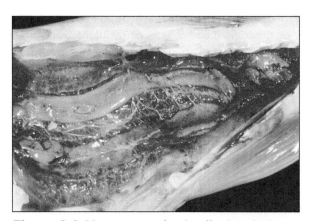

Figure 8.6 Numerous coelomic adhesions in a common carp (*Cyprinus carpio*) as a result of a systemic infection of *Aeromonas hydrophila*. (Image courtesy of S.A. Smith.)

perished or sacrificed specimen. Histopathological examination of the peritoneum as well as other coelomic organs involved may also be useful in the identification of the infectious agent as well as characterization of the inflammatory response. If circumstances warrant, predisposing factors such as traumatic injury to the body wall, peritoneum, or coelomic organs should also be ruled out.

Management/control: Management is based on the nature of the infectious agent identified and circumstances unique to the case, but cases of bacterial infection would generally involve antimicrobial therapy as warranted.

Vaccine-associated peritonitis

Overview: Intracoelomic vaccination with oil-adjuvanted vaccines may produce a sterile granulomatous peritonitis at or near the injection site. A phenomenon observed primarily among farmed salmonids, particularly Atlantic salmon, vaccine-associated peritonitis has also been noted in Atlantic cod (*Gadus morhua*).[27,28] Although this peritonitis is generally not fatal and often only noted incidentally at slaughter or necropsy, it is of concern from the perspectives of both poor animal husbandry practices and reduced quality of fillets in food fish.[29]

Etiology: Mineral oils that are not readily metabolized and are used as adjuvants for intraperitoneal vaccination of fish can produce strong localized inflammatory reactions at or near the site of injection.

Clinical presentation: This disorder may not be clinically apparent until an internal examination of the fish is performed. Nonspecific clinical signs such as anorexia or lethargy have not typically been reported, although poor feed uptake and reduced growth have been reported in association with oil-adjuvanted vaccination among salmonids.[30] Internally, a granulomatous peritonitis may be accompanied by fibrous adhesions between coelomic organs and the peritoneum, as well as melanization of affected tissues (**Figure 8.7**). Hyperemia due to hemorrhage and fibrinous exudate may sometimes be apparent.[31] Pigmented foci in the musculature of the body wall may also be associated with the peritonitis and appear microscopically as granulomatous inflammatory lesions in the white muscle tissue.[29] Extracoelomic effects are also possible such

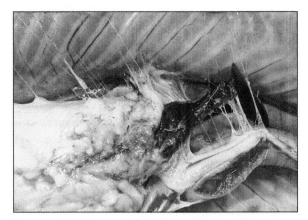

Figure 8.7 Post-vaccination adhesions with melanization comprising the spleen and pyloric caeca in an Atlantic salmon (*Salmo salar*). (Image courtesy of T. Poppe.)

as granulomatous uveitis as reported among Atlantic salmon (*Salmo salar*) or systemic autoimmunity manifested as multisystemic inflammation and production of autoantibodies.[32–34] Uncomplicated cases of vaccine-associated peritonitis may be self-limiting and not overly problematic, and lesions may regress over months to years.[35]

Differential diagnosis: Differential diagnoses will include other causes of peritonitis that produce similar lesions or masses within the coelomic cavity, such as parasitism with encysted helminths, diseases associated with focal granulomatous inflammation such as mycobacteriosis, and neoplasia.

Diagnosis: Diagnosis is based upon a combination of signalment (e.g., fish previously vaccinated with an oil adjuvant vaccine), clinical and histological presentation, and ruling out other differential diagnoses (i.e., lack of presence of infectious agents in association with the peritonitis).

Management/control: There are no management options after the peritonitis has been noted.

Coelomic parasitism (helminths)

Overview: Parasitism by helminths is frequently observed among fish, and the coelomic cavity is a common location for their occurrence. As a general rule, the presence and severity of lesions associated with helminths in the coelomic cavity is dependent upon both the life stage and pathogenic nature of the parasite species as well as upon the number of

organisms present. For developmental stages of helminths that rapidly encyst within the coelomic cavity, host lesions and associated impacts may be minimal, whereas those parasites that migrate extensively in the coelomic cavity are more likely to produce significant lesions and even mortality.

Numerous fish species serve as intermediate, paratenic, or definitive hosts for helminth parasites. Both larval and adult stages of nematodes can parasitize the coelomic cavity of fish. Larval stages of cestodes (i.e., pleurocercoids) are generally among the most harmful metazoan parasites of fish, and may heavily damage coelomic organs and tissues. This is especially true for those species that migrate for a length of time within the host rather than encysting. For many species of trematodes, fish serve as an intermediate host for development from the cercarial stages through the encysted metacercarial stage in target organs or tissues. This development often involves tissue migration through the coelomic cavity and its organs. Lesions and organ dysfunction may result from large numbers of metacercarial cysts displacing normal tissue. Acanthocephalan are generally gastrointestinal adult parasites of fish that embed in the lumen wall of the host's gut. Effects of an infestation are mostly contained to the gastrointestinal tract, however, in severe cases perforation of the gut wall by the parasite may cause peritonitis and associated lesions in the coelomic cavity.

Etiology: Larvae are generally the most pathogenic stages of nematodes among fish. Larval ascarid nematodes such as *Anasakis* spp. may be problematic among marine fishes, whereas larval *Eustronylides* spp. may affect freshwater fishes. *Contracaecum* species utilize a variety of fresh water and marine fishes as intermediate hosts. Adult life stages generally inhabit the gastrointestinal tract of fish, although adults of some dracunculoidean species may occupy the coelomic cavity.[36] Examples include *Philomena* spp. among salmonid fishes, and *Philometra* spp. that impact striped bass and other species. The cestode *Ligula* sp. has a global distribution and is particularly harmful among catfish, suckers and minnows in freshwater environments. They may grow from the larval pleurocercoid to the adult stage within the body of the fish, reaching over 20 cm in length and a body weight that may exceed that of its fish host.[37]

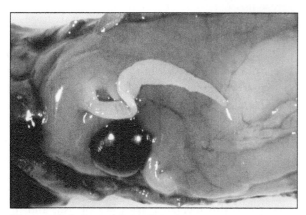

Figure 8.8 Larval *Diphyllobothrium* sp. in coelomic cavity of an Alaska blackfish (*Dallia pectorali*). (Image courtesy of S.A. Smith.)

Diphyllobothrium spp. affect many types of fishes, including salmonids in particular. These cestodes may be long lived and therefore may be most pathogenic among older fish (**Figure 8.8**). *Proteocephalus ambloptis*, the bass tapeworm, is likewise problematic among centrarchid species including largemouth bass (*Micropterus salmoides*) and smallmouth bass (*Micropterus dolomieu*). Multiple species of trematodes may produce coelomic disease among fishes. *Posthodiplostomum* spp., the so-called white grub, is a common complex of various trematodes species affecting freshwater fishes to the point of lethality, particularly among centrarchids and cyprinids. *Clinostomum marginatum*, the yellow grub, is another example of a trematode that affects many freshwater fish species and may be damaging to viscera due to its coelomic migration. Acanthocephalans are also known to cause infestations of many types of freshwater and marine fishes. Important genera in fishes include *Acanthocephalus*, *Paragorgorhynchus*, *Termisentic* and *Neoechinorhynchus*.[38]

Clinical presentation: Clinical signs will vary considerably in coelomic nematode infestations. Oftentimes fish are completely asymptomatic. Signs may be as benign as the observed presence of roundworms either encysted or free in the coelomic cavity or within the coelomic viscera with no apparent host tissue reactions associated. At the other end of the spectrum, a clinical presentation of fulminant peritonitis with fibrosis and adhesions is also possible. Appearance varies with the nematode species and life stage. For instance, *Eustrongyloides* spp. are generally deep red in color, whereas *Anisakis* spp. usually appear whitish. Larval stages of *Eustrongyloides* may be quite large and damaging to coelomic organs, especially the gonads, of freshwater fish. Larval *Anisakis spp.* may encyst in various coelomic organs or tissues, including muscle, of marine fishes and there is zoonotic potential when undercooked fish containing the parasite is consumed by humans. Philometrids may be highly pathogenic to a variety of fish in both fresh and salt water. *Philometra* species that affect the gonads are particularly damaging.[39] Adult stages of *Philometra* may also encapsulate in the coelom and produce an associated peritonitis.[37] A mild infestation of cestode pleurocercoids in the coelomic cavity may not present with clinical signs, especially if the parasites are encysted. In greater numbers, encystment in viscera may be associated with inflammation, generalized peritonitis with adhesions, and even death. For instance, *Diphyllobothrium* pleurocercoids may produce a chronic granulomatous peritonitis among salmonid fishes with fibrous coelomic adhesions and nodular lesions throughout the viscera.[40] Severe infestations of *Ligula* sp. may be accompanied by peritonitis, gross coelomic distension, and organ compression or distortion, potentially resulting in multiple organ dysfunction and death of the host. In smaller fish, rupture of the body wall may also be a potential sequelae of *Ligula* sp. infestation.[41] Clinical indications of trematode-associated coelomic disease depend upon the specificity of the target organs. In many cases, encysted trematodes and associated host tissue reactions are apparent as small pinpoint or larger multifocal discolorations either externally, internally, or both. Within the coelomic cavity, these visceral cysts may be apparent in the muscle of the body wall or on organs and may also be associated with inflammation and fibrosis.[42] Visceral migration of the cercarial stage prior to encystment may also produce associated inflammatory or degenerative changes in tissues characteristic of peritonitis. While mild cases of larval trematodes may be virtually asymptomatic, severe infestations with highly pathogenic species may be fatal. Acanthocephalans parasitizing the intestines of fish are sometimes visible or palpable within the intestine upon examination at surgery or necropsy. Secondary impacts to the coelomic cavity generally only occur in severe infestations due to perforation of the gut wall and secondary fibrous peritonitis.[43] Leakage of gastrointestinal contents into the coelomic cavity may produce additional complications of peritonitis such as hemorrhage, inflammation, effusion, or necrosis of serosal surfaces of the intestine or other coelomic organs.

Differential diagnosis: Differentials include the various forms of coelomic parasitism as well as other causes of peritonitis.

Diagnosis: Diagnosis is based on observation and identification of the parasite, generally upon surgery or necropsy. Perforation of the gut wall may be evident grossly with acanthocephalan parasites and clinical signs of peritonitis may also be apparent. Parasite identification is based on taxonomical identification using morphological features and/or molecular identification to genus/species.

Management/control: Management options are often limited for control of helminths within the coelomic cavity. Oftentimes in the case of few to no accompanying symptoms, no treatment or control is warranted. Anthelminthic treatment may not be effective or advisable for control of parasites that are free or encysted within the body cavity, as opposed to parasites found within the gastrointestinal tract.[44] Control of alternative host populations may help to break the parasite's life cycle in some cases. Culling of affected fish within a population may also be necessary if significant disease is noted.

REFERENCES

1. Austin, B. and Austin, D.A. *Bacterial Fish Pathogens: Disease of Farmed and Wild Fish*, 3rd ed. Springer Science & Business Media/Praxis Publishing, Chichester, UK, 1999.
2. Kumar, D., Mishra, B.K. and Dey, R.K. Dropsy in *Catla catla* (Ham.) caused by mixed infection of *Aeromonas hydrophila* and *Myxosporidian* sp. *Aquacultura Hungarica* 1986;5:107–112.
3. Fijan, N., Petrinec, Z., Sulimanovic, D. and Zwillenberg, L.O. Isolation of the viral causative agent from the acute form of infectious dropsy of carp. *Veterinarski Arhiv* 1971;41(5–6):125–138.
4. Wolf, K. *Fish Viruses and Fish Viral Diseases*. Comstock Publishing Associates/Cornell University Press, Ithaca, NY, 1988.
5. Lumsden, J.S. Gastrointestinal tract, swimbladder, pancreas and peritoneum. In: *Systemic Pathology of Fish*, 2nd ed. pp. 168–199, 2006.
6. Lewisch, E., Dressler, A., Menanteau-Ledouble, S., Saleh, M. and El-Matbouli, M. Francisellosis in ornamental African cichlids in Austria. *Bulletin of the European Association of Fish Pathologists* 2014;34(2):63.
7. Dixon, B.A., Straub, D. and Truscott, J. Isolation of *Clostridium difficile* (Prevot) from the African cichlid, *Nimbochromis venustus* (Boulenger), with "Malawi bloat". *Journal of Aquariculture and Aquatic Sciences* 1997;8(2):35–38.
8. Staurnes, M., Andorsdottir, G. and Sundby, A. Distended, water-filled stomach in sea-farmed rainbow trout. *Aquaculture* 1990;90(3–4):333–343.
9. Kent, M.L. Diseases of seawater netpen-reared salmonid fishes in the Pacific Northwest. *Canadian Special Publication of Fisheries and Aquatic Sciences* 1992;116:76.
10. Bruno, D., Noguera, P.A. and Poppe, T.T. *A Colour Atlas of Salmonid Diseases*. Vol. 91. Academic Press, London, 2013.
11. Hicks, B. *British Columbia Salmon Farming Manual. British Columbia Salmonid Disease Handbook*. Ministry of Agriculture and Fisheries, British Columbia, Canada, 1989.
12. Goodwin, A.E. Steatitis, fin loss and skin ulcers of channel catfish, *Ictalurus punctatus* (Rafinesque), fingerlings fed salmonid diets. *Journal of Fish Diseases* 2006;29(1):61–64.
13. Herman, R.L. and Kircheis, F.W. Steatitis in Sunapee trout, *Salvelinus alpinus oquassa* Girard. *Journal of Fish Diseases* 1985;8(2):237–239.
14. Roberts, R.J. and Agius, C. Pan-steatitis in farmed northern bluefin tuna, *Thunnus thynnus* (L.), in the eastern Adriatic. *Journal of Fish Diseases* 2008;31(2):83–88.
15. Miyazaki, T., Kubota, S., Kaige, N. and Miyashita, T. A histopathological study of streptococcal disease in tilapia. *Fish Pathology (Japan)* 1984;19(3):167–172.
16. Decostere, A., Hermans, K. and Haesebrouck, F. Piscine mycobacteriosis: A literature review covering the agent and the disease it causes in fish and humans. *Veterinary Microbiology* 2004;99(3):159–166.
17. Schmidtke, L.M. and Carson, J. Characteristics of *Vagococcus salmoninarum* isolated from diseased salmonid fish. *Journal of Applied Bacteriology* 1994;77(2):229–236.
18. Roberts, R.J. The bacteriology of teleosts. In: *Fish Pathology*, 3rd ed. R.J. Roberts, ed. W.B. Saunders, London, 2001; p. 472.
19. Fryer, J.L. and Hedrick, R.P. *Piscirickettsia salmonis*: A Gram-negative intracellular bacterial pathogen of fish. *Journal of Fish Diseases* 2003;26(5):251–262.
20. Steckler, N.K., Yanong, R.P., Pouder, D.B., Nyaoke, A., Sutton, D.A., Lindner, J.R., Wickes, B.L., Frasca Jr., S., Wolf, J.C. and Waltzek, T.B. New disease records for hatchery-reared sturgeon. II. Phaeohyphomycosis due to *Veronaea botryosa*. *Diseases of Aquatic Organisms* 2014;111(3):229–238.
21. Ostland, V.E., Ferguson, H.W., Armstrong, R.D., Asselin, A. and Hall, R. Granulomatous peritonitis in

fish associated with *Fusarium solani. Veterinary Record* 1987;121(25–26):595–596.

22. Borucinska, J., Kohler, N., Natanson, L. and Skomal, G. Pathology associated with retained fishing hooks in blue sharks, *Prionace glauca* (L.), with implications for their conservation. *Journal of Fish Diseases* 2002;25(9):515–521.

23. Rummer, J.L. and Bennett, W.A. Physiological effects of swim bladder overexpansion and catastrophic decompression on red snapper. *Transactions of the American Fisheries Society* 2005;134(6):1457–1470.

24. Leatherland, J.F. and Ferguson, H.W. Endocrine and reproductive systems. In: *Systemic Pathology of Fish*, H.W. Ferguson, ed. Iowa State University Press, Ames, IA, 1989;pp. 195–214.

25. Gardiner, C.H. and Bunte, R.M. Granulomatous peritonitis in a fish caused by a flagellated protozoan. *Journal of Wildlife Diseases* 1984;20(3):238–240.

26. Jones, M.W. and Cox, D.I. Clinical disease in sea-farmed Atlantic salmon (*Salmo salar*) associated with a member of the family Pasteurellaceae-a case history. *Bulletin of the European Association of Fish Pathologists* 1999;19:75–78.

27. Lillehaug, A., Lunder, T. and Poppe, T.T. Field testing of adjuvanted furunculosis vaccines in Atlantic salmon, *Salmo salar* L. *Journal of Fish Diseases* 1992;15(6):485–496.

28. Gjessing, M.C., Falk, K., Weli, S.C., Koppang, E.O. and Kvellestad, A. A sequential study of incomplete Freund's adjuvant-induced peritonitis in Atlantic cod. *Fish & Shellfish Immunology* 2012;32(1):141–150.

29. Koppang, E.O., Haugarvoll, E., Hordvik, I., Aune, L. and Poppe, T.T. Vaccine-associated granulomatous inflammation and melanin accumulation in Atlantic salmon, *Salmo salar* L., white muscle. *Journal of Fish Diseases* 2005;28(1):13–22.

30. Poppe, T.T. and Breck, O. Pathology of Atlantic salmon *Salmo salar* intraperitoneally immunized with oil-adjuvanted vaccine. A case report. *Diseases of Aquatic Organisms* 1997;29(3):219–226.

31. Simko, E., El-Mowafi, A., Bettger, W.J., Ostland, V.E., Ferguson, H.W. and Hayes, M.A. Alterations in iron, zinc and major plasma proteins of rainbow trout, *Oncorhynchus mykiss* (Walbaum), and brook trout, *Salvelinus fontinalis* (Mitchill), with sterile peritonitis induced by oil-adjuvanted multivalent bacterin vaccination. *Journal of Fish Diseases* 1999;22(2):81–90.

32. Koppang, E.O., Haugarvoll, E., Hordvik, I., Poppe, T.T. and Bjerkås, I. Granulomatous uveitis associated with vaccination in the Atlantic salmon. *Veterinary Pathology Online* 2004;41(2):122–130.

33. Koppang, E.O., Bjerkås, I., Haugarvoll, E. et al. Vaccination-induced systemic autoimmunity in farmed Atlantic salmon. *The Journal of Immunology* 2008;181(7):4807–4814.

34. Haugarvoll, E., Bjerkås, I., Szabo, N.J., Satoh, M. and Koppang, E.O. Manifestations of systemic autoimmunity in vaccinated salmon. *Vaccine* 2010;28(31):4961–4969.

35. Midtlyng, P.J. A field study on intraperitoneal vaccination of Atlantic salmon (*Salmo salar* L.) against furunculosis. *Fish & Shellfish Immunology* 1996;6(8):553–565.

36. Hoffman, G.L. *Parasites of North American Freshwater Fishes*, 2nd ed. Cornell University Press, Ithaca, NY, 1999.

37. Roberts, R.J. The parasitology of teleosts. In: *Fish Pathology*, 3rd ed. R.J. Roberts, ed. W.B. Saunders, London, 2001; chap. 7.

38. Iyaji, F.O. and Eyo, J.E. Parasites and their freshwater fish host. *Bio-Research* 2008;6(1):328–338.

39. Moravec, F. and de Buron, I. A synthesis of our current knowledge of philometrid nematodes, a group of increasingly important fish parasites. *Folia Parasitologica* 2013;60(2):81.

40. Van Kruiningen, H.J., Placke, M.E. and Wojan, L.D. *Diphyllobothrium plerocercoid* infestation in landlocked salmon. *Veterinary Pathology Online* 1987;24(3):285–286.

41. Hoffman, G.L. Lesions due to internal helminths of freshwater fishes. In: *The Pathology of Fishes*, Ribelin W.E. and G. Migaki, eds. The University of Wisconsin Press, Madison, WI, 1975; pp. 151–188.

42. Paperna, I. Diseases caused by parasites in the aquaculture of warm water fish. *Annual Review of Fish Diseases* 1991;1:155–194.

43. Rajeshkumar, S., Gomathinayagam, S., Ansari, A. and Munuswamy, N. Infection of acanthocephalan parasite *Neoechinorhynchus agilis* sp. in the grey mullet, (*Mugil cephalus*) a candidate species from-Corentyne coast, Berbice, Guyana. *International Journal of Current Research and Review* 2013;5(5):53.

44. Yanong, R.P.E. *Nematode (roundworm) Infections in Fish*. Cooperative Extension Service Circular 91, Institute of Food and Agricultural Sciences, University of Florida, Gainesville, FL, 2011.

CHAPTER 9

GASTROINTESTINAL DISORDERS

STEPHEN A. SMITH

Few infectious agents specifically target the gastrointestinal tract of fish. However, the gastrointestinal tract often becomes secondarily involved as a systemic extension from the primary organ infected.

ORAL AND BRANCHIAL CAVITY

Goiter

Overview: An endocrine disorder resulting in a nodular mass or masses of nonneoplastic thyroid epithelial cell proliferation in the oral and branchial cavity of fish.[1]

Etiology: A deficiency of iodine or the presence of goiterogenic materials in the diet or water presumably leads to a decrease in thyroid hormone production, which stimulates an increase in thyroid stimulating hormone. This in turn leads to an increase in the size and number of thyrocytes, which results in the stimulation and enlargement of diffuse, ectopic follicles of thyroid tissue present along the floor of the branchial chamber.

Route of transmission: Deficiency of iodine in diet or water column.

Host range: Goiter has been reported in numerous species of wild and captive freshwater, brackish and marine fishes.[2,3] Sharks in captivity appear to be predisposed to goiter.[4,5]

Clinical presentation: Single or multiple growths of light, cream to tan colored, lobular mass or masses within the oral and branchial cavity (**Figure 9.1**). Large growth may interfere with ingestion of prey items or affect the flow of water over the gills and thus interfere with respiration.

Pathology: Distinguishing thyroid hyperplasia from thyroid adenoma or carcinoma can often be challenging. Thyroid tissue in fish lacks a discrete fibrous capsule, is capable of ectopic growth to nonpharyngeal sites, and is frequently predisposed to hyperplastic proliferation.[6] A diagnosis of goiter is represented by nodular follicular cell hyperplasia, which does not have the characteristics of neoplastic growth (i.e., presence of cellular atypia, cellular pleomorphism and/or a high mitotic index).

Differential diagnosis: The primary differentials for goiter are tumors, granulomatous masses and nodular foreign body reactions (**Figure 9.2**).

Diagnosis: Clinical observation of individual or multiple nodular growths most commonly at the base of the gills and sometimes extending upward along the gill arches, and histopathology demonstrating thyroid hyperplasia, which often appears invasive.

Management/control: Supplemental iodine in diet or water. Removal of goiterogenic substances such as adulterated feeds, therapeutics, pesticides and elevated nitrites in the water.[5]

Enteric redmouth disease

Overview: Enteric redmouth disease (ERM), or yersiniosis, is an acute or chronic bacterial systemic infection of wild and cultured salmonids and has caused significant economic losses in both freshwater and marine aquaculture. The disease has been reported in North America, South America, Europe, Africa, China and Australia.[7]

Etiology: The causative agent is *Yersinia ruckeri*, a Gram-negative, motile, cytochrome oxidase–negative, rod-shaped enterobacterium.

Route of transmission: The bacterium can be transmitted horizontally by direct contact with an infected host or shed in the feces where the bacterium can survive in the environment for up to 4 months.[7] The spread of *Y. ruckeri* has also been associated with vectors such as aquatic invertebrates and birds.[8] The bacteria initially infect the gill lamellae, then spread via the blood to the intestine, kidney, liver, spleen, brain and heart.

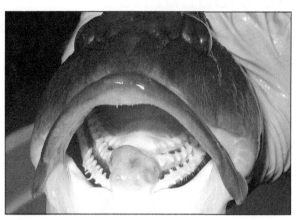

Figure 9.1 Captive black sea bass (*Centropristis striata*) with proliferative thyroid tissue (i.e., goiter) along ventral gill arches. (Image courtesy of S. Bolan.)

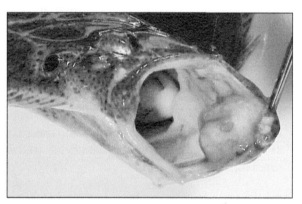

Figure 9.2 Nodular oral lesion in a summer flounder (*Paralichthys dentatus*) due to *Mycobacterium* sp.

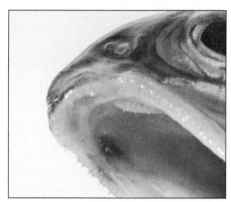

Figure 9.3 Submucosal hemorrhage in the oral cavity of a rainbow trout (*Oncorhynchus mykiss*) infected with *Yersinia ruckeri*. Also note the hemorrhage in the eye, which is commonly associated with enteric redmouth disease.

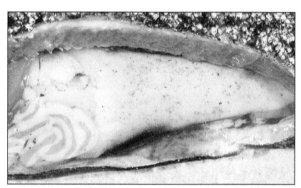

Figure 9.4 Petechial hemorrhage of the adipose tissues in a rainbow trout infected with enteric redmouth disease (i.e., *Yersinia ruckeri*).

Host range: This is primarily a disease of cultured salmonids, with rainbow trout (*Oncorhynchus mykiss*) being particularly susceptible. However, the bacterium has also been isolated from a number of other species of diseased fish including farmed turbot (*Scophthalmus maximus*), European sea bass (*Dicentrarchus labrax*), sea bream (*Sparus auratus*), sturgeon (*Acipenser sturio*), common carp (*Cyprinus carpio*), channel catfish (*Ictalurus punctatus*) and Nile tilapia (*Oreochromis niloticus*); and muskrats, turtles and sea gulls.[7,9–11]

Clinical presentation: The disease is characterized by subcutaneous hemorrhages of the jaw, oral cavity, fins, and eyes, in addition to hemorrhages on the body surface and vent (**Figure 9.3**).[7] Internally there may be petechial hemorrhages of the liver,

swim bladder and adipose tissue, and necrosis of the hematopoietic tissues of the kidney (**Figure 9.4**).[12] Survivors often exhibit exophthalmia, darkening of the skin and anorexia, and generally become chronic carriers of the bacteria.

Pathology: The bacterium causes a generalized septicemia with petechial hemorrhage and inflammation occurring in the gills, kidney, spleen, liver and heart. There may be areas of focal necrosis in the spleen, kidney and liver.

Differential diagnosis: Other enteric bacterial infections (e.g., *Proteus* sp. and *Citrobacter* sp.), intestinal parasites, other diseases that cause anorexia.[13]

Diagnosis: A presumptive diagnosis can be made from a history of low-level, chronic losses and clinical signs, while a definitive diagnosis is made on bacterial identification using standard culture techniques, fluorescent antibody test (FAT), serological (i.e., ELISA) and molecular methods. The species is subdivided into two biotypes, five serotypes and five outer membrane protein types.[14]

Management/control: Clinical outbreaks of ERM are often stress-mediated as a result of poor water quality or increased water temperatures. Thus, maintaining optimal water quality and reducing stocking densities are essential for disease prevention. Antibiotic therapy is standard treatment for a clinical outbreak, and several commercial vaccines are available for control.

Tumors

A variety of tumors have been reported from the oral and branchial cavity of fishes and include spontaneous neoplasia in addition to those caused by exposure to environmental agents (i.e., chemicals) and infectious agents (i.e., viruses). These include branchioblastomas in wild salmonids, odontomas in clownfish (*Amphiprion ocellaris*), osteochodromas in gilthead sea bream (*Sparus aurata*), osteosarcoma in Italian barbels (*Barbus barbus plebejus*), papillomas and carcinomas in brown bullheads (*Ictalurus nebulosus*), and fibromas in wild cod (*Gadus* spp.) and other gadoid fishes.[15–19] Though most are benign, some may be locally invasive. The majority of these growths are easily observed either along the margins of the mouth, in the oral cavity of the fish or protruding from under the operculum (**Figure 9.5**).

STOMACH

Salmon water belly

Water belly occurs among saltwater pen-reared salmonids, including Atlantic salmon (*Salmo salar*), Chinook salmon (*Oncorhynchus tshawytscha*) and rainbow trout (*Oncorhynchus mykiss*) (see Chapter 8). This condition is idiopathic and presents clinically as a fluid distention of the gastrointestinal tract primarily due to the accumulation of seawater in the stomach of the fish. The condition is associated with intensive feeding regimes and dietary composition of production feeds[20,21] (see Chapter 8, **Figure 8.4**).

Parasitism

There are a number of different parasite species that infest the stomach of fishes. *Cryptobia iubilans* is a flagellate parasite of discus (*Symphysodon* spp.) and other cichlids that causes a granulomatous reaction in the stomach wall and sometimes the anterior intestine. Affected fish often present with emaciation, lethargy, hyperpigmentation and a history of increasing mortality. Internally the stomach, and sometime anterior intestine, has a plicated or corrugated appearance (**Figure 9.6**).[22,23] The apicomplexan parasite *Cryptosporidium* sp. has been reported from a number of wild and cultured fish species including the freshwater angelfish (*Pterophyllum scalare*), catfish (*Plecostomus* spp.), gilthead sea bream (*Sparus aurata*), turbot (*Scophthalmus maximus)* and European sea bass (*Dicentrarchus labrax*).[24–28] A number of adult and larval nematode species can often

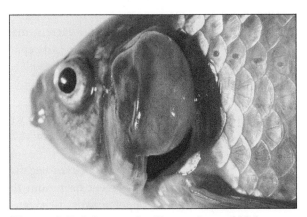

Figure 9.5 Subopercular fibroma in a goldfish (*Carassius auratus*).

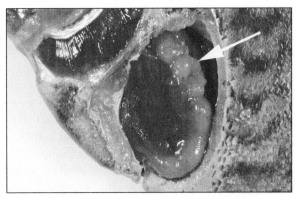

Figure 9.6 Corrugated appearance of the stomach (arrow) of a discus (*Symphysodon* sp.) infected with *Cryptobia iubilans*.

be found encysted in the tissue or attach to the luminal wall of the esophagus or stomach of fishes. Larval nematodes belonging to the genera *Anisakis, Eustrongylides, Pseudoterranove, Contracaecum* and *Hysterothylacium* are commonly observed in cod, hake, horse mackerel, sardines, anchovies, salmon, herring, tuna, whiting, turbot, halibut and Pollack, and can be a consumption zoonotic hazard. Adult nematodes of the stomach include Ascaridoidea, Spirurida, Camellanoidea and Anguillicolidae.[29–31]

INTESTINE

Visceral toxicosis of catfish

Overview: A syndrome characterized by sudden mortality in apparently healthy market-sized and brood stock-sized channel catfish (*Ictalurus punctatus*) that primarily occurs in the spring and fall when water temperatures are below 20°C.[32]

Etiology: This syndrome is caused by Gram-positive *Clostriudium botulinum* type E neurotoxin.

Route of transmission: Unknown.

Host range: A similar syndrome and etiology has been reported in cultured rainbow trout (*Oncorhynchus mykiss*) and coho salmon (*O. kisutch*), and experimentally in the round goby (*Neogobius melanostomas*), walleye (*Stizostedion vitreum*), yellow perch (*Perca flavescens*) and tilapia (*Oreochromis mossambicus*).[33–36]

Clinical presentation: Clinical signs include erratic swimming behavior and progressive muscular weakness leading to paralysis, lethargy and death. Gross lesions include exophthalmia, gastric eversion, intussusception of the intestine, pallor of the proximal intestinal tract, chylous ascites, splenic congestion and a reticular pattern to the liver (**Figures 9.7 and 9.8**).

Pathology: Histopathological findings include cerebral, splenic and hepatic congestion; vascular dilatation and edema of the gastrointestinal tract; and perivascular edema of the spleen and kidney.[32]

Differential diagnosis: A similar syndrome causing intussusception of the intestine in cultured channel catfish but a different etiology (i.e., *Hafnia alvei*) has been reported in China, Israel and Mexico.[37–39]

Diagnosis: A presumptive diagnosis can be made from clinical signs (i.e., abnormal swimming and

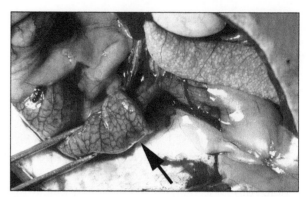

Figure 9.7 Intussusception (arrow) in a channel catfish (*Ictalurus punctatus*) with visceral toxicosis. (Image courtesy of L. Khoo.)

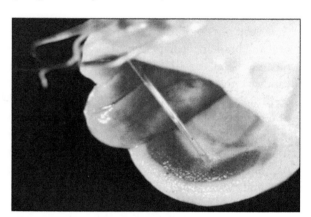

Figure 9.8 Gastric eversion in a channel catfish (*Ictalurus punctatus*) with visceral toxicosis. (Image courtesy of L. Khoo.)

listless behavior), gross observations, negative bacterial cultures and lack of microscopic evidence of an infectious process. A definitive diagnosis requires a serum bioassay or mass spectrometry.[40]

Management/control: There are no current management or control recommendations as the epidemiology of the disease has not been elucidated.[32]

Dissecting enteritis of flounder

Overview: A bacterial enteritis associated with cultured, juvenile summer flounder (*Paralichthys dentatus*).

Etiology: *Vibrio carchariae* is a Gram-negative, motile, rod-shaped, bioluminescent bacterium that may act as a primary or opportunistic pathogen of many marine organisms. Some consider this a synonym of *V. harveyi*.[41]

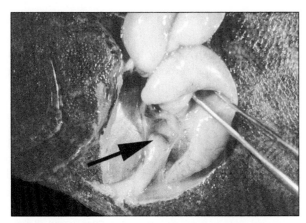

Figure 9.9 Dissecting enteritis and atresia of posterior intestine (arrow) caused by *Vibrio carchariae* in a summer flounder (*Paralichthys dentatus*).

Route of transmission: The bacteria is most likely shed into the water through the feces of infected fish and acquired by ingestion of water or contaminated feed.

Host range: Though the clinical syndrome has only been reported from summer flounder, the bacterium has been isolated from grouper (*Epinephelus coioides*), red drum (*Sciaenops ocellatus*), sharks, octopus, squid and abalone.[41-45]

Clinical presentation: Fish initially develop coelomic distention and redness around the vent. The coelom is filled with a serosanguinous fluid, and there is enteritis and necrosis of the posterior intestine. In later stages of the infection, the posterior intestine may rupture and become separated from the vent (**Figure 9.9**). Survivors may have a posterior intestine that becomes a blind-end sack filled with food and fluid, which often results in regurgitation of food and abdominal distention of the affected fish. However, affected fish may continue to feed, though their growth is severely stunted.[42]

Pathology: Lesions are restricted mostly to the posterior intestine and the peritoneum and include necrosis, hemorrhage, fibrin deposition, and an inflammatory cell infiltration consisting predominantly of lymphocytes and granulocytes. Bacterial colonies were also observed in the perivascular regions and capsule of the spleen.[42]

Differential diagnosis: A similar syndrome of enteritis has been reported in other flounder species but caused by *Vibrio* spp. FINE, i.e., "flounder infectious

necrotizing enteritis."[46] Differentials include other bacterial or viral diseases causing primary or secondary enteritis.

Diagnosis: Standard isolation of the bacteria from the peritoneal fluid or posterior intestine on marine culture medium, blood agar or a selective *Vibrio* agar such as TCBS (thiosulfate-citrate-bile salts-sucrose) agar.

Management/control: Antibiotic therapy is standard treatment for a clinical outbreak, while maintaining optimal water quality, reducing stocking densities and culling affected individuals are essential for disease control.

Intestinal gas

Overview: An abnormal accumulation of air/gas within the intestinal tract.

Etiology: There are a number of reported causes of air/gas within the intestinal tract. Some bacterial pathogens, such as *Streptococcus iniae* or *Clostridium difficile* (i.e., cichlid bloat or Malawi bloat, see Chapter 8) may cause enteric gas production during to the pathogenesis of the disease (**Figure 9.10**).[47] Supersaturation of the water column with abnormally high levels of atmospheric gases can also cause the accumulation of gases within the capillaries of the fins and gills, under the skin, within the anterior chamber of the eye, and in the lumen of the intestinal tract of fish (**Figure 9.11**).[48-50] Some fish, such as goldfish, may ingest abnormal amounts of air by gulping air at the surface of the water. In addition, some poorer quality fish feeds may produce gases

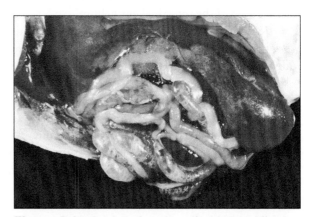

Figure 9.10 Intestinal gas in a tilapia (*Oreochromis* sp.) infected with *Steptococcus iniae*.

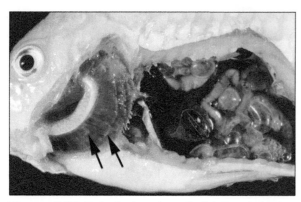

Figure 9.11 Intestinal gas in a tilapia (*Oreochromis* sp.) affected by elevated gas levels in the water column, i.e., supersaturation. Also note blanched areas of the gill (arrows) as a result of air/gas in the lamellar capillaries.

during the digestion process allowing gas bubbles to form in the lumen of the intestine.[51]

Route of transmission: Depends on etiology, but mostly through the water or diet.

Host range: Probably any fish is susceptible to the development of abnormal accumulation of air/gas within the intestinal tract.

Clinical presentation: The fish may appear to have a bloated appearance or abdominal distention. The fish may have problems controlling buoyancy within the water column. In severe cases the fish may be found floating at the surface, sometimes on one side or completely upside down.

Pathology: Depends on the etiology. Most bacterial diseases directly affecting the intestinal tract cause an initial enteritis followed by necrosis and exfoliation of the intestinal epithelium.

Differential diagnosis: Differentials would include ascites, tumors within the coelom, polycystic kidney disease in goldfish, gravid fish, and cystic ovaries in koi and others species of fish.

Diagnosis: This syndrome needs to be differentiated from overinflation of the swim bladder and other swim bladder disorders. Radiography will often clearly demonstrate the air/gas within the intestinal tract as opposed to the swim bladder or other cause of abdominal distention.

Management/control: Depends on the etiology. Antibiotic therapy for an infectious agent may help to control a disease outbreak, while reducing

saturated gases within the water column would help to eliminate the cause of "gas bubble disease." Feeding goldfish sinking feeds rather than floating feeds often helps to reduce the incidence of air being ingested by goldfish during feeding.

Parasitism

Overview: Parasitism by a variety of protozoan and metazoan parasites may be commonly observed within and around the intestinal tract of fish. A multitude of fish species can serve as intermediate, paratenic or definitive hosts for the adult and larval stages of these parasites (see also Chapter 8).[29–31,52,53]

Etiology: These include ciliates, flagellates, microsporidians, apicomplexans, myxosporidians, digenetic trematodes, nematodes, cestodes and acanthocephalans. Most of the protozoan parasites can be found in the lumen and/or epithelial cells lining the intestinal tract. The adult stages of the metazoan parasites commonly inhabit the lumen of the intestinal tract, while the larval stages encyst within the tissues or on the serosal surface of the intestine.

Route of transmission: With such a diversity of parasites, there are a number of different pathways depending on the species of parasites that may be used to infect another host. Some parasites may have direct fish-to-fish life cycles, or indirect life cycles that may involve one of more invertebrate or vertebrate intermediate hosts.

Host range: Presumably all fish are susceptible to a variety of protozoan and metazoan parasite species.

Clinical presentation: Generally, the presence and severity of clinical signs associated with parasites of the intestinal tract is dependent upon the life stage, the number and the pathogenicity of the parasite. Thus, fish may show no noticeable symptoms for parasites that are few in number, become encysted as larval stages or which do not cause much pathology. Conversely, a heavy infestation of protozoan or metazoan parasites may result in hyperpigmentation, emaciation, lethargy, enteritis, abdominal distention, rectal prolapse, stunted growth and significant mortality in a population.

Pathology of disease: Some enteric protozoans such as the flagellate *Spironucleus* sp. and various coccidian parasites may cause widespread necrosis and sloughing of the epithelial cells lining the intestinal

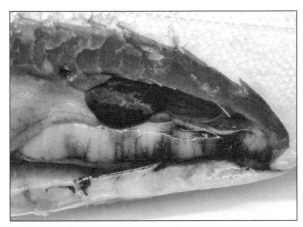

Figure 9.12 Pale, swollen posterior intestine of rainbow trout (*Oncorhynchus mykiss*) due to an extensive late-stage *Ceratonova shasta* infection. (Image courtesy of S. Atkinson.)

tract. *Glugea anomala*, a microsporidian parasite of killifishes, may cause the proliferation of epithelial cells and the formation of xenomas in the intestinal wall.[54] *Ceratonova* (~*Ceratomyxa*) *shasta*, a myxosporean parasite of salmonids, causes necrosis and sloughing of the epithelial cells of the intestinal tract followed by penetration of the muscularis and serosa (**Figure 9.12**) and invasion of adjacent tissue in the coelomic cavity.[55] *Enteromyxum leei*, a myxosporidian parasite of the Japanese flounder (*Paralichthys olivaceus*), parrotfish (*Sparisoma cretense*), Red Sea bream (*Pargus major*), spotted knifefish (*Oplegnathus punctatus*), turbot (*Scophthalmus maximus*) and the tiger puffer (*Takifugu rubripes*) may cause hyperplasia, exfoliation and progressive destruction of the intestinal epithelium.[56–60] Large numbers of nematodes or cestodes may cause physical occlusion of the intestinal tract, migrating larval stages of many of the metazoan parasites may cause an intense inflammatory response by the host, and some nematodes and acanthocephalans may cause a focal host reaction at the site of attachment and in rare cases perforation of the intestinal wall.

Differential diagnosis: As the clinical signs of these parasitic infections are so variable, differentials could include multiple viral and bacterial diseases, as well as noninfectious problems.

Diagnosis: A presumptive diagnosis can often be made by observation of nonspecific clinical signs (e.g., weight loss, abdominal distention, fecal cast), or the results of a fecal examination or wet mount for live or encysted protozoan stages or metazoan eggs. A definitive diagnosis is based on identification of the parasite by taxonomic methods using morphological features or molecular identification.

Management/control: Controlling intestinal parasites in wild fish populations is not feasible nor appropriate in most cases, however, managing economically important intestinal parasites in captive fish populations can sometimes be accomplished depending on the type of parasite involved. Antiparasitic treatment for both protozoan and metazoan parasites that are free within the lumen of the intestinal tract has afforded variable results, and most treatments are ineffective for the encysted tissue stages. Alternative control methods may include filtration of water to eliminate infectious stages in the water, elimination of the intermediate hosts (e.g., snail, other fish) to interrupt the life cycle of the parasite, or the exclusion of piscivorous birds or mammalian hosts harboring the adult stages of parasites that have fish as an intermediate host.

Neoplasia

Neoplasms of the intestinal tract of fish are extremely rare.[15] Invasive adenomas and adenocarcinomas have been reported in laboratory fish exposed to chemicals, and carcinomas and mixed malignant neoplasms have been reported in laboratory zebrafish in association with the parasitic nematode *Pseudocapillaria tomentosa*.[61,62]

REFERENCES

1. Hoover, K.L. Hyperplastic thyroid lesions in fish. *National Cancer Institute Monographs* 1984;65:275–289.
2. Sonstegard, R. and Leatherland, J.F. The epizootiology and pathogenesis of thyroid hyperplasia in Coho Salmon (Oncorhynchuskisutch) in Lake Ontario. *Cancer Research* 1976;36:4467–4475.
3. Wolf, J.C., Ginn, P.E. and Francis-Floyd, R. Goitre in a colony of African cichlids. *Journal of Fish Diseases* 1998;21:139–143.
4. Crow, G.L., Luer, W.H. and Harshbarger, J.C. Histological assessment of goiters in elasmobranch fishes. *Journal of Aquatic Animal Health* 2001;13:1–7.
5. Morris, A.L., Hamilin, H.J., Francis-Floyd, R., Sheppard, B.J. and Guillette, L.J. Nitrate-induced goiter

in captive whitespotted bamboo sharks *Chilosryllium pla-giosum. Journal of Aquatic Animal Health* 2011;23:92–99.

6. Fournie, J.W., Wolfe, M.J., Wolf, J.C., Courtney, L.A., Johnson, R.D. and Hawkins, W.E. Diagnostic criteria for proliferative thyroid lesions in bony fishes. *Toxicologic Pathology* 2005;33:540–551.

7. Kumar, G., Menanteau-Ledouble, S., Saleh, M. and El-Matbouli, M. Yersinia ruckeri, the causative agent of enteric redmouth disease in fish. *Veterinary Research* 2015;46(1):103–113.

8. Willumsen, B. Birds and wild fish as potential vectors of *Yersinia ruckeri. Journal of Fish Diseases* 1989;12:275–277.

9. Tobback, E., Decostere, A., Hermans, K., Haesebrouck, F. and Chiers, K. *Yersinia ruckeri* infections in salmonid fish. *Journal of Fish Diseases* 2007;30(5):257–268.

10. Eissa, A.E., Moustafa, M., Abdelaziz, M. and Ezzeldeen, N.A. *Yersinia ruckeri* infection in cultured Nile tilapia, *Oreochromis niloticus*, at a semi-intensive fish farm in lower Egypt. *African Journal of Aquatic Science* 2008;33(3):283–286.

11. Willumsen, B. Birds and wild fish as potential vectors of *Yersinia ruckeri. Journal of Fish Diseases* 1989;12:275–277.

12. Wobeser, G. An outbreak of redmouth disease in rainbow trout (*Salmo gairdneri*) in Saskatchewan. *Journal of the Fisheries Research Board of Canada* 1993;30:571–575.

13. Daly, J.D. Other bacterial pathogens. In: *Fish Diseases and Disorders*. P.T.K. Woo and D.W. Bruno, eds. CABI, Wallingford, UK, 1999; pp. 577–598.

14. Davies, R.L. Clonal analysis of *Yersinia ruckeri* based on biotypes, serotypes and outer membrane protein-types. *Journal of Fish Diseases* 1991;14(2):221–228.

15. Groff, J.M. Neoplasia in fishes. *Veterinary Clinics of North America: Exotic Animal Practice* 2004;7:705–756.

16. Vorbach, B.S., Wolf, J.C. and Yanong, R.P. Odontomas in two long-finned ocellaris clownfish (*Amphiprion ocellaris*). *Journal of Veterinary Diagnostic Investigation* 2018;30:36–139.

17. Poulet, F.M., Wolfe, M.J. and Spitsbergen, J.M. Naturally occurring orocutaneous papillomas and carcinomas of brown bullheads (*Ictalurus nebulosus*) in New York State. *Veterinary Pathology* 1994;31:8–18.

18. Roberts, R.J. Oral carcinomata in a salmon (*Salmo salar* L.). *The Veterinary Record* 1972;91:199.

19. Nash, G. and Porter, C. Branchial osteochondroma in a gilthead sea bream, *Sparus aurata* L., cultured in the Gulf of Aqaba. *Journal of Fish Diseases* 1985;8:333–336.

20. Staurnes, M., Andorsdottir, G. and Sundby, A. Distended, water-filled stomach in sea-farmed rainbow trout. *Aquaculture* 1990;90:333–343.

21. Kent, M.L. Diseases of seawater netpen-reared salmonid fishes in the Pacific Northwest. *Canadian Special Publication of Fisheries and Aquatic Sciences* 1992;116.

22. Nohynkova, E. A new pathogenic Cryptobia from freshwater fishes: A light and electron microscopic study. *Protistologica* 1984;20:181–195.

23. Yanong, R.P.E., Curtis, E., Russo, R., Francis-Floyd, R., Klinger, R., Berzins, I., Kelley, K. and Poynton,

S.L. *Cryptobia iubilans* infection in juvenile discus. *Journal of the American Veterinary Medical Association* 2004;224:1644–1650.

24. Koinari, M., Karl, S., Ng-Hublin, J., Lymbery, A.J. and Ryan, U.M. Identification of novel and zoonotic *Cryptosporidium* species in fish from Papua New Guinea. *Veterinary Parasitology* 2013;198:1–9.

25. Muench, T.R. and White, M.R. Cryptosporidiosis in a tropical freshwater catfish (*Plecostomus* spp.). *Journal of Veterinary Diagnostic Investigation* 1997;9:87–90.

26. Sitja-Bobadilla, A., Pujalte, M.J., Macian, M.C., Pascual, J., Alverez-Pellitero, P. and Garay, E. Interactions between bacteria and *Cryptosporidium molnari* in gilthead sea bream (*Sparus aurata*) under farm and laboratory conditions. *Veterinary Parasitology* 2006;142:248–259.

27. Alvarez-Pellitero, P., Quiroga, M.I., Sitja-Bobadilla, A., Redondo, M.J., Palenzuela, O., Padros, F., Vazquez, S. and Nieto, J.M. *Cryptosporidium scophthalmi* n. sp. (Apicomplexa: Cryptosporidiidae) from cultured turbot *Scophthalmus maximus*: Light and electron microscope description and histopathological study. *Diseases of Aquatic Organisms* 2004;62:133–145.

28. Alvarez-Pellitero, P. and Sitja-Bobadilla, A. *Cryptosporidium molnari* n. sp. (Apicomplexa: Cryptosporidiidae) infecting two marine fish species, *Sparus aurata* L. and *Dicentrarchus labrax* L. *International Journal for Parasitology* 2002;32:1007–1021.

29. Hoffman, G.L. *Parasites of North American Freshwater Fishes*, 2nd ed. Cornell University Press, Ithaca, NY, 1999.

30. Dick, T.A. and Choudhury, A. Phylum nematoda. In: *Fish Diseases and Disorders, Vol. 1: Protozoan and Metazoan Infections*. P.T.K. Woo, ed. CABI, Wallingford, UK, 1995; pp. 415–446.

31. Molnar, K., Buchmann, K. and Szekely, C. Phylum nematoda. In: *Fish Diseases and Disorders, Vol. 1: Protozoan and Metazoan Infections*, 2nd ed. P.T.K. Woo, ed. CABI, Wallingford, UK, 2006; pp. 414–440.

32. Khoo, K.H., Goodwin, A.E., Wise, D.J., Holmes, W.E., Hanson, L.A., Steadman, J.M., McIntyre, L.M. and Guant, P.S. The pathology associated with visceral toxicosis of catfish. *Journal of Veterinary Diagnostic Investigation* 2011;23:1217–1221.

33. Cann, D.C. and Taylor, L.Y. An outbreak of botulism in rainbow trout, *Salmo gairdneri* Richardson, farmed in Britain. *Journal of Fish Diseases* 1982;5:393–399.

34. Eklund, M.W., Poysky, F.T., Peterson, M.E., Peck, L.W. and Brunson, W.D. Type E botulism in salmonids and conditions contributing to outbreaks. *Aquaculture* 1984;41:293–309.

35. Huss, H.H. and Eskildsen, U. Botulism in farmed trout caused by *Clostridium botulinum* type E; a preliminary report. *Nordisk Veterinary Medicine* 1974;26:733–738.

36. Yule, A.M., Barker, I.K., Austin, J.W. and Moccia, R.D. Toxicity of *Clostridium botulinum* type E neurotoxin to Great Lakes fish: Implications for avian botulism. *Journal of Wildlife Diseases* 2006;42(3):479–493.

37. Jin-Yu, L., Wu-Ming, Y., Ai-Hua, L. and Guang-Wen, H. Preliminary study on the etiology of channel catfish intussusception disease. *Acta Hydrobiologica Sinica* 2008;32:824–831.

38. Cao, H., He, S., Li, Y., Yang, Y. and Ai, X. *Hafnia alvei*: A pathogen causing infectious intussusception syndrome (IIS) in farmed channel catfish *Ictalurus punctatus*. *Israeli Journal of Aquaculture – Bamidgeh* 2016;68:1305–1311.

39. Montelongo-Alfaro, I.O., Rabago-Castro, J.L., Sanchez-Martunez, J.G., Benavides-Gonzalez, F. and De La Cruz-Hernandez, N.I. Report on intussusception in channel catfish *Ictalurus punctatus* (Rafinesque, 1818) from commercial farms in Mexico: A case study. *Indian Journal of Fisheries* 2018;65:119–122.

40. Gaunt, P.S., Kalb, S.R. and Barr, J.R. Detection of botulinum type E toxin in channel catfish with visceral toxicosis syndrome using catfish bioassay and endopep mass spectrometry. *Journal of Veterinary Diagnostic Investigation* 2007;19:349–354.

41. Liu, P.C., Chuang, W.H. and Lee, K.K. Infectious gastroenteritis caused by *Vibrio harveyi* (*V. carchariae*) in cultured red drum, *Sciaenops ocellatus*. *Journal of Applied Ichthyology* 2003;19:59–61.

42. Soffientinol, B., Gwaltney, T., Nelson, D.R., Specker, J.L., Mauel, M. and Gomez-Chiarri, M. Infectious necrotizing enteritis and mortality caused by *Vibrio carchariae* in summer flounder *Paralichthys dentatus* during intensive culture. *Diseases of Aquatic Organisms* 1999;38:201–210.

43. Yii, K.C., Yang, T.I. and Lee, K.K. Isolation and characterization of *Vibrio carchariae*, a causative agent of gastroenteritis in the groupers, *Epinephelus coioides*. *Current Microbiology* 1997;35(2):09–115.

44. Lee, K.K., Lui, P.C. and Chuang, W.H. Pathogenesis of gastroenteritis caused by *Vibrio carchariae* in cultured marine fish. *Marine Biotechnology (NY)* 202;4(3):267–277.

45. Nicolas, J.L., Basuyaux, O., Mazurie, J. and Thebault, A. *Vibrio carchariae*, a pathogen of the abalone *Haliotis tuberculata*. *Diseases of Aquatic Organisms* 2002;50(1):35–43.

46. Muroga, K., Yasunobu, H., Okada, N. and Masumura, K. Bacterial enteritis of cultured flounder *Paralichthys olivaceus* larvae. *Diseases of Aquatic Organisms* 1990;9:121–125.

47. Dixon, B.A., Straub, D. and Truscott, J. Isolation of *Clostridium difficile* (Prevot) from the African cichlid, *Nimbochromis venustus* (Boulenger), with "Malawi bloat." *Journal of Aquariculture and Aquatic Sciences* 1997;8(2):35–38.

48. Machado, J.P., Garling Jr, D.L., Kevern, N.R., Trapp, A.L. and Bell, T.G. Histopathology and the pathogenesis of embolism (gas bubble disease) in rainbow trout (*Salmo gairdneri*). *Canadian Journal of Fisheries and Aquatic Sciences* 1987;44:1985–1994.

49. Bouck, G.R. Etiology of gas bubble disease. *Transactions of the American Fisheries Society* 1980;119:703–707.

50. Weitkamp, D.E. and Katz, M. A review of dissolved gas supersaturation literature. *Transactions of the American Fisheries Society* 1980;109:659–702.

51. D'Abramo, L.R. and Frinsko, M.O. *Hybrid striped bass: Pond production of food fish*. Southern Regional Aquaculture Center, Stoneville, Mississippi, 2008, #303.

52. Smith, S.A. and Noga, E.J. General parasitology of fish. In: *Clinical Fish Medicine*. M.K. Stoskopf, ed. W.B. Saunders, Philadelphia, 1992; pp. 131–148.

53. Paperna, I. Diseases caused by parasites in the aquaculture of warm water fish. *Annual Review of Fish Diseases* 1991;1:155–194.

54. Lom, J., Noga, E.J. and Dykova, I. Occurrence of a microsporean with characteristics of *Glugea anomala* in ornamental fish of the family Cyprinodontidae. *Diseases of Aquatic Organisms* 1993;21:239–242.

55. Bartholomew, J.L., Smith, C.E. and Rohovec, J.S. Characterization of a host response to the myxosporean parasite, *Ceratomyxa shasta* (Noble), by histology, scanning electron microscopy and immunological techniques. *Journal of Fish Diseases* 1989;12:509–522.

56. Yasuda, H., Ooyama, T., Nakamura, A., Iwata, K., Palkenzuela, O. and Yokoyama, H. Occurrence of the myxosporean emaciation disease caused by *Enteromyxum leei* in cultured Japanese flounder *Paralichthys olivaceus*. *Fish Pathology* 2005;40:175–180.

57. Katharios, P., Kokkari, C., Sterioti, A., Smyrli, M. and Kalatzis, P.G. *Enteromyxum leei* infection in parrotfish, *Sparisoma cretense*: Histopathological, morphological and molecular study. *Veterinary Parasitology* 2014;199:136–143.

58. Yanagida, T., Palenzuela, O., Hirae, T., Tanaka, S., Yokoyama, H. and Ogawa, K. Myxosporean emaciation disease of cultured Red Sea bream *Pagrus major* and spotted knifejaw *Oplegnathus punctatus*. *Fish Pathology* 2008;43:45–48.

59. Quiroga, M.I., Redondo, M.J., Sitja-Bobadilla, A., Palenzuela, O., Riaza, A., Macias, A., Vazquez, S., Perez, A., Nieto, J.M. and Alvarez-Pellitero, P. Risk factors associated with *Enteromyxum scophthalmi* (Myxozoa) infection in cultured turbot, *Scophthalmus maximus* (L.). *Parasitology* 2006;133:433–442.

60. Yasuda, H., Ooyama, T., Iwata, K., Tun, T., Yokoyama, H. and Ogawa, K. Fish-to-fish transmission of *Myxidium* spp. (Myxozoa) in cultured tiger puffer suffering from emaciation disease. *Fish Pathology* 2002;37:29–33.

61. Grizzle, J.M. and Goodwin, A.E. Neoplasms and related lesions. In: *Fish Diseases and Disorders, Vol. 2: Non-Infectious Disorders*. A.F. Leatherland and P.T.K. Woo, eds. CABI, Wallingford, UK, 1998; pp. 37–104.

62. Kent, M.L., Bishop-Stewart, J.K., Matthews, J.L. and Spitsbergen, J.M. Pseudocapillaria tomentosa, a nematode pathogen, and associated neoplasms of zebrafish (*Danio rerio*) kept in research colonies. *Comparative Medicine* 2002;52:354–358.

CHAPTER 10

CARDIAC DISEASES

TRYGVE T. POPPE

Both farmed and wild fish can suffer from numerous infectious and noninfectious conditions that may compromise cardiac function and survival of the fish. In recent years, increasing focus has been put on the cardiac health of farmed fish. In farmed salmonids, and in particular Atlantic salmon (*Salmo salar*), three viral diseases affecting the heart represent a serious challenge for profitability and fish welfare. In addition, some bacterial and fungal diseases may occasionally cause severe cardiac disease in salmonids, and in cleaner fish used for delousing salmon in aquaculture farms. The significance of cardiac diseases in farmed salmonids is not restricted to acute mortality; chronic manifestations may result in poor growth and reduced capacity to handle stressful management operations like handling, transport and treatments.

CARDIOMYOPATHY SYNDROME

Overview: Cardiomyopathy syndrome (CMS) is a slowly developing serious cardiac disease culminating in acute death affecting large Atlantic salmon (*Salmo salar*) in good body condition and close to harvest size. The disease was first recorded in 1985 in Norway and later diagnosed in Scotland, Faroe Islands and Canada.[1,2]

Etiology: Cardiomyopathy syndrome is caused by piscine myocarditis virus (PMCV), a double-stranded RNA virus belonging to the family Totiviridae. Presence of the virus is associated with clinical disease, but the reservoir(s) and route of transmission of the virus has not been identified.

Clinical presentation: Depending on the extent of cardiac lesions, CMS may manifest itself with circulatory dysfunction with ascites, skin edema and lethargy. Even severely affected fish may continue to eat until they die. Cardiac dysfunction typically culminates in rupture of the atrium and/or sinus venosus resulting in cardiac tamponade and death.

Pathology: Gross external lesions may include ascites, ventral hemorrhage/petechiation and scale-pocket edema. Internally, hemopericardium is the most consistent finding along with ascitic fluid and a fibrinous cast on the liver surface (**Figure 10.1**). Histologically, multifocal to diffuse endocarditis and myocarditis with myolysis, comprising most of the spongy myocardium and atrium, are hallmarks of the disease (**Figure 10.2**). A cellular or fibrinous epicarditis is frequently present. In the liver, hypoxic necrosis resulting from circulatory collapse typically leave the hepatic parenchyma close to the central veins intact.

Differential diagnosis: Both pancreas disease (PD) and heart and skeletal muscle inflammation (HSMI) may occur concurrently and even in the same individuals. CMS can be differentiated from these by the absence of pancreatic and red muscle lesions.

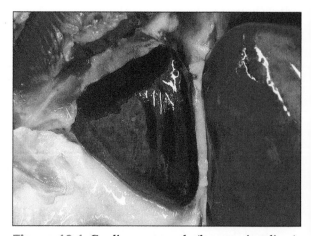

Figure 10.1 **Cardiac tamponade (hemopericardium) in farmed Atlantic salmon (*Salmo salar*) suffering from cardiomyopathy syndrome (CMS). The heart itself is completely hidden within the clot.**

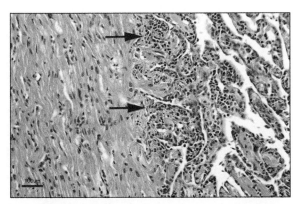

Figure 10.2 Inflammation of the ventricular myocardium (arrows) of farmed Atlantic salmon (*Salmo salar*) suffering from cardiomyopathy syndrome (CMS). Note the sharp demarcation between heavily affected spongy layer (right) and the unaffected compact layer. H&E stain.

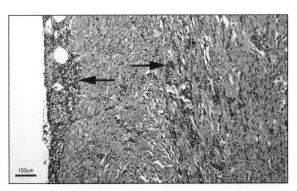

Figure 10.3 Myocardium of farmed Atlantic salmon (*Salmo salar*) suffering from heart and skeletal muscle inflammation (HSMI). Note inflammation (arrow) in both muscular layers and epicardium. H&E stain.

Diagnosis: Histopathology is the primary diagnostic tool supplemented by polymerase chain reaction (PCR) for piscine myocarditis virus in complex cases.

Management/control: No treatment or vaccine exists for CMS. Gentle handling and a minimum of operational disturbance will reduce stress and therefore reduce mortality in affected fish. Some farms have experienced good results by moving sea cages to locations with better environmental qualities.

HEART AND SKELETAL MUSCLE INFLAMMATION

Overview: Heart and skeletal muscle inflammation (HSMI) is a serious viral disease of Atlantic salmon (*Salmo salar*). The disease was first recorded in Norway in 1999 and is now widespread in Norwegian aquaculture.[3,4] The causative virus has also been found in several other salmon-farming countries. Experimentally, the disease has been transferred by injection of tissue homogenates and virus-containing erythrocytes from diseased fish. Transmission is both waterborne and with transportation of subclinically infected fish.

Etiology: HSMI is caused by a naked double-stranded RNA-virus called piscine orthoreovirus (PRV). The virus is widespread in farmed fish populations (Atlantic salmon, *Salmo salar*; and rainbow trout, *Oncorhynchus mykiss*), but also commonly occurs in wild salmonids.

Clinical presentation: Affected fish show nonspecific clinical behavior with increasing mortality.

Pathology: Gross external lesions are few and nonspecific. Internal lesions may include hemopericardium, orange-colored liver and petechiation of visceral organs. Microscopic lesions include diffuse inflammation of both layers of the myocardium and a highly cellular epicarditis (**Figure 10.3**).[5] Red skeletal muscle shows focal to multifocal degeneration and inflammation.

Differential diagnosis: Cardiomyopathy syndrome (CMS) and pancreas disease (PD) are both relevant differential diagnoses and both may occur simultaneously and in the same fish.

Diagnosis: Histopathology and PCR for the virus are the standard methods used in the diagnosis of HSMI.

Management/control: No treatment or vaccine is currently available for HSMI.

PANCREAS DISEASE

Overview: Pancreas disease is a serious viral disease of farmed Atlantic salmon (*Salmo salar*), rainbow trout (*Oncorhynchus mykiss*) and brown trout (*Salmo trutta*). The disease was first described in Scottish aquaculture in 1975, but a viral etiology was not confirmed until 1995.[4,6]

Etiology: Pancreas disease is caused by salmonid alphavirus (SAV), a single-stranded alphavirus in

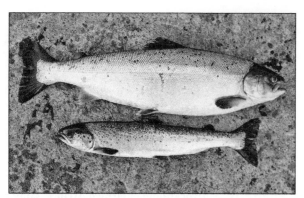

Figure 10.4 Emaciation in Atlantic salmon (*Salmo salar*) suffering from salmonid alphavirus (SAV) (lower fish) compared to unaffected sibling (upper fish).

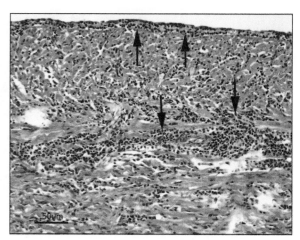

Figure 10.5 Compact myocardium of Atlantic salmon (*Salmo salar*) suffering from salmonid alphavirus. Note severe inflammation (arrows) of compact myocardium and epicardium. H&E stain.

the family Togaviridae. Six different subtypes of the virus have been identified, with SAV1 causing PD in Ireland and Scotland.

Route of transmission: Both live and dead infected salmon can shed SAV into the water, where the virus can survive for extended periods in the marine environment.

Clinical presentation: Acutely affected fish show nonspecific clinical signs with aberrant swimming behavior and increased mortality. Fish may congregate near the surface with heads oriented toward the current and close to the net. Rainbow trout (*Oncorhynchus mykiss*) may be found on the bottom of tanks in lateral recumbency (i.e., "sleeping disease"). Acute outbreaks are typically followed by lethargy and loss of appetite. After weeks and months off feed, classical "pin-head" fish develop (**Figure 10.4**).

Pathology: External pathological changes are nonspecific. Cachexia that develops after a few weeks is characteristic. Histopathological changes include myocarditis and loss of exocrine pancreatic tissue following acute necrosis, inflammation and hemorrhage (**Figure 10.5**). Myositis of red muscle and degeneration of white muscle may occur in cachectic fish.

Differential diagnosis: CMS and HSMI are differential diagnoses as well as any other condition leading to emaciation and cachexia.

Diagnosis: Histopathology and PCR for the virus are the standard methods used in the diagnosis of this disease.

Management/control: No treatment or vaccine exists for SAV. Management of the disease is by preventing horizontal spread to naïve fishes. On a national scale, prevention is through the establishment of epidemiological zones and strict regulation of traffic including well-boats and movement of other biological material.

BACTERIAL DISEASES

Overview: Few, if any bacterial diseases are specific to the heart, but a number of systemic infections may manifest themselves in different parts of the heart in addition to lesions in other organs. Transmission routes may be diverse depending on the agent, but most cases appear to be waterborne or through transportation of subclinically infected fish. Cardiac involvement of systemic bacteremias is not limited to any particular fish families.

Etiology: In salmonids, good examples of bacterial infections causing cardiac disease are *Aeromonas* spp., *Pseudomonas* spp., *Vibrio* spp., *Allivibrio salmonicida* and *Yersinia ruckeri*. In addition, *Aeromonas* spp., *Pseudomonas* spp., *Vibrio* spp. and *Mycobacterium* spp. can all cause cardiac disease in various freshwater and marine species of fish. In farmed Atlantic cod (*Gadus morhua*), *Francisella noatunensis* is a major pathogen causing granulomatous lesions in many organs, including the heart.

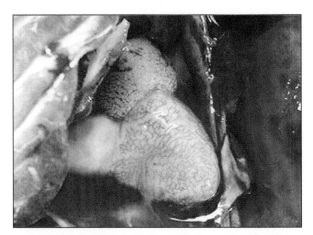

Figure 10.6 Bacterial epicarditis in Atlantic salmon (*Salmo salar*).

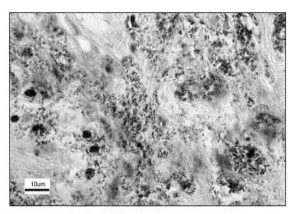

Figure 10.7 Numerous bacterial aggregates in the spongy/compact interface of the myocardium in Atlantic salmon (*Salmo salar*) suffering from cold-water vibriosis (Giemsa stain).

Clinical presentation: Gross lesions will depend on the species of bacteria, the fish species infected, the general presentation and organ distribution of the disease, but will often involve aberrant swimming, exophthalmia, ascites and hemorrhage at the base of the pectoral and pelvic fins, and increased mortality.

Pathology: At necropsy, ascitic fluid and petechiation of internal organs are common. Gross cardiac lesions may involve a pale fibrinous cast on the surface of the ventricle and fluid in the pericardium (**Figure 10.6**). Microscopic lesions may include diffuse infiltration with bacteria (e.g., *Vibrio* spp., *Allivibrio salmonicida*, *Yersinia ruckeri*) in the myocardium and in particular at the compactum/spongiosum interface (**Figure 10.7**). Dense, bacterial aggregates (i.e., "microcolonies") in the myocardium are characteristic for both typical and atypical strains of *Aeromonas salmonicida* subspecies *salmonicida* (**Figure 10.8**). An inflammatory response is typically absent or sparse in the previously mentioned infections. Bacterial epicarditis with fibrinous thickening and an inflammatory response may be seen in infections caused by *Aeromonas salmonicida* subspecies *salmonicida* and *Pseudomonas* spp. (**Figure 10.9**). Granulomatous inflammation and/or discrete granulomas may be seen with mycobacteriosis depending on the species of bacteria and species of fish infected.[1]

Diagnosis: Standard bacteriological methods and histopathology are the classical methods for the diagnosis of bacterial septicemias.

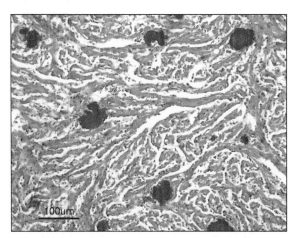

Figure 10.8 Microcolonies in the myocardium of lumpfish (*Cyclopterus lumpus*) suffering from atypical furunculosis. H&E stain.

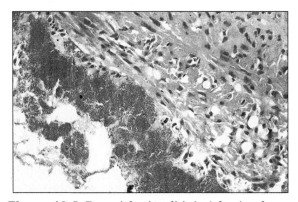

Figure 10.9 Bacterial epicarditis in Atlantic salmon (*Salmo salar*) suffering from atypical furunculosis. H&E stain.

Management/control: Routine health surveillance, vaccination programs if available and strict control of the movement of biological material are key elements to control of bacterial infections in fish. Medicated feed may be an option in ongoing outbreaks of certain bacterial diseases.

PARASITIC DISEASES

Overview: Larval trematodes and several protozoans may be associated with cardiac disease, particularly in wild fishes. With the exception of *Spironucleus salmonicida*, these parasites are generally not considered serious pathogens.

Etiology: Many trematodes, such as *Apatemon gracilis* and *Ichthyocotylurus* spp., have their larval stages in a variety of fish species, while the adult stages are generally found in the intestines of a number of fish-eating birds. *Spironucleus salmonicida* (Sarcomastigophora), a flagellate, may cause systemic infection in salmonids and serious involvement of the heart.[7,8] The reservoir is found in the intestines of wild salmonids. *Ichthyophonus hoferi* (Mesomycetozoa) is a commonly occurring protist pathogen in several marine fish species and has a preference for active muscle (e.g., cardiac muscle).

Clinical presentation: Encysted larval trematodes of the heart seldom result in any clinical presentation. Both *Spironucleus salmonicida* and *Ichthyophonus hoferi* may cause serious pathological changes that may compromise cardiac function and subsequently result in mortality. Both may present themselves in fish as signs of cardiac dysfunction like ascites, congestion and dilated atrium. Swimming stamina may be severely compromised in Pacific salmon (*Oncorhynchus* spp.) infected with *Ichthyophonus hoferi*.[9]

Pathology: Encysted trematode larvae are typically found on the ventricular surface and are seen as small, rounded structures, sometimes accompanied by fibrinous epicarditis that may restrict normal cardiac movement (**Figures 10.10** and **10.11**).[10] Microscopically, *Spironucleus salmonicida* will typically cause a significant purulent epicarditis in addition to pathological changes in many organ systems (**Figure 10.12**). *Ichthyophonus hoferi* can be found as multifocal, periodic acid-Schiff (PAS)–positive,

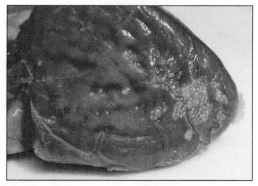

Figure 10.10 Encysted metacercariae of *Ichthyocotylurus* spp. on the ventricular wall of wild Atlantic salmon (*Salmo salar*).

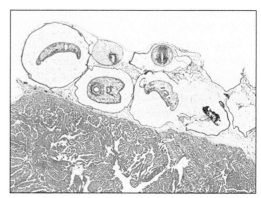

Figure 10.11 Encysted larval trematodes on the outside of the ventricular wall in a pumpkinseed (*Lepomis gibbosus*). H&E stain. (Image courtesy of S.A. Smith.)

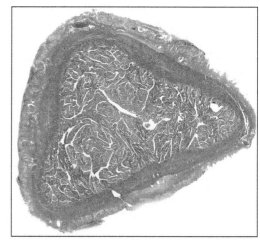

Figure 10.12 Fibro-purulent epicarditis of farmed Atlantic salmon (*Salmo salar*) infected with the flagellate *Spironucleus salmonicida*. H&E stain.

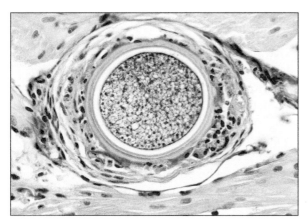

Figure 10.13 *Ichthyophonus hoferi* in the heart of an Atlantic salmon (*Salmo salar*). H&E stain.

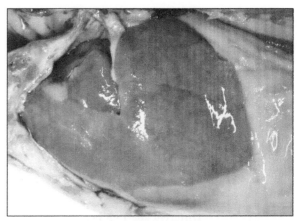

Figure 10.14 Aplasia of septum transversum in farmed Atlantic salmon (*Salmo salar*). Note impression of the heart in the hepatic parenchyma.

well-circumscribed double-walled structures in cardiac muscle and other organs as well (**Figure 10.13**).

Diagnosis: The diagnosis is based on characteristic gross and histopathological lesions. On the species level, PCR is a useful tool for differentiation.

Management/control: No treatments are currently approved for these parasites.

NONINFECTIOUS CARDIAC DISEASES AND ABNORMALITIES

Overview: Farmed salmonids may suffer from numerous noninfectious conditions that may compromise normal cardiac function. These include malformations, anatomical abnormalities, inflammation and metabolic abnormalities. Their etiology is complex and in some cases unknown.

Etiology: Developmental, environmental and genetic factors may contribute to this complex entity.[11,12] For example, elevated temperature (>9°C) during incubation of salmon eggs may result in aplasia or hypoplasia of septum transversum (**Figure 10.14**). As a result, the heart will be found in the abdominal cavity, typically under or in front of the liver. The normal triangular shape of the ventricle will be altered resembling a flattened bean, sac or cylinder resulting in compromised function and reduced swimming stamina. This condition leads to atrial natriuretic peptide (ANP) expression during the development of the embryonic heart.[13] The size and shape of the heart may also be altered following severe chronic gill inflammation with the amoeba *Paramoeba perurans*.[14]

Situs inversus or situs ambiguous is a condition where the position of the heart is altered within an otherwise normal pericardial cavity. The alignment of bulbus arteriosus and proximal part of the ventral aorta will be altered and the shape of the ventricle will deviate from the normal triangular shape. The etiology is not known.

Epicarditis (visceral pericarditis) and fat infiltration of the epicardium are very common findings in farmed salmonids and other fishes. The conditions may be idiopathic or associated with infectious cardiac diseases like HSMI.

Clinical presentation: These conditions may never manifest themselves clinically in farmed fish unless the fish is stressed and challenged, e.g., during crowding, transportation, treatments and suboptimal environmental conditions. Affected fish typically will be the first to succumb and turn belly-up. Chronic gill inflammation and/or frayed fins/fin rot will further aggravate the problems in these fish.

Pathology: Gross pathological changes are typically restricted to the ventricle where shape and location are key factors. Affected fish will have ventricles that deviate in shape and size from the normal triangular shape (**Figure 10.15**).[15] Fish with extensive epicarditis and or/fat infiltration may present with a pale appearance of the ventricle. Histopathologically, the epicardium will be thickened and often extensively vascularized. The epicarditis may be highly cellular with extensive

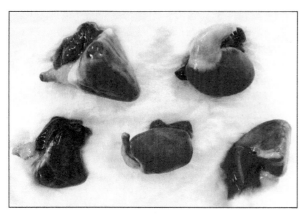

Figure 10.15 Different aberrant heart shapes in farmed Atlantic salmon (*Salmo salar*). The heart in the upper left has a normal shape.

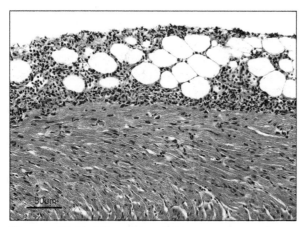

Figure 10.16 Idiopathic cellular epicarditis and fat infiltration in farmed Atlantic salmon (*Salmo salar*). H&E stain.

invasion of mononuclear inflammatory cells, or chronic with layered fibrinous coats, particularly on the caudal side of the ventricle (**Figure 10.16**).

Differential diagnosis: There are no relevant differential diagnoses.

Diagnosis: Aberrant shape and location is diagnosed based on gross findings that require knowledge of the normal shape and location of the heart. Epicarditis and fat infiltration are diagnosed based on standard histological methods.

Management/control: No treatment is available. Stressful operational practices will challenge fish with subclinical abnormalities, including such factors as handling, bath treatments and transportation.

ARTERIOSCLEROSIS

Overview: This condition is one of the first pathological conditions of the salmonid heart described. The condition commonly occurs in both wild and farmed salmonids and has been characterized as "a fact of life," as most fish over a certain size and age develop some degree of lesions. Lesions protruding into the vascular lumen are typical for this condition.[16]

Etiology: The pulsation of the highly compliable bulbus arteriosus is believed to be the direct cause of lesions inside the coronary artery. The stress on the bulbus arteriosus has been reported to increase with fast growth. Sexual maturation may also affect the development of lesions.

Clinical presentation: No lesions are grossly visible.

Pathology: Histologically, characteristic lesions develop inside the wall of the coronary artery, in particular where it runs on the ventral side of bulbus arteriosus. Lesions are characterized by multifocal myointimal hyperplasia arranged in "pads" (**Figure 10.17**). These will, to a variable degree, obstruct the lumen of the vessel and thereby the blood flow to the outer compact myocardium. If full occlusion of the vessel occurs, this may result in degenerative changes/necrosis of the outer compact myocardium followed by dystrophic calcification of the affected tissue (**Figure 10.18**).

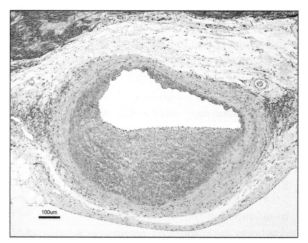

Figure 10.17 Arteriosclerosis of the coronary artery of Atlantic salmon (*Salmo salar*). The ventral part of the vessel lumen is obliterated by the myointimal hyperplasia. H&E stain.

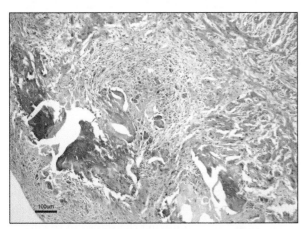

Figure 10.18 Dystrophic calcification of the outer compact myocardium following occlusion of the coronary artery in Atlantic salmon (*Salmo salar*) with arteriosclerosis. H&E stain.

Diagnosis: The diagnosis is based on characteristic histopathological lesions.

Management/control: No control measures are relevant.

REFERENCES

1. Poppe, T.T. and Ferguson, H.W. Cardiovascular system. In: *Systemic Pathology of Fish*, 2nd ed. H.W. Ferguson, ed. Scotian Press, London, 2006; pp. 141–167.
2. Fritsvold, C., Kongtorp, R.T., Taksdal, T., Ørpetveit, I., Heum, M. and Poppe, T.T. Experimental transmission of cardiomyopathy syndrome (CMS) in Atlantic salmon *Salmo salar*. *Diseases of Aquatic Organisms* 2009;87:225–234.
3. Kongtorp, R.T., Kjerstad, A., Taksdal, T., Guttvik, A. and Falk, K. Heart and skeletal muscle inflammation in Atlantic salmon *Salmo salar* L.: A new infectious disease. *Journal of Fish Diseases* 2004;27:351–358.
4. Bruno, D.W., Noguera, P.A. and Poppe, T.T. Bacterial diseases. In: *A Colour Atlas of Salmonid Diseases*, 2nd ed. Springer, London, 2013; pp. 73–96.
5. Yousaf, M.N., Koppang, E.O., Skjødt, K., Hordvik, I., Zou, J., Secombes, C. and Powell, M.D. Cardiac pathological changes of Atlantic salmon (*Salmo salar* L.) affected with heart and skeletal muscle inflammation

(HSMI), cardiomyopathy syndrome (CMS) and pancreas disease (PD). *Veterinary Immunology and Immunopathology* 2012;151:49–62.
6. Graham, D.A., Fringuelli, E., Rowley, H.M., Cockerill, D., Cox, D.I., Turnbull, T., Rodger, D., Morris, D. and McLoughlin, M.F. Geographical distribution of salmonid alphavirus subtypes in marine farmed Atlantic salmon *Salmo salar* L. in Scotland and Ireland. *Journal of Fish Diseases* 2012;35:755–765.
7. Poppe, T.T., Mo, T.A. and Iversen, L. Disseminated hexamitosis in sea-caged Atlantic salmon, *Salmo salar*. *Diseases of Aquatic Organisms* 1992;14:91–97.
8. Sterud, E., Mo, T.A. and Poppe, T.T. Systemic spironucleosis in sea-farmed Atlantic salmon *Salmo salar* L, caused by Spironucleus barkhanus transmitted from feral Arctic char *Salvelinus alpinus*? *Diseases of Aquatic Organisms* 1988;33:63–66.
9. Kocan, R.P., Hershberger, P. and Winton, J. Ichthyophoniasis: An emerging disease of Chinook salmon in the Yukon river. *Journal of Aquatic Animal Health* 2004;16:58–72.
10. Watson, J.J., Pike, A.W. and Priede, I.G. Cardiac pathology associated with the infection of *Oncorhynchus mykiss* Walbaum with *Apatemon gracilis* Rud. 1819. *Journal of Fish Biology* 1992;41:163–167.
11. Graham, M.S. and Farrell, A.P. Environmental influences on cardiovascular variables in rainbow trout *Oncorhynchus mykiss* (Walbaum). *Journal of Fish Biology* 1992;41:851–858.
12. Gamperl, A.K. and Farrell, A.P. Cardiac plasticity in fishes: Environmental influences and intraspecific differences. *Journal of Experimental Biology* 2004;207:2539–2550.
13. Takle, H., Bæverfjord, G., Helland, S., Kjørsvik, E. and Andersen, Ø. Hyperthermia induced natriuretic peptide expression and deviant heart development in Atlantic salmon *Salmo salar* embryos. *General and Comparative Endocrinology* 2006;147:118–125.
14. Powell, M.D., Nowak, B.F. and Adams, M.B. Cardiac morphology in relation to amoebic gill disease history in Atlantic salmon, *Salmo salar* L. *Journal of Fish Diseases* 2002;25:209–215.
15. Poppe, T.T., Johansen, R., Gunnes, G. and Tørud, B. Heart morphology in wild and farmed Atlantic salmon *Salmo salar* and rainbow trout *Oncorhynchus mykiss*. *Diseases of Aquatic Organisms* 2003;57:103–108.
16. Farrell, A.P. Coronary arteriosclerosis in salmon: Growing old or growing fast? *Comparative Biochemistry and Physiology—Part A* 2002;132:723–735.

CHAPTER 11

HEPATIC, BILIARY, AND PANCREATIC DISEASES

JEFFREY C. WOLF

EPIZOOTIC HEMATOPOIETIC NECROSIS

Overview: Epizootic hematopoietic necrosis (EHN) is an iridoviral disease (*Ranaviridae*) that causes systemic infections in fish such as redfin perch (*Perca fluviatilis*), rainbow trout (*Oncorhynchus mykiss*), catfish (*Ictalurus melas*) and sheatfish (*Silurus glanis*).[1-4] Additional fish species have demonstrated susceptibility to experimental infection.

Etiology: The virus responsible for EHN in redfin perch and rainbow trout is epizootic hematopoietic necrosis virus, and related viruses that cause similar disease are European catfish virus (ECV) and European sheatfish virus (ESV). EHN is endemic in Australia, whereas ECV and ESV are currently restricted to Europe. Direct transmission via water or fomites is likely.

Clinical presentation: The disease typically presents as sudden high mortality in redfin perch, whereas in rainbow trout it is characterized by more gradual losses. EHN and related viruses typically cause focal necrosis and hemorrhage in a wide variety of tissues, and depending on the fish species, the liver may or may not be the predominantly affected organ.[5]

Pathology: Macroscopic changes in the liver usually consist of variably sized areas of pale discoloration that correspond microscopically with localized to extensive hepatocellular necrosis. Intact hepatocytes proximate to necrotic foci may contain ovoid basophilic cytoplasmic inclusions.

Differential diagnosis: Diseases with similar presentations include infectious hematopoietic necrosis and viral hemorrhagic septicemia.

Diagnosis: Isolation in cell culture with ELISA or polymerase chain reaction (PCR) confirmation from samples collected of liver, kidney, heart, and/or spleen.[6,7]

Management/control: There is currently no vaccination or treatment available for EHN. Prevention measures such as disinfection, quarantine, and culling are key to minimizing the spread of the disease, and improving husbandry conditions may limit fish losses in endemic populations, especially in trout. This is currently an Office Internationale des Epizooties (OIE) reportable disease.

HEPATIC LIPIDOSIS

Overview: Hepatic lipidosis (steatosis) is characterized by excessive fat accumulation within the cytoplasm of hepatocytes.[8,9] For this diagnosis to have meaning in the context of fish health, lipidosis should be considered a degenerative condition that is, by definition, deleterious to the host. Although prospective studies in fish are limited, it may be the case that, as in mammals, excess hepatic lipid storage may result in oxidative stress that damages subcellular membranous structures. Occasional misuse of the term *lipidosis* throughout the fish literature has resulted from a failure to define what constitutes "excessive." The amount of hepatocellular fat in a given fish, as visualized by light or electron microscopy with or without special lipid stains, is dependent on myriad factors that include species, age, physical exercise, gender and reproductive state, various stressors, and the type and availability of feed. The injudicious use of lipidosis as a fallback diagnosis for otherwise unexplained morbidity is problematic for two main reasons: (1) for clinically ill fish, ascribing their disease incorrectly to hepatic lipidosis may cause the true etiology to remain undetected; (2) in toxicological investigations, test substances may be inaccurately characterized as inducing liver disease.

Etiology: Causes of lipidosis include malnutrition (excessive caloric intake and/or inappropriate nutrient composition) and possibly toxicosis.[10] The latter is especially difficult to establish because many diagnoses of hepatic lipidosis in published reports are of questionable accuracy.

Clinical presentation: Lipidosis typically presents as the sudden death of an individual fish, or low-level mortalities in a fish population. Affected fish may exhibit normal, excessive or depleted body condition. Macroscopically, fatty livers are comparatively large, pale tan or yellow, and friable (**Figure 11.1**).

Pathology: In histologic sections, lipidotic livers are usually affected diffusely, and fat-laden hepatocytes are characterized by single large (macrovesicular) or multiple small (microvesicular), round, clear cytoplasmic vacuoles, and eccentric nuclei (**Figures 11.2** and **11.3**).

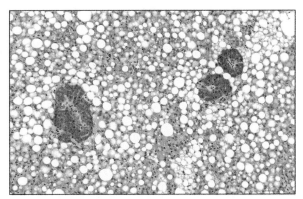

Figure 11.3 Hybrid striped bass (*M. saxatilis* × *M. chrysops*) liver with abundant lipid vacuolation. Extensive hepatic lipid storage may be observed in many captive fish fed high energy diets. In this case, lipid droplets are beginning to coalesce, which can be an early indication of the degenerative condition termed lipidosis. H&E stain.

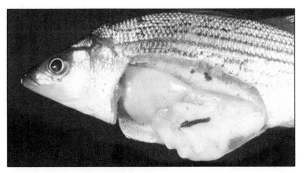

Figure 11.1 Hepatic lipidosis as demonstrated by the cream-colored lipid-laden liver in a cultured hybrid striped bass (*Morone saxatilis* × *M. chrysops*). (Image courtesy of S.A. Smith.)

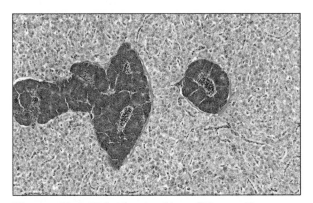

Figure 11.2 Hybrid striped bass (*M. saxatilis* × *M. chrysops*) liver with minimal energy storage typical of many wild-caught fish. Note the existence of the intra-hepatic pancreas in this species. H&E stain.

Differential diagnosis: Because of ready access to high caloric foods that require minimal foraging activity, captive reared or maintained fish typically have greater amounts of stored hepatic lipid than their wild fish counterparts. However, even certain wild fishes, such as elasmobranchs and sturgeon, normally have abundant fat stores. Consequently, the observation of a lipid-laden liver should not automatically confer a diagnosis of hepatic lipidosis. That terminology is more appropriately reserved for cases in which there is visible histologic evidence of cellular deterioration, such as coalescence of lipid vacuoles in neighboring hepatocytes, fat necrosis, and/or fat calcification (saponification). Fat calcification typically manifests as pale basophilic concretions in hematoxylin and eosin-stained sections.

Diagnosis: Lipidotic livers may float when placed in a fixative solution; however, the diagnosis is more commonly established via histopathological examination of the liver. Special histologic stains applied to frozen sections, such as Sudan stains or Oil Red O, may be used to confirm the fat content of cytoplasmic vacuoles.

Management/control: This disease may be managed by providing limited quantities of natural and commercially prepared foods of a variety and composition that is nutritionally appropriate for the species, age, and physical activity of a particular captive fish population.

INFECTIOUS PANCREATIC NECROSIS

Overview: Infectious pancreatic necrosis (IPN) is an economically important, contagious acute viral disease of young salmonids that can be associated with high levels of mortality.[11]

Etiology: Infectious pancreatic necrosis is caused by an aquabirnavirus. Since the time of its original discovery, a diverse array of serologically related aquabirnaviruses (IPNV and IPNV-like aquatic birnaviruses) with different host specificity have been isolated from a wide variety of both diseased and non-diseased salmonid and non-salmonid fish. Fish that survive the initial infection can become subclinically infected adult carriers that are capable of transmitting the disease both vertically in the eggs and horizontally via virus-infected feces. The disease may also be transmitted via infected water, blood-feeding parasites, and piscivorous birds.

Clinical presentation: The characteristic presentation is a sudden explosive outbreak with variable to high mortality. Signs and macroscopic lesions in salmonid fry may include darkened skin, rotational motion while swimming (i.e., "rolling"), exophthalmia, abdominal swelling, petechial hemorrhage, pale gills and viscera (anemia), and white or mucoid fecal casts.[12,13] External lesions in post-smolt salmonids may be less apparent. The stomach and anterior intestines may contain gelatinous material, and there may be intestinal hemorrhage.

Pathology: Microscopically, predominant features include necrosis of pancreatic acinar tissue, intestinal enterocytes, renal hematopoietic tissue, and, on occasion, the liver (**Figure 11.4**). The pattern of necrosis in the pancreas and elsewhere tends to be focal and of the individual cell type. Unlike pancreas disease, the necrotic cells are associated with an inflammatory response. Focal brain vacuolation has also been observed.

Differential diagnosis: Rule-outs generally include diseases caused by other viral agents, such as infectious hematopoietic necrosis, infectious salmon anemia, viral hemorrhagic septicemia, and pancreas disease.

Diagnosis: In addition to histopathology and immunohistochemistry, a broad variety of immune-based and molecular diagnostic methods are available for the diagnosis of IPNV.[13,14]

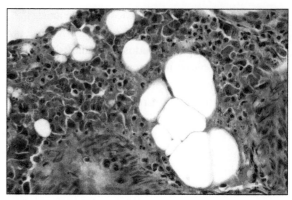

Figure 11.4 Acinar cell (exocrine pancreas) necrosis in a rainbow trout (*Oncorhynchus mykiss*) infected with infectious pancreatic necrosis (IPN) birnavirus. H&E stain.

Management/control: Management tools for IPN generally include pathogen avoidance, basic biosecurity measures designed to prevent the transport of infected biological materials, the use of disinfectant chemicals, and the application of commercially available vaccines. Vaccination, which is primarily focused on protecting the post-smolt stage of marine-cultured salmonids, has met with variable success.

MYCOBACTERIOSIS AND NOCARDIOSIS

Overview: *Mycobacterium* spp. and *Nocardia* spp. are genera of Gram-positive, acid-fast positive (partially for *Nocardia* spp.), rod-shaped actinobacteria that cause localized or systemic infections in fish. Review of the literature suggests that mycobacteriosis is more common in fish than nocardiosis. Systemically infected fish can have hepatic and/or pancreatic involvement, although organs such as the kidney and spleen tend to be more common internal targets.

Etiology: The causative agents of mycobacteriosis and nocardiosis encompass a variety of species, but those most commonly isolated from fish include *M. marinum*, *M. chelonei*, *M. fortuitum*, *M. abscessus*, *M. peregrinum*, *N. seriolae* (formerly known as *N. kampachi*), *N. asteroides*, *N. salmonicida* and *N. crassostreae*. Transmission of these agents, some of which are ubiquitous, is thought to occur via infected water, sediment, biofilms, and via the cannibalism of contaminated carcasses.

Clinical presentation: Virtually all wild and captive fishes can become infected, although certain species appear to be more susceptible than others, e.g., striped bass (*Morone saxatilis*) as compared to tilapia (*Oreochromis* spp.).[15] The incidence of infection can be high and thus have economic impact in wild caught or farmed marine fish such as mycobacteriosis in Chesapeake Bay striped bass (*Morone saxatilis*) and nocardiosis in Japanese yellowtail (*Seriolae quinqueridiata*).[16,17] There also tends to be a high incidence of mycobacterial infection in ornamental fish kept in public or private aquaria. The disease generally has a long latent period and frequently manifests as chronic low-level mortalities in affected populations. Fish may present thin, with or without dermal ulcers. Internal examination often reveals splenomegaly and renomegaly, with multiple small irregular foci of pale discoloration that may be slightly raised (**Figure 11.5**).

Pathology: Microscopically, both of these diseases present as multiple, variably sized granulomas in various tissues, often with necrotic centers. Few to numerous bacteria may be present freely or within granulomas, and such bacilli may be difficult or impossible to visualize without special acid-fast staining. In certain fish species, such as Japanese medaka (*Oryzias latipes*) and summer flounder (*Paralichthys dentatus*), mycobacterial infections tend to manifest as diffuse granulomatous inflammation without necrosis.[18,19] Ultimately, the microscopic appearance of the disease may be subject to a variety of factors such as the species, age, and general health of the infected fish; the species, strain, and virulence of the bacteria; the ambient water temperature; the magnitude of the initial exposure; and the chronicity of the infection. Granulomatous inflammation induced by mycobacteria and other agents should be distinguished from pigmented macrophage aggregates (e.g., melanomacrophage centers), which are constitutive noninflammatory foci that may be present in the liver and mesenteric pancreas of some fish.

Differential diagnosis: Other bacterial, fungal, and parasitic infections can cause granulomatous inflammation in the liver that strongly resembles lesions caused by mycobacteriosis or nocardiosis, e.g., *Francisella noatunensis* infections in tilapia (*Oreochromis* spp.) and other fishes.

Diagnosis: A variety of techniques are used to diagnose these diseases, the most common of which include acid-fast stained impression smears of infected tissues, bacterial culture, histopathology and PCR. Successful culture of these organisms typically requires special agar and can be challenging due to non-target bacterial overgrowth that can occur during the extended culture period.

Management/control: These agents tend to be persistent and recurring in aquaculture settings, especially in closed systems, as the organisms can be difficult to eradicate from biofilms. Management tools may include all-in–all-out culture practices, bleach and alcohol disinfection of entire systems, limited introduction of fish from outside sources, frequent health screening, selective culling of suspect and infected fish, immediate removal of carcasses, ultraviolet (UV)-sterilization of circulated water, and other general biosecurity measures. Although the disease can be responsive to pharmaceutical intervention (e.g., valuable non-food fish), this is generally not attempted as both mycobacteriosis and nocardiosis are potential zoonotic diseases. Thus care must be taken when handling suspect fish to prevent contamination of skin breaks and other routes of entry.

MICROCYSTINS AND NET PEN LIVER DISEASE

Overview: Microcystins are cyclic heptapeptide hepatotoxic molecules that are produced by

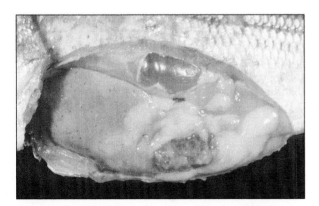

Figure 11.5 Patchy, pale yellow liver in a hybrid striped bass (*Morone saxatilis* × *M. chrysops*) with systemic mycobacteriosis. Note the pale, mottled nodular spleen characteristic of this disease. (Image courtesy of S.A. Smith.)

various cyanobacteria. Although commonly called blue-green algae, cyanobacteria are actually photosynthetic prokaryotes rather than plants. These organisms tend to proliferate episodically in freshwater or marine habitats that have high levels of nutrients. "Net pen liver disease" was a term used to describe outbreaks of microcystin-induced hepatotoxicosis in net pen–raised Atlantic salmon (*Salmo salar*) and other salmonids off the northwest and northeast coasts of the United States in the late 1980s.

Etiology: Wild fish may be exposed to microcystins via gill absorption and also through dietary intake, as these toxins can bioaccumulate in the flesh of forage animals and thus may be transferred up the food chain. The most commonly produced and potent hepatotoxin of the microcystin family is microcystin-LR, which contains L-Leu and L-Arg. Key mechanisms of microcystin-induced liver toxicity are thought to include inhibition of protein phosphatases 1 and 2A, and lipid peroxidation caused by oxidative stress.[20,21]

Clinical presentation: Experimentally, fish administered microcystin-LR exhibit nonspecific signs such as lethargy, frenetic swimming, color changes, buoyancy control issues and death.[22] The magnitude of morbidity and mortality appear to be dependent on the fish species and exposure level. At necropsy, exposed fish typically have soft, pale, tan livers with red blotches (i.e., ecchymotic hemorrhage).

Pathology: The extent and character of microscopic liver lesions are dependent on the level of exposure and duration of disease post-exposure. The acute stages are characterized by severe diffuse liquefactive and/or apoptotic hepatocellular necrosis, hepatocyte dissociation, and hemorrhage (**Figure 11.6**). By contrast, histopathologic features during the subacute to chronic phases are consistent with liver regeneration and include patchy areas of megalocytosis (polyploid hepatocytes with abundant cytoplasm, enlarged irregularly shaped nuclei, and prominent nucleoli), marked hepatocyte anisokaryosis, streaming bile ductular and precursor cells, histiocytic cells, and variable amounts of cellular debris. Remarkably fish that survive the acute insult may virtually regenerate their livers within days to weeks following the exposure.

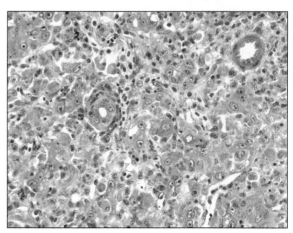

Figure 11.6 **Liver of Atlantic salmon (*Salmo salar*) with hepatic megalocytosis, characteristic of the early repair phase of salmonid "net pen liver disease," which has been attributed to algal microcystin toxicity. H&E stain.**

Differential diagnosis: Rule-outs for microcystin toxicity include other potent hepatotoxicants.

Diagnosis: Diagnostic evidence for this disease can include a history of exposure to cyanobacterial blooms, identification of the characteristic histopathologic changes, and measurements of microcystins in fish tissues by chromatography or mass spectrometry.

Management/control: Reduction of nutrient levels in freshwater and marine environments should lead to less frequent cyanobacterial blooms.

NEOPLASIA

Overview: The fish liver is a comparatively common location for both primary and secondary (metastatic) neoplasia. Primary neoplasia refers to benign and malignant versions of tumors originating from hepatocytes, bile duct epithelial cells, or pancreatic exocrine or endocrine tissues. These chiefly include benign hepatocellular or cholangiocellular adenomas, and malignant hepatocellular or cholangiocellular carcinomas (**Figures 11.7** and **11.8**). Mixed hepatobiliary tumors are also possible. Exocrine pancreatic tumors in fish tend to be of the malignant variety (adenocarcinomas), and benign or malignant islet cell tumors appear to be quite rare. Secondary neoplasms that have metastasized from distant

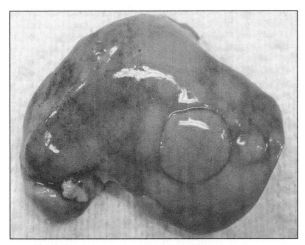

Figure 11.7 Hepatocellular adenoma in a common dab (*Limanda limanda*). Other patchy nodular areas may represent additional hepatocellular tumors, or foci of cellular alteration.

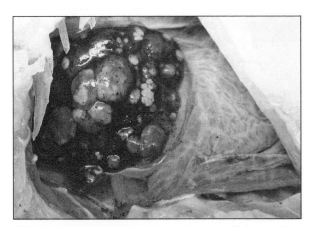

Figure 11.8 Multiple primary hepatocellular and/or biliary tumors throughout the liver of a kissing gourami (*Helostoma temminckii*). (Image courtesy of J. Shelley.)

locations are infrequently observed. Unlike their mammalian counterparts, malignant fish tumors have less of a tendency to spread systemically; however, when such tumors do travel they tend to locate in the liver.

Etiology: Fish liver neoplasms may arise spontaneously (i.e., with no apparent cause) or they may be produced by exposure to a variety of tumor-inducing agents such as aflatoxins. The ability of various direct- or indirect-acting chemical carcinogens to induce primary liver, biliary and pancreatic tumors

in fish is well-documented. Certain fish species may be predisposed to the formation of these neoplasms as a result of genetic factors, preferential exposure to environmental carcinogens (e.g., as a function of specific dietary or habitat requirements), or a combination of both. Certain viruses and parasites have been implicated as potential causes of neoplastic transformation, e.g., a hepadnavirus associated with liver tumors in white suckers (*Catostomus commersonii*), and *Pseudocapillaria tomentosa* associated with biliary tumors in zebrafish, although definitive causality is often difficult to establish.[23] Tumors may also be produced by intentional manipulation of oncogenes or tumor suppressor genes in experimental models, such as zebrafish engineered to overexpress *myc* oncogenes.[24]

Clinical presentation: Fish with liver, biliary, or pancreatic tumors may be emaciated, or such neoplasms may be encountered as incidental findings during health screenings or discovered while investigating other concurrent diseases. Macroscopically, such tumors typically present as single or multiple, spherical or irregular, domed or flattened masses that are often raised and discolored when compared to the surrounding tissue. Malignant tumors are more commonly accompanied by adhesions to surrounding abdominal mesenteric and visceral tissues.

Pathology: Microscopically, adenomas typically present as single, well-circumscribed, expansile masses in which the cells bear at least moderate resemblance to normal hepatocytes or bile ducts. In contrast, primary carcinomas are generally characterized by increased cellular pleomorphism and atypical cytologic features, in addition to invasive tendencies. Metastatic tumors may bear some resemblance to the distant tissue of origin, or they may be difficult to categorize.

Differential diagnosis: Macroscopically, larger parasitic cysts or nodular inflammatory foci may be mistaken for tumors. Histopathologically, primary liver neoplasms must be distinguished from foci of hepatocellular alteration, which are localized, nonneoplastic proliferations of hepatocytes that differ from the surrounding liver in terms of cytoplasmic coloration and cell size. Unlike adenomas, such altered foci do not compress adjacent liver parenchyma, nor do the cells have atypical cytologic features and growth patterns characteristic of hepatocellular carcinomas. Categories of altered foci in fish have been known to include eosinophilic, basophilic, and clear cell varieties, and it is thought that at least some of these may represent preneoplastic lesions.[13] Occasionally, primary liver tumors may have to be distinguished from regenerative hyperplasia, which can similarly have a nodular appearance, cytologic atypia, and frequent mitotic figures. Regenerative hyperplasia can be a chronic consequence of exposure to cytotoxic chemicals such as ketoconazole.

Diagnosis: Diagnosis is typically based on macroscopic and/or microscopic detection of tumors, followed by histopathologic confirmation of the tumor type. Ultrastructural and/or immunohistochemical investigations may be used to support the diagnosis.

Management/control: Tumors from public aquarium or pet specimens may be excised surgically, and because of the low metastatic potential, removal of even malignant tumors may be effectively curative. Cleanup of chemical contamination in waterways has proven effective at decreasing the occurrence of hepatic, biliary, and/or pancreatic tumors in some fish species, and the incidence of such tumors in repeated survey studies has been used to monitor the success of remediation efforts in some localities.

PANCREAS DISEASE/SLEEPING DISEASE

Overview: Pancreas disease (PD) and sleeping disease (SD) are economically important viral diseases that primarily affect farmed Atlantic salmon and rainbow trout, respectively, in Europe and North America.[25–27]

Etiology: The agent of both PD and SD is salmonid alphavirus (SAV), a member of the Togaviridae family, but the two closely related isolates responsible for these diseases are often referred to separately as pancreas disease virus (PDV) and sleeping disease virus (SDV). Transmission of the virus is thought to occur horizontally through infected water in which the virus can survive for extended periods, and via the transport of infected fish or equipment. Vertical egg transmission is considered unlikely.

Clinical presentation: Clinical signs associated with experimental alphavirus infections are mostly nonspecific and include lethargy and inappetence, bilateral exophthalmia, abdominal swelling, and a tendency to lie sideways on the bottom of the tank (hence the "sleeping sickness" moniker for affected trout).

Pathology: Microscopic lesions are consistently represented by necrosis of the exocrine pancreas, heart, and both red and white skeletal muscle, with occasional kidney involvement represented by increased eosinophilic granular cells. The pancreatic lesions often precede those in the heart and skeletal muscle.[28] In the pancreas, individual cell necrosis of acinar cells predominates, which depletes the acinar cells while sparing the endocrine tissue (**Figure 11.9**). Although the pancreatic necrosis is typically unaccompanied by inflammation (unlike IPN), increased mononuclear cell infiltrates are common sequelae of necrosis in the heart and skeletal muscle. Additionally, while the cardiac and skeletal muscle lesions may resolve in surviving fish, there is usually minimal if any regeneration of the pancreatic tissue.

Differential diagnosis: Other diseases and conditions that may resemble pancreas disease, at least in part, include IPN, cardiomyopathy syndrome (CMS; which has a possible togavirus etiology), and a condition known as heart and skeletal muscle inflammation (HSMI) that has been loosely associated with piscine orthoreovirus infection.

Diagnosis: In addition to recognition of the characteristic histopathologic lesions, serologic and molecular assays are available.

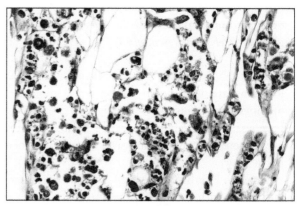

Figure 11.9 Widespread necrosis of the exocrine pancreas in an Atlantic salmon (*Salmo salar*) experimentally infected with salmonid alphavirus, i.e., "pancreas disease."

Management/control: Management is aimed primarily at controlling horizontal spread of the disease by limiting transport of live fish and equipment; disinfection of equipment and tissues from slaughtered fish; and vaccination, which has been demonstrated to decrease cumulative mortality.[29]

PARASITES

Overview: The livers of wild and ornamental aquarium fish are common locations for a wide variety of metazoan and protozoan parasites.[30,31] In contrast, parasites are less commonly encountered in the livers of laboratory fish used for research when those test subjects are obtained from legitimate laboratory animal vendors.

Etiology: Typical parasites observed in the hepatic parenchyma include larval digenetic trematodes, larval cestodes, and migrating nematodes. Such organisms may be observed macroscopically as small focal nodules that may or may not be surrounded by host-derived pigment ("black grubs" or "white grubs," respectively), or as single or multiple cyst-like structures (e.g., digenetic trematodes) (**Figure 11.10**). Microscopically, it is not unusual to find the plasmodial stages of myxozoan protozoans within bile duct lumina in some fish species; these sporozoan stages can be mistaken for metazoan parasites due to their elongated, and sometimes coiled, vermiform appearance. Microsporidia, which were once thought to be protozoan but are actually more appropriately classified as fungi, are observed infrequently. A similar array of organisms can be found in the abdominal mesentery adjacent to or directly affecting pancreatic tissue.

Clinical presentation: Fish with hepatic, biliary, or pancreatic parasites may be thin or, in many cases, overtly unaffected. The host inflammatory response to such parasites tends to be modest, especially for digenetic trematodes, and often these infections appear well-tolerated, even in individuals with heavy parasite burdens, if the fish are otherwise healthy.

Pathology: Inflammatory reactions that do occur are generally of the granulomatous type, either presenting as discrete spherical granulomas in which the outer layers consist of flattened macrophages, or as more diffuse, irregular granulomatous foci. Hepatic pigmented macrophage aggregates (melanomacrophage centers) may be relatively more numerous, larger, and more heavily pigmented in parasite-laden fish. In zebrafish (*Danio rerio*) there is anecdotal evidence to suggest that the capillarid parasite *Pseudocapillaria tomentosa* may be associated with the formation of malignant bile duct neoplasia in addition to intestinal adenocarcinomas.

Differential diagnosis: Parasitic cysts that form large nodules may be mistaken for neoplasms based on macroscopic inspection alone. Patterns of granulomatous inflammation resembling parasite reactions may be observed in some hyphal fungal infections, for example.

Diagnosis: Most hepatic parasites can be diagnosed by finding the organisms via macroscopic examination, liver squash preparations, and/or histopathological evaluation. Definitive identification of certain parasites in histologic sections can be challenging because only a portion of the parasite may be evident in a given section; in the case of migrating parasites such as nematodes, the sole evidence of parasite involvement may be linear tracts surrounded by inflammation. In other instances, distinctive morphologic characteristics of a parasite may be obscured or eliminated by the host inflammatory response. In histologic sections, myxozoan parasites are often best visualized using a Giemsa stain, and a superior technique for detecting and visualizing tiny microsporidian organisms is the Luna stain.

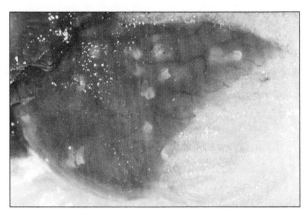

Figure 11.10 **Liver of bluegill (*Lepomis macrochirus*) containing multiple encysted trematode metacercariae. (Image courtesy of S.A. Smith.)**

Management/control: A number of chemical anthelmintic agents of veterinary origin have been used to treat fish parasites, although none are approved for use in food fish, and their efficacy for encysted liver, biliary, and pancreatic parasites may be questionable. More efficacious management can be achieved through disease prevention, which is usually achieved by minimizing exposure to parasites. Biosecurity measures for captive fish populations include isolation from stocks of parasite-infected fish, rigorous decontamination of clothing and equipment that might promote parasite transmission, and the control of intermediate hosts such as snails, copepods, and in the case of myxozoan sporozoans, oligochaete worms.

PASTEURELLOSIS (*PHOTOBACTERIA DAMSELAE* SSP. *PISCICIDA*)

Overview: Pasteurellosis (pseudotuberculosis) is a systemic bacterial disease that manifests as hemorrhagic septicemia and causes massive mortalities in various species of commercially important marine fishes, and is especially problematic for fisheries in European Mediterranean countries and Japan.

Etiology: Previously known as *Pasteurella piscicida*, the agent of pasteurellosis, which is now called *Photobacteria damselae* ssp. *piscicida*, is a nonmotile, Gram-negative coccobacillus. Another subspecies, *Photobacteria damselae* ssp. *damselae*, is another fish pathogen that occasionally causes zoonotic infections in people. These organisms are ubiquitously present and widely distributed. Transmission is thought to occur through invasion of epithelial cells of the skin and intestinal tract via infected water.

Clinical presentation: The relatively few external signs may include darkened skin, anorexia, focal gill necrosis, and petechial hemorrhage.

Pathology: Internally, acute lesions consist of multifocal necrosis affecting the liver, spleen, and kidney, with bacteria evident intracellularly within phagocytes and extracellularly in vascular and interstitial spaces. The chronic disease is characterized by raised nodular white foci (i.e., granulomas) in the spleen, kidney, liver, and skeletal muscle. Histologically, the multiple, large, irregular, coalescing granulomas frequently have necrotic centers.

Differential diagnosis: A variety of bacterial agents (e.g., *Aeromonas* spp., *Edwardisella* spp., *Streptococcus* spp., *Vibrio* spp., and *Yersinia ruckeri*) may induce lesions in freshwater and marine fish that resemble

the acute phase of pasteurellosis, including infections that spread to the liver hematogenously from primary sites of infection (**Figures 11.11** and **11.12**). Rule-outs for chronic pasteurellosis include systemic bacterial diseases that induce granuloma formation, such as mycobacteriosis, nocardiosis, and francisellosis, in addition to systemic fungal infections.

Diagnosis: Diagnostic tools, including methods for distinguishing the *P. piscicida* from *P. damselae*

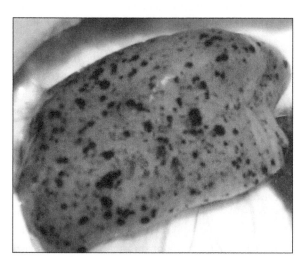

Figure 11.11 Myriad petechial and ecchymotic hemorrhages in the liver of a channel catfish (*Ictalurus punctatus*) infected with *Edwardsiella ictalurid*, i.e., "enteric septicemia of catfish." (Image courtesy L. Khoo.)

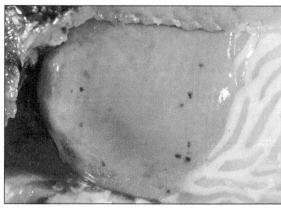

Figure 11.12 Coalescing pale foci (necrosis) and multiple hemorrhages in the liver of a rainbow trout (*Onchorynchus mykiss*) infected with *Yersinia ruckeri*, i.e., "enteric redmouth disease." (Image courtesy of S.A. Smith.)

subspecies, rely on bacterial culture and isolation plus biochemical characterization, and immunologic and molecular assays form the basis for most diagnoses of this disease.

Management/control: Control of pasteurellosis is highly challenging. Because of the ability of the organism to survive in intracellular locations (e.g., macrophages) and the emergence of broad antibiotic resistance, antibiotic therapy is often unsuccessful. Bacterial vaccines have also demonstrated limited efficacy, and recent attention has been given to the administration of dietary probiotics.[32]

SALMON RICKETTSIAL SEPTICEMIA

Overview: Salmonid rickettsial septicemia (SRS; piscirickettsiosis) is a commercially important systemic disease of salmon reared in saltwater, freshwater rainbow trout, and occasionally other species of aquacultured fishes. Outbreaks have occurred in North America, South America, and Europe.

Etiology: The etiologic agent of SRS is the Gram-negative, nonencapsulated, nonmotile facultative intracellular pathogen *Piscirickettsia salmonis*. SRS is thought to be spread horizontally by absorption through the skin or gills of water contaminated with bacteria-laden urine or feces.

Clinical presentation: Clinical features of SRS include lethargy, erratic swimming, darkened skin, raised scales, and dermal hemorrhage, although some infected fish may not display any of those signs. Findings observed at necropsy can include pale gills, ascitic abdominal fluid, and fibrinous epicarditis, but the most consistent macroscopic characteristic of SRS is multifocal pale nodules beneath the liver capsule, and similar foci in spleen and kidney that may be enlarged.

Pathology: Microscopic changes are widespread and include necrosis and focal granulomatous inflammation affecting the liver, spleen, kidney, pancreas, brain, gill, renal hematopoietic tissue, intestinal lamina propria, and peritoneal surfaces. Vasculitis and thrombosis may also be observed in multiple tissues.

Differential diagnosis: Few diseases closely resemble SRS, but one major differential diagnosis is viral hemorrhagic septicemia.

Diagnosis: The piscirickettsial organisms can be observed within macrophage vacuoles in histologic sections stained with hematoxylin and eosin, new methylene blue, or Giemsa stain. Immunohistochemistry and PCR are also commonly employed.

Management/control: Although antibiotics and commercial vaccines have thus far met with very limited success, newer vaccine strategies may prove more promising.

REFERENCES

1. Langdon, J.S. Experimental transmission and pathogenicity of epizootic haematopoietic necrosis virus (EHNV) in redfin perch, *Perca fluviatilis* L., and 11 other teleosts. *Journal of Fish Diseases* 1989;12:295–310.
2. Langdon, J.S., Humphrey, J.D. and Williams, L.M. Outbreaks of an EHNV-like iridovirus in cultured rainbow trout, *Salmo gairdneri* Richardson, in Australia. *Journal of Fish Diseases* 1988;11:93–96.
3. Whittington, R.J. and Reddacliff, G.L. Influence of environmental temperature on experimental infection of redfin perch (*Perca fluviatilis*) and rainbow trout (*Oncorhynchus mykiss*) with epizootic haematopoietic necrosis virus, an Australian iridovirus. *Australian Veterinary Journal* 1995;72:421–424.
4. Whittington, R.J., Philbey, A., Reddacliff, G.L. and MacGown, A.R. Epidemiology of epizootic haematopoietic necrosis virus (EHNV) infection in farmed rainbow trout, *Oncorhynchus mykiss* (Walbaum): Findings based on virus isolation, antigen capture ELISA and serology. *Journal of Fish Diseases* 1994;17:205–218.
5. Reddacliff, L.A. and Whittington, R.J. Pathology of epizootic haematopoietic necrosis virus (EHNV) infection in rainbow trout (*Oncorhynchus mykiss*, Walbaum) and redfin perch (*Perca fluviatilis* L). *Journal of Comparative Pathology* 1996;115(2):103–115.
6. Steiner, K.A., Whittington, R.J., Petersen, R.K., Hornitzky, C. and Garnett, H. Purification of epizootic haematopoietic necrosis virus and its detection using ELISA. *Journal of Virological Methods* 1991;33:199–210.
7. Whittington, R.J. and Steiner, K.A. Epizootic haematopoietic necrosis virus (EHNV): Improved ELISA for detection in fish tissues and cell cultures and an efficient method for release of antigen from tissues. *Journal of Virological Methods* 1993;43:205–220.
8. Ørpetveit, I., Mikalsen, A.B., Sindre, H., Evensen, Ø., Dannevig, B.H. and Midtlyng, P.J. Detection of infectious pancreatic necrosis virus in subclinically infected Atlantic salmon by virus isolation in cell culture or real-time reverse transcription polymerase chain reaction: Influence of sample preservation and storage. *Journal of Veterinary Diagnostic Investigation* 2010;22:886–895.
9. Speare, D.J. Liver diseases of tropical fish. *Seminars in Avian and Exotic Pet Medicine* 2000;9(3):174–178.

10. Wolf, J.C. and Wolfe, M.J. A brief overview of non-neoplastic hepatic toxicity in fish. *Toxicologic Pathology* 2005;33(1):75–85.

11. Genc, E., Yilmaz, E. and Akyurt, I. Effects of dietary fish oil, soy-acid oil, and yellow grease on growth and hepatic lipidosis of hybrid tilapia fry. *Israeli Journal of Aquaculture – Bamidgeh* 2005;57(2):90–96.

12. McAllister, P.E. Infectious pancreatic necrosis (IPN) of salmonid fishes. 1983. US Fish & Wildlife Publications 141. http://digitalcommons.unl.edu/usfwspubs/141.

13. Roberts, R.J. and Pearson, M.D. Infectious pancreatic necrosis in Atlantic salmon. *Salmo salar* L. *Journal of Fish Diseases* 2005;28(7):383–390.

14. Rodriguez Saint-Jean, S., Borrego, J.J. and Perez-Prieto, S.I. Infectious pancreatic necrosis virus: Biology, pathogenesis, and diagnostic methods. *Advances in Virus Research* 2003;62:113–165.

15. Wolf, J.C. and Smith, S.A. Comparative severity of experimentally induced mycobacteriosis in striped bass *Morone saxatilis* and hybrid tilapia *Oreochromis* spp. *Diseases of Aquatic Organisms* 1999;38(3):191–200.

16. Kane, A.S., Cynthia, B., Stine, C.B., Laura Hungerford, L., Mark Matsche, M., Cindy Driscoll, C., Ana, M., Baya, A.M. Mycobacteria as environmental portent in Chesapeake Bay fish species. *Emerging Infectious Diseases* 2007;13(2):329–331.

17. Labrie, L., Ng, J., Tan, Z., Komar, C., Ho, E. and Grisez, L. Nocardial infections in fish: An emerging problem in both freshwater and marine aquaculture systems in Asia. In: *Diseases in Asian Aquaculture VI*. M.G. Bondad-Reantaso, C.V. Mohan, M. Crumlish and R.P. Subasinghe, eds. Fish Health Section, Asian Fisheries Society, Manila, Philippines, 2008; pp. 297–312.

18. Sanders, G.E. and Swaim, L.E. Atypical piscine mycobacteriosis in Japanese medaka (*Oryzias latipes*). *Comparative Medicine* 2001;51(2):171–175.

19. Hughes, K.P., Duncan, R.B. and Smith, S.A. Renomegaly associated with a mycobacterial infection in summer flounder *Paralichthys dentatus*. *Fish Pathology* 2002;37(2):83–86.

20. Fischer, W.J., Hitzfeld, B.C., Tencalla, F., Eriksson, J.E., Mikhailov, A. and Dietrich, D.R. Microcystin-LR toxicodynamics, induced pathology, and immuno-histochemical localization in livers of blue-green algae exposed rainbow trout (*Oncorhynchus mykiss*). *Toxicological Sciences* 2000;54(2):365–373.

21. Jos, A., Pichardo, S., Prieto, A.I., Repetto, G., Vázquez, C.M., Moreno, I. and Cameán, A.M. Toxic cyano-bacterial cells containing microcystins induce oxidative stress in exposed tilapia fish (*Oreochromis* sp.) under laboratory conditions. *Aquatic Toxicology* 2005;72(3):261–271.

22. Kotak, B.G., Semalulu, S., Fritz, D.L., Prepas, E.E., Hrudey, S.E. and Coppock, R.W. Hepatic and renal pathology of intraperitoneally administered microcystin-LR in rainbow trout (*Oncorhynchus mykiss*). *Toxicon* 1996;34(5):517–525.

23. Hahn, C.M., Iwanowicz, L.R., Cornman, R.S., Conway, C.M., Winton, J.R. and Blazer, V.S. Characterization of a novel hepadnavirus in the white sucker (*Catostomus commersonii*) from the Great Lakes Region of the United States. *Journal of Virology* 2015;89(23):11801–11811.

24. Sun, L., Nguyen, A.T., Spitsbergen, J.M. and Gong, Z. Myc-induced liver tumors in transgenic zebrafish can regress in tp53 null mutation. *PLOS ONE* 2015;10(1):e0117249.

25. Taksdal, T., Olsen, A.B., Bjerkas, I., Hjortaas, M.J., Dannevig, B.H., Graham, D.A. and McLoughlin, M.F. Pancreas disease in farmed Atlantic salmon, *Salmo salar* L. and rainbow trout, *Oncorhynchus mykiss* (Walbaum) in Norway. *Journal of Fish Diseases* 2007;30:545–558.

26. Jansen, M.D., Jensen, B.B., Loughlin, M.F., Rodger, H.D., Taksdal, T., Sindre, H., Graham, D.A. and Lillehaug, A. The epidemiology of pancreas disease in salmonid aquaculture: A summary of the current state of knowledge. *Journal of Fish Diseases* 2017;40:141–155.

27. Villoing, S., Bearzotti, M., Chilmonczyk, S., Castric, J. and Bremont, M. Rainbow trout sleeping disease virus is an atypical alphavirus. *Journal of Virology* 2000;74:173–183.

28. Boscher, S.K., McLoughlin, M., Le Ven, A., Cabon, J., Baud, M. and Castric, J. Experimental transmission of sleeping disease in one-year-old rainbow trout, *Oncorhynchus mykiss* (Walbaum), induced by sleeping disease virus. *Journal of Fish Diseases* 2006;29(5):263–273.

29. Jensen B, B., Kristoffersen, A.B., Myr, C. and Brun, E. Cohort study of effect of vaccination on pancreas disease in Norwegian salmon aquaculture. *Diseases of Aquatic Organisms* 2012;102(1):23–31.

30. Hoffman, G.L. *Parasites of North American Freshwater Fishes*, 2nd ed. Cornell University Press, Ithaca, NY, 1999.

31. Woo, P.T.K. and Buchmann, K. *Fish Parasites: Pathobiology and Protection*. CABI, Wallingford, Oxfordshire, UK, 2012.

32. Andreoni F. and Magnani M. Photobacteriosis: Prevention and diagnosis. *Journal of Immunology Research* 2014; Article ID 793817, 7 pages, http://dx.doi.org/10.1155/2014/793817.

CHAPTER 12

RENAL DISEASES AND DISORDERS

LESTER KHOO

BACTERIAL KIDNEY DISEASE

Overview: Bacterial kidney disease (BKD) is a systemic, slowly progressing, often chronic disease of wild and cultured salmonids that manifests predominately as white nodular lesions in the kidney and sometimes also in the spleen and liver. The disease was first described in Atlantic salmon in the Dee and Spey Rivers of Scotland.[1] Due to the appearance of the gross lesions and where the disease was first observed, it is sometimes referred to as white boil disease or Dee disease.[1,2]

Etiology: *Renibacterium salmonarium* is a small, Gram-positive, nonmotile, asporogenous diplobacillus that was originally classified as a *Corynebacterium*.

Route of transmission: The disease can be transmitted both horizontally and vertically with subclinical or latent carriers being reservoirs of infection. Clinically affected fish can shed the bacterium in the feces and the bacterium can survive up to 21 days in the feces or pond sediment. High numbers of *R. salmonarium* are also found in the coelomic fluid of affected fish, which is the main source of infection for eggs. The organism is small enough to enter the egg through the micropyle and is transmitted internally within the egg thereby limiting the effectiveness of typical disinfection.[2]

Host range: The disease has a worldwide distribution in both freshwater and saltwater salmonids including Pacific (Chinook salmon, *Oncorhynchus tshawytscha*; coho salmon, *O. kisutch*) and Atlantic salmon (*Salmo salar*), grayling (*Thymallus thymallus*) and trout species (brook, lake, brown and rainbow trout [*Salvelinus fontinalis*, *S. namaycush*, *Salmo trutta* and *Oncorhynchus mykiss*, respectively]).[2] In addition, *R. salmonarium* has also been found in Pacific hake (*Merluccius productus*), Pacific herring (*Clupea harengus pallasi*) and most recently in sea lamprey (*Petromyzon marinus*).[3,4] However, the role that these non-salmonid species play in the spread of this disease has yet to be determined.

Clinical presentation: Gross clinical presentation of the disease may differ among the susceptible salmonid species, environmental temperature and stage of the disease. Affected fish tend to be hyperpigmented or darker in color, and may also have petechial hemorrhages at the base of the pectoral fins.[1] Exophthalmia, which may be present in some fish, may be the only clinical sign in others such as in the early stages of infection in Chinook salmon before it becomes systemic.[2] In coho salmon, exophthalmia with massive numbers of bacteria may be the only lesion with no other lesions or bacteria present in the visceral organs. Affected fish may also have distended abdomens as well as ulcerated or nonulcerated raised dermal lesions containing necrotic tissue, bacteria and blood cells.[2]

Pathology: The kidney is the organ that is most commonly affected, although lesions may also be present in the heart, spleen, liver, gill and muscle. Other gross internal lesions include hemorrhagic lesions in the posterior intestine, liver, peritoneum and visceral fat. The kidneys are swollen and often have discrete gray-white nodular lesions (**Figure 12.1**). On histopathology, these granulomatous lesions often have a necrotic core and bacteria around the periphery of the granuloma. In advanced cases, most of the renal tissue may be destroyed affecting both excretory and hematopoietic functions. The skeletal muscle lesions are often large cavitations in the muscles adjacent to the kidney.[1] A pseudodiphtheritic membrane may cover the liver, spleen and organs of affected Atlantic salmon at temperatures below 8.3°C, with similar membranes seen in trout but at higher temperatures 12°C–13°C.[2]

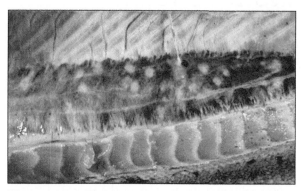

Figure 12.1 Discrete gray-white nodular lesions in the posterior kidney of an Atlantic salmon (*Salmo salar*) due to bacterial kidney disease, i.e., *Renibacterium salmoninarum*. (Image courtesy of T. Poppe.)

Differential diagnoses: Differential diagnoses include other bacterial diseases such as mycobacteriosis, which causes systemic granulomatous disease. However, the cavernous muscle lesions are only seen in piscirickettsiosis and not in these other bacterial diseases.

Diagnosis: Presumptive diagnosis is based on clinical signs and demonstration of Gram-positive diplobacillus in the infected tissue. Serological, immunological and molecular methods, as well as culture and biochemical characterization of the bacteria are used for confirmation of this disease. This bacterium is a notoriously slow grower even at optimal temperatures (15°C–18°C) and requires specialized media and methods (e.g., nurse culture and spent media) to decrease the culture time.

Management/control: Currently, there are no approved antibiotics for treating the disease. A bacterin consisting of live *Arthrobacter davidanieli*, a related bacteria, has been used to help control the disease in some aquaculture situations. Transmission by feeding infected fish carcasses and/or viscera should be avoided or can be prevented by pasteurization of infected material.[5]

ENTERIC SEPTICEMIA OF CATFISH

Overview: This is a systemic bacterial disease predominately of cultured catfish especially in the southeastern United States occurring during the optimal temperature range (22°C–28°C) of the bacterium. The etiological agent was first recognized in 1981 and the disease incidence increased with the growth of the channel catfish industry from 1982 to 1986.[6] The chronic form of the disease is often associated with the raised or ulcerative lesion along the dorsal midline of the head overlying the open fontanel that has led to the colloquial term "hole-in-the-head" disease.

Etiology: The etiological agent of enteric septicemia of catfish (ESC) is *Edwardsiella ictaluri*, a Gram-negative, peritrichous, oxidase-negative and fermentative bacillus. The bacteria is most closely related to *E. tarda* in the Enterobacteriacae family, but is negative for motility at 37°C, indole test, Jordan tartrate test, gas production in glucose at 37°C, and H$_2$S production in triple sugar iron agar.

Route of transmission: This disease is only known to be transmitted horizontally most notably by the fecal–oral route, though the bacteria is also known to enter via the gills, nares and skin.[7–10]

Host range: Historically, *E. ictaluri* has been considered a host-specific pathogen with most disease outbreaks limited to the catfish producing states in the southeastern United States. It now appears that this pathogen's host range extends beyond the commonly cultured and wild catfish in the region, for example, channel catfish, hybrid catfish (*Ictalurus punctatus* ♀ × *Ictalurus fucatus* ♂), blue catfish (*I. furcatus*), white catfish (*Ameiurus catus*), and brown bullhead (*A. nebulosus*). The pathogen has been isolated from outbreaks in the walking catfish (*Clarias batachus*) and other *Clarias* hybrids, Vietnamese freshwater catfish (*Pangasius hypophthalmus*), Chinese yellow catfish (*Pelteobagrus fluvidraco*), Japanese ayu (*Plecoglossus altevelis*), Nile tilapia (*Oreochromis niloticus*), Green knifefish (*Eigemannia virescens*), rosy barb (*Puntius conchonius*), danios (*Danio devario*) and zebrafish (*D. rerio*).[11–20]

Clinical presentation: The acute form of the disease has few clinical signs/lesions but is usually associated with high mortalities, whereas the subacute form has a slower onset, more obvious external lesions and a cumulative mortality that may be high. The chronic form has an even slower onset with typically lower mortalities but has more central nervous system signs, as well as the associated raised or ulcerative lesion along the dorsal midline of the head, and exhibits abnormal swimming behavior (i.e., spinning or spiraling near the surface of the water). Affected fish also go off feed. Fish may have a pendulous abdomen containing serosanguinous to straw-colored ascites, uni- or bilateral exophthalmia that is sometimes accompanied with periorbital tissue swelling, petechial hemorrhages on the skin particularly in the buccal region, and hemorrhage around the base of fins.

Pathology: In most species, the disease is systemic with renal involvement. Lesions may be present in the kidney whether the disease is acute, subacute or chronic. The posterior kidney often exhibits renomegaly with rounded edges and rises above the level of the swim bladder in all three forms of the disease. Multiple, small, tan-white foci may be visible on the surface of the kidney with these being more common in the subacute or chronic forms (**Figure 12.2**). In the more acute stages, the liver may have hemorrhages that become granulomatous foci of inflammation (**Figure 12.3**). Segmental hemorrhage can be

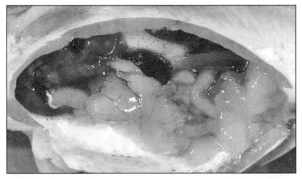

Figure 12.2 Coelomic cavity of a channel catfish (*Ictalurus punctatus*) with enteric septicemia of catfish. Note the straw-colored ascitic fluid surrounding the viscera, the swollen posterior kidney and the nodular appearance of the liver.

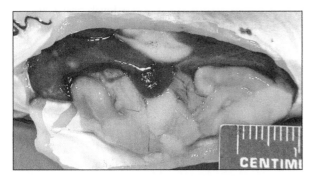

Figure 12.3 Coelomic cavity of a channel catfish (*I. punctatus*) with enteric septicemia of catfish. Note the white/tan foci in the liver as well as the slightly swollen posterior kidney.

seen in the gastrointestinal tract and the spleen may be congested. The renal lesions are mainly interstitial with multifocal to regionally extensive necrosis and mononuclear inflammation that may also extend to the glomeruli and surrounding tubules. There is also an interstitial nephritis in the anterior kidney, although the gross lesions are usually less apparent. Renal lesions have also been reported in ayu (i.e., swelling and softening) and Nile tilapia (i.e., enlarged anterior kidney with nodules).[15,16]

Differential diagnoses: *Edwardsiella piscicida*, a closely related bacterium, also causes similar gross lesions in cultured catfish.[21,22] Channel catfish virus (CCV) is another possible differential, but CCV does not cause nodular lesions in the kidney or liver, nor does it cause segmental intestinal hemorrhage.

Diagnosis: Presumptive diagnosis is based on lesions and bacterial cultures. Confirmation of diagnosis is via immunological or molecular methods.

Management/control: Management of this disease in catfish during outbreaks involves the use of approved medicated feeds to control mortalities and taking the fish off feed to reduce the fecal–oral route of transmission, especially when the environmental temperature is above the optimal temperature of the bacterium. A modified live bacterin is available to limit outbreaks of the disease, although current vaccination strategies involve vaccinating fry that may not be fully immunocompetent.

PISCIRICKETTSIOSIS

Overview: A septicemic condition of farmed salmon and marine fish caused by an intracellular bacterial pathogen. Initial reports of the disease were from Chile in 1989 from coho salmon (*O. kisutch*) that had been recently introduced into saltwater.[23] Since then, the disease has been observed in other salmonids and a few non-salmonid species.

Etiology: *Piscirickettsia salmonis* is a Gram-negative, nonmotile, highly fastidious, aerobic, obligate intracellular coccoid bacterium.

Route of transmission: Infections are horizontally transmitted with other fish species and aquatic animals as possible reservoirs.[24] While horizontal transmission can occur with or without fish-to-fish contact in freshwater and saltwater, the source and reservoir in the natural environment as well as the mode of transmission remain unknown.[24,25] Vertical transmission has also been shown to be possible with experimentally inoculated males and female broodstock.[25] However, the disease is less frequently observed in salmonids in freshwater compared to the marine environment suggesting that vertical transmission of this disease is less common in nature.[23]

Host range: The disease has been reported in numerous salmonid species including coho salmon (*O. kisutch*), Atlantic salmon (*Salmo salar*), cherry salmon (*O. masou*), Chinook salmon (*O. tshawytscha*), pink salmon (*O. gorbuscha*) and rainbow trout (*O. mykiss*).[23] It has also been isolated from hatchery-reared white seabass (*Atractoscion nobilis*).[26] A similar rickettsial-like-organism isolated from European seabass (*Dicentrarchus labrax*) has been found to be another strain of *P. salmonis* that is closely related to the salmon pathogen.[27]

Clinical presentation: Clinical signs include darker colored fish with pale gills, inappetence, lethargy and swimming near the water surface or edges of cages. Affected fish often have small dermal lesions, slightly raised white patches that ulcerate to form shallow, hemorrhagic ulcers.[23,28] Some fish may also have ascites.[28] Less affected fish may show no abnormal external signs. Erratic swimming behavior has also been reported and the bacterium has been isolated from the brain. However, the most consistent external sign is the pale gills due to the profound anemia.[23]

Pathology: One of the most common internal lesions of this disease is a swollen and gray discolored kidney. Affected fish can also have an enlarged spleen; ascites; and hemorrhages on the visceral fat, stomach, swim bladder and body musculature. Livers of severely affected fish are pale with cream-colored opaque nodules. Microscopic kidney lesions include necrosis of hematopoietic cells during the acute phase with necrosis followed by granulomatous inflammation in the kidney interstitium as the disease progresses resulting in anemia.[23] These changes are also seen in the spleen of affected fish. Vascular and perivascular necrosis is also present in the liver. Recent cases of piscirickettsiosis have mainly reported dermal ulcerations and cavernous lesions in the musculature rather than the classical

lesions of renomegaly, white nodular hepatic lesions and splenomegaly.[25]

Differential diagnoses: Francisellosis (*Francisella noatunensis*), furunculosis (*Aeromonas salmonicida*), mycobacteriosis, viral hemorrhagic septicemia, marine fungi and various parasites are possible differential diagnoses in freshwater, brackish water and saltwater fishes.

Diagnosis: Diagnosis is made on clinical signs, isolation of *P. salmonis* in cell culture, and detection of the dark blue Giemsa-stained organism in tissue impressions or sections. Confirmation is by indirect florescent antibody testing.[23]

Management/control: Control of the disease involves using management practices, as there are no current bacterins available and antibiotics have limited effectiveness.[25] Fallowing a production site following an outbreak has been used to limit the spread of the disease.[29]

FRANCISELLOSIS

Overview: This is a systemic bacterial disease caused by various *Fransicella* species in fresh, brackish and saltwater species of farmed and wild fish.[30,31]

Etiology: All piscine francisellosis is attributed to *Francisella noatunensis* with two subspecies *F. noatunensis* subsp. *noatunensis* in coldwater fish, and *F. noatunensis* subsp. *orientalis* in warmwater fish.[32] These organisms are Gram-negative, small pleomorphic or coccobacilli that are strictly aerobic, facultatively intracellular and nonmotile.[30]

Route of transmission: The disease is transmitted horizontally primarily via the fecal–oral route.[31] It is highly unlikely that fish pathogenic *Francisella* sp. has any zoonotic potential, although *F. noatunensis* is most closely related to *F. philomiragia*, which is opportunistic but less virulent than *F. tularensis* and causes pneumonia and systemic infections.[31]

Host range: Francisellosis has been reported in Atlantic cod, Atlantic salmon, tilapia, threeline grunt, hybrid striped bass, several species of fairy wrasses (*Cirrhilabrus* spp.) and blue-green damsel fish (*Chromis viridis*), though this list is likely to grow with time.[30,33–37]

Clinical presentation: No matter the subspecies of *F. noatunensis* or diverse array of susceptible species, the clinical signs and lesions associated with piscine francisellosis are similar, i.e., there are both acute and chronic morbidity and mortalities associated with nonspecific clinical signs such as lethargy, anorexia, abnormal swimming, dermal ulcerations and darken coloration.[38,39]

Pathology: The most prominent internal lesions are splenomegaly and renomegaly, although other organ systems such as the gills or gastrointestinal tract system can also be affected.[38,39] In some tilapia cases, the spleens are often 10 times normal size and the renomegaly is especially severe in the anterior kidney.[40] Multiple pale tan, often coalescing nodules are present in both the spleen and kidney of affected fish. Histologically, these nodules correspond to granulomas that have vacuolated macrophages with intracellular bacteria and are often circumscribed by lymphocytic cuffs.[39] Chronic or mature granulomas may have necrotic cores and fibrous encapsulation in which the intracellular bacteria may be less apparent.[30,31] Granulomas can also be present in other organ systems that do not have macroscopic lesions and may even extend into the musculature.[30,33,40] In addition, there may be a focal to diffuse necrotizing vasculitis in both the spleen and kidney.[30]

Differential diagnoses: Mycobacteriosis, nocardiosis, piscirickettsiosis, furunculosis, fungi and various parasites are differential diagnoses for this disease.

Diagnosis: Diagnosis of the disease is by cultures incubated at 22°C–25°C, macroscopic lesions and histologic observations consistent with the disease.[31] Specialized selective media containing elevated levels of cysteine and glucose are required, often with the addition of antibiotics, as the organism is readily inhibited by other bacteria.[31] *Francisella* sp. can also be cultured in several different cell lines, (i.e., salmon head kidney [SHK-1], Atlantic salmon kidney [ASK] and Chinook salmon embryo [CHSE-214]). Molecular means are utilized to definitively determine the piscine pathogenic species since *Francisella* spp. are considered biochemically unreactive and there are only a few phenotypical tests available for differentiating the different *Francisella* spp.[31]

Management/control: Several therapeutics have been experimentally shown to be efficacious in controlling the disease.[36,39,41] There are currently no commercial bacterins available for this disease.[31]

MYCOBACTERIOSIS

Overview: Piscine mycobacteriosis is a systemic, globally distributed disease of a wide range of cultured and wild, freshwater and marine fish. Piscine mycobacteriosis is in most instances a chronic debilitative disease, although there are also acute forms.[42,43]

Etiology: Historically, three mycobacterial species were considered mainly responsible for piscine mycobacteriosis, namely, *Mycobacterium marinum*, *M. fortuitum* and *M. chelonae*. However, there is a growing array of *Mycobacterium* spp. that have been isolated from fish, and although many of these isolates have been assigned to recognized species, caution must be applied in accepting these species designations.[43]

Route of transmission: The transmission of mycobacteria in fish is primarily by consumption of contaminated feed, water or detritus, as well as cannibalism of infected fish.[42,43] Injuries or skin abrasions, and external parasites may also be possible routes of infection. Vertical transmission has been reported in a viviparous fish (i.e., transovarian infection) but not in ovaparious.[44,45] Other vertebrates (e.g., frogs, snakes, turtles) and invertebrates may serve as reservoirs or as contaminated prey.[42]

Host range: First described in carp (*Cyprinus carpio*), there have been more than 167 susceptible fish species listed by 2009.[46] Virtually all fish are considered susceptible, but several families of freshwater fish appear to be disproportionately represented, including the Anabantidae (bettas and gouramis), Characidae (tetras and piranhas), Cichlidae (angelfish and other cichlids) and Cyprinidae (danios and barbs).[45] The disease is also commonly seen in wild and cultured striped bass (*Morone saxatilis*) and cultured cobia (*Rachycentron canadum*) and southern flounder (*Paralichthys dentatus*).[46–49]

Clinical presentation: Acute, fulminating mycobacteriosis is rare and seen with high bacterial loads resulting in relatively rapid morbidity and mortality with few clinical signs. Chronic presentations usually result in listlessness, lethargy, anorexia and emaciation. Affected fish often separate from other individuals. Fish may have scale loss and dermal ulcerations with pigment alterations (i.e., darker or lighter). They may develop

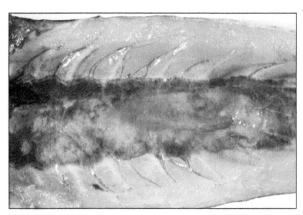

Figure 12.4 Mycobacteriosis in the kidney of a cultured cobia, *Rachycentron canadum*. (Image courtesy of S.A. Smith.)

spinal curvature, be stunted in growth and may not develop sexually. Uni- or bilateral exophthalmos is also common.[42,43]

Pathology: Typical internal lesions include renomegaly, splenomegaly and hepatomegaly together with multiple or singular gray-white, miliary nodules or plaques on these and other organs (**Figures 12.4 and 12.5**).[50,51] Histologically, granulomas typically consist of concentrically arranged epithelioid macrophages surrounding a core of necrotic cells and variable numbers of peripherally located acid-fast bacilli.

Differential diagnoses: The same differential list that would be considered for piscirickettsiosis (i.e., raised, nodular lesions) should be considered, including francisellosis (*F. noatunensis*), furunculosis

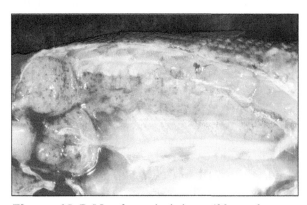

Figure 12.5 Mycobacteriosis in a wild-caught striped bass, *Morone saxatilis*. Note the pale appearance to the kidney and the swollen anterior kidney. (Image courtesy of S.A. Smith.)

(*A. salmonicida*), fungal pathogens and encysted metazoan parasites.

Diagnosis: Presumptive diagnosis is based on gross lesions and visualization of acid-fast organisms in impression smears or tissue sections. Bacterial cultures, which may take weeks to months even on specialize media (e.g., Löwenstein Jensen or Middlebrook 7H10), coupled with phenotypic characterization (via biochemical tests, high performance liquid chromatography or capillary gas chromatography for fatty-acid methyl esters) and molecular techniques can provide definitive diagnosis.[42,46] Cultures of external lesions may result in the mycobacteria being outcompeted by environmental bacterial contaminants, whereas molecular techniques using tissues or whole fish may indicate the presence of mycobacterial DNA due to environmental contamination and not infection.

Management/control: In light of the zoonotic potential of piscine mycobacteriosis, there are no widely accepted antimicrobial treatments for mycobacteriosis in fish.[43] The disease in humans is often referred to as "fish tank granuloma," "fish handler's disease" or "fish fancier's finger syndrome," and is often limited to the extremities due to the thermal tolerance of piscine mycobacteria.[43] Control of mycobacteriosis in aquariums (e.g., recirculating systems or reuse systems) generally involves depopulation of the infected stock and disinfection. Several commonly used chemical disinfectants in aquaculture have been found to be ineffective even with extended contact times, and this is further complicated by the presence of biofilms, which can serve as natural protective habitats for mycobacteria.[52]

PROLIFERATIVE KIDNEY DISEASE

Overview: Proliferative kidney disease (PKD) is an economically important systemic parasitic disease of salmonids. The disease primarily affects first season freshwater salmonids and is linked to increased water temperatures (>15°C) with outbreaks typically seen in summer and autumn when fingerlings are stocked into infected waters.

Etiology: The causative agent is the myxozoan *Tetracapsuloides bryosalmonae* (syn. *Tetracapsula bryosalmonae*, *T. renicola*) in the class Malacosporean of the phylum Myxozoa.[53] Prior to its identification, the causative agent was known as "PKX" or "PKD organism unknown." The primary host for this parasite is the freshwater bryozoan, *Federicella sultana*, in which spores develop and become infectious to fish. There is also vertical transmission of this parasite in *F. sultana*, thus this coelomate invertebrate plays an important role in the maintenance of PKD.[54]

Route of transmission: The route of transmission in the fish is indirect requiring a bryozoan host to release the infective parasite stage.

Host range: PKD is primarily restricted to the family Salmonidae, however, not all salmonids are equally susceptible. While the disease has been reported once in brook trout (*Salvelinus fontainalis*), there have been no additional reports in this species even when reared in the same site where other salmonids are afflicted.[55]

Clinical presentation: Clinical signs are mainly exhibited in severe infections where there may be nonspecific signs including darken body, bilateral exophthalmos, abdominal distension, pale gills due to anemia and up to 100% mortality.[55]

Pathology: Swelling, especially of the posterior kidney, is characteristic but not pathognomonic for the disease. The kidney may be 10 times or greater than normal size and may be discolored dark purple to red/pink or mottled gray, which is dependent on the stage and extent of vascular disruption of the various regions of the kidney caused by the parasite. Blood-tinged ascites may be present, especially in chronic infections, and the spleen may be enlarged, rough or knobbly. Presporogenic stages infect the kidney interstitium where the initial response is hematopoietic hyperplasia and reduction of glomeruli and renal tubules. This progresses to chronic inflammation with coalescing whorls of inflammatory cells (primarily macrophages) surrounding the parasite. The parasite also infects vascular walls of the kidney, gills, liver, spleen and pancreas eliciting a necrotizing vasculitis.[55] Mortality levels are chronic and variable. Healing or recovery begins as early as 12 weeks postexposure as evidenced by degeneration of the parasite, although sporogenic stages of the parasite may continue to be present several months following recovery from clinical signs.[55]

Differential diagnoses: Piscirickettsiosis is a differential for this disease, but fish infected with PKD do not have the dermal lesions associated with *P. salmonis* infection.

Diagnosis: Presumptive diagnosis is based on demonstrating the presence of *T. bryosalmonae* on Giemsa-stained impression smears of the kidney or spleen, or on wet mounts of kidney. Definitive diagnosis is based on identifying the parasite in histological sections or in tissue imprints stained with the GS-1 specific lectin.[56]

Management/control: There are no approved therapeutics, although increasing salinity (8–12 ppt) decreases morbidity and mortality. Other management tools include controlling secondary infections (e.g., bacterial and parasitic), reducing stocking densities and feeding rates may reduce mortalities. Survivors have increased immunity against the parasite, but may continue to shed the organism.[55]

KIDNEY ENLARGEMENT DISEASE OF GOLDFISH

Overview: Kidney enlargement disease (KED) of goldfish (i.e., kidney bloater disease, papillary cystic hyperplasia) is a slowly progressive parasitic disease of the renal tissue of goldfish and gibel carp that is invariably fatal.

Etiology: The disease is caused by the myxozoan parasite *Hoferellus carassii*.[57,58] The closely related *Hoferellus cyprinii* (syn. *Mitraspora cyprinii*) was incorrectly implicated in the past as the causative agent.[57,59–61]

Route of transmission: Like other myxozoans, this parasite has a complex life cycle that can include two different aquatic oligochaete worms, *Branchiura sowerbyi* and *Nais eligius* as intermediate hosts.[58,62] Fish are infected by the aurantiactinomyxon spore released by the oligochaete worm in the summer, but do not show clinical signs until the following spring.

Host range: *Hoferellus carassii* is a common parasite of *Carassius* species and can infect both gibel carp (*C. gibello*) and goldfish (*C. auratus*), unlike *H. cyprinii* that only affects common carp (*C. carpio*).[60,63] Due to the life cycle of the parasite requiring an oligochaete intermediate host, the disease is more common in pond-reared fish.

Clinical presentation: Affected goldfish have markedly uni- or bilaterally distended abdomens during the later stages of disease. The swelling may be large enough to affect buoyancy and swimming. There are usually no major symptoms in gibel carp.

Pathology: The parasite elicits cystic papillomatous hyperplasia of the renal tubular epithelium forming intraluminal papillary projections resulting in degeneration of the renal interstitium.[64] Glomeruli are rarely involved and the anterior kidney appears to be spared.[131] During the early stages of the disease, there are no gross visible kidney changes, but plasmodia and spores can be detected microscopically. In the late stages, the tubules become markedly dilated and contain a yellow fluid.[64]

Differential diagnoses: *Hoferellus carassii* invades individual renal tubular cells that develop an adenoma-like appearance, whereas *Hoferellus cyprinii* causes syncytial fusion of epithelial cells forming nodules.[60] Additional differentials for this disease would include bacterial and fungal causes of kidney enlargement, renal tumors and other causes of cystic dilation of tubules including polycystic kidney disease or obstruction of collecting ducts and ureters.

Diagnosis: Presumptive diagnosis is based on identification of the myxozoan trophozoites in the lesions. A definitive diagnosis is by identifying the miter-like myxospores in the lesions, although typically only a few are present. Microscopic examination of impression smears of the kidney, ureters and urinary bladder should be performed, as spores are likely to be lost during histological processing. This is also useful for detecting disease in the early stages, as the parasite is difficult to discern even in Giemsa-stained sections.[60]

Management/control: Management of the disease involves disinfection of ponds and restocking with uninfected fish, as there are no proven therapeutics. Culture in systems lacking soil/sediment substrate (e.g., concrete ponds) to eliminate the aquatic oligochaete host may help control the parasite similar to management techniques for whirling disease caused by different myxozoan parasite (i.e., *Myxobolus cerebralis*).

ACOLPENTERON URETEROECETES

Overview: *Acolpenteron ureteroecetes* is a parasitic infestation of the urinary bladder and ureters of largemouth bass (*Micropterus salmoides*).

Etiology: *Acolpenteron ureteroecetes* is a monogenean that infects the urinary bladder of largemouth bass. Reports of monogenean urinary tract infestations are limited, although there are more than 10 species that are known to infect fish, including *Acolpenteron catostomi*, *A. austral*, *A. nephriticum*, *A ureteronectes*, *A. willfordensis*, *Kritskyia annakohnae*, *K. boegeri*, *K. eirasi*, *K. moraveci*, *Philureter trigoniopsis* and *Urogyrus cichlidarum*.[65–76]

Route of transmission: As a monogenean, *Acolpenteron ureteroecetes* has a direct mode of transmission and does not require an intermediate host.

Host range: *Acolpenteron ureteroecetes* has been reported in largemouth bass (*M. salmoides*), smallmouth bass (*M. dolomieu*), spotted bass (*M. punctulatus*) and redbreast sunfish (*Lepomis auritus*).[72]

Clinical presentation: Affected fish have abdominal distention, epidermal darkening, inappetence, and are often disoriented with intermittent muscular spasms prior to death (**Figure 12.6**).[65,66] The parasite is often an incidental pathologic finding, but heavy infestations due to cumulative reinfestations in closed systems (i.e., ponds and recirculation systems) may result in clinical disease.[65,66]

Pathology: Fish have pale, enlarged kidneys with variable numbers of adult monogeneans and eggs on wet mount preparations of the renal tissue (**Figure 12.7**).[65] There is extensive necrosis of the renal interstitial tissue with marked eosinophilia due to the influx and degranulation of eosinophilic granular cells. The presence of adult monogeneans and eggs in the collecting ducts and ureter as well as

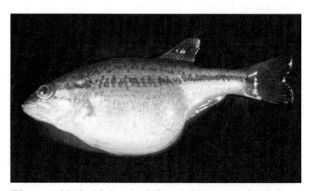

Figure 12.6 Abdominal distention in a cultured juvenile largemouth bass (*Micropterus salmoides*) due to *Acolpenteron ureteroecetes*. (Image courtesy of S.A. Smith.)

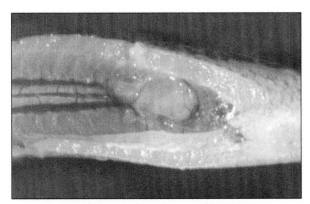

Figure 12.7 Renal enlargement and dilatation in a cultured juvenile largemouth bass (*M. salmoides*) due to *Acolpenteron ureteroecetes*. (Image courtesy of S.A. Smith.)

the host response is dependent on the chronicity and intensity of the infection. This ranges from hyperplasia of the luminal epithelium and dilation of the tubules to an intense inflammatory response with fibrosis. In the latter stages, the eggs are surrounded by granulomatous inflammation.[76]

Differential diagnoses: Differentials should include conditions that cause abdominal distention and gross enlargement of the kidney.

Diagnosis: Diagnosis of the condition is by the identification of the adult monogeneans and eggs on wet mount preparations of the renal tissue.[65] The location (i.e., in the ureters and collecting ducts of the posterior kidney) and distinctive morphological features of the monogenean (i.e., the absence of head lappets, the presence of 14 marginal hooks, and the blunt process on the egg) allow for the identification of this parasite.

Management/control: No therapeutics are currently approved for food fish species, although several anthelmintics have been used in non-food fish species. Surviving infected fish appear to develop immunity and/or have adapted to the parasite and become carrier fish.[76] Quarantine procedures with frequent health inspections of fish can help minimize the clinical manifestations of the disease in a population of fish.

HERPESVIRAL HEMATOPOIETIC NECROSIS OF GOLDFISH

Overview: Herpesviral hematopoietic necrosis (HVHN) produces severe epizootics in all ages of goldfish and can affect other cyprinids and has been reported to cause mortalities in gibel carp.[77] The disease was initially recognized in the early 1990s with mortalities in goldfish *Carassius auratus* in Japan. Because the virus mainly targets the hematopoietic cells of the kidney and spleen, it was initially designated as herpesviral hematopoietic necrosis virus.[78] This virus appears to be globally distributed with clinical disease seen during permissive water temperatures (20°C–25°C) during the spring and autumn with mortalities subsiding outside this temperature range.[79,80]

Etiology: Herpesviral hematopoietic necrosis of goldfish is caused by *cyprinid herpesvirus 2* (CyHV-2) and is an alloherpesvirus in the family Herpesviridae.[81]

Route of transmission: Horizontal transmission is the primary route of infection with survivors being carriers. There is some on-farm evidence for vertical transmission, but this has not been proven in laboratory experiments.[79]

Host range: Both goldfish (*C. auratus*) and gibel carp (*C. gibello*) are susceptible to this disease.[77,78]

Clinical presentation: Fish may be anorexic and lethargic, with fish lying listlessly at the bottom of the pond due to the profound anemia. Fish have pale gills and may have a pendulous abdomen due to fluid accumulation in the coelom.

Pathology: Affected fish have swollen kidneys and splenomegaly with white nodules.[79] Microscopically, there is necrosis in multiple tissues, including the hematopoietic tissue within the kidney, the pancreas, spleen and intestinal submucosa. Large amphophilic intranuclear inclusion bodies are present in areas of necrosis.[79] Gross and histologic lesions in the gills have been reported to resemble koi herpesvirus (*cyprinid herpevirus-3*) including intranuclear inclusions.[79]

Differential diagnoses: Differentials should include conditions causing anemia in goldfish, such as the hemoparasite *Trypanosoma danilewskyi*, external parasites (i.e., leeches) or chronic high levels of nitrites in the water.

Diagnosis: The virus has been difficult to culture with established cell lines and does not produce cytopathic effect on commonly used cell lines. Molecular methods have been developed for the diagnosis of this disease.[82,83] A permissive cell line from the brain of gibel carp has also been developed that will allow for the replication of the virus and formation of cytopathic effects (CPE).[84]

Management/control: Avoidance is the best line of defense against this disease. Thermal treatment regimens have been suggested as a means for managing this disease (i.e., to raise the water temperature to 27°C, which causes cessation of mortalities due to this disease). It has also been suggested that carriers that are placed in temperatures higher than the permissive temperature be subjected to a slow drop in water temperature to the permissive range or a drop in the temperature followed by raising the temperature above the permissive range to allow for immunity to develop.[79] Alternatively, the use of goldfish–carp hybrids, which are more resistant to this disease, has also been suggested.[85]

CHANNEL CATFISH VIRUS

Overview: Channel catfish virus (CCV) disease is an acute infection of channel catfish fry or young-of-the-year fingerlings less than 4 months old usually during the summer months when temperatures are 27°C or higher.[86,87] The disease was initially isolated from channel catfish in Alabama, Arkansas and Kentucky experiencing massive mortalities due to a hemorrhagic disease. This disease is primarily confined to catfish populations in the southern United States but has also been reported in Central America.[87]

Etiology: Channel catfish virus disease is caused by *ictalurid herpesvirus I*, which is an alloherpesvirus.[88]

Route of transmission: This highly contagious disease can easily be spread horizontally by cohabitation and via fomites, and is exacerbated by environmental stress and crowding resulting in reduced growth, secondary bacterial infections and massive mortalities. It is thought to be endemic in aquacultured channel catfish populations in the southern United States and maintained in these populations via vertical transmission.[88]

Host range: The virus is host specific, and natural outbreaks have only been reported in channel catfish (*Ictalurus punctatus*), blue catfish (*Ictalurus furcatus*) and hybrid catfish (*Ictalurus punctatus* ♀ × *Ictalurus fucatus* ♂).[88] Experimental challenges have shown that other catfish, i.e., black bullhead (*Ameiurus melas*), brown bullhead (*A. nebulosus*), yellow bullhead (*A. natalis*), African catfish (*Claris gariepinus*), Asian walking catfish (*C. batrachus*) and European wels catfish (*Silurus glanis*), are resistant to the disease.

Clinical presentation: Infected fish exhibit exophthalmia, distended abdomens, pale or hemorrhagic gills, hemorrhage on fins, and erratic swimming including spiraling along the long axis and hanging vertically with their head at the water surface (**Figure 12.8**). This latter clinical presentation was once thought to be characteristic for the disease.[89]

Pathology: Although CCV is a systemic infection with generalized viremia, the kidney is the first and most severely affected organ.[87] Infected fish have a general hyperemia in the viscera of the coelomic cavity and a straw-/yellow- colored ascites, which results in abdominal distension (**Figure 12.9**). The fish may also have pale livers with eosinophilic intracytoplasmic inclusion bodies in hepatocytes, pale enlarged posterior kidneys, enlarged hemorrhagic and congested spleens, and gastrointestinal tracts devoid of food but filled with a yellow mucoid fluid. Increased numbers of lymphoid cells have been observed in the posterior kidney, in addition to hemorrhage and necrosis of epithelial cells of the proximal tubules as well as extensive necrosis of the hematopoietic tissue.[90] There is also necrosis of the epithelium surrounding the pancreatic acinar cells with limited or minimal pancreatic acinar cell necrosis. Infected fish have vacuolation of neurons with edema of surrounding nerve fibers in the brain.[91] Younger naturally

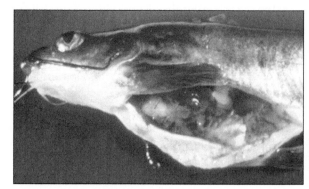

Figure 12.8 Coelomic cavity of a cultured channel catfish (*I. punctatus*) fingerling with channel catfish virus (CCV). Note the abdominal distention (i.e., due to ascites), and the hyperemia of the visceral tissues.

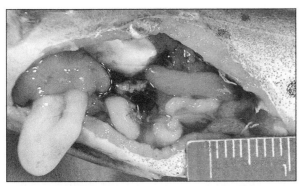

Figure 12.9 Coelomic cavity of a cultured channel catfish (*I. punctatus*) with CCV. The stomach has been reflected cranially to reveal the generalized hyperemia of the viscera and the markedly congested/hemorrhagic spleen.

infected fish have hepatocellular necrosis, whereas edema (i.e., kidney, heart, spinal cord and gastrointestinal tract) and necrosis were more common in the older fish.

Differential diagnoses: Differential diagnoses include enteric septicemia of catfish (ESC) and infestations with the digenetic trematode *Bolbophorus damnificus*. Fish infected with CCV will lack the hole-in-the-head lesion, hemorrhagic lesions in the gastrointestinal tract and nodular granulomatous renal lesions seen in ESC infected fish or the raised papular lesions of the skin observed in *Bolbophorus damnificus* infected fish.

Diagnosis: Presumptive diagnosis can be based on clinical signs at temperatures above 27°C or virus isolation on channel catfish ovary or brown bullhead cell lines, and observation of cytopathic effects of cell fusion and syncytial formation. Definitive diagnosis requires virus isolation with serum neutralization.

Management/control: There is no treatment for channel catfish virus infections. Avoidance followed by quarantine and disinfection are the best means of controlling the disease, while decreasing stress during warmer months is the best prevention strategy.

PHAEOHYPHOMYCOSIS

Overview: Phaeohyphomycosis is a mycotic infection caused by dematiaceous (brown pigmented or melanized) fungi where the tissue morphology of the causative agent is mycelial.

Etiology: Several different genera of black yeast (e.g., *Exophiala*, *Ochroconis*, *Phoma*) are known to cause systemic infections in fish and occur in the kidney as one of their predilection sites.[92,93] At least five species of *Exophiala* are known to cause renal lesions: *Exophiala psychrophila*, *E. salmonis*, *E. pisciphila* (syn. *E. pisciphilus*), *E. angulospora* and *E. aquamarina*.[94–100] There are three *Ochroconis* species that have been implicated in phaeohyphomycosis with renal lesions: *O. tshawytschae* (syn. *Heterosporium tshawytschae*, *Scolecobasidium tshawytschae*), *O. humicola* and an unnamed species closely related to *O. tshawytschae*.[101–104] *Phoma hebarium* is also known to cause kidney lesion.[105–107]

Route of transmission: Transmission is usually through direct environmental contamination or orally. Infections are generally considered secondary when immune function is compromised due to water quality problems, trauma, metabolic factors, or other systemic infections or stresses due to captivity or housing.[93]

Host range: *Exophilia* infections have been reported in Atlantic salmon (*Salmo salar*), channel catfish (*Ictalurus punctatus*), cod (*Gadus morhua*), Japanese flounder (*Paralichthys olivaceus*), and weedy and leafy seadragons (*Phyllopteryx taeniolatus* and *Phycodurus eques*).[89,96,97,100,108] *Ochroconis* infections have been reported in salmonids, i.e., Chinook salmon (*Oncohynchus tshawytschae*), coho salmon (*O. kisutch*), rainbow trout (*O. mykiss*) and masou salmon (*O. masou*), as well as non-salmonid species, i.e., striped jack (*Pseudocarnax dentex*), red sea bream (*Pagrus major*) and marbled rockfish (*Sebastiscus marmoratus*).[98,101–104,109,110] *Phoma* infections were reported in coho (*O. kisutch*), Chinook (*O. tshawytschae*) and ayu (*Plecoglossus altivelis*).[105–107]

Clinical presentation: Clinical presentations for phaeohyphomycosis with renal involvement varies slightly with the different fungi and fish species. Salmon infected with *Exophilia salmonis* have been reported to have erratic swimming followed by whirling behavior. Fish have distended abdomens and cutaneous cranial ulcers. The kidney is enlarged with an opaque capsule with raised off-white nodules. Similar lesions are present in the heart, liver, spleen and muscle.[105] Channel catfish infected with *Exophiala* have dermal ulcers and soft nodules of varying sizes in the kidney and on other abdominal organs.[87] *Phoma*-infected Chinook salmon exhibited abnormal swimming behavior, exophthalmia, abdominal swelling, rounded areas of muscle softening and protruding hemorrhagic vents.[107]

Pathology: The renal nodules seen in Atlantic salmon infected with *Exophiala* sp. were granulomas with giant cell formation, though the amount of fungus present did not correlate to the extent of granulomas formed.[105] In phaeohyphomycosis caused by *E. salmonis* in Atlantic salmon, the posterior kidneys were swollen with an opaque capsule and raised areas on the surface that oozed a white opaque fluid when cut.[97] Histologically, the lesions resembled microabscesses rather than granulomas and contained fungal hyphae. In catfish infected with *Exophiala* sp., abscesses were present with fungal hyphae penetrating radially from the necrotic cores, although a surrounding granulomatous response was described with the presence of histiocytes and giant cells. The kidneys were the most frequently affected organ in cod infected with *Exophiala* sp. and contained well-organized granulomas with fungal hyphae radiating from the center.[100] The skin and kidney were the most frequently affected organs of weedy and leafy seadragons infected with *Exophiala* sp. and were characterized by well-demarcated dermal ulcers with raised, black margins and multiple well-demarcated black foci in the kidney, swim bladder, gills and intestinal wall. The kidneys were friable with extensive renal necrosis and intralesional pigmented hyphae.[99] *Ochroconis* sp.–infected fish had lesions similar to those caused by *Exophiala* sp. The primary site for *Phoma* appears to be the swim bladder, which is usually filled with fungal mycelium. It is hypothesized that the route of this systemic fungal infection is by the gastrointestinal tract to the swim bladder via the pneumatic duct with subsequent hematogenous distribution or direct extension to other organs.

Differential diagnoses: Several of the bacterial diseases resulting in granulomatous lesions such as bacterial kidney disease, mycobacteriosis and francisellosis with renal and systemic nodular lesions and cutaneous ulcers are differentials for phaeohyphomycosis. The pigmented lesions seen in some of the fungal infections may help differentiate them from the bacterial lesions.

Diagnosis: The diagnosis of phaeohyphomycosis is based on microscopic examination of the tissues. Etiological confirmation requires fungal cultures and possibly molecular methods if there are no distinguishing morphological fungal features.

Management/control: There are no approved antifungal agents for food fish. Several different antifungal agents have been tried in non-food fish but with limited results.[99] Phaeohyphomycosis is difficult to treat due to it recalcitrant nature, which may be enhanced by the melanin in the cell wall.[93] Since phaeohyphomycosis is usually secondary to stress and compromised immunity, management practices that reduce stress such as proper handling and optimal water quality may help reduce the incidence of phaeohyphomycosis.

NEPHROCALCINOSIS

Overview: Nephrocalcinosis results from the deposition of minerals (mainly calcium phosphate) in the collecting ducts and ureters of fish usually cultured in intensive systems.

Etiology: There are multiple noninfectious etiologies for nephrocalcinosis. There is an increased incidence and severity of nephrocalcinosis with hypercapnia or increased carbon dioxide in the water, with diets low in magnesium or high in minerals, as well as with diets high in selenium.[111–114] Nephrocalcinosis has also been reported in rainbow trout secondary to proliferative kidney disease.[115]

Route of transmission: Not applicable.

Host range: Nephrocalcinosis has been reported in salmonids (i.e., trout and salmon), wolffish and tilapia.[111,112,116,117]

Clinical presentation: Affected fish generally have no external lesions, although occasionally some may have abdominal distension and exophthalmos.[118]

Pathology: The kidneys of mildly affected fish have normal color and texture, but in the advanced cases of severely affected fish, the kidneys are swollen, gray with white mottling, and are firm and gritty in texture. Varying lengths of one or both ureters may be prominent due to off-white mineral casts (**Figure 12.10**). Severely affected fish usually also present with ascites and edema. There may be swelling caused by edema of the epaxial musculature

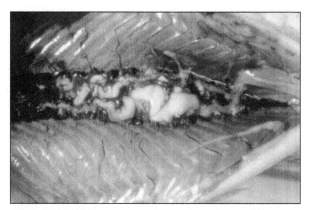

Figure 12.10 Nephrocalcinosis in the posterior kidney of a cultured Gila trout, *Oncorhynchus gilae*, where the ureters are dilated with a white granular material. (Image courtesy of S.A. Smith.)

with white granular foci and focal thickening of the stomach wall.[118] The earliest histological lesions are precipitation of calcium salts within the tubules and collecting ducts leading to tubular dilation and granuloma formation. Muscle lesions are only present in the most severely affected fish and consist of calcareous bodies or granulomas. The lesions in the muscle, stomach and renal interstitium are thought to be the result of deranged calcium metabolism.[118]

Differential diagnoses: Although fish with severe nephrocalcinosis may have kidneys that are swollen and discolored (i.e., mottled white and gray), which could be mistaken for several bacterial or fungal diseases. The prominence of the affected ureters and the grittiness of tissues due to deposition of minerals makes the gross clinical appearance of this disease unique.

Diagnosis: The diagnosis of nephrocalcinosis is based on gross and microscopic examination of the tissues.

Management/control: Prevention or management of the condition is by eliminating the cause(s) such as ensuring proper carbon dioxide levels as well as correct levels of minerals in the diets of fish.

NEPHROBLASTOMA

Overview: Primary renal neoplasms are relatively rare in fish but like higher vertebrates, the two most common forms are nephroblastomas and adenocarcinomas/adenomas.[119] Traditional nephroblastomas are embryonal tumors that arise in primitive nephrogenic blastema, however nephroblastomas in fish are not always embryonal and most (for instance, those in eel and koi) arise from the opistonephros or modified mesonephros.[120,121]

Etiology: Most fish nephroblastomas arise spontaneously, whereas others can be induced experimentally using carcinogens.[122,123] The exception is in the Japanese eel in which there are reported epizootics where carcinogens and other environmental factors as well as a viral etiology have been suspected but remain unproven.[120,123,124]

Route of transmission: Not applicable or unknown, as infectious etiology has not been proven.

Host range: Nephroblastomas have been reported in a wide variety of fish including Japanese eels, European eels, rainbow trout, striped bass, smelt, koi carp, crucian carp, Japanese dace, Siamese fighting fish, rose bitterling, banded cichlid and sockeye salmon.[119–121,125–129]

Clinical presentation: Fish with nephroblastomas may present with vertebral abnormalities such as lordosis as well as abdominal distension.

Pathology: Internally the visceral organs may be displaced by a large, firm, pale renal mass that may be attached to the dorsal body wall. Nephroblastomas are white to pale beige in color, and are firm or cystic with a granular texture.[119] Nephroblastomas are expansile, and in rare cases metastasis has been reported in crucian carp, Japanese dace, Japanese eels and rainbow trout. The tumor is frequently an unencapsulated, poorly demarcated mass with epithelial, mesenchymal and blastemal components that infiltrate the interstitium and replace the glomeruli and tubules. The blastemal component is usually small polygonal cells with scant cytoplasm and dense nuclei with indistinct nucleoli arranged in large rafts or islands. The mesenchymal elements are composed of whorls of stellate cells with scant cytoplasm and spindle-shaped nuclei. The mesenchymal component is sometimes differentiated into striated muscle, cartilage or bone.

Differential diagnoses: Differentials that might be higher on the list would be other renal neoplasms such as adenomas and carcinomas. However, any bacterial, fungal or metabolic disease that causes nodular lesions is a possible differential for nephroblastomas. Red oscars (*Astronotus ocellatus*) appear to have a predisposition for renal adenomas.[119]

Diagnosis: The diagnosis of nephroblastomas is based on histopathological examination of the tumor, which allows differentiation from other renal neoplasms (e.g., lymphoma/lymphosarcoma, carcinomas and adenomas) that have been reported in fish.[119]

Management/control: There are no management or control techniques, as most of these neoplasms are spontaneous except for those that are chemically induced.

POLYCYSTIC KIDNEY

Overview: Polycystic kidney disease in fish can be genetic, induced by pollutants or the sequelae of obstruction caused by parasites or space-occupying lesions. Some have suggested that the cystic lesions might actually be a precursor to cystadenomas seen in crucian carp.[130]

Etiology: This condition can be inherited, induced by chemicals or a result of physical obstruction.

Route of transmission: Inherited or induced by exposure to chemicals/pollutants.

Host range: Polycystic kidney disease has been reported in goldfish (*Carassius auratus*), medaka (*Oryzias latipes*), zebrafish (*Danio rerio*), flowerhorn fish (crossbred cichlid–three spot cichlid, *Cichlasoma trimaculatum*), guayas cichlid (*C. festae*) and Jingang blood parrot hybrid cichlid.[131–134]

Clinical presentation: Affected fish may display progressive anorexia and buoyancy problems. Fish may have distended abdomens and other fluid imbalance signs such as dermal edema with scale protrusion and exophthalmia.[134]

Pathology: Abdominal distension is caused by renomegaly and the affected kidneys are composed of large fluid-filled or empty cysts lined by attenuated epithelial cells. The other visceral organs are displaced and compressed by the enlarged kidney. Both the medaka and zebrafish models of polycystic kidney disease have altered cilia within the mesonephros and pronephros, respectively, that slow urine flow leading to cyst formation. This results in swollen renal tubules, fluid-filled cysts and abdominal distension that can be marked.

Differential diagnoses: Polycystic kidney disease in goldfish can be differentiated from kidney enlargement disease (KED) of goldfish by the absence of the causative agent, *Hoferellus carassii*, as well as the glomerular involvement in PKD. In KED the glomeruli are rarely if ever involved, whereas in PKD the glomeruli become cystic, although remnants of glomeruli are often found attached to the inner wall in these markedly dilated cystic structures.

Diagnosis: The diagnosis of PKD requires both gross and microscopic examination of the kidney and ruling out the other causes of polycystic kidney such as obstructions caused by parasites or space-occupying lesions.

Management/control: There are no management or control techniques for this condition except to avoid exposure to toxicants that can possibly induce the condition.

REFERENCES

1. Roberts, R.J. *The Bacteriology of Teleosts. Fish Pathology*, 3rd ed. Harcourt, London, 2001; pp. 297–331.
2. Bullock, G.L. and Herman, R.L. *Bacterial Kidney Disease of Salmonid Fishes Caused by Renibacterium Salmoninarum. Fish Disease Leaflet #78*. US Fish and Wildlife Service, Washington DC, 1988.
3. Kent, M.L., Traxler, G.S., Kieser, D., Richard, J., Dawe, S.C., Shaw, R.W., Prosperi-Porta, G., Ketcheson, J. and Evelyn, T.P. Survey of salmonid pathogens in ocean-caught fishes in British Columbia, Canada. *Journal of Aquatic Animal Health* 1998;10(2):211–219.
4. Paclibare, J.O., Albright, L.J. and Evelyn, T.P. Investigations on the occurrence of the kidney disease bacterium *Renibacterium salmoninarum* in non-salmonids on selected farms in British Columbia. *Bulletin of Aquaculture Association of Canada* 1988 July;88:113–115.
5. Fryer, J.L. and Sanders, J.E. Bacterial kidney disease of salmonid fish. *Annual Reviews in Microbiology* 1981;35(1):273–298.
6. Hawke, J.P., McWhorter, A.C., Steigerwalt, A.G. and Brenner, D.J. *Edwardsiella ictaluri* sp. nov., the causative agent of enteric septicemia of catfish. *International Journal of Systematic and Evolutionary Microbiology* 1981;31(4):396–400.
7. Baldwin, T.J. and Newton, J.C. Pathogenesis of enteric septicemia of channel catfish, caused by *Edwardsiella ictaluri*: Bacteriologic and light and electron microscopic findings. *Journal of Aquatic Animal Health* 1993;5(3):189–198.
8. Nusbaum, K.E. and Morrison, E.E. Entry of 35S-labeled *Edwardsiella ictaluri* into channel

catfish. *Journal of Aquatic Animal Health* 1996;8(2): 146–149.

9. Morrison, E.E. and Plumb, J.A. Olfactory organ of channel catfish as a site of experimental *Edwardsiella ictaluri* infection. *Journal of Aquatic Animal Health* 1994;6(2):101–109.

10. Menanteau-Ledouble, S., Karsi, A. and Lawrence, M.L. Importance of skin abrasion as a primary site of adhesion for *Edwardsiella ictaluri* and impact on invasion and systematic infection in channel catfish *Ictalurus punctatus*. *Veterinary Microbiology* 2011; 148(2):425–430.

11. Kasornchandra, J., Rogers, W.A. and Plumb, J.A. *Edwardsiella ictaluri* from walking catfish, *Clarias batrachus* L., in Thailand. *Journal of Fish Diseases* 1987; 10(2):137–138.

12. Suanyuk, N., Rogge, M., Thune, R., Watthana-phiromsakul, M., Champhat, N. and Wiangkum, W. Mortality and pathology of hybrid catfish, *Clarias macrocephalus* (Günther) × *Clarias gariepinus* (Burchell), associated with *Edwardsiella ictaluri* infection in southern Thailand. *Journal of Fish Diseases* 2014;37(4): 385–395.

13. Crumlish, M., Dung, T.T., Turnbull, J.F., Ngoc, N.T. and Ferguson, H.W. Identification of *Edwardsiella ictaluri* from diseased freshwater catfish, *Pangasius hypophthalmus* (Sauvage), cultured in the Mekong Delta, Vietnam. *Journal of Fish Diseases* 2002;25(12):733–736.

14. Liu, J.Y., Li, A.H., Zhou, D.R., Wen, Z.R. and Ye, X.P. Isolation and characterization of *Edwardsiella ictaluri* strains as pathogens from diseased yellow catfish *Pelteobagrus fulvidraco* (Richardson) cultured in China. *Aquaculture Research* 2010;41(12):1835–1844.

15. Sakai, T., Kamaishi, T., Sano, M., Tensha, K., Arima, T., Iida, Y., Nagai, T., Nakai, T. and Iida, T. Outbreaks of *Edwardsiella ictaluri* infection in ayu *Plecoglossus altivelis* in Japanese rivers. *Fish Pathology (Japan)* 2008; 43(4):152–157.

16. Soto, E., Griffin, M., Arauz, M., Riofrio, A., Martinez, A. and Cabrejos, M.E. *Edwardsiella ictaluri* as the causative agent of mortality in cultured Nile tilapia. *Journal of Aquatic Animal Health* 2012;24(2):81–90.

17. Kent, M.L. and Lyons, J.M. *Edwardsiella ictaluri* in the green knifefish, *Eigemannia virescens*. *Fish Health News* 1982;2, p. ii.

18. Humphrey, J.D., Lancaster, C., Gudkovs, N. and McDonald, W. Exotic bacterial pathogens *Edwardsiella tarda* and *Edwardsiella ictaluri* from imported ornamental fish *Betta splendens* and *Puntius conchonius*, respectively: Isolation and quarantine significance. *Australian Veterinary Journal* 1986;63(11):369–371.

19. Waltman, W.D., Shotts, E.B. and Blazer, V.S. Recovery of *Edwardsiella ictaluri* from danio (*Danio devario*). *Aquaculture* 1985;46(1):63–66.

20. Hawke, J.P., Kent, M., Rogge, M., Baumgartner, W., Wiles, J., Shelley, J., Savolainen, L.C., Wagner, R., Murray, K. and Peterson, T.S. Edwardsiellosis caused

by *Edwardsiella ictaluri* in laboratory populations of zebrafish *Danio rerio*. *Journal of Aquatic Animal Health* 2013;25(3):171–183.

21. Griffin, M.J., Ware, C., Quiniou, S.M., Steadman, J.M., Gaunt, P.S., Khoo, L.H. and Soto, E. *Edwardsiella piscicida* identified in the southeastern USA by gyrB sequence, species-specific and repetitive sequence-mediated PCR. *Diseases of Aquatic Organisms* 2014;108:23–35.

22. Reichley, S.R., Ware, C., Greenway, T.E., Wise, D.J. and Griffin, M.J. Real-time polymerase chain reaction assays for the detection and quantification of *Edwardsiella tarda*, *Edwardsiella piscicida*, and *Edwardsiella piscicida*–like species in catfish tissues and pond water. *Journal of Veterinary Diagnostic Investigation* 2015;27(2):130–139.

23. Fryer, J.L. and Hedrick, R.P. *Piscirickettsia salmonis*: A Gram-negative intracellular bacterial pathogen of fish. *Journal of Fish Diseases* 2003;26(5):251–262.

24. Almendras, F.E., Fuentealba, I.C., Jones, S.R., Markham, F. and Spangler, E. Experimental infection and horizontal transmission of *Piscirickettsia salmonis* in freshwater-raised Atlantic salmon, *Salmo salar* L. *Journal of Fish Diseases* 1997;20(6):409–418.

25. Rozas, M. and Enríquez, R. Piscirickettsiosis and *Piscirickettsia salmonis* in fish: A review. *Journal of Fish Diseases* 2014;37(3):163–188.

26. Chen, M.F., Yun, S., Marty, G.D., McDowell, T.S., House, M.L., Appersen, J.A., Guenther, T.A., Arkush, K.D. and Hedrick, R.P. A *Piscirickettsia salmonis*-like bacterium associated with mortality of white seabass *Atractoscion nobilis*. *Diseases of Aquatic Organisms* 2000;43(2):117–126.

27. McCarthy, U., Steiropoulos, N.A., Thompson, K.D., Adams, A., Ellis, A.E. and Ferguson, H.W. Confirmation of *Piscirickettsia salmonis* as a pathogen in European sea bass *Dicentrarchus labrax* and phylogenetic comparison with salmonid strains. *Diseases of Aquatic Organisms* 2005;64(2):107–119.

28. Mauel, M.J. and Miller, D.L. Piscirickettsiosis and piscirickettsiosis-like infections in fish: A review. *Veterinary Microbiology* 2002;87(4):279–289.

29. Olivares, J. and Marshall, S.H. Determination of minimal concentration of *Piscirickettsia salmonis* in water columns to establish a fallowing period in salmon farms. *Journal of Fish Diseases* 2010;33(3):261–266.

30. Birkbeck, T.H., Feist, S.W. and Verner–Jeffreys, D.W. *Francisella* infections in fish and shellfish. *Journal of Fish Diseases* 2011;34(3):173–187.

31. Colquhoun, D.J. and Duodu, S. *Francisella* infections in farmed and wild aquatic organisms. *Veterinary Research* 2011;42(45):1–5.

32. Ottem, K.F., Nylund, A., Karlsbakk, E., Friis-Møller, A. and Kamaishi, T. Elevation of *Francisella philomiragia* subsp. *noatunensis* Mikalsen et al. (2007) to *Francisella noatunensis* comb. nov. [syn. *Francisella piscicida* Ottem et al. (2008) syn. nov.] and characterization of *Francisella noatunensis* subsp. *orientalis* subsp.

nov., two important fish pathogens. *Journal of Applied Microbiology* 2009;106(4):1231–1243.

33. Olsen, A.B., Mikalsen, J., Rode, M., Alfjorden, A., Hoel, E., Straum-Lie, K., Haldorsen, R. and Colquhoun, D.J. A novel systemic granulomatous inflammatory disease in farmed Atlantic cod, *Gadus morhua* L., associated with a bacterium belonging to the genus *Francisella*. *Journal of Fish Diseases* 2006;29(5): 307–311.

34. Hsieh, C.Y., Tung, M.C., Tu, C., Chang, C.D. and Tsai, S.S. Enzootics of visceral granulomas associated with Francisella-like organism infection in tilapia (*Oreochromis* spp.). *Aquaculture* 2006;254(1): 129–138.

35. Kamaishi, T., Fukuda, Y., Nishiyama, M., Kawakami, H., Matsuyama, T., Yoshinaga, T. and Oseko, N. Identification and pathogenicity of intracellular *Francisella* bacterium in three-line grunt *Parapristipoma trilineatum*. *Fish Pathology* 2005;40(2):67–71.

36. Ostland, V.E., Stannard, J.A., Creek, J.J., Hedrick, R.P., Ferguson, H.W., Carlberg, J.M. and Westerman, M.E. Aquatic *Francisella*-like bacterium associated with mortality of intensively cultured hybrid striped bass *Morone chrysops* × *M. saxatilis*. *Diseases of Aquatic Organisms* 2006;72(2):135–145.

37. Camus, A.C., Dill, J.A., McDermott, A.J., Clauss, T.M., Berliner, A.L., Boylan, S.M. and Soto, E. *Francisella noatunensis* subsp. *orientalis* infection in Indo-Pacific reef fish entering the United States through the ornamental fish trade. *Journal of Fish Diseases* 2013;36(7):681–684.

38. Soto, E., Hawke, J.P., Fernandez, D. and Morales J, A. *Francisella* sp., an emerging pathogen of tilapia, *Oreochromis niloticus* (L.), in Costa Rica. *Journal of Fish Diseases* 2009;32(8):713–722.

39. Mauel, M.J., Soto, E., Moralis, J.A. and Hawke, J. A piscirickettsiosis-like syndrome in cultured Nile tilapia in Latin America with *Francisella* spp. as the pathogenic agent. *Journal of Aquatic Animal Health* 2007;19(1): 27–34.

40. Soto, E., Baumgartner, W., Wiles, J. and Hawke, J.P. *Francisella asiatica* as the causative agent of piscine francisellosis in cultured tilapia (*Oreochromis* sp.) in the United States. *Journal of Veterinary Diagnostic Investigation* 2011;23(4):821–825.

41. Chern, R.S. and Chao, C.B. Outbreak of a disease caused by rickettsia-like organism in cultured tilapias in Taiwan. *Fish Pathology* 1994;29:61–71.

42. Decostere, A., Hermans, K. and Haesebrouck, F. Piscine mycobacteriosis: A literature review covering the agent and the disease it causes in fish and humans. *Veterinary Microbiology* 2004;99(3):159–166.

43. Gauthier, D.T. and Rhodes, M.W. Mycobacteriosis in fishes: A review. *The Veterinary Journal* 2009;180(1): 33–47.

44. Conroy, D.A. Observaciones sobre cases espontáneos de tuberculosis ictica. *Microbiologia Española* 1966;19:93–113.

45. Astrofsky, K.M., Schrenzel, M.D., Bullis, R.A., Smolowitz, R.M. and Fox, J.G. Diagnosis and management of atypical *Mycobacterium* spp. infections in established laboratory zebrafish (*Brachydanio rerio*) facilities. *Comparative Medicine* 2000;50(6):666–672.

46. Jacobs, J.M., Stine, C.B., Baya, A.M. and Kent, M.L. A review of mycobacteriosis in marine fish. *Journal of Fish Diseases* 2009;32(2):119–130.

47. Hedrick, R.P., McDowell, T. and Groff, J. Mycobacteriosis in cultured striped bass from California. *Journal of Wildlife Diseases* 1987;23(3):391–395.

48. Hughes, K.P., Duncan, R.B. and Smith, S.A. Renomegaly associated with a mycobacterial infection in summer flounder, *Paralichthys dentatus*. *Fish Pathology* 2002;37:83–86.

49. Lowry, T.L. and Smith, S.A. *Mycobacterium* sp. in cultured cobia. *Bulletin of the European Association of Fish Pathologists* 2006;26(2):87–92.

50. Frerichs, G.N. Mycobacteriosis: Nocardiosis. In: *Bacterial Diseases of Fish*. V. Inglis, R.J. Roberts and N.R. Bromage, eds. Blackwell, Oxford, UK, 1993; pp. 219–233.

51. Wolf, J.C. and Smith, S.A. Comparative severity of experimentally induced mycobacteriosis in striped bass *Morone saxatilis* and hybrid tilapia *Oreochromis* spp. *Diseases of Aquatic Organisms* 1999;38(3): 191–200.

52. Mainous, M.E. and Smith, S.A. Efficacy of common disinfectants against *Mycobacterium marinum*. *Journal of Aquatic Animal Health* 2005;17(3):284–288.

53. Canning, E.U., Tops, S., Curry, A., Wood, T.S. and Okamura, B. (Ecology, development and pathogenicity of *Buddenbrockia plumatellae* Schröder, 1910 (Myxozoa, Malacosporea)(syn. *Tetracapsula bryozoides*) and establishment of *Tetracapsuloides* n. gen. for *Tetracapsula bryosalmonae*. *Journal of Eukaryotic Microbiology* 2002;49(4):280–295.

54. Abd-Elfattah, A., Fontes, I., Kumar, G., Soliman, H., Hartikainen, H., Okamura, B. and El-Matbouli, M. Vertical transmission of *Tetracapsuloides bryosalmonae* (Myxozoa), the causative agent of salmonid proliferative kidney disease. *Parasitology* 2014;141(4): 482–490.

55. Hedrick, R.P., MacConnell, E. and De Kinkelin, P. Proliferative kidney disease of salmonid fish. *Annual Review of Fish Diseases* 1993;3:277–290.

56. Hedrick, R.P., Marin, M., Castagnaro, M., Monge, D. and de Kinkelin, P. Rapid lectin-based staining procedure for the detection of the myxosporean causing proliferative kidney disease in salmonid fish. *Diseases of Aquatic Organisms* 1992;13(2):129–132.

57. Molnár, K., Csaba, G. and Kovacs-Gayer, E. Study of the postulated identity of *Hoferellus cyprini* (Doflein, 1898) and *Mitraspora cyprini* Fujita, 1912. *Acta Veterinaria Hungarica* 1986;34:175–181.

58. Trouillier, A., El-Matbouli, M. and Hoffman, R.W. A new look at the life cycle of *Hoferellus carassii* in the goldfish (*Carassius auratus auratus*) and its

relation to "kidney enlargement disease" (KED). *Folia Parasitologica* 1996;43:173–187.

59. Ahmed, A.T.A. Kidney enlargement disease in goldfish in Japan. *Japanese Journal of Zoology* 1973;17:37–57.

60. El-Matbouli, M., Fischer-Scherl, T. and Hoffmann, R.W. Present knowledge on the life cycle, taxonomy, pathology, and therapy of some Myxosporea spp. important for Freshwater Fish. *Annual Review of Fish Diseases* 1992;2:367–402.

61. Alama-Bermejo, G., Jirků, M., Kodádková, A., Pecková, H., Fiala, I. and Holzer, A.S. Species complexes and phylogenetic lineages of *Hoferellus* (Myxozoa, Cnidaria) including revision of the genus: A problematic case for taxonomy. *Parasites & Vectors* 2016;9:13.

62. Yokoyama, H., Ogawa, K. and Wakabayashi, H. Involvement of *Branchiura sowerbyi* (Oligocheta: Annelida) in the transmission of *Hoferellus carassii* (Myxosporea: Myxozoa) the causative agent of kidney enlargement disease (KED) of goldfish *Carassius auratus*. *Gyobo Kenkyu* 1993;28(3):135–139.

63. Molnár, K., Fischer-Scherl, T., Baska, F. and Hoffmann, R.W. Hoferellosis in goldfish *Carassius auratus* and gibel carp *Carassius auratus gibelio*. *Diseases of Aquatic Organisms* 1989;7:89–95.

64. Feist, S.W. Pathogenicity of renal myxospreams of fish. *Bulletin of the European Association of Fish Pathologists* 1997;17(6):209–212.

65. Petrie-Hanson, L. First reported mortality and associated pathology attributed to *Acolpenteron ureteroecetes* in largemouth bass. *Journal of Aquatic Animal Health* 2001;13(4):364–367.

66. Du Plessis, S.S. A gyrodactyloid parasite from the ureters of largemouth bass at the Jonkershoek Inland Fish Hatchery, South Africa. *Transactions of the American Fisheries Society* 1948;75(1):105–109.

67. Fischthal, J.H. and Allison, L.N. *Acolpenteron catostomi* n. sp. (Gyrodactyloidea: Calceostomatidae), a monogenetic trematode from the ureters of suckers, with observations on its life history and that of *A. ureteroecetes*. *Transactions of the American Microscopical Society* 1942;61(1):53–56.

68. Viozzi, G.P. and Brugni, N.L. *Acolpenteron australe* sp. n. (Dactylogyridae: Dactylogyrinae), a new species from the ureters of *Percichthys trucha* (Perciformes: Percichthyidae) in Patagonia (Argentina). *Folia Parasitologica* 2003;50(2):105–108.

69. Fischthal, J.H. and Allison, L.N. *Acolpenteron ureteroecetes* ng, n. sp., a monogenetic trematode from the ureters of black basses. *Journal of Parasitology* 1940;26(Suppl.):34–35.

70. Boeger, W.A., Tanaka, L.K. and Pavanelli, G.C. Neotropical Monogenoidea. 39: A new species of *Kritskyia* (Dactylogyridae, Ancyrocephalinae) from the ureters and urinary bladder of *Serrasalmus marginatus* and *S. spilopleura* (Characiformes, Serrasalmidae) from southern Brazil with an emended generic diagnosis. *Zoosystema-Paris* 2001;23(1):5–10.

71. Takemoto, R.M., Lizama, M.D. and Pavanelli, G.C. A new species of *Kritskyia* (Dactylogyridae, Ancyrocephalinae) parasite of urinary bladder of *Prochilodus lineatus* (Prochilodontidae, Characiformes) from the floodplain of the high Paraná river, Brazil. *Memórias do Instituto Oswaldo Cruz* 2002;97(3):313–315.

72. Fayton, T.J. and Kritsky, D.C. *Acolpenteron willifordensis* n. sp. (Monogenoidea: Dactylogyridae) parasitic in the kidney and ureters of the spotted sucker *Minytrema melanops* (Rafinesque) (Cypriniformes: Catostomidae) from Econfina Creek, Florida. *Comparative Parasitology* 2013;80(1):1–8.

73. Guidelli, G.M., Takemoto, R.M. and Pavanelli, G.C. A new species of *Kritskyia* (Dactylogyridae, Ancyrocephalinae), parasite of urinary bladder and ureters of *Leporinus lacustris* (Characiformes, Anostomidae) from Brazil. *Acta Scientiarum* 2003;25(2):279–282.

74. Kohn, A. *Kritskyia moraveci* n. g., n. sp. (Monogenea: Dactylogyridae) from the urinary bladder and ureters of *Rhamdia quelen* (Quoy and Gaimard, 1824) (Pisces: Pimelodidae) in Brazil. *Systemic Parasitology* 1990;17:81–85.

75. Viozzi, G. and Gutiérrez, P. *Philureter trigoniopsis*, a new genus and species (Dactylogyridae, Ancyrocephalinae) from the ureters and urinary bladder of *Galaxias maculatus* (Osmeriformes: Galaxiidae) in Patagonia (Argentina). *Journal of Parasitology* 2001;87:392–394.

76. Gieseker, C.M., Serfling, S.G., Poynton, S.L. and Reimschuessel, R. Laboratory transmission of the monogenean *Acolpenteron ureteroecetes* infecting the posterior kidneys of largemouth bass: Time course and pathology. *Journal of Aquatic Animal Health* 2007;19(3):141–150.

77. Ito, T. and Maeno, Y. Susceptibility of Japanese Cyprininae fish species to cyprinid herpesvirus 2 (CyHV-2). *Veterinary Microbiology* 2014;169(3):128–134.

78. Jung, S.J. and Miyazaki, T. Herpesviral haematopoietic necrosis of goldfish, *Carassius auratus* (L.). *Journal of Fish Diseases* 1995;18(3):211–220.

79. Goodwin, A.E., Sadler, J., Merry, G.E. and Marecaux, E.N. Herpesviral haematopoietic necrosis virus (CyHV-2) infection: Case studies from commercial goldfish farms. *Journal of Fish Diseases* 2009;32(3):271–278.

80. Ito, T. and Maeno, Y. Effects of experimentally induced infections of goldfish *Carassius auratus* with cyprinid herpesvirus 2 (CyHV-2) at various water temperatures. *Diseases of Aquatic Organisms* 2014;110:193–200.

81. Waltzek, T.B., Kelley, G.O., Stone, D.M., Way, K., Hanson, L., Fukuda, H., Hirono, I., Aoki, T., Davison, A.J. and Hedrick, R.P. Koi herpesvirus represents a third cyprinid herpesvirus (CyHV-3) in the family Herpesviridae. *Journal of General Virology* 2005;86(6):1659–1667.

82. Goodwin, A.E., Merry, G.E. and Sadler, J. Detection of the herpesviral hematopoietic necrosis disease

agent (Cyprinid herpesvirus 2) in moribund and healthy goldfish: Validation of a quantitative PCR diagnostic method. *Diseases of Aquatic Organisms* 2006;69:137–143.

83. Waltzek, T.B., Kurobe, T., Goodwin, A.E. and Hedrick, R.P. Development of a polymerase chain reaction assay to detect cyprinid herpesvirus 2 in goldfish. *Journal of Aquatic Animal Health* 2009;21(1):60–67.

84. Ma, J., Jiang, N., LaPatra, S.E., Jin, L., Xu, J., Fan, Y., Zhous, Y. and Zeng, L. Establishment of a novel and highly permissive cell line for the efficient replication of cyprinid herpes virus 2 (CyHV-2). *Veterinary Microbiology* 2015;177:315–325.

85. Hedrick, R.P., Waltzek, T.B. and McDowell, T.S. Susceptibility of koi carp, common carp, goldfish, and goldfish × common carp hybrids to cyprinid herpesvirus-2 and herpesvirus-3. *Journal of Aquatic Animal Health* 2006;18(1):26–34.

86. Plumb, J.A. Effects of temperature on mortality of fingerling channel catfish (*Ictalurus punctatus*) experimentally infected with channel catfish virus. *Journal of the Fisheries Research. Board of Canada* 1973;30:568–570.

87. Plumb, J.A. Epizootiology of channel catfish virus disease. *Marine Fisheries Review* 1978;40(3):26–29.

88. Hanson, L., Dishon, A. and Kotler, M. Herpesviruses that infect fish. *Viruses* 2011;3(11):2160–2191.

89. Fijan, N.N. Systemic mycosis in channel catfish. *Bulletin of the Wildlife Disease Association* 1969;5(2):109–110.

90. Plumb, J.A., Gaines, J.L., Mora, E.C. and Bradley, G.G. Histopathology and electron microscopy of channel catfish virus in infected channel catfish, *Ictalurus punctatus* (Rafinesque). *Journal of Fish Biology* 1974;6:661–664.

91. Major, R.D., McCraren, J.P. and Smith, C.E. Histopathological changes in channel catfish (*Ictalurus punctatus*) experimentally and naturally infected with channel catfish virus disease. *Journal of the Fisheries Board of Canada* 1975;32(4):563–567.

92. Hoog GS, D., Vicente, V.A., Najafzadeh, M.J., Harrak, M.J., Badali, H. and Seyedmousavi, S. Waterborne *Exophiala* species causing disease in cold-blooded animals. *Persoonia-Molecular Phylogeny and Evolution of Fungi* 2011;27(1):46–72.

93. Seyedmousavi, S., Guillot, J. and De Hoog, G.S. Phaeohyphomycoses, emerging opportunistic diseases in animals. *Clinical Microbiology Reviews* 2013;26(1):19–35.

94. Langvad, F., Pedersen, O. and Engjom, K. A fungal disease caused by *Exophiala* sp. nova in farmed Atlantic salmon in Western Norway. In: *Fish and Shellfish Pathology*. F. Langvad, O. Pederson and K. Engjom, eds. Academic Press, London, 1985; pp. 323–328.

95. Pedersen, O.A. and Langvad, F. *Exophiala psychrophila* sp. nov., a pathogenic species of the black yeasts isolated from farmed Atlantic salmon. *Mycological Research* 1989;92(2):153–156.

96. Richards, R.H., Holliman, A. and Helgason, S. *Exophiala salmonis* infection in Atlantic salmon *Salmo salar* L. *Journal of Fish Diseases* 1978;1(4):357–368.

97. Otis, E.J., Wolke, R.E. and Blazer, V.S. Infection of *Exophiala salmonis* in Atlantic salmon (*Salmo salar* L.). *Journal of Wildlife Diseases* 1985;21(1):61–64.

98. McGinnis, M.R. and Ajello, L. A new species of *Exophiala* isolated from channel catfish. *Mycologia* 1974;66(3):518–520.

99. Nyaoke, A., Weber, E.S., Innis, C. et al. Disseminated phaeohyphomycosis in weedy seadragons (*Phyllopteryx taeniolatus*) and leafy seadragons (*Phycodurus eques*) caused by species of *Exophiala*, including a novel species. *Journal of Veterinary Diagnostic Investigation* 2009;21(1):69–79.

100. Gjessing, M.C., Davey, M., Kvellestad, A. and Vrålstad, T. *Exophiala angulospora* causes systemic inflammation in Atlantic cod *Gadus morhua*. *Diseases of Aquatic Organisms* 2011;96(3):209.

101. Doty, M.S. and Slater, D.W. A new species of *Heterosporium* pathogenic on young chinook salmon. *American Midland Naturalist* 1946;36(3):663–665.

102. Ross, A.J. and Yasutake, W.T. *Scolecobasidium humicola*, a fungal pathogen of fish. *Journal of the Fisheries Board of Canada* 1973;30(7):994–995.

103. Ajello, L., McGinnis, M.R. and Camper, J. An outbreak of phaeohyphomycosis in rainbow trout caused by *Scolecobasidium humicola*. *Mycopathologia* 1977;62(1): 15–22.

104. Hatai, K. and Kubota, S.S. A visceral mycosis in cultured masu salmon (*Oncorhynchus masou*) caused by a species of *Ochroconis*. *Journal of Wildlife Diseases* 1989;25(1):83–88.

105. Ross, A.J., Yasutake, W.T. and Leek, S. *Phoma herbarum*, a fungal plant saprophyte, as a fish pathogen. *Journal of the Fisheries Board of Canada* 1975;32(9): 1648–1652.

106. Hatai, K., Fujimaki, Y., Egusa, S. and Jo, Y. A visceral mycosis in ayu fry, *Plecoglossus altivelis* Temminck & Schlegel, caused by a species of *Phoma*. *Journal of Fish Diseases* 1986;9(2):111–116.

107. Faisal, M., Elsayed, E., Fitzgerald, S.D., Silva, V. and Mendoza, L. Outbreaks of phaeohyphomycosis in the chinook salmon (*Oncorhynchus tshawytscha*) caused by *Phoma herbarum*. *Mycopathologia* 2007;163(1):41–48.

108. Kanchan, C., Muraosa, Y. and Hatai, K. *Exophiala angulospora* infection found in cultured Japanese flounder *Paralichthys olivaceus* in Japan. *Bulletin of the European Association of Fish Pathologists* 2014;34(5):187–194.

109. Munchan, C., Kurata, O., Hatai, K., Hashiba, N., Nakaoka, N. and Kawakami, H. Mass mortality of young striped jack *Pseudocaranx dentex* caused by a fungus *Ochroconis humicola*. *Fish Pathology (Japan)* 2006;41(4):179–182.

110. Wada, S., Hanjavanit, C., Kurata, O. and Hatai, K. *Ochroconis humicola* infection in red sea bream *Pagrus major* and marbled rockfish *Sebastiscus marmoratus* cultured in Japan. *Fisheries Science* 2005;71(3):682–684.

111. Smart, G.R., Knox, D., Harrison, J.G., Ralph, J.A., Richard, R.H. and Cowey, C.B. Nephrocalcinosis in

rainbow trout *Salmo gairdneri* Richardson; the effect of exposure to elevated CO_2 concentrations. *Journal of Fish Diseases* 1979;2(4):279–289.

112. Foss, A., Røsnes, B.A. and Øiestad, V. Graded environmental hypercapnia in juvenile spotted wolffish (*Anarhichas minor* Olafsen): Effects on growth, food conversion efficiency and nephrocalcinosis. *Aquaculture* 2003;220(1):607–617.

113. Cowey, C.B., Knox, D., Adron, J.W., George, S. and Pirie, B. The production of renal calcinosis by magnesium deficiency in rainbow trout (*Salmo gairdneri*). *British Journal of Nutrition* 1977;38(1):127–135.

114. Hicks, B.D., Hilton, J.W. and Ferguson, H.W. Influence of dietary selenium on the occurrence of nephrocalcinosis in the rainbow trout, *Salmo gairdneri* Richardson. *Journal of Fish Diseases* 1984;7(5):379–389.

115. Ferguson, H.W. and Needham, E.A. Proliferative kidney disease in rainbow trout *Salmo gairdneri* Richardson. *Journal of Fish Diseases* 1978;1(1):91–108.

116. Chen, C.Y., Wooster, G.A., Getchell, R.G., Bowser, P.R. and Timmons, M.B. Blood chemistry of healthy, nephrocalcinosis-affected and ozone-treated tilapia in a recirculation system, with application of discriminant analysis. *Aquaculture* 2003;218(1):89–102.

117. Fivelstad, S., Olsen, A.B., Kløften, H., Ski, H. and Stefansson, S. Effects of carbon dioxide on Atlantic salmon (*Salmo salar* L.) smolts at constant pH in bicarbonate rich freshwater. *Aquaculture* 1999; 178(1):171–187.

118. Harrison, J.G. and Richards, R.H. The pathology and histopathology of nephrocalcinosis in rainbow trout *Salmo gairdneri* Richardson in fresh water. *Journal of Fish Diseases* 1979;2(1):1–12.

119. Lombardini, E.D., Hard, G.C. and Harshbarger, J.C. Neoplasms of the urinary tract in fish. *Veterinary Pathology* 2014;51(5):1000–1012.

120. Masahito, P., Ishikawa, T., Okamoto, N. and Sugano, H. Nephroblastomas in the Japanese eel, Anguilla japonica Temminck and Schlegel. *Cancer Research* 1992;52(9):2575–2579.

121. Stegeman, N., Heatley, J.J., Rodrigues, A. and Pool, R. Nephroblastoma in a koi (*Cyprinus carpio*). *Journal of Exotic Pet Medicine* 2010;19(4):298–303.

122. Kimura, I. Studies on carcinogenesis and tumors of lower animals. *Igakuno-ayumi* 1976;96:216–225.

123. Miyazaki, T. and Hyakkoku, N. A histopathological study on nephroblastomas of the Japanese eel. *Bulletin of the Faculty of Fisheries, Mie University* 1978;14: 21–32.

124. Ueno, Y., Chen, S.N., Kou, G.H., Hedrick, R.P. and Fryer, J.L. Characterization of a virus isolated from Japanese eels (*Anguilla japonica*) with nephroblastoma. *Bulletin of the Institute of Zoology, Academa Sinica* 1984;23(1):47–55.

125. Odense, P.H., Logan, V.H. and Baker, S.R. Spontaneous nephroblastoma in a rainbow trout (*Salmo gairdneri*). *Journal of the Fisheries Board of Canada* 1973;30(4):549–551.

126. Helmsoldt, C. and Wyand, D.S. Nephroblastoma in a striped bass. *Journal of Wildlife Diseases* 1971;7(3): 162–165.

127. Huizinga, H.W. and Budd, J. Nephroblastoma in the smelt, *Osmerus mordax* (Mitchill). *Journal of Fish Diseases* 1983;6(4):389–391.

128. Lombardini, E.D., Law, M. and Lewis, B.S. Nephroblastoma in two Siamese fighting fish *Betta splendens*. *Fish Pathology* 2010;45(3):137–139.

129. Grizzle, J.M., Bunkley-Williams, L. and Harshbarger, J.C. Renal adenocarcinoma in Mozambique tilapia, neurofibroma in goldfish, and osteosarcoma in channel catfish from a Puerto Rican hatchery. *Journal of Aquatic Animal Health* 1995;7(2):178–183.

130. Hoole, D., Bucke, D., Burgess, P. and Wellby, I. Noninfectious diseases. In: *Diseases of Carp and Other Cyprinid Fishes*. Blackwell Science, Oxford, UK, 2001; pp. 134–135.

131. Munkittrick, K.R., Moccia, R.D. and Leatherland, J.F. Polycystic kidney disease in goldfish (*Carassius auratus*) from Hamilton Harbour, Lake Ontario, Canada. *Veterinary Pathology Online* 1985;22(3):232–237.

132. Mochizuki, E., Fukuta, K., Tada, T., Harada, T., Watanabe, N., Matsuo, S., Hashimoto, H., Ozato, K. and Wakamatsu, Y. Fish mesonephric model of polycystic kidney disease in medaka (*Oryzias latipes*) pc mutant. *Kidney International* 2005;68(1):23–34.

133. Gill, J.M. Polycystic kidney disease in goldfish (*Carassius auratus*). *New Zealand Veterinary Journal* 1994;42(2):77.

134. Rahmati-Holasoo, H., Ebrahimzadeh Mousavi, H., Vajhi, A., Shokrpoor, S., Tavakkoli, A., Mirdamadi, M.A. and Fayyaz, S. Polycystic liver in flower horn fish, hybrid cichlid. *Journal of Fish Diseases* 2015; 38(3):325–328.

CHAPTER 13

SWIM BLADDER DISORDERS

ALISA L. NEWTON

INFECTIOUS DISEASES OF THE SWIM BLADDER

General bacterial and fungal infections

Overview: The swim bladder is a common target of infectious disease conditions. Primary bacterial and fungal infections due to direct invasion of the pneumatic duct occur in physostomes. The highly vascular gas gland (i.e., rete mirabile) present in physoclists and many physostomes can serve as a site of bacterial entrapment or thromboembolism, making the swim bladder a common site of secondary bacterial and fungal spread during systemic infection.[1]

Etiology: A wide variety of Gram-negative and Gram-positive bacteria have been implicated in infections of the swim bladder including acid-fast *Mycobacterium* spp. Swim bladder infection is a common feature of primary *Nocardia seriolae* infection of cultured Japanese yellowtail (*Seriola quinqueradiata*).[2] Reports of opportunistic fungal infection with a similarly wide variety of ubiquitous hyphomycetes, coelomycetes, eumycetes and oomycetes abound in the literature.

Route of transmission: Primary pneumatic duct exposure can occur secondary to ingestion of bacteria or fungal spores/hyphae in food, detritus, cannibalism of infected fish, airborne aspiration, or aspiration of contaminated water.[3] Within aquaculture facilities, management practices that move fish too rapidly to a larger pellet size can result in esophageal obstructions in smaller fish at the level of the pneumatic duct promoting access to the swim bladder.[4] Trauma or the practice of intentional puncture of the swim bladder to relieve distention secondary to barometric pressure shifts can result in direct infection of the swim bladder lumen.[5] Many bacterial and fungal opportunists demonstrate a propensity for vascular invasion, which can lead to local thrombosis and thromboembolic showers that allow seeding of the gas gland.

Host range: All species of fish are potentially susceptible to infection of the swim bladder. Infections are more common in fishes intensively raised in aquaculture due to the frequent presence of other environmental stressors that alter physiology and immune function making fish more susceptible to disease.[1]

Exophiala sp., *Paecilomyces* sp. and *Saprolegnia* sp. are commonly reported systemic fungal pathogens that can result in secondary aerocystitis in marine and freshwater fishes. Primary swim bladder infection with *Verticillum lecanii*, Amylomyces sp., *Rhizopus* sp., *Absidia* sp. and *Mucor* sp. has been reported in Atlantic salmon (*Salmo salar*).[3,6] A case report of primary *Exophiala xenobiotica* aerocystitis has been published in a captive Queensland grouper (*Epinephelus lanceolatus*).[7] Other reported primary and secondary systemic infections resulting in fungal aerocystitis include *Cladosporium cladosporiodes*, *Scopulariopsis brumptii* and *Ochroconis humicola* in Australian barramundi cod (*Cromileptes altivelis*), *Penicillium corylophilum* and *Cladosporium spharospermum* in wild caught red snapper (*Lutjanus campechanus*).[5,8] *Sporobolomyces salmonicolor* has been reported to cause aerocystitis as part of visceral mycosis in Chinook salmon fry (*Oncorhynchus tshawytscha*) from a cold-water hatchery.[9] *Phialophora* spp. infection is reported in Atlantic salmon and rainbow trout (*Oncorhynchus mykiss*) as primary and secondary infections at low temperatures.

Clinical presentation: Nonspecific signs such as anorexia, lethargy, and abnormal or negative buoyancy are the most frequent clinical presentations. Coelomic distention and skin hyperpigmentation are also common findings. Fish may lay on the bottom and only swim when stimulated. They may also

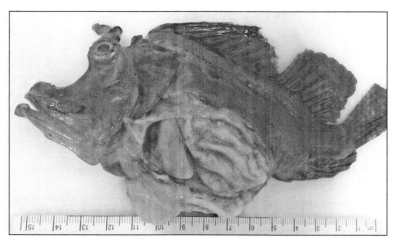

Figure 13.1 Bacterial aerocystitis in a weedy scorpionfish (*Rhinopias frondosa*). Diffuse thickening, yellow discoloration, opacification, and distention of the swim bladder due to a secondary bacterial infection. (Image courtesy of K. Heym.)

be unable to surface to feed. Signs of bacterial sepsis or systemic fungal infection may also be present including multifocal petechial hemorrhages of the skin and fins.[1,2,4]

Pathology: Chronic bacterial and fungal aerocystitis results in diffuse thickening and opacification of the swim bladder wall, filling of the swim bladder lumen with tan to yellow inflammatory debris, and serosanguineous coelomic effusion due to extension of the inflammatory process through the swim bladder wall (**Figure 13.1**). In acute infections, a progression of changes from minimal multifocal serosal hemorrhage, to mild fluid accumulation and luminal fibrin deposition, to accumulations of inflammatory debris and gas gland and mucosal proliferation may be seen (**Figures 13.2** through **13.6**). With fungal infections, a green to brown to black discoloration of the luminal debris or overt fungal mats may sometimes be seen (**Figure 13.7**). An exception is *Phialophora* spp. fungal infection in Atlantic salmon parr, which results in minimal secondary inflammation.[10] The infectious agent may be evident within inflammatory cells, cellular infiltrates or the swim bladder lumen. Fibrosis, fibroplasia and neovascularization within the swim bladder wall all contribute to increased opacity (**Figure 13.8**).

Differential diagnosis: Differential diagnoses include other diseases that result in buoyancy abnormalities such as swim bladder rupture, neoplasia, or other causes of coelomic distention and effusion

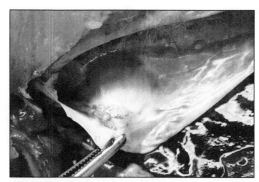

Figure 13.2 Bacterial aerocystitis in a French grunt (*Haemulon flavolineatum*) with mild swim bladder inflammation. A thin exudate overlies the vascular rete. (Image courtesy of C. Rodrigues.)

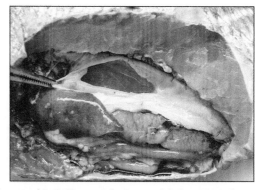

Figure 13.3 Bacterial aerocystitis in a French grunt (*Haemulon flavolineatum*) with severe swim bladder infection and effusion. (Image courtesy of C. Rodrigues.)

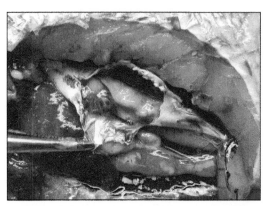

Figure 13.4 Bacterial aerocystitis in a French grunt (*Haemulon flavolineatum*) with severe swim bladder infection and caseous luminal exudate due to primary infection and *Photobacterium damselae*. (Image courtesy of C. Rodrigues.)

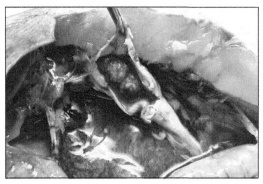

Figure 13.5 Bacterial aerocystitis in a blue striped grunt (*Haemulon sciurus*) with severe granulomatous inflammation of the vascular rete. (Image courtesy of C. Rodrigues.)

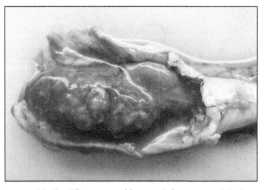

Figure 13.6 Close-up of bacterial aerocystitis in a blue striped grunt (*Haemulon sciurus*) with severe granulomatous inflammation. (Images courtesy of C. Rodrigues.)

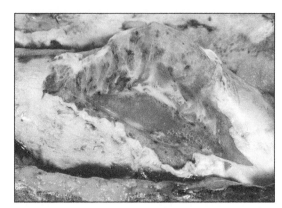

Figure 13.7 Fungal infections with effusion in swim bladder of an adult striped catfish (*Pangasius hypothalamus*). (Image courtesy of S.A. Smith.)

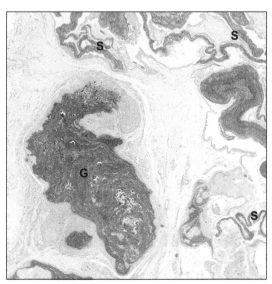

Figure 13.8 Fungal aerocystitis in an amberjack (*Seriola spp.*) showing severe granulomatous inflammation (G) of the swim bladder wall (S) with marked proliferation of the swim bladder lining. H&E stain. (Image courtesy of K. Conley.)

such as cardiac, renal, or hepatic disease and organ failure.

Diagnosis: Radiography may reveal a distended swim bladder with variable radiodensity/decreased radiolucency and potentially a detectable fluid line with horizontal beam projections. Ultrasound may reveal similar changes in echogenicity and can facilitate guided aspiration of the swim bladder lumen. Specialized techniques such as magnetic resonance imaging (MRI) and computer assisted tomography (CAT scan) are possible but infrequently performed.[11] Swim bladder aspiration may be a useful diagnostic tool for any swim bladder disease with and without other diagnostic imaging. Except for some deep water species that utilize lipids for buoyancy, aspiration of an uninfected swim bladder should recover only gas. Recovery of any type of fluid should be considered abnormal and the recovered fluid should be utilized for bacterial and fungal culture as well as direct microscopy and stained cytology. Culture in Sabouraud dextrose broth and plating onto Sabouraud dextrose agar (SDA), Mycosel agar (MAT), potato dextrose agar (PDA), or polymerase chain reaction (PCR) of the internal transcribed spacer (ITS) and D1/D2 regions may allow for definitive bacterial or fungal identification.

Management/control: Treatment of individual fish should employ appropriate antifungal or antibiotic therapies based on culture and sensitivity results. In acute bacterial infections prognosis is favorable in the absence of signs of sepsis. Prognosis is generally poor with chronic infections despite appropriate antimicrobial treatments.[4] Fungal infections are often more refractory to treatment. Removal of the inflammatory effusion and direct introduction of antimicrobial treatments into the swim bladder lumen may provide a method of direct access of the antibiotic to the site of infection. With chronic infections, surgical exploration, aerocystotomy and removal of inflammatory debris from the swim bladder lumen may be required. Within hatchery populations the focus is on prevention versus antimicrobial treatment. This includes keeping raceways clean, using appropriate-sized feed, proper frequent cleaning of mechanical feeders and proper storage of feeds.[3]

Phomamycosis

Overview: Phomamycosis is a primary fungal infection reported sporadically in hatchery-reared young Chinook salmon (*Oncorhyncus tshawytscha*), coho salmon (*Oncorhyncus kisutch*) and rainbow trout (*Oncorhyncus mykiss*) in the Pacific Northwest.[12] Synonyms for this infection include coelomycosis, swim bladder disease, air bladder disease and swollen vent disease.[4]

Etiology: *Phoma herbarum* is a coelomycete fungus known to be a saprophyte of a wide range of organic materials including soil, plants and sewage. It is a rare cause of phaeohyphomycosis in humans and animals.

Route of transmission: The distribution of lesions in infected fish suggests that the swim bladder is the primary site of exposure.[3,12,13] The route of infection is hypothesized to be aspiration of fungal spores through the pneumatic duct during the initial filling of the swim bladder.

Host range: The host range includes hatchery-reared young Chinook and coho salmon and rainbow trout in the Pacific Northwest. Infection has also been reported in farmed ayu (*Plecoglossues altivelis*).[14] The disease generally impacts only fry and fingerlings less than 100 days old and morbidity is typically low.[2]

Clinical presentation: In the acute infection, fish may be seen resting on their side and will swim only when stimulated. Abnormal swimming behavior (swimming on the side or semi-vertical), loss of equilibrium, exophthalmia, focal body wall discoloration/myonecrosis, protrusion of the vent and red discoloration are all consistent clinical signs.[1,2,12,13]

Pathology: Gross lesions are confined to the swim bladder with evidence of local and visceral spread in advanced cases. Numerous small white foci may be present early in the infection at the anterior pole of the swim bladder near the entry of the pneumatic duct. In advanced infections, the swim bladder lumen is filled with a gelatinous to caseous white mass within which irregularly branching, septate, hyaline mycelia may be readily evident.[13,15] Gastric distention with yellow fluid and adhesions between the swim bladder and the intestinal tract may also be present in advanced infection. In ayu fry extensive visceral spread was also reported.[2,13,14]

Differential diagnoses: Differential diagnoses include paecilomycosis and other swim bladder mycoses, though the host range, clinical signs and gross findings are relatively characteristic.

Diagnosis: Aspiration of the swim bladder will often recover fluid for culture and cytology. Fungal culture utilizing Sabouraud dextrose, potato dextrose or oatmeal agars will produce growth of brown-pigmented hyphae. Sequencing segments of the 18S SSU rDNA and ITS1, 5.8S and ITS 2 regions has been used for molecular confirmation.[13,15]

Management/control: There are no therapeutic or control measures, though some fish can recover spontaneously from infection. Hatcheries focus on prevention through maintenance of runway cleanliness, proper feed storage, appropriate-sized feed and frequent cleaning of mechanical feeders.[3]

Paecilomycosis (isariamycosis)

Overview: Paecilomycosis (isariamycosis) is an ascomycete fungal infection of the swim bladder, which causes sporadic low mortality in farmed Atlantic salmon (*Salmo salar*) in Scotland and Norway.[15–17]

Etiology: *Isaria farinosa* (~*Paecilomyces farinosus*).

Route of transmission: *Isaria farinosa* has been used as a biological control for insects, and swim bladder infection in salmon is hypothesized to be through consumption of insect larvae containing spores.[4,18]

Host range: Atlantic salmon fry and parr.

Clinical presentation: Fish demonstrate generalized hyperpigmentation, abnormal buoyancy/balance, coelomic distention, red discoloration of the vent and low levels of mortality.

Pathology: Gross necropsy reveals a distended swim bladder, mural and local hemorrhage, and a lumen filled by a white mass of branching, septate, hyaline hyphae that infiltrates and effaces the wall of the swim bladder. Local coelomitis may be evident, but visceral spread is not common.[15]

Differential diagnoses: Differential diagnoses include phomamycosis and other swim bladder mycoses, though the host range, clinical signs, gross and histologic findings are characteristic.

Diagnosis: Fungal culture of swim bladder aspirates or necropsy samples on Sabouraud maltose agar will result in white colonies producing conidiophores and conidia. Molecular confirmation is via amplification and sequencing of the ITS region.[4,15,18]

Management/control: No therapeutic or control measures are available.

METAZOAL INFECTIONS

Anguillicolidae infection

Overview: Nematodes of the family Anguillicolidae are parasites of the swim bladder of eels. Species described include *Anguillicoloides australensis* in the Australian eel (*Anguilla reinhardtii*), and *Anguillicola*

globiceps and *Anguillicoloides crassus* in the Pacific (Japanese) (*Anguilla japonica*), European (*Anguilla anguilla*) and American (*Anguilla rostrata*) eels.[19,20] *Anguillicoloides crassus* infection is believed to be a cause or initiating factor in eel population collapses in Europe and the United States.[21,22]

Etiology: *Anguillicolidae* are dracunculoid nematodes with a life cycle that involves an eel definitive host and a crustacean intermediate host or small fish or invertebrate paratenic hosts.[19,23]

Route of transmission: Transmission is through direct oral exposure. Sexual reproduction occurs in the swim bladder lumen with embryonated eggs. Larvae leave the swim bladder through the pneumatic duct and enter the digestive system where they are released into the water with feces.[24,25] At least 11 species of copepods and two species of ostracods can act as an intermediate host for the parasite, and numerous aquatic snails, amphibians, insects and freshwater fish have been identified as paratenic hosts.[23,26] The larval parasites undergo a series of molts in the hemocoel, and after the intermediate host or paratenic host is ingested the larvae penetrate the intestinal tract of the definitive eel host and migrate to the swim bladder where they become adults (**Figure 13.9**).[26]

Host range: The natural hosts of *Anguillicoloides crassus* are Pacific (Japanese) eels throughout Asia; in European eels in Europe (Netherlands, Belgium, Spain, Portugal, France, England, Denmark, Italy, Greece, Austria, Czech Republic, Hungary, Poland, Sweden, Estonia, Russia and Egypt) and North Africa; and in American eels (*Anguilla rostrata*) from

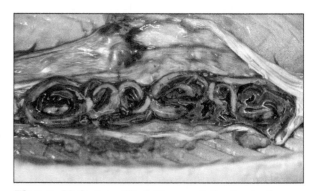

Figure 13.9 *Anguillicoloides* spp. infection in the swim bladder of a silver eel *Ariosoma mellissii*. (Image courtesy of J. Simon.)

the Southeastern United States (North and South Carolina) through New England (Rhode Island, Massachusetts, Maine) and eastern Canada (New Brunswick and Northern Nova Scotia).[20,22,26–28]

Clinical presentation: *Anguillicoloides crassus* is not normally pathogenic in Pacific eels, however in European and American eels it may generate a significant host response.[29] Eels demonstrate hyporexia, decreased swimming speeds, coelomic distention and skin ulcers along the posterior abdomen.[30] Infected swim bladders have decreased elasticity and a higher likelihood of rupture due to fibrosis.[21,26]

Pathology: *Anguillicolidae* consume blood from the host via the wall of the swim bladder.[19] Gross lesions include luminal hemorrhage and diffuse inflammation and thickening of the swim bladder wall. The lumen is often filled with fluid containing degenerate eggs and larvae as well as digested blood and debris.[22,26] With repeat infection and severe chronic inflammation, the swim bladder may completely collapse and atrophy.[31,32]

Differential diagnoses: None in *Anguilla* spp. eels.

Diagnosis: Radiology and gross necropsy are the two primary methods of detecting and scoring *Anguillicolidae* infection. A Length Ratio Index (LRI) has been described that uses radiographic evidence as a correlate for disease severity.[30,31] Scoring is based on alterations in the length and regularity of the swim bladder silhouette, dilation and gas distention of the pneumatic duct, and discernable worm contours within the swim bladder lumen.[32,33]

Management/control: Drug treatment in aquaculture is possible, but no treatment exists for wild populations. Antihelminthics, such as levamisole, metrifonate and emamectin benzoate have been shown to be efficacious.[26,34,35] Control of parasites in eel ponds can be difficult, and reducing densities of copepods, increasing water flow, using chemicals to eliminate copepods and increasing salinity are not considered practical.[26]

Cystidicola infection

Overview: Spirurid nematodes of the genus *Cystidicola* are parasites of the swim bladder of physosomous fishes.[36]

Etiology: The two species recognized are *C. cristivomeri* and *C. faronis*.[2,36]

Route of transmission: Transmission is through direct oral exposure. *C. cristivomeri* utilizes an

opossum shrimp (*Mysis relicta*) intermediate host, whereas *C. farionis* utilizes freshwater amphipod (*Gammarus*, *Hyalella* and *Pontoporeia* spp.) intermediate hosts.[36] Following ingestion of an infected intermediate host, larvae migrate through the pneumatic duct via retrograde migration from the stomach to the esophagus.[37,38] Adult nematodes of *C. cristomeri* may live up to 10 years.[38]

Host range: *Cystidicola cristivomeri* is a parasite of arctic char (*Salvelinus alpinus*) and lake trout (*Salvelinus namaycush*) and its distribution is restricted to North America. *Cystidicola faronis* infects a variety of North American, Asian and Eurasian salmonids.[2,36]

Clinical presentation: There are no reported clinical signs associated with infection. Despite heavy worm burdens, mortality is low in all but arctic char, which may have long-term infections and increased mortality.[38]

Pathology: The degree of swim bladder damage depends on the host species infected and the nematode burden with damage most likely related to chronic irritation.[39] Rainbow trout (*Oncorhynchus mykiss*) infected with *C. farionis* have raised ulcers consisting of a central plaque of ochre-colored material overlying a central crater.[39,40] Lake trout infected with *C. cristivomeri* show evidence of ulceration only with massive worm burdens.[40] Lesions on the ventrolateral surface of the swim bladder appear as raised ulcers surrounded by hyperemic mucosa and covered by a hard, ochre-colored material over a central crater.[39] Histopathology of *C. farionis* infection shows multifocal inflammation of the submucosa and muscularis of the swim bladder with epithelial erosion occurring in more severe infections.[41]

Differential diagnoses: None.

Diagnosis: Gross necropsy and parasite identification are the only described methods of diagnosis.[37] Similar to other swim bladder infections, radiography and ultrasound may be able to detect filling of the swim bladder lumen particularly in heavy worm burdens.

Management/control: No treatments or management practices are described for natural infections.

Sphaerosporosis

Overview: Swim bladder inflammation of carp (SBI) or cyprinid swim-bladder inflammation is an economically important protozoal disease of common carp associated with the intermediate stage of a myxosporean.

Etiology: Intermediate stage of the renal myxosporean (sphaerosporan) *Sphaerospora renicola*.[2,42]

Route of transmission: The route of transmission is currently undetermined. Direct transmission by contact with spore-releasing carp and direct transmission through oral administration of infected kidney tissue have been unsuccessful.[43]

Host range: Swim bladder inflammation is a disease of farmed common carp (*Cyprinus carpio*) throughout Asia, North America and Europe. Frequency and occurrence varies between carp farms and seasons with peak prevalence of disease in July.

Clinical presentation: Clinical signs are often absent in early stages of the disease. With chronic disease, carp show abnormal buoyancy/balance and will swim on their back or side with the head pointed downward. The caudal fin may stand out of the water and fish will attempt to dive unsuccessfully. Abdominal distention is also common involving either just the anterior coelom or caudal coelom depending on whether one or both chambers of the swim bladder are affected.

Pathology: Gross lesions are similar to other inflammatory causes of aerocystitis. Early lesions include loss of transparency of the inner wall of the swim bladder with petechial hemorrhages associated with congested vessels. Later in the disease process there is thickening of the swim bladder wall (2–3 mm) and accumulation of a red-brown exudate.[2] The posterior sac of the swim bladder is rarely involved.[41] One differentiating feature from other causes of aerocystitis is the development of marked multifocal hemorrhage and layers of fibrin on the outer surface of the swim bladder in severe cases.[1] In the final stages of inflammation cysts may form in the wall of the swim bladder, the lumen will be filled with seropurulent material, and inflammation can spread to local organs.[42] Organisms are localized predominantly extravascularly within the fibrous tissue of the tunica interna and are most often seen at the border between hemorrhagic and healthy tissues.[44,45] Pansporoblasts and spores will be seen concurrently in renal tubules, though the biological significance of the SBI stages of the parasite remain unclear.[1,45] The disease is also frequently complicated by secondary bacterial infection.[42]

Differential diagnoses: Clinical signs and gross features are similar to other causes of aerocystitis barring characteristic multifocal hemorrhage and fibrin accumulation on the serosa of the swim bladder.

Diagnosis: Cytology and histology of the affected swim bladder are the primary methods of diagnosis. Impression smears of the anterior swim bladder will contain Giemsa-positive, multicellular stages of the parasite.[44,45]

Management/control: No treatment is currently available. Fumagillin is the only medication reported to be effective experimentally for prevention of sphaerosporosis. Antibiotic medicated feed can be used to control secondary bacterial infections in actively infected carp. Drying and disinfecting ponds will effectively destroy spores.[42,46]

VIRAL INFECTIONS

Largemouth bass virus

Overview: Initially isolated from asymptomatic largemouth bass (*Micropterus salmoides*) collected in Florida, largemouth bass virus (LMBV) can result in mortality events of wild fish.[47,48] Outbreaks typically impact adult, trophy-size fish and frequently occur during the summer with water temperatures above 30°C.[49]

Etiology: LMBV is an iridovirus and can be isolated from clinically normal fish, suggesting there could be different strains of LMBV circulating in populations.[48,49]

Route of transmission: Transmission is believed to be through waterborne exposure or consumption of infected prey.[50,51] The virus retains infectivity in water after 2 days and can still be detected after 7 days.

Host range: Clinical and subclinical infection is most commonly reported in largemouth bass, though smallmouth bass (*Micropterus dolomieu*) can also be affected. Subclinical infection is possible in other cetrarchid species but is considered rare.[49,52] The geographic distribution includes fish populations in the central and eastern portions of the United States and as far west as Texas, Oklahoma, Minnesota and Southern Michigan. It is predominantly a disease of wild fish though the virus has been detected in hatchery stocks with no evidence of disease.[50]

Clinical presentation: Clinical signs include loss of equilibrium and floating at the water surface due to swim bladder overinflation.

Pathology: Gross lesions reported in wild fish are minimal and include only red discoloration and/or distention of the swim bladder with a yellow or brown exudate occasionally present in the lumen.[49,52] Gross lesions reported with experimental infections included multifocal pale foci in the liver, bright red discoloration of the spleen, mild congestion of the mesentery and abdominal fat near intestinal ceca, and fibrinous coelomitis. Inflammation and necrosis of the exocrine pancreas and focal necrosis of the mucosa of the stomach, intestine and intestinal ceca were also noted.

Differential diagnoses: Due to the subtle gross lesions and clinical signs, mass mortality events involving environmental stressors (hypoxia, algal blooms or other toxins, lightening) would need to be considered, but the species-specific nature of the mortality should be considered a hallmark.

Diagnosis: Diagnosis is challenging because distinctive, easily recognized lesions are often not present, and not all fish infected with the virus develop disease.[49] Virus isolation, using bluegill fry (BF-2) or fathead minnow (FHM) cell lines, confirmed by PCR specific for the LMBV iridovirus along with documentation of anatomical and behavior changes that are consistent with the disease are diagnostic for LMBV.[49]

Management/control: No treatment options have been reported in the literature. Geographic spread may have been the result of transport of infected fish or water in the wells of fishing boats or through stocking.[49] The risk of transmission between fish shedding virus and naïve fish during catch and release tournaments has also been suggested as a link.[52]

NEOPLASIA

Swim bladder sarcoma

Overview: Epizootic swim bladder tumors have been described in marine-farmed Atlantic salmon (*Salmo salar*) and offspring of North American wild Atlantic salmon.[53–55] Single spontaneous tumors of the swim bladder have also been reported and include similar leiomyosarcomas and fibromas/fibrosarcomas.

Etiology: Swim bladder sarcoma virus (SSSV), an exogenous piscine retrovirus in the *Epsilonretroviradae* family, is the suspected etiology of epizootic leiomyosarcomas in farmed Atlantic salmon. Retroviral particles were observed by electron microscopy in the cases of epizootic neoplasia.[56]

Route of transmission: The route of natural transmission of this virus is unknown.

Host range: Cultured and wild Atlantic salmon between 1 and 4 years of age are typically impacted.[53,54]

Clinical presentation: This disease results in chronic low-level morbidity and mortality in affected populations. Fish with advanced neoplasia show signs of lethargy, poor body condition and buoyancy problems.[53,54]

Pathology: In both epizootic and spontaneous neoplasia, multifocal to coalescing, firm tan masses are observed emanating from the external and internal surface wall of the swim bladder both encroaching into the coelom and filling the swim bladder lumen (**Figure 13.10**). Immunohistochemistry of the North American epizootic confirmed positive staining for muscle markers (desmin and actin) in a pattern consistent with a leiomyosarcoma.[53–55]

Differential diagnoses: None.

Diagnosis: Although theoretically detectable by radiography and ultrasound, gross necropsy

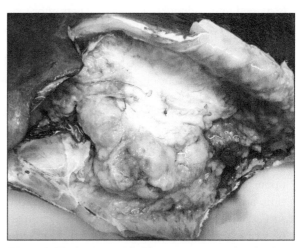

Figure 13.10 Swim bladder sarcoma in a blackfish (*Tautog onitis*).

and histopathology are necessary to confirm the diagnosis.

Management/control: No management or control techniques have been described.

MECHANICAL DISEASES OF THE SWIM BLADDER

Barotrauma/catastrophic decompression disease

Overview: Overinflation of the swim bladder with and without rupture can occur in fish secondary to the rapid reduction of bariatric pressure experienced when animals are caught at depth and rapidly surfaced due to angling or scientific sampling.[57]

Etiology: Decreases in barometric pressure associated with a rapid decrease in depth. A change in depth of as little as 10–20 feet can result in acute distention in some fishes.[1] As fish are surfaced they experience a progressive decrease in ambient pressure, resulting in an increase in partial pressure of dissolved gases within the blood and tissues (Boyle's law). Therefore, the blood and tissues become supersaturated, gases may leave solution and form emboli in blood vessels and bubbles in various tissues and organs including eyes, brain, heart, arteries, gills, spleen, fins, skeletal muscle and dermis beneath the scales.[57]

Route of transmission: Not applicable.

Host range: Both physoclists and physostomes can be affected by rapid depressurization, but the lack of a pneumatic duct in physoclists, particularly Gadids (e.g., cod and haddock), may make them more vulnerable due to their inability to rapidly adjust gas volume.[4,57]

Clinical presentation: Acute barotrauma may result in abdominal distention, exophthalmia, respiratory distress, abnormal buoyancy, external hemorrhage, gastric eversion and intestinal herniation.[4,58] Positive buoyancy is seen in fish with acute distention, whereas negative buoyancy is seen in fish with swim bladder rupture. Fish are unable to submerge upon release and have poor survival due to predation, stress of increased surface water temperature, sun exposure and boat trauma. The chronic impacts of swim bladder rupture include inefficient swimming due to an inability to control swim bladder volume, increased energy expenditure, higher oxygen consumption and potentially increase susceptibility to predation. Some fishes may lose the ability to appropriately orient within the water column.[58]

Pathology: Fish that suffer barotrauma experience a wide range of serious, permanent and debilitating injuries. Over 70 injuries are reported to occur associated with overexpansion of the swim bladder alone and many barotrauma injuries are unaffected by recompression (e.g., stomach and intestinal prolapse, torsion and volvulus, multiorgan hemorrhage, and severe exophthalmia). The swim bladder can fill a significant amount of the coelomic space causing severe organ compression.[58] Additional physiological impacts of barotrauma include alterations in plasma coagulation proteins, erythrocyte lysis and increase in concentrations of tissue-damaging enzymes.[57]

Differential diagnoses: None.

Diagnosis: Diagnosis is made primarily due to the circumstances of capture of the fish as well as clinical signs.

Management/control: Puncture of the swim bladder (i.e., venting or "fizzing") with a needle or other instrument is one of the most common therapeutic techniques used and can result in immediate correction of overinflation, however, it also allows for contamination of the swim bladder lumen, inflammation and is considered controversial.[57–59] A review of relative risk of this procedure under experimental conditions as well as capture-release studies determined that this procedure did not improve survival in either freshwater or marine fishes.[57] This review discouraged venting as a fishery practice and believed it should be prohibited.[57] Alternatives to venting include baskets and cages where fish are lowered to a depth (often the bottom) and the use of shot weights. Low cost hyperbaric chambers have also been described and used to rapidly recompress fish once they are brought to the surface and then decompress them over a series of days.[60]

Overinflation

Overview: Swim bladder distention and associated buoyancy disorders are one of the most common conditions of fish, particularly ornamental fish and goldfish (*Carrasius auratus*).[2,61]

Etiology: Alterations in acid base balance are likely the most common causes of overinflation of the swim bladder but are not well characterized clinically.[1] Pneumatic duct obstruction secondary to fungal infections, bacterial infections, or nutritional disease with metaplasia of the lining and blockage by squamous epithelial cells and mucus can also occur.[2,61] Altered body conformation through selective breeding (e.g., goldfish and cyprinids) is thought to also be a contributing factor.[61]

Route of transmission: Not applicable.

Host range: Any species can be impacted but overinflation is common in fancy goldfish and can be very difficult to resolve.[61]

Clinical presentation: Clinical signs are often acute resulting in abnormal positive buoyancy and the animal floating either upside down, head up or tail up.[2,62] Some fish may also demonstrate coelomic distention (**Figure 13.11**).[2] Skin damage due to exposure and desiccation can result in secondary infections and complicate recovery.

Pathology: No consistent external lesions or environmental factors are noted in ornamental fishes.[62]

Differential diagnoses: Gastrointestinal gas distention can present with similar clinical signs.

Diagnosis: Radiography can detect a number of abnormalities including overinflation, displacement, and rupture, and can rule out fluid accumulation or gastrointestinal gas accumulation.[62] Aspiration of the swim bladder can establish the presence of gas within the lumen and may prove temporarily therapeutic though the underlying cause of the problem is not addressed.

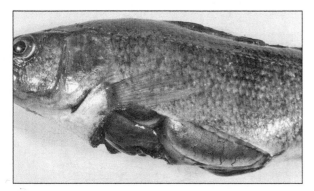

Figure 13.11 **Abdominal distention due to swim bladder overinflation in cultured yellow perch (*Perca flavescens*). (Image courtesy of S.A. Smith.)**

Management/control: Aspiration of gas from the swim bladder can provide relief but distention may recur. Penetration of the body wall and swim bladder with an appropriate gauge needle, butterfly catheter or extension set can allow for gradual removal of gas from the lumen and return of the fish to neutral rather than negative buoyancy. Although fish can function at negative buoyancy, neutral buoyancy is preferred. There are anecdotal reports of fish being fed fresh or undercooked peas resulting in resolution of the issue. Surgical removal or reduction of the swim bladder have occasionally been performed to relieve chronic overinflation.[63,64] Adding ballast to the coelom of fish with chronic swim bladder distention has also been suggested.[65]

Swim bladder torsion

Overview: A rarely reported condition in both ornamental fish and farmed rainbow trout fed during cold weather. Torsion is midviscus causing caudal distention of the coelom and dilation of the swim bladder.[2,66]

Etiology: A clear cause is not evident in ornamental fishes, which is similar for most buoyancy disorders in ornamental fishes.

Route of transmission: Not applicable.

Host range: The condition has been reported primarily in ornamental goldfish and in small numbers of rainbow trout.

Clinical presentation: Fish present with abnormal positive buoyancy and often distention of the coelom particularly caudally.[66]

Pathology: Clinical and gross findings typically demonstrate distention of the caudal chamber of the swim bladder due to gas entrapment following torsion, with secondary marked dilation and frequently with displacement.

Differential diagnoses: Other causes of swim bladder distention or gas retention within the gastrointestinal tract.

Diagnosis: Similar to swim bladder overinflation, radiography can reveal gas distention with possibly displacement of the caudal chamber.

Management/control: Aspiration of the affected caudal chamber may provide temporary relief. Torsions may spontaneously resolve, or coeliotomy with either pneumocystoplasty (i.e., removal of the affected chamber) or surgical correction of the torsion is required.[66]

DEVELOPMENTAL DISEASES OF THE SWIM BLADDER

Aplasia/hypoplasia/failure to fill/anatomic variation

Overview: Lack of inflation or abnormal development of the swim bladder in larval fish had been a major issue in the intensive culture of marine and freshwater fish larvae.

Etiology: A variety of contributory factors have been described including autogenous oil/surface films due to decomposition of feed/eggs/larvae, aeration, light, temperature and salinity. High salinity has been associated with hypertrophy of the swim bladder in European bass (*Morone labrax*).[67–69] Swim bladder hypoplasia in seadragons was described as having a possible association with calcium hydroxide supplementation of the tank water.[70] In estuarine larvae, salinity also appears to affect inflation through interactions between water density and larval buoyancy.[68]

Route of transmission: Not applicable.

Host range: Failure of swim bladder development has been reported in at least 27 physoclistous fish species in families including Gadidae, Cyprinodontiidae, Poeciliidae, Syngnathidae, Gasterosteidae, Mornidae, Percichthydiae, Percidae, Sciaenidae, Silaginidae, Sparidae, Cichlidae and Pleuronectidae.[71]

Clinical presentation: Developmental anomalies of the swim bladder can result in specific behavioral and morphological abnormalities, particularly with the lack of swim bladder development. These include slowed growth rate due to increased energy demand when swimming, stereotypic upward swimming or side swimming, spinal deformities (lordosis, kyphosis) likely due to the abnormal swimming behavior, and in some fish abrasions and contortion of the pectoral fins.[71,72]

Pathology: Initial filling of the swim bladder in larval fishes often occurs through gulping of air at the surface and transmittal to the swim bladder by the pneumatic duct. Following regression of the pneumatic duct, the swim bladder's volume is maintained by the vascular rete and gas gland.[73] Other developmental abnormalities of the swim bladder that have resulted in side swimming in Atlantic salmon include pneumatic duct entry that was ventral and at the caudal pole of the swim bladder, underinflation, *S*-shaped deviation, tortuous malformation and cranial retroflexion.[1,72]

Differential diagnoses: Not applicable.

Diagnosis: Gross examination of larvae with a dissecting microscope will reveal lack of swim bladder filling and other abnormalities (**Figure 13.12** and **13.13**). Abnormal larvae can also be separated based on their lack of buoyancy while under anesthesia or by their buoyancy in various gradients of salt water.[74] Radiography has also been useful for detecting swim bladder inflation in walleye and hybrid striped bass (**Figure 13.14**).[75]

Management/control: Oil film removal using inlet sprayer pipes and polypropylene oil-absorbent pads has been successful in improving swim bladder filling in striped bass larvae.[69]

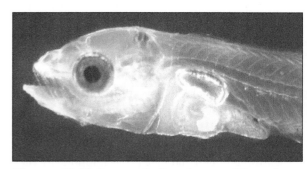

Figure 13.12 Larvae of a French grunt (*Haemulon flavolineatum*) with normally developed swim bladder. (Image courtesy of R.P.E. Yanong.)

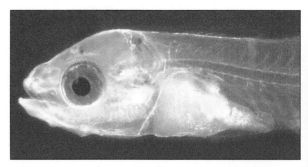

Figure 13.13 Larvae of a French grunt (*Haemulon flavolineatum*) with swim bladder hypoplasia/lack of filling. (Image courtesy of R.P.E. Yanong.)

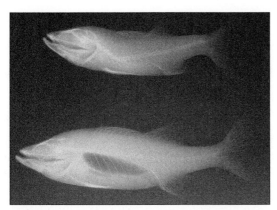

Figure 13.14 Radiograph of cultured juvenile hybrid striped bass. Fish with normal swim bladder (bottom) and fish with no swim bladder development due to lack of initial swim bladder inflation at the fry stage. Note the severe lordosis due to chronic compensation of swimming behavior. (Image courtesy of S.A. Smith.)

REFERENCES

1. Lumsden, J.S. Gastrointestinal tract, swim bladder, pancreas and peritoneum. In: *Systemic Pathology of Fish: A Text and Atlas of Normal Tissues in Teleosts and Their Responses in Disease*, 2nd ed. H.W. Ferguson, ed. Scotian Press, London, 2006; 187–193.

2. Roberts, R.J. and H.D. Rodger. The pathophysiology and systematic pathology of teleosts. In: *Fish Pathology*, 4th ed. R.J. Roberts, ed. Wiley-Blackwell, West Sussex, 2012; 62–143.

3. Burton, T.O., Meyers, T.R., Starkey, N.S. and Follett, J.E. Experimental transmission of the fungus *Phoma herbarum* to chinook salmon. *Journal of Aquatic Animal Health* 16: 2004;4:251–257.

4. Stoskopf, M.K. *Fish Medicine*. W.B. Saunders, Philadelphia, 1993.

5. Blaylock, R.B., Overstreet, R.M. and Klich, M.A. Mycoses in red snapper (*Lutjanus campechanus*) caused by two deuteromycete fungi (*Penicillium corylophilum* and *Cladosporium sphaerospermum*). *Hydrobiologia* 2001;460:221–228.

6. Aho, R., Koski, P., Salonen, A. and Rintamaki, P. Fungal swim bladder infection in farmed Baltic salmon (*Salmo salar* L.) caused by *Verticillium lecanii*. *Mycoses* 1988;31(4):208–212.

7. Camus, A., Berliner, A., Hatcher, N. and Clauss, T. *Exophiala xenobiotica* aerocystitis in a Queensland grouper *Epinephelus lanceolatus* (Bloch). *Journal of Fish Diseases* 2015;38:221–225.

8. Bowater, R.O., Thomas, A., Shivas, R.G. and Humphrey, J.D. Deuteromycotic fungi infecting barramundi cod, *Cromileptes altivelis* (Valenciennes), from Australia. *Journal of Fish Diseases* 2003;26:681–686.

9. Meunch, T.M., White, M.R. and Wu, C.C. Visceral mycosis in chinook salmon (*Oncorhynchus tschawytscha*) due to *Sporobolomyces salmonicolor*. *Veterinary Pathology* 1996;33:238–241.

10. Ellis, A.E., Waddell, I.F. and Minter, D.W. A systemic fungal disease in Atlantic salmon parr, *Salmo salar* L., caused by a species of *Phialophora*. *Journal of Fish Diseases* 1983;6:511–523.

11. Stetter, M.D. Diagnostic imaging and endoscopy. In: *BSAVA Manual of Ornamental Fish*, 2nd ed. W.H. Wildgoose, ed. British Small Animal Veterinary Association, Gloucester, 2001; 103–108.

12. Ross, A.J. and Yasutake, W.T. *Phoma herbarum*, a fungal plant saprophyte, as a fish pathogen. *Journal of the Fish Research Board of Canada* 1975;32(9):1648–1652.

13. Faisal, M., Elsayed, E., Fitzgerald, S.D., Silva, V. and Mendoza, L. Outbreaks of phaeohyphomycosis in the chinook salmon (*Oncorhynchus tshawytscha*) caused by *Phoma herbarum*. *Mycopathologia* 2007;163:41–48.

14. Hatai, K., Fujimaki, Y. and Egusa, S. A visceral mycosis in ayu fry, *Plecoglossus altivelis* Temmininck & Schlegel, caused by a species of *Phoma*. *Journal of Fish Diseases* 1986;9:111–116.

15. Bruno, D., Noguera, P.A. and Poppe, T.T. *A Colour Atlas of Salmonid Diseases*, 2nd ed. Springer, Dordrecht, 2013.

16. Lehmann, J., Mock, D. and Schafer, W. Swim bladder infection of farmed Atlantic salmon (*Salmo salar* L.) by a fungus: A case report. *Bulletin of the European Association of Fish Pathologists* 1999;19(2):83–84.

17. Kirk, R.S. The impact of *Anguillicola crassus* on European eels. *Fisheries Management and Ecology* 2003;10:385–394.

18. Bruno, D.W. Observations on a swim bladder fungal infection of farmed Atlantic salmon, *Salmo salar* L. *Bulletin of the European Association of Fish Pathologists* 1989;9(1):7–8.

19. Peters, G. and Hartmann, F. *Anguillicola*, a parasitic nematode of the swim bladder spreading among eel populations in Europe. *Diseases of Aquatic Organisms* 1986;1:229–230.

20. Fries, L.T., Williams, J.D. and Johnson, S.K. Occurrence of *Anguillicola crassus*, an exotic parasitic swim bladder nematode of eels in the southeastern United States. *Transactions of the American Fisheries Society* 1996;125(5):794–797.

21. Barry, J., McLeish, J., Dodd, J.A., Turnbull, J.F., Boylan, P. and Adams, C.E. Introduced parasite *Anguillicola crassus* infection significantly impedes swim bladder function in the European eel *Anguilla anguilla* (L.). *Journal of Fish Diseases* 2014;37:921–924.

22. Aieta, A.E. and Olivieira, K. Distribution, prevalence, and intensity of the swim bladder parasite *Anguillicola crassus* in New England and eastern Canada. *Diseases of Aquatic Organisms* 2009;84:229–235.

23. Moravec, F. and Konecny, R. Some new data on the intermediate and paratenic hosts of the nematode *Anguillicola crassu* Kuwahara, Niimi et Itagaki 1974 (Dracunculoidea), a swim bladder parasite of eels. *Folia Parasitologica* 1994;41:65–70.

24. Moravec, F., Di Cave, D., Orecchia, P. and Paggi, I. Experimental observations on the development of *Anguillicola crassus* (Nematoda: Dracunculoidea) in its definitive host *Anguilla anguilla* (Pisces). *Folia Parasitologica* 1994;41:138–148.

25. De Charleroy, D., Grisez, L., Thomas, K., Belpaire, C. and Ollevier, F. The life cycle of Anguillicola crassus. *Diseases of Aquatic Organisms* 1990;8:77–84.

26. Kennedy, C.R. The pathogenic helminth parasites of eels. *Journal of Fish Diseases* 2007;30:319–334.

27. Barse, A.M. and Sector, D.H. An exotic nematode parasite of the American eel. *Fisheries* 1999;24(2):6–10.

28. Moser, M.L., Patrick, W.S. and Crutchfield, J.U. Infection of American eels, *Anguillicola rostrata*, with the introduced nematode parasite, *Anguillicola crassus*, in North Carolina. *Copeia* 2001;3:848–853.

29. Knopf, K. and Mahnke, M. Difference in susceptibility of the European eel (*Anguilla anguilla*) and the Japanese eel (*Anguilla japonica*) to the swim-bladder nematode *Anguillicola crassus*. *Parasitology* 2004;129:491–496.

30. Palstra, A.P., Heppener, D.F.M., Van Ginneken, V.J.T., Szekeley, C. and Van den Thillart, G.E.E.J.M. Swimming performance of silver eels severely impaired by the swim bladder parasite *Anguillicola crassus*. *Journal of Experimental Marine Biology and Ecology* 2007;352:244–256.

31. Berengi, A., Molnar, K., Bekesi, L. and Szekely, C.S. Radiodiagnostic method for studying swim bladder inflammation caused by *Anguillicola crassus* (Nematoda:Draculuncoidea). *Diseases of Aquatic Organisms* 1998;34:155–160.

32. Lefebvre, F., Fazio, G., Palstra, A.P., Szekely, C. and Crivelli, A.J. An evaluation of gross indices of pathology associated with the nematode *Anguillicola crassus* in eels. *Journal of Fish Diseases* 2011;34:31–45.

33. Lefebvre, F., Contournet, P. and Crivelli, A.J. The health state of the eel swim bladder as a measure of parasite pressure by *Anguillicola crassus*. *Parasitology* 2002;124:457–463.

34. Taraschewski, H., Renner, C. and Mehlhorn, H. Treatment of fish parasites 3. Effects of levamisole HCl, metrifonate, fenbendazole, mebendazole and ivermectin on *Anguillicola crassus* (nematodes) pathogenic in the air bladder of eels. *Parasitology Research* 1988;74:281–289.

35. Larrat, S., Marvin, J. and Lair, S. Safety and efficacy of emamectin benzoate to treat *Anguillicola crassus* (Kuwahara, Niimi, and Itagaki) infections in American eels, *Anguilla rostrata* (Lesueur). *Journal of Fish Diseases* 2012;35:467–470.

36. Smith, J.D. and Lankester, M.W. Development of swim bladder nematodes (*Cystidicola* spp.) in their intermediate hosts. *Canadian Journal of Zoology* 1979;57:1736–1744.

37. Black, G.A. and Lankester, M.W. Migration and development of swim bladder nematodes, *Cystidicola* spp. (Habronematoidea) in their definitive hosts. *Canadian Journal of Zoology* 1980;58:1997–2005.

38. Black, G.A. and Lankester, M.W. The transmission, life span, and population biology of *Cystidicola cristivomeri* White, 1947 (Nematoda: Habronematoidea) in char, *Savelinus* spp. *Canadian Journal of Zoology* 1981;59:498–509.

39. Black, G.A. Swimbladder lesions in lake trout (*Salvelinus namaycush*) associated with mature *Cystidicola stigmatura* (Nematoda). *Journal of Parasitology* 1984;70(3):441–443.

40. Lankester, M.W. and Smith, J.D. Host specificity and distribution of the swim-bladder nematodes *Cystidicola farionis* Fischer, 1978 and *C. cristivomeri* White, 1941 (Habronematoidea), in salmonid fishes in Ontario. *Canadian Journal of Zoology* 1980;58:1298–1305.

41. Willers, W.B., Dubielzig, R.R. and Miller, L. Histopathology of the swim bladder of cisco due to the presence of the nematode *Cystidicola farionis* Fischer. *Journal of Aquatic Animal Health* 1991;3(2):130–133.

42. Jenney, Z. and Jenney, G. Recent achievements in studies on diseases on diseases of the common carp (*Cyprinus carpio* L.). *Aquaculture* 1995;129:397–420.

43. GroBheider, G. and Korting, W. Experimental transmission of *Sphaeorspora renicola* to common carp *Cyprinus carpio* fry. *Diseases of Aquatic Organisms* 1993;16:91–95.

44. Csaba, G., Kovaks-Gayer, E., Bekeshi, L., Bucsek, M., Szakolcza, J. and Molnar, K. Studies into the possible protozoan etiology of swim bladder inflammation in carp fry. *Journal of Fish Diseases* 1984;7:39–56.

45. Dykova, I., Lom, J. and Korting, W.K. Light and electron microscopic observations on the swimbladder stages of *Sphaerospora renicola* a parasite of carp (*Cyprinus carpio*). *Parasitology Research* 1990;76:228–237.

46. Molnar, K., Basca, F. and Szekely, C. Fumagillin, an efficacious drug against renal spharosporosis of the common carp *Cyprinus carpio*. *Diseases of Aquatic Organisms* 1987;2:187–190.

47. Plumb, J.A., Grizzle, J.M., Young, H.E. and Noyes, A.D. An iridovirus isolated from wild largemouth bass. *Journal of Aquatic Animal Health* 1996;8:265–270.

48. Grizzle, J.M., Altinok, I., Fraser, W.A. and Francis-Floyd, R. First isolation of largemouth bass virus. *Diseases of Aquatic Organisms* 2002;50:233–235.

49. Grizzle, J.M. and Brunner, C.J. Review of largemouth bass virus. *Fisheries 28*: 2003b;11:10–14.

50. Woodland, J.E., Noyes, A.D. and Grizzle, J.M. A survey to detect largemouth bass virus among fish from hatcheries in the Southeastern USA. *Transactions of the American Fisheries Society* 2002;131:308–311.

51. Grizzle, J.M., Altinook, I. and Noyes, A.D. PCR method for detection of largemouth bass virus. *Diseases of Aquatic Organisms* 2003a;54:29–33.

52. Beck, B.H., Bakal, R.S., Brunner, C.J. and Grizzle, J.M. Virus distribution and signs of disease after immersion

exposure to largemouth bass virus. *Journal of Aquatic Animal Health* 2006;18:176–183.

53. McKnight, I.J. Sarcoma of the swim bladder of Atlantic salmon (*Salmo salar* L.). *Aquaculture* 1978;13:55–60.

54. Bowser, P.R., Casey, J.W., Casey, R.N., Quackenbush, S.L., Lofton, L., Coll, J.A. and Cipriano, R.C. Swimbladder leiomyosarcoma in Atlantic salmon (*Salmo salar*) in North America. *Journal of Wildlife Diseases* 2012;48(3):795–798.

55. Paul, T.A., Quakenbush, S.L., Sutton, C., Casey, R.N., Bowser, P.R. and Casey, J.W. Identification and characterization of an exogenous retrovirus from Atlantic salmon swim bladder sarcomas. *Journal of Virology* 2006;8(6):2941–2948.

56. Duncan, I.B. Evidence for an oncovirus in swim bladder fibrosarcoma of Atlantic salmon *Salmo salar* L. *Journal of Fish Diseases* 1978;1:127–131.

57. Wilde, G.R. Does venting promote survival of released fish? *Fisheries* 2009;34:20–28.

58. Rummer, J.L. and Bennet, W.A. Physiological effects of swim bladder overexpansion and catastrophic decompression on red snapper. *Transactions of the American Fisheries Society* 2005;134(6):1457–1470.

59. Jarvis, E.T. and Lowe, C.G. The effects of barotrauma on the catch-and-release survival of southern nearshore and shelf rockfish (Scorpaenidae, *Sebastes* spp.). *Canadian Journal of Fisheries and Aquatic Sciences* 2008;65(7):1286–1296.

60. Smiley, J.E. and Drawbridge, M.A. Techniques for live capture of deep water fishes with special emphasis on design and application of a low cost hyperbaric chamber. *Journal of Fish Biology* 2007;70(3):867–878.

61. Lewbart, G.A. Green peas for buoyancy disorders. *Exotic DVM* 2000;2:7.

62. Wildgoose, W.H. Buoyancy disorders of ornamental fish: A review of cases seen in private practice. *Fish Veterinary Journal* 2007;9:22–37.

63. Lewbart, G.A., Stone, E.A. and Love, N.E. Pneumocystectomy in a Midas cichlid. *Journal of the American Veterinary Medical Association* 1995;207:319–321.

64. Britt, T., Weisse, C., Weber, E.S., Matzkin, Z. and Klide, A. Use of pneumocystoplasty for over-inflation

of the swim bladder in a goldfish. *Journal of the American Veterinary Medical Association* 2002;221(5):690–693.

65. Werkman, P. Fish surgery: How to ballast a fish. *Aquatic Vet News* 2009;3(3):12–14.

66. Lewbart, G.A. *Self-Assessment Color Review of Ornamental Fish*. Iowa State University Press, Ames, 1998.

67. Johnson, D.W. and Katavic, I. Mortality, growth and swim bladder stress syndrome of sea bass (*Dicentrarchus labrax*) larvae under varied environmental conditions. *Aquaculture* 1984;38:67–78.

68. Battaglene, S.C. and Talbot, R.B. Effects of salinity and aeration on survival of and initial swim bladder inflation in larval Australian bass. *The Progressive Fish-Culturalist* 1993;55:35–39.

69. Friedman, B.R. and Shutty, K.M. Effect of timing of oil film removal and first feeding on swim bladder inflation success among intensively cultured striped bass larvae. *North American Journal of Aquaculture* 1999;61(1):43–46.

70. Bonar, C.J., Garner, M.M., Weber, E.S., Keller, C.J., Murray, M., Adams, L.M. and Frasca Jr. S. Pathologic findings in weedy (*Phyllopteryx taeniolatus*) and leafy (*Phycodurus eques*) seadragons. *Veterinary Pathology* 2013;50(3):368–376.

71. Egloff, M. Failure of swim bladder inflation of perch, *Perca fluviatilis* L. found in natural populations. *Aquatic Sciences* 1996;58(1):15–23.

72. Good, C., Davidson, J., Kinman, C., Kenney, P.B., Baeverfjord, G. and Summerfelt, S. Observations on side-swimming rainbow trout in water recirculation aquaculture systems. *Journal of Aquatic Animal Health* 2014;26(4):219–224.

73. Steen, J.B. The swim bladder as a hydrostatic organ. In: *Fish Physiology*, W.J. Hoar and D.J. Randall, eds. Academic Press, New York, 1970; 413–443.

74. Chapman, D.C., Jackson, U.T. and Hubert, W.A. Method for separating normal striped bass larvae from those with uninflated gas bladders. *The Progressive Fish-Culturalist* 1988;50(3):166–169.

75. Barrows, F.T., Kindschi, G.A. and Zitzow, R.E. Detecting swim bladder inflation in fingerling walleyes. *The Progressive Fish-Culturalist* 1993;55(2):90–94.

CHAPTER 14

REPRODUCTIVE DISORDERS

LESTER KHOO

DYSTOCIA/EGG BINDING/ EGG RETENTION

Overview: Dystocia or egg binding/egg retention is the pathologic condition/disorder that occurs when there is a failure to spawn. This condition is often seen in cultured fish but can also be seen in wild fish.[1,2]

Etiology: There are several factors that have been associated with egg retention in female fish including small body size, obesity, overcrowding, environmental acidity, elevated concentrations of heavy metals, imbalances in sex ratios of fish, and stress.[1] In cultured fish, especially those raised indoors, there may be a lack of environmental cues (i.e., photoperiod or temperature) that might lead to dystocia or egg binding.[2] Failed or delayed spawning can lead to over-ripening of eggs, which can lead to decreased egg quality.[3] It may also result in increased follicular and oocyte atresia and in some species death.[1,4–6]

Route of transmission: Not applicable except where egg retention may be due to exposure to contaminated waters containing heavy metals.

Host range: Egg binding/egg retention occurs in oviparious fish. It has been reported in multiple species including koi and carp, three-spined stickleback, white suckers, salmon, and zebrafish.[1,2,7–10]

Clinical presentation: Fish with dystocia will have a markedly distended abdomen (**Figure 14.1**).[10] Other organs within the coelomic cavity may have compromised function due to compression or obstruction caused by the enlarged ovaries (**Figure 14.2**). Fish may show signs of lethargy and anorexia. Prolapse of the ovary through the genital pore may also occur concurrently with dystocia.[2]

Pathology: When there is relatively short-term egg retention, there may be changes in the eggs due

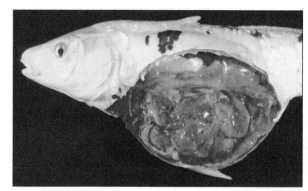

Figure 14.1 Severe abdominal distention and organ compression in a koi, *Cyprinus carpio*, with dystocia due to enlarged cystic ovaries. (Image courtesy of S.A. Smith.)

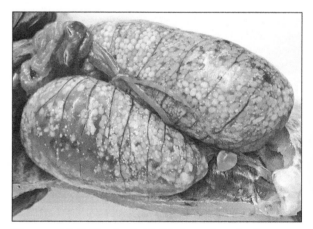

Figure 14.2 Cystic, fluid-filled ovaries of unknown etiology in a cultured hybrid tilapia, *Oreochromis* sp. (Image courtesy of S.A. Smith.)

to over-ripening of the eggs. The morphological changes seen in over-ripen eggs include increased translucency (i.e., semitransparent yolk), aggregation of the cortical cytoplasm, cortical alveloli and oil droplets at the animal pole. There may also be swelling of the eggs with increased water content.[11] Other biochemical changes include a significant decrease in the ovarian fluid pH, and an increase in proteins and esterified and nonesterified fatty acids, as well as decreased activity of aspartate aminotransferase and acid phosphatase.[3] Atresia is the highly regulated process by which ovarian follicles recruited into the vitellogenesis pool fail to complete maturation and proceed through ovulation and ultimately undergo degeneration and resorption. This is an essential part of ovarian homeostasis in fish, and normally occurs at the end of each reproductive cycle.[4] However, there are conditions like dystocia or egg binding where there may be an increase in follicular and oocyte atresia. Early signs of atresia include disintegration of the oocyte nucleus and other cytoplasmic organelles, which is followed by the fragmentation of the zona pellucida and hypertrophy of follicular cells. These follicular cells become phagocytic engulfing the oocyte yolk and organelles. In some cases, there is recruitment of eosinophilic granular leukocytes and macrophages, which digests the degenerating oocyte. Finally, both the follicular cells and inflammatory cells degenerate leaving lipofuscin deposits.[4,5,12,13] It is hypothesized that egg retention and the consequent increased atresia may lead to the condition known as "egg associated inflammation and fibroplasia" in zebrafish.[10,14] While some have not found infectious agents within the acute granulomatous inflammation seen with this condition, others have been able to demonstrate the presence of acid-fast bacilli within the inflammation.[14,15]

Differential diagnosis: The most likely differential diagnosis would be other conditions that have space-occupying lesions such as neoplasms, with granulomatous inflammation of coelomic organs lower on the list of differentials.

Diagnosis: The presumptive diagnosis of dystocia can be made in female fish that retain a markedly distended abdomen after the spawning season has passed. Although physical examination, palpation and ballottement might aid in the determination that the fish has an abdomen full of mature eggs, the diagnosis of dystocia is still subjective.[2,16] An extended period between the spawning season and clinical presentation and the presence of related conditions, such as a prolapsed ovary, may also aid in the

diagnosis. Imaging modalities such as radiography, ultrasonography and computer-aided tomography can be used to confirm involvement of and characterize the coelomic mass prior to resorting to invasive procedures such as an exploratory coeliotomy.[2]

Management/control: Providing the correct conditions for natural spawning helps prevent occurrence of dystocia. Correcting environmental problems, if identifiable, would be the first approach in attempting to resolve the condition. This may also include medical intervention by providing hormone injections of human chorionic gonadotrophin by itself or in combination with carp pituitary extract.[2] Surgical resection might be required if the protruding tissue is necrotic after reduction of the egg mass with a purse string suture around the genital pore to reduce the possible recurrence of prolapse.[2] Another possible surgical intervention might be an ovariectomy to prevent recurrence.

BACTERIAL DISEASES

Overview: Although usually not the primary site for bacterial diseases, some systemic bacterial diseases such as mycobacterial and streptococcal infections that result in granulomatous inflammation can also affect the gonads. Usually the lesions are microscopic, but some may form granulomas and be large enough to be visualized grossly.[17–20]

Etiology: Although *Mycobacterium marinum, M. salmoniphilum, M. fortuitum, M. chelonae* and *M. abscessus* have been the main species implicated in fish mycobacteriosis, there has been an ever-growing array that have been isolated from fish.[21,22] Like mycobacteria, there are several streptococcal species that have been implicated in piscine streptococcosis including *S. iniae* (syn. *S. shiloi*), *S. agalactiae* (syn. *S. difficile*), *S. parauberis, S. dysgalactiae, Lactococcus garvieae* (syn. *Enterococcus sericolicida*), *L. piscium* and *Vagococcus salmoninarium*.[23–26] Most of these organisms cause systemic infections resulting in lesions especially in the central nervous system; however, both *S. iniae* and *S. agalactiae* have been reported as causing infections in the gonads of tilapia (**Figure 14.3**).[27,28]

Route of transmission: For mycobacteriosis, it is presumed that fish are infected by consumption of contaminated food or water. Water and biofilms

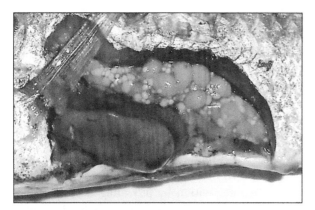

Figure 14.3 Ovaries of tilapia with *Steptococcus iniae* infection. (Image courtesy S.A. Smith.)

are natural habitats for the bacterium that not only infect fish but can survive and replicate in protozoans, which thus serve as vectors for this disease.[22] Mycobacteria may also gain entry via damaged skin or gills due to injury or parasite infection.[29,30] Since the bacteria can been found in the ovary, vertical transmission seems likely and transovarian infection has been reported in oviparous (e.g., Siamese fighting fish) and viviparous fish.[31,32] Similarly, the main route of transmission (intraspecies and interspecies, and between cultured and wild populations) for streptococcosis is horizontally through direct contact with dead or diseased fish, or indirectly through contaminated water. Although natural outbreaks of streptococcosis suggests that vertical transmission is unlikely, with larvae and juvenile tilapia less than 20 g appearing not to be susceptible, evidence for vertical transmission has been demonstrated.[26]

Host range: There is a broad host range of freshwater and marine fish susceptible to mycobacterial infections, and some freshwater families of fish (e.g., Anabantidae, Characidade and Cyprinidae) appear to be especially susceptible. In addition, mycobacteriosis has become a serious problem for cultured food fish such as the European sea bass, striped bass, cobia and tilapia that are raised in intensive aquaculture systems. However, while the literature is replete with systemic mycobacteriosis in fish, there are few reports that specify gonadal involvement with perhaps the exception of angelfish and zebrafish.[17,19,20,33–36] Streptococcosis also involves multiple species of fish including numerous important

aquaculture species such as rainbow trout, tilapia, yellowtail, flounder, European sea bass, red drum and barramundi.[25] However, tilapia are the species that streptococcal gonadal involvement has been most often reported.[27,28]

Clinical presentation: Fish with mycobacteriosis may display abnormal behavior and pigmentary changes. External lesions are also nonspecific and include scale loss, hemorrhage, dermal ulceration, abdominal distention due to ascites, spinal defects and emaciation. Typical internal lesions include splenomegaly, renomegaly and hepatomegaly with gray-white nodules on visceral organs and sometimes the gonads.[19,22,25,30] Although clinical signs and lesions of streptococcosis may vary with fish species infected, there are often abnormal swimming behaviors due to central nervous system (CNS) involvement including loss of orientation and anorexia. External lesions include exophthalmia, corneal opacity, hemorrhages around the anus and base of fins, abdominal distension, and hyperpigmentation.[26]

Pathology: In both bacterial diseases, there can be miliary nodules present on the surface of the reproductive organs.[19,37] In mycobacteriosis, these nodules histologically, depending on chronicity, can range from highly organized lesions with thick layers of epithelioid macrophages to poorly organized inflammation with minimal epithelioid macrophages. These may have cores of caseous necrosis with rare dystrophic calcification. Multinucleate giant cells, a common feature in mammalian mycobacterial granulomas, are occasionally present. Frequently, a fibrotic and/or leucocyte-rich capsule surrounds these inflammatory foci. Extracellular and intracellular (i.e., in macrophages) acid-fast bacilli may be evident in these foci.[17,22,30] In zebrafish with "egg-associated inflammation and fibrosis," the affected fish have distended abdomens, and acid-fast bacteria are present within the chronic inflammation lesions associated with atresia and degeneration of ova.[10,15,38] In streptococcosis, the bacteria appear to replicate more in the testes and ovaries than in other organs. These organs display either exudative or granulomatous inflammation. The exudative inflammation is characterized by extracellular bacterial, tissue necrosis, congestion of capillaries, edema, and infiltrates of bacteria-laden macrophages and neutrophils. The granulomatous inflammation is characterized by granuloma formation with central cores of coagulative or caseous necrosis and bacteria.[18,28]

Differential diagnosis: The differential diagnosis for the granulomatous form of mycobacteria would be streptococcosis and vice versa. Also, some of the parasitic (e.g., myxozoans and microsporidian) granulomas or xenomas and neoplasia could also be viable differentials for gonadal disease caused by bacteria.

Diagnosis: For mycobacteriosis, the presumptive diagnosis is based on the presence of gross lesions and the identification of acid-fast bacilli in touch impressions or histologic sections of the affected organ. Serological and molecular techniques have been employed to provide a definitive diagnosis. Bacterial cultures on selective media such as Lowenstein-Jensen agar or Middlebrook agar can be attempted, but most mycobacterial species are notoriously fastidious and slow growing.[22,25,30] The presumptive diagnosis of streptococcosis is by the identification of Gram-positive cocci on touch impressions or histologic sections of affected organs. Confirmation can be achieved via culture and biochemical profiles, serological tests (i.e., slide agglutination or immunofluorescent antibody) and molecular methods.[25,28]

Management/control: Mycobacteriosis has zoonotic potential, and as such, there are no widely accepted antimicrobial treatments for this disease in fish.[20,22] Control of this disease in recirculating systems, including aquariums, usually involves culling or depopulation and disinfection. Unfortunately, commonly used aquaculture disinfectants are generally ineffective.[39] In addition, with the possibility of vertical transmission, enhanced biosecurity procedures, especially in aquaculture and biomedical facilities, such as obtaining fish from sources certified specific pathogen free (SPF), incorporation of screening/detection during the quarantine period, utilizing successively smaller diameter filters prior to ultraviolet sterilization and proper disinfection, should be incorporated.[35] Although several streptococcal diseases of fish are zoonotic, antibiotics have been used for treating disease in warmwater fish caused by *S. iniae*. Accurate identification of the bacterium, as well as susceptibility testing is recommended.[40,41] Vaccines have been developed for *S. iniae*, but they

should contain both serotypes I and II for effectiveness.[41,42] Since vertical transmission is possible, obtaining fish from certified sources and incorporation of screening/detection during the quarantine period is warranted.

PARASITIC DISEASES

Overview: A number of parasites are known to infect the reproductive system of fish resulting in grossly visible lesions. Some of these have the reproductive tract as their primary predilection site, whereas others are less tissue-specific infecting the different visceral organs including the gonads or reproductive tracts. Infestations can have detrimental results on reproduction and in severe cases can lead to parasitic castration of their host.

Etiology: The most commonly reported types of parasites that infect the reproductive system of fish are microsporidia, myxozoans and nematodes. Most often, lesions caused by these parasites are microscopic, but with severe infestations the lesions can become grossly visible. Both xenoma-forming microsporidia such as *Obruspora papernae* and several *Glugea* species including *G. anomala*, *G. hertwigi* and *G. malabaricii*, and non-xenoma-forming microsporidia such as *Ovipleistophora ovariae* (syn. *Pleistophora ovariae*) and *Ovipleistophora mirandallae* (syn. *Pleistophora mirandallae*, *P. elegans*, *P. oolytica*) have been reported to infect the gonads.[43–52] Myxosporeans that have been implicated include *Sphaerospora testicularis*, *Myxobolus dahomeyensis*, *M. kainjiae*, *M. djoudjensis*, *Kudoa azevedoi* and *Myxidium* sp.[53–61] There are at least 16 species of *Philometra* nematodes that have been reported to infect the reproductive tracts of fish including *P. carolinensis*, *P. cynoscionis*, *P. charlestonensis*, *P. lateolabracis*, *P. pellucida* and *P. saltatrix*.[62–66]

Route of transmission: All three groups of parasites can have complex life cycles. The microsporidian *O. ovariae* can be transmitted horizontally (i.e., orally) as well as vertically (i.e., transovarian).[67,68] There is also autotransmission or intrahost transmission from one oocyte of the fish to another, which increases the intensity of infection within the same individual.[69] Microsporidian parasites of the genus *Glugea* are acquired by the host fish when they either ingest free spores from the water column or consume infected aquatic invertebrates.[44] Myxozoans have complex life cycles that involve an invertebrate definitive host (usually an oligochaete) and a fish as the intermediate host.[70] *Philometra* sp. are thought to use aquatic invertebrates, such as copepods, as an intermediate host, and the fish becomes infected by consuming an infected copepod or a paratenic fish host.[66,71]

Host range: The type host for *Ovipleistophora ovariae* is the golden shiner (*Notemigonus crysoleucas*), whereas fathead minnows (*Pimephales promelas*) are considered incidental hosts.[44] *Ovipleistophora miriandellae* has been reported in cypinids including barbel (*Barbus barbus*), common bleak (*Alburnus alburnus*), roach (*Rutilus rutilus*), chub (*Leuciscus cephalus*), common dace (*L. leucicsus*), carp bream (*Abramis bramus*) and gudgeon (*Gobio gobio*). The parasite has also been reported in Eurasian ruffe (*Gymnocephalus cernuus*) and only rarely in northern pike (*Esox luciu*).[49,52] *Obruspora papernae* has been reported in the blotch-fin dragonet (*Callionymus filamentosus*).[43] *Glugea anomala* has been reported in three-spined stickleback (*Gasterosteus aculeatus*), nine- or ten-spined stickleback (*Pungitius pungitius*), and the southern nine-spined stickleback (*Pungitius platygaster*); and in the killifish (*Nothobranchius eggersi, N. korthausae, N. rachowii, N. rubripinnis, N. annectens, Fundulopanchax filamentosus*, and *Austrolebias nigripinnis*).[52] *Glugea hertwigi* has been reported in smelt (*Osmerus eperlanus eperlanus* and *O. eperlanus mordax*), and *G. malabaricii* has been reported in Malabar trevally (*Carangoides malabaricus*).[45,46,52] The myxozoan *Sphaerospora testicularis* has been reported in both wild and cultured gilthead seabream (*Dicentrarchus labrax*).[72] *Kudoa azevedoi* has been reported in Atlantic horse mackerel (*Trachurus trachurus*), and a *Myxidium* sp. has been reported in the one-spot snapper (*Lutjanus monostigma*).[60,61] *Myxobolus dahomeyensis* has been reported in the upside-down catfish (*Synodontis ansorgii*), African sharptooth catfish (*Clarias gariepinus*) and several species of tilapia (*Tilapia zillii, T. guineensis, Sarotherodon melanotheron* and hybrids *Oreochromis mossambicus × O. niloticus*).[55–57] *Myxobolus kainjiae* and *M. djoudjensis* have also been reported in tilapia.[58,59] There are several species of philometrids that are known to display a high degree of specificity for the gonads of fish and are found mainly in marine percids such as bluefish, snapper and grouper.[73] However, there are also reports of this parasite in non-perciforms such as the three-spotted flounder (*Pseudorhombus triocellatus*) and red cusk-eel (*Genypterus chilensis*).[74,75]

Clinical presentation: The gross clinical presentation of fish that have gonads infected by microsporidia is dependent on whether they are xenoma- or non-xenoma-forming microsporidia. With *Ovipleistorphora ovariae*, no behavioral or external gross lesions are usually evident.[47] The infected ovaries have white marbling or whitish opaque streaks unlike uninfected ovaries that are uniformly colored and translucent (**Figure 14.4**). Roach ovaries infected with *O. miriandellae* can be discolored and may be white to red and dark brown. Infected ovaries may also be smaller than uninfected ovaries.[50] In xenoma-forming microsporidia like *O. parpernae*, there may be multiple white xenomas that may cause abdominal distension that are visible through the skin.[43] The gross clinical presentation of a myxozoan infection in the gonads is also varied and dependent on the myxozoan species. *Sphaerospora testicularis*, a coelozoic myxozoan parasite in the seminiferous tubules, does not generally incite a host reaction in mild infections, but in heavy infections can cause inflammation of adjacent testicular tissues resulting in abdominal distension due to hypertrophy and hyalinization of the testes as well as the accumulation of ascites.[53] *Myxobolus djoudjensis*–infected ovaries have small, white or yellow cysts that are spherical, elongated or have an irregular shape.[59] Other

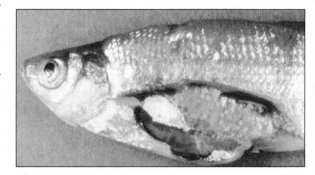

Figure 14.4 *Ovipleistophora* (~*Pleistophora*) *ovariae* infected ovaries of a golden shiner, *Notemigonus crysoleucas*. (Image courtesy of A. Mitchell.)

visible indications of myxozoan-infected ovaries are white oocytes that have a soft consistency and may progress to nodular lesions.[55,60] The presentation of *Myxidium* sp.–infected ovaries of one-spot snapper is atypical of most myxozoan with black digitiform cysts filled with myxospores projecting from the surface of the ovaries.[61] *Philometra* nematodes, depending on the stage and severity of infection, as well as host species, can cause partial or complete atrophy of the gonads, with testes more commonly affected than ovaries.[64] There can be complete destruction of both testes or ovaries with replacement by a mass of nematodes (**Figures 14.5** and **14.6**).[76] In some cases, philometrid infections are evidenced by the presence of red slender vermiform nematodes on the surface of the ovary, which sometimes is associated with

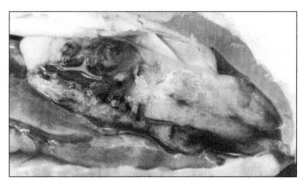

Figure 14.7 **Hemorrhage in ovaries of spotted grunter, *Pomadasys argenteus*, due to *Philometra barnesi*. (Image courtesy of B. Diggles.)**

hemorrhage in the surrounding connective tissues (**Figure 14.7**). Live nematodes can be found in well-developed gonads during the spawning season, but after spawning these parasites die and often become encapsulated in a fibrous sheath produced by the host fish.[64]

Pathology: There is minimal cell reaction to the developing non-xenoma-forming microsporidia and it is only when mature spores are released from the ruptured oocyte that phagocytosis occurs. The proliferating connective tissue does not tend to delineate spores from affected oocytes and spores may spread to the lumen of the ovary.[77] This is seen in *O. ovariae* where the initial reaction is minimal until it causes oocyte atresia characterized by an influx of macrophages that digest the spores and atretic oocytes.[47] Similarly, there is granuloma formation in the later stages of *O. miriandellae*–infected roach ovaries together with the presence of pigmented macrophages (i.e., melanomacrophages).[50] The tissue reaction to xenoma-inducing microsporidians occurs relatively quickly making most xenomas short-lived.[77] In the initial reactive stage, the xenomas, which are thin walled and contain only schizonts, undergo massive hypertrophy and can impinge on adjacent tissues causing pressure atrophy. This elicits the proliferation of connective tissue and hyperplasia of collagen fibers resulting in multiple thin concentric layers of connective tissue around the xenoma. The productive stage occurs when the xenoma is gradually filling with spores displacing the host cell cytoplasm and nucleus to the periphery, which results in a mature xenoma where nothing

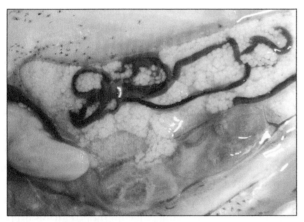

Figure 14.5 *Philometra johni* in ovary of croaker, *Johnius* sp. (Image courtesy of B. Diggles.)

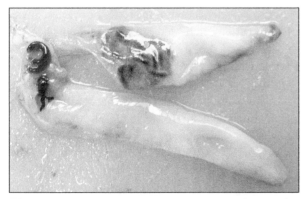

Figure 14.6 *Philometra barnesi* in testes of spotted grunter, *Pomadasys argenteus*. (Image courtesy of B. Diggles.)

remains of the host cell components except for the xenoma wall. Granulation tissue surrounding this mature xenoma consists of proliferating fibroblasts, histiocytes and newly formed capillaries.[77] In severe myxosporidian infections of *Sphaerospora testicularis*, the parasite spills over from the seminiferous tubules to the adjacent testicular tissues, followed by hypertrophy of the affected serosa together with a leukocytic infiltrate consisting mainly of granulocytes. This results in the swelling of the testes and ascites formation leading to the distention of the abdomen. At the end of the spawning season, the tubular lumen of the infected testes is often occluded by parasites encapsulated by a fibrotic host reaction.[53] In other myxozoan infections, the parasites appear to parasitize mature rather than immature oocytes, and are less pathogenic in ovarian and testicular stroma than in oocytes and seminiferous tubules. As the infection of the mature oocytes progresses, swelling of the oocytes causes them to become white with a soft consistency. These parasitized oocytes finally rupture releasing the spores and remnants of the host cell debris. The destruction of the mature oocytes can lead to cavity formation in the ovary, or the ovaries fill with thick, viscous, suppurative fluid.[54,55] The cysts in the *Myxidium* sp. infected fish consist of a capsule with a relatively thick layer of fibrous connective tissue of host cell origin and is followed by a distinct internal black layer composed of melanomacrophages. Smaller cysts may be scattered in the connective tissue between the follicles. Degenerative changes may also be noted in adjacent ovarian tissue.[61] In *Philometra*-infected ovaries of blue fish a moderate lymphocytic infiltration and hemorrhage in the connective tissues occurs with hemorrhage sometimes extending to the lumen. There is also swelling and necrosis of the connective tissue and oocytes. Granulomatous inflammation and fibrosis, when present, is associated with dead worms and occasionally atretic follicles. The fibrotic capsules are multilayered and melanized.[66]

Differential diagnoses: The differential diagnosis for microsporidian infections in the gonads would be myxozoan infections and vice versa. Other differentials would be neoplasms and infectious etiologies that cause granuloma formation, especially for xenoma-forming microsporidians.

Diagnosis: A presumptive diagnosis of an *O. ovariae* infection in the ovary would be a white marbling appearance of the ovaries of golden shiners and the observation of spores in wet mounts of macerated ovarian tissue.[47] Histological examination of tissues is required to confirm the presence of other life stages (i.e., meront and sporoblasts) or to ascertain if the fish are not infected. Molecular assays (i.e., quantitative polymerase chain reaction [qPCR]) can be performed to determine both clinical and subclinical infections.[78] Similarly, diagnosis of other microsporidian infections can be based on microscopic examination of macerated gonadal tissue and/or histological examination of tissues. Microsporidian spores are Giemsa positive, variably Gram positive, acid-fast positive and refractile when viewed using dark phase microscopy. The polar cap at the spore apex stains red with period acid–Schiff positive.[79] A practical key and a variety of ultrastructural studies are available for determining genera and species of the microsporidian.[52,80,81] Detection of spores in tissue smears can also be used to diagnose myxozoan infection. Although morphology of these mature spores can be used to differentiate the genus involved, specific identification is generally not possible.[82] Better visualization of the spores can be obtained by using Giemsa stains. Several monoclonal and polyclonal antibodies have been developed to diagnose a number of fish myxozoan pathogens, however, these do not include the myxozoans that affect the gonads. Molecular methods can be useful in providing a definitive diagnosis.[83] Diagnosis and identification of *Philometra* infection in the gonads is by observation of the nematode on the surface of the organ or by dissection of the testes or ovaries. Species identification can be determined using morphological characteristics. Microscopic examination of the tissue for nematodes is warranted to detect male or juvenile worms.[64,66]

Management/control: Since there can be direct transmission of microsporidia and due to the longevity of their spores, implementation of control measures for this parasite in natural or aquaculture facilities is difficult.[77] Several compounds have been suggested for the treatment of *G. anomala* and *O. ovariae*, but none have been approved for food fish.[84–86] There are several chemical and biological controls that have been used to lessen the impact of myxozoan parasites. However, many of these treatment recommendations were prior to elucidation of the life cycles of the myxozoans, and the effectiveness of these treatments may need to be reexamined against the actinosporean stage that might be more susceptible. Several different drugs have been explored for treating myxozoans, but again none of the compounds are approved for food fish.[83] Proper biosecurity, such as a secure water source and restriction of movement of potentially infected fish, can help stop the spread of myxozoan infections. Philometrid infections are primarily a problem in wild fish. Control of other fish nematodes have centered on control of the intermediate hosts, establishment of quarantine procedures and the use of anthelmintics.[87] The latter may be a viable option for philometrid-infected feral fish being maintained in display aquariums.

NEOPLASIA

Overview: Neoplasia of the male and female reproductive organs are generally considered rare but have been reported in a diverse variety of fish.[88–90] Those that have been reported are gonadal germ cell tumors (e.g., dysgerminomas or seminomas), gonadal stromal tumors (e.g., Sertoli-Leydig cell tumors, granulosa cell tumors, theca cell tumors), mesenchymal tumors (e.g., fibromas, fibroleiomyoma, leiomyomas, leiomyosarcomas) or epithelial tumors (e.g., cystadenomas, carcinomas).

Etiology: Most if not all of these neoplasms occur spontaneously and are of unknown etiology. Although chemical carcinogenesis has been suspected because of the high prevalence of gonadal tumors in goldfish hybrids in the Great Lakes, this has not been conclusively proven.[91] In fact, it has been shown that these tumors were also as common in areas that were less polluted.[92] Though seminomas have been reported in Japanese medaka exposed to N-methyl-N′-nitro-N-nitrosoguanidine, spontaneous formation of seminomas has also been reported in both negative control and chemically exposed male and female medaka.[90,93] It appears that genetics and age may play a role because of the disproportionally high incidence in some species.[91,94] In zebrafish, it has been postulated that

female fish with egg-associated inflammation and fibroplasia, which may result from being egg bound, may lead to the development of fibromas and fibrosarcomas.[94]

Route of transmission: Chemical induction or unknown.

Host range: Gonadal germ cell tumors have been reported in African lungfish species (*Protopterus aethiopicus*, *P. dolloi*, *P. annectens*), bagrid catfish (*Mystus macropterus*), barbel (*Barbus barbus*), black sea bass (*Centropristis striata*), carp (*Cyprinus carpio*), goldfish (*Carassius auratus*), hybrid catfish, Japanese medaka (*Oryzias latipes*), Japanese dace (*Tribolodon hakonesis*), largemouth bass (*Micropterus salmoides*), platyfish (*Xiphophorus maculatus*), yellow perch (*Perca flavescens*) and zebrafish (*Danio rerio*).[88,90–93,95–107] Gonadal stroma tumors such as Sertoli-Leydig cell tumors, granulosa cell tumors and theca cell tumors have been described in carp and channel catfish.[89,91,92,101,108] Gonadal tumors of mesenchymal origin have been reported in African lungfish (*Protopterus dolloi*), Atlantic cod (*Gadus morhua*), numerous cyprinids, largemouth bass (*Micropterus salmoides*), and yellow perch (*Perca flavescens*).[97,101,105,109–111] Those of epithelial origin include cystadenoma in the European ling (*Molva molva*), embryonal carcinoma in pike (*Esox lucius*) and ovarian carcinoma in medaka.[93,112,113]

Clinical presentation: The clinical presentation is variable and dependent on the size of the tumor, chronicity of the condition and the degree of malignancy (i.e., if there is metastasis), and the resultant effects on other visceral organs. Gonadal neoplasms can compress surrounding visceral organs causing loss of function, e.g., obstruction of the gastrointestinal tract.[98] Anorexia and cachexia are also common presentations.[88,96,100,102,110] Abdominal distension, a sequelae of massive tumor size may also result in loss of mobility, thinning of the overlying tissues, loss of scales and even death (**Figure 14.8**).[94,100] In some tumors, the onset of tumor growth may be hormonally regulated and seen at time of sexual maturity resulting in relatively rapid growth of the tumor.[91] In other tumors, there may be no gross external lesions.[108]

Pathology: Replacement or obliteration of normal gonadal tissue by benign or malignant neoplastic cells can result in presumed partial or complete loss of function of the gonads. Benign tumors also

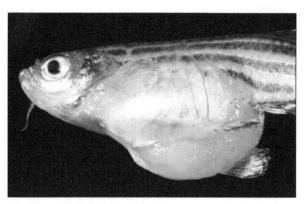

Figure 14.8 Seminoma of the testes of a zebrafish, *Danio rerio*. (Image courtesy of L. Craig.)

may result in compression necrosis due to size and/ or compromised vascular circulation. Depending on tumor type, these tumors can vary in appearance, color and texture. Although most are solid, some can result in cystic structures.[94]

Differential diagnosis: Any infectious diseases (i.e., bacterial or parasitic) resulting in grossly visible granulomas should be differentials for gonadal neoplasms.

Diagnosis: Observation of tumors during radiography, ultrasonography, exploratory surgery or necropsy provides a tentative diagnosis. Definitive diagnosis requires fixed tissues or biopsy, and confirmation via microscopic examination and histopathological identification.

Management/control: Not applicable.

REFERENCES

1. Trippel, E.A. and Harvey, H.H. Ovarian atresia and sex ratio imbalance in white sucker, *Catostomus commersoni*. *Journal of Fish Biology* 1990;36(2):231–239.
2. Lewbart, G.A. Reproductive medicine in koi (*Cyprinus carpio*). *Veterinary Clinics of North America: Exotic Animal Practice* 2002;5(3):637–648.
3. Lahnsteiner, F. Morphological, physiological and biochemical parameters characterizing the over-ripening of rainbow trout eggs. *Fish Physiology and Biochemistry* 2000;23(2):107–118.
4. Lubzens, E., Young, G., Bobe, J. and Cerdà, J. Oogenesis in teleosts: How fish eggs are formed. *General and Comparative Endocrinology* 2010;165(3):367–389.
5. Miranda, A.C., Bazzoli, N., Rizzo, E. and Sato, Y. Ovarian follicular atresia in two teleost species: A histological and ultrastructural study. *Tissue and Cell* 1999;31(5):480–488.
6. Mills, C.A. Spawning and rearing eggs of the dace *Leuciscus leuciscus* (L.). *Aquaculture Research* 1980;11(2):67–72.
7. Lam, T.J., Nagahama, Y., Chan, K. and Hoar, W.S. Overripe eggs and postovulatory corpora lutea in the three-spine stickleback, *Gasterosteus aculeatus* L., form *trachurus*. *Canadian Journal of Zoology* 1978;56(9):2029–2036.
8. McFarlane, G.A. and Franzin, W.G. Elevated heavy metals: A stress on a population of white suckers, *Catostomus commersoni*, in Hamell Lake, Saskatchewan. *Journal of the Fisheries Board of Canada* 1978;35(7):963–970.
9. Quinn, T.P., Eggers, D.M., Clark, J.H. and Rich Jr, H.B. Density, climate, and the processes of prespawning mortality and egg retention in Pacific salmon (*Oncorhynchus* spp.). *Canadian Journal of Fisheries and Aquatic Sciences* 2007;64(3):574–582.
10. Kent, M.L., Harper, C. and Wolf, J.C. Documented and potential research impacts of subclinical diseases in zebrafish. *ILAR Journal* 2012;53(2):126–134.
11. Formacion, M.J., Hori, R. and Lam, T.J. Overripening of ovulated eggs in goldfish: I. Morphological changes. *Aquaculture* 1993;114(1–2):155–168.
12. Sharma, R.K. and Bhat, R.A. Histomorphology of atretic follicles in rainbow trout (*Oncorhynchus mykiss*) from Kashmir. *Journal of Entomology and Zoology Studies* 2014;2(4):21–26.
13. Besseau, L. and Faliex, E. Resorption of unemitted gametes in *Lithognathus mormyrus* (Sparidae, Teleostei): A possible synergic action of somatic and immune cells. *Cell and Tissue Research* 1994;276(1):123–132.
14. Rossteuscher, S., Schmidt-Posthaus, H., Schäfers, C., Teigeler, M. and Segner, H. Background pathology of the ovary in a laboratory population of zebrafish *Danio rerio*. *Diseases of Aquatic Organisms* 2008;79(2):169–172.
15. Kent, M.L., Whipps, C.M., Matthews, J.L., Florio, D., Watral, V., Bishop-Stewart, J.K., Poort, M. and Bermudez, L. Mycobacteriosis in zebrafish (*Danio rerio*) research facilities. *Comparative Biochemistry and Physiology Part I* 2004;138(3):383–396.
16. Raidal, S.R., Shearer, P.L., Stephens, F. and Richardson, J. Surgical removal of an ovarian tumor in a koi carp (*Cyprinus carpio*). *Australian Veterinary Journal* 2006;84(5):178–181.
17. Gómez, S. Prevalence of microscopic tubercular lesions in freshwater ornamental fish exhibiting clinical signs of non-specific chronic disease. *Diseases of Aquatic Organisms* 2008;80(2):167–171.
18. Miyazaki, T., Kubota, S.S., Kaige, N. and Miyashita, T. A histopathological study of streptococcal disease in tilapia. *Fish Pathology* 1984;19(3):167–172.
19. Abernethy, C.S. and Lund, J.E. Mycobacteriosis in mountain whitefish (*Prosopium williamsoni*) from the Yakima River, Washington. *Journal of Wildlife Diseases* 1978;14(3):333–336.
20. Smith, S.A. Mycobacterial infections in pet fish. *Seminars in Avian and Exotic Pet Medicine* 1997;6:40–45.

21. Jacobs, J.M., Stine, C.B., Baya, A.M. and Kent, M.L. A review of mycobacteriosis in marine fish. *Journal of Fish Diseases* 2009;32(2):119–130.

22. Gauthier, D.T. and Rhodes, M.W. Mycobacteriosis in fishes: A review. *The Veterinary Journal* 2009;180(1): 33–47.

23. Eldar, A., Frelier, P.F., Assenta, L., Varner, P.W., Lawhon, S. and Bercovier, H. *Streptococcus shiloi*, the name for an agent causing septicemic infection in fish, is a junior synonym of *Streptococcus iniae*. *International Journal of Systematic and Evolutionary Microbiology* 1995;45(4):840–842.

24. Kawamura, Y., Itoh, Y., Mishima, N., Ohkusu, K., Kasai, H. and Ezaki, T. High genetic similarity of *Streptococcus agalactiae* and *Streptococcus difficilis*: *S. difficillis* Eldar et al. 1995 is a later synonym of *S. agalactiae* Lehmann and Neumann 1896 (Approved Lists 1980). *International Journal of Systematic and Evolutionary Microbiology* 2005;55:961–965.

25. Toranzo, A.E., Magarinos, B. and Romalde, J.L. A review of the main bacterial fish diseases in mariculture systems. *Aquaculture* 2005;246(1):37–61.

26. Pradeep, P.J., Suebsing, R., Sirthammajak, S., Kampeera, J., Jitrakorn, S., Saksmerprome, V., Turner, W. et al. Evidence of vertical transmission and tissue tropism of streptococcosis from naturally infected red tilapia (*Oreochromis* spp.). *Aquaculture Reports* 2016;3: 58–66.

27. Suebsing, R., Kampeera, J., Tookdee, B., Withyachumnarnkul, B., Turner, W. and Kiatpathomchai, W. Evaluation of colorimetric loop-mediated isothermal amplification assay for visual detection of *Streptococcus agalactiae* and *Streptococcus iniae* in tilapia. *Letters in Applied Microbiology* 2013;57(4): 317–324.

28. Jantrakajorn, S., Maisak, H. and Wongtavatchai, J. Comprehensive investigation of streptococcosis outbreaks in cultured Nile tilapia, *Oreochromis niloticus*, and red tilapia, *Oreochromis* sp., of Thailand. *Journal of the World Aquaculture Society* 2014;45(4):392–402.

29. Lewis, S. and Chinabut, S. Mycobacteria and nocardiosis. In: *Fish Diseases and Disorders*, Vol. 3: *Bacterial and Fungal Infections*, 2nd ed. P.T.K. Woo and D.W. Bruno, eds. CABI Publishing, Wallingford, Oxfordshire, UK, 2006; pp. 397–423.

30. Decostere, A., Hermans, K. and Haesebrouck, F. Piscine mycobacteriosis: A literature review covering the agent and the disease it causes in fish and humans. *Veterinary Microbiology* 2004;99(3):159–166.

31. Chinabut, S., Kanayati, Y. and Pungkachonboon, T. Study of transovarian transmission of mycobacteria in *Betta splendens* Regan. In: *Proceedings of the Third Asian Fisheries Forum*, October 26–30, 1992, Singapore. L.M. Chou, A.D. Munro, T.J. Lam, T.W. Chen, L.K.K. Cheong, J.K. Ding, K.K. Hooi et al., eds. 1994; pp. 339–341.

32. Frerichs, G.N. Mycobacteriosis: Nocardiosis. In: *Bacterial Diseases of Fish*. V. Inglis, R.J. Roberts and N.R. Bromage, eds. Blackwell Scientific Publications, London, 1993; pp. 219–235.

33. Novotny, L., Halouzka, R., Matlova, L., Vavra, O., Bartosova, L., Slany, M. and Pavlik, I. Morphology and distribution of granulomatous inflammation in freshwater ornamental fish infected with mycobacteria. *Journal of Fish Diseases* 2010;33(12):947–955.

34. Astrofsky, K.M., Schrenzel, M.D., Bullis, R.A., Smolowitz, R.M. and Fox, J.G. Diagnosis and management of atypical *Mycobacterium* spp. infections in established laboratory zebrafish (*Brachydanio rerio*) facilities. *Comparative Medicine* 2000;50(6):666–672.

35. Sanders, S.E. and Swain, L.E. Atypical piscine mycobacteriosis in Japanese medaka (*Oryzias latipes*). *Comparative Medicine* 2001;51(2):171–175.

36. Kent, M.L., Watral, V.G., Kirchoff, N.S., Spagnoli, S.T. and Sharpton, T.J. Effects of subclinical *Mycobacterium chelonae* infections on fecundity and embryo survival in zebrafish. *Zebrafish* 2016;13(S1):S88–95.

37. Miyazaki, T., Kubota, S.S., Kaige, N. and Miyashita, T. A histopathological study of streptococcal disease in tilapia. *Fish Pathology* 1984;19(3):167–172.

38. Whipps, C.M., Matthews, J.L. and Kent, M.L. Distribution and genetic characterization of *Mycobacterium chelonae* in laboratory zebrafish (*Danio rerio*). *Diseases of Aquatic Organisms* 2008;82:45–54.

39. Mainous, M.E. and Smith, S.A. Efficacy of common disinfectants against *Mycobacterium marinum*. *Journal of Aquatic Animal Health* 2005;17(3):284–288.

40. Weinstein, M.R., Litt, M., Kertesz, D.A., Wyper, P., Rose, D., Coulter, M., McGeer, A. et al. Invasive infections due to a fish pathogen, *Streptococcus iniae*. *New England Journal of Medicine* 1997;337(9):589–594.

41. Agnew, W. and Barnes, A.C. *Streptococcus iniae*: An aquatic pathogen of global veterinary significance and a challenging candidate for reliable vaccination. *Veterinary Microbiology* 2007;122(1):1–5.

42. Bachrach, G., Zlotkin, A., Hurvitz, A., Evans, D.L. and Eldar, A. Recovery of *Streptococcus iniae* from diseased fish previously vaccinated with a streptococcus vaccine. *Applied and Environmental Microbiology* 2001; 67(8):3756–3758.

43. Diamant, A., Rothman, S.B., Goren, M., Galil, B.S., Yokes, M.B., Szitenberg, A. and Huchon, D. Biology of a new xenoma-forming gonadotropic microsporidium in the invasive blotchfin dragonet *Callionymus filamentosus*. *Diseases of Aquatic Organisms* 2014;109(1): 35–54.

44. Weissenberg, R. Intracellular development of the microsporidan *Glugea anomala* Moniez in hypertrophying migratory cells of the fish *Gasterosteus aculeatus* L., an example of the formation of "xenoma" tumors. *Journal of Eukaryotic Microbiology* 1968;15(1):44–57.

45. Haley, A.J. Microsporidian parasite, *Glugea hertwigi*, in American smelt from the Great Bay region, New Hampshire. *Transactions of the American Fisheries Society* 1954;83(1):84–90.

46. Narasimhamurti, C., Kalavati, C. and Sandeep, B. A new microsporidian *Glugea malabaricii* sp. n. from the viscera of *Carangoides malabaricus*. *Protozoologica* 1985; 24(2):153–164.

47. Summerfelt, R.C. and Goodwin, A.E. 2010. Ovipleistophoriasis: A Microsporidian disease of the golden shiner ovary. In *Fish Health Section Blue Book: Suggested Procedures for the Detection and Identification of Certain Finfish and Shellfish Pathogens*. 2014. American Fisheries Society-Fish Health Section. http://afs-fhs.org/bluebook/bluebook-index.php.

48. Nagel, M.L. and Hoffman, G.L. A new host for *Pleistophora ovariae* (Microsporida). *Journal of Parasitology* 1977;76:160–162.

49. Pekkarinen, M., Lom, J. and Nilsen, F. Ovipleistophora gen. n., a new genus for *Pleistophora mirandellae*-like microsporidians. *Diseases of Aquatic Organisms* 2002;48: 133–142.

50. Wiklund, T., Lounasheimo, L., Lom, J. and Bylund, G. Gonadal impairment in roach *Rutilus rutilus* from Finnish coastal areas of the northern Baltic Sea. *Diseases of Aquatic Organisms* 1996;26(3):163–171.

51. Maurand, J., Loubes, C., Gasc, C., Pelletier, J. and Barral, J. *Pleistophora mirandellae* Vaney & Conte, 1901, a microsporidian parasite in cyprinid fish of rivers in Hérault: Taxonomy and histopathology. *Journal of Fish Diseases* 1988;11:251–258.

52. Lom, J. A catalogue of described genera and species of microsporidians parasitic in fish. *Systematic Parasitology* 2002;53(2):81–99.

53. Alvarez-Pellitero, P. and Sitja-Bobadilla, A. Pathology of myxosporea in marine fish culture. *Diseases of Aquatic Organisms* 1993;17:229–238.

54. Gbankoto, A., Tossavi, N.D., Sindété, M., Sakiti, G.N., Moutaïrou, K. and Ribou, A.-C. Some pathophysiological insights into ovarian infestation by *Myxobolus* sp. (Myxozoa: Myxosporea) in *Clarias gariepinus* (Clariids: Silurids) from Bénin (West Africa). *Parasitology Research* 2015;114:2941–2949.

55. Grankoto, A., Pampoulie, C., Marques, A. and Sakiti, G.N. *Myxobolus dahomeyensis* infection in ovaries of Tilapia species from Benin (West Africa). *Journal of Fish Biology* 2001;58(3):883–886.

56. Sakiti, G.N., Blanc, E., Marques, A. and Bouix, G. Myxosporidies (Myxozoa, Myxosporea) du genre *Myxobolus* Bütschli, 1882 parasites de poissons Cichlidae du lac Nokoué au Bénin (Afrique de l'Ouest). *Journal of African Zoology* 1991;105:173–186.

57. Siau, Y. Myxosporidies de *Synodontis ansorgii* Boulenger 1911 et de *Eleotris (Kribia) kribiensis* Boulenger, 1964, poissons des eaux saumâtres de la lagune de Porto-Novo (Dahomey). *Bulletin de la Société Zoologique de France* 1971;96:563–570.

58. Obiekezie, A.I. and Okaeme, A.N. Myxosporea (Protozoa) infections of cultured tilapias in Nigeria. *Revue de Zoologie Africaine* 1990;104(1):77–91.

59. Damanka, A., Faye, N., Fall, M. and Toguebaye, B.S. Myxosporidian parasites of the genus *Myxobolus*

butschli, 1882 found for the first time in Cichlid fishes from Senegal River (West Africa). *Acta Protozoologica* 2007;46(3):257–262.

60. Mansour, L., Thabet, A., Chourabi, K., Harrath, A.H., Gtari, M., Al Omar, S.Y. and Hassine, O.K.B. *Kudoa azevedoi* n. sp. (Myxozoa, Multivalvulida) from the oocytes of the Atlantic horse mackerel *Trachurus trachurus* (Perciformes, Carangidae) in Tunisian coasts. *Parasitology Research* 2013;112(4):1737–1747.

61. Al-Jahdali, M.O. and Hassanine, R. Ovarian abnormality in a pathological case caused by *Myxidium* sp. (Myxozoa, Myxosporea) in one spot snapper fish *Lutjanus monostigma* (Teleostei, Lutjanidae) from Red Sea. *Acta Parasitologica* 2010;55(1):1–7.

62. Moravec, F., de Buron, I. and Roumillat, W.A. Two new species of Philometra (Nematoda: Philometridae) parasitic in the perciform fish *Cynoscion nebulosus* (Sciaenidae) in the estuaries of South Carolina, USA. *Folia Parasitologica* 2006;53(1):63–70.

63. Moravec, F., de Buron, I., Baker, T. and González-Solís, D. Some gonad-infecting species of Philometra (Nematoda, Philometridae) from offshore fishes of South Carolina and Georgia, USA, including *Philometra charlestonensis* sp. nov. from the scamp *Mycteroperca phenax*. *Acta Parasitologica* 2008;53(4): 382–391.

64. Hesp, S.A., Hobbs, R.P. and Potter, I.C. Infection of the gonads of *Glaucosoma hebvaicum* by the nematode *Philometva lateolabracis*: Occurrence and host response. *Journal of Fish Biology* 2002;60(3):663–673.

65. Hooper, J.N. Parasites of estuarine and oceanic flathead fishes (Family Platycephalidae) from northern New South Wales. *Australian Journal of Zoology Supplementary Series* 1983;31(90):1–69.

66. Clarke, L.M., Dove, A.D. and Conover, D.O. Prevalence, intensity, and effect of a nematode (*Philometra saltatrix*) in the ovaries of bluefish (*Pomatomus saltatrix*). *Fishery Bulletin* 2006;104(1):118–124.

67. Summerfelt, R.C. *Studies on the transmission of Plistophora ovariae, an ovary parasite of the golden shiner*. Final Report: Project, 1972; pp. 4–66.

68. Phelps, N.B.D. and Goodwin, A.E. Vertical transmission of *Ovipleistophora ovariae* (Microspora) within the eggs of the golden shiner. *Journal of Aquatic Animal Health* 2008;20:45–53.

69. Summerfelt, R.C. and Warner, M.C. Geographical distribution and host-parasite relationships of *Plistophora ovariae* (Microsporida, Nosematidae) in *Notemigonus crysoleucas*. *Journal of Wildlife Diseases* 1970;6:457–465.

70. Lom, J. and Dyková, I. Myxozoan genera: Definition and notes on taxonomy, life-cycle terminology and pathogenic species. *Folia Parasitologica* 2006;53(1):1–36.

71. Moravec, F. Some aspects of the taxonomy and biology of dracunculoid nematodes parasitic in fishes: A review. *Folia Parasitologica* 2004;51(1):1–13.

72. Sitja-Bobadilla, A. and Alvarez-Pelliterio, P. *Sphaerospora testicularis* sp. nov. (Myxosporea: Sphaerosporidae)

in wild and cultured sea bass, *Dicentrarchus labrax* (L.), from the Spanish Mediterranean area. *Journal of Fish Diseases* 1990;13(3):193–203.

73. Moravec, F., Chaabane, A., Neifar, L., Gey, D. and Justine, J.-L. Species of Philometra (Nematoda, Philometridae) from fishes off the Mediterranean coast of Africa, with a description of *Philometra rara* n. sp. from *Hyporthodus haifensis* and a molecular analysis of *Philometra saltatrix* from *Pomatomus saltatrix*. *Parasite* 2017;24(8):1–12.

74. Selvakumar, P., Gopalakrishnan, A., Sakthivel, A. and Bharathirajan, P. Ovarian nematode (Nematoda: *Philometra* sp.) infestation on Pseudorhombus triocellatus (Paralichthydiadae). *Asian Pacific Journal of Tropical Disease* 2016;6(10):793–796.

75. Moravec, F., Rosa, A.C. and Oliva, M.E. A new gonad-infecting species of *Philometra* (Nematoda: Philometridae) from the red cusk-eel *Genypterus chilensis* (Osteichthyes: Ophidiidae) off Chile. *Parasitology Research* 2011;108:227–232.

76. Grau, A., Riera, F. and Carbonell, E. Some protozoan and metazoan parasites of the amberjack from the Balearic Sea (western Mediterranean). *Aquaculture International* 1999;7(5):307–317.

77. Dyková, I. and Lom, J. Tissue reactions to microsporidian infections in fish. *Journal of Fish Diseases* 1980;3(4):265–283.

78. Phelps, N.B. and Goodwin, A.E. Validation of a quantitative PCR diagnostic method for detection of the microsporidian *Ovipleistophora ovariae* in the cyprinid fish *Notemigonus crysoleucas*. *Diseases of Aquatic Organisms* 2007;76(3):215–221.

79. Dyková, I. Phylum Microspora. In: *Fish Diseases and Disorders, Vol. 1: Protozoan and Metazoan Infections*, 2nd ed. P.T.K. Woo, ed. CABI, Wallingford, Oxfordshire, UK, 2006; pp. 205–229.

80. Canning, E.U., Lom, J. and Dykova, I. *The Microsporidia of Vertebrates*. Academic Press, London, 1986; p. 304.

81. Lom, J. and Dykova, I. *Protozoan Parasites of Fish: In Developments in Aquaculture and Fisheries Science*, Vol. 26. Elsevier Science, Amsterdam, 1992; pp. 129–135.

82. Lom, J. and Arthur, J.R. A guideline for the preparation of species descriptions in Myxosporea. *Journal of Fish Diseases* 1989;12(2):151–156.

83. Feist, S.W. and Longshaw, M. Phylum myxozoa. In: *Fish Diseases and Disorders, Vol. 1: Protozoan and Metazoan Infections*, 2nd ed. P.T.K. Woo, ed. CABI, Wallingford, Oxfordshire, UK, 2006; pp. 230–296.

84. Schmahl, G. and Mehlhorn, H. Treatment of fish parasites: 6. Effects of sym. triazinone (toltrazuril) on developmental stages of *Glugea anomala*, Moniez, 1887 (Microsporidia): A light and electron microscopic study. *European Journal of Protistology* 1989;24(3):252–259.

85. Schmahl, G., El Toukhy, A. and Ghaffar, F.A. Transmission electron microscopic studies on the effects of toltrazuril on *Glugea anomala*, Moniez, 1887 (Microsporidia) infecting the three-spined stickleback *Gasterosteus aculeatus*. *Parasitology Research* 1990; 76(8):700–706.

86. Nagel, M.L. and Summerfelt, R.C. Nitrofurazone for control of the microsporidan parasite *Pleistophora ovariae* in golden shiners. *The Progressive Fish-Culturist* 1977;39(1):18–23.

87. Molnár, K., Buchmann, K. and Székley, C. Phylum Nematoda. In: *Fish Diseases and Disorders, Vol. 1: Protozoan and Metazoan Infections*, 2nd ed. P.T.K. Woo, ed. CABI, Wallingford, Oxfordshire, UK, 2006; pp. 417–443.

88. Sirri, R., Mandrioli, L., Grieco, V., Bacci, B., Brunetti, B., Sarli, G. and Schmidt-Posthaus, H. Seminoma in a koi carp *Cyprinus carpio*: Histopathological and immunohistochemical findings. *Diseases of Aquatic Organisms* 2010;92:82–88.

89. Groff, J. Neoplasia in fishes. *Veterinary Clinics of North America Exotic Animal Practice* 2004;7:705–756.

90. Hawkins, W.E., Fournie, J.W., Ishikawa, T. and Walker, W.W. Germ cell neoplasms in Japanese medaka. *Journal of Aquatic Animal Health* 1996;8:120–129.

91. Leatherland, J.F. and Sonstegard, R.A. Structure of normal testis and testicular tumors in cyprinids from Lake Ontario. *Cancer Research* 1978;38:3164–3173.

92. Down, N.E. and Leatherland, J.F. Histopathology of the gonadal neoplasms in cyprinid fish from the lower Great Lakes of North America. *Journal of Fish Diseases* 1989;12:415–437.

93. Bunton, T.E. and Wolfe, M.J. N-methyl-N′-nitro-N-nitrosoguanidine-induced neoplasms in medaka (*Oryzias latipes*). *Toxicologic Pathology* 1996;24:323–330.

94. Ishikawa, T. and Takayama, S. Ovarian neoplasms in ornamental hybrid carp (Nishikigoi) in Japan. *Annals of the New York Academy of Science* 1977;298:330–341.

95. Nigrelli, R.F. and Jakowska, S. Spontaneous neoplasms in fishes. VII: A spermatocytoma and renal melanoma in an African lungfish *Protopterus annectens* (Owen). *Zoologica* 1953;38:109–112.

96. Masahito, P., Ishikawa, T. and Takayama, S. Spontaneous spermatocytic seminoma in African lungfish, *Protopterus aethiopicus* Heckel. *Journal of Fish Diseases* 1984;7:169–172.

97. Hubbard, G.B. and Fletcher, K.C. A seminoma and a leiomyosarcoma in an albino African lungfish (*Protopterus dolloi*). *Journal of Wildlife Diseases* 1985;21:72–74.

98. Majeed, S.K. and Wang, D.S. Tumours in the gonads of bagrid catfish, *Mystus macropterus* (Bleeker). *Journal of Fish Diseases* 1994;17:527–532.

99. Palikova, M., Navratil, S., Svobodova, Z., Tichy, L., Recek, L. and Pikula, J. Skin and gonadal tumours in a barbel *(Barbus barbus)*: A case report. *Bulletin of the European Association Fish Pathologists* 2007;27:236–238.

100. Weisse, C., Weber, S.E., Matzkin, Z. and Klide, A. Surgical removal of a seminoma from a black sea bass.

Journal of the American Veterinary Medical Association 2002;221:280–283.

101. Granado-Lorencio, C., Garcia-Novo, F. and Lopez-Campos, J. Testicular tumors in carp-funa hybrid: Annual cycle and effect on a wild population. *Journal of Wildlife Diseases* 1987;23:422–427.

102. Sahoo, P.K., Sahoo, S.K., Giri, S.S., Swain, T. and Sahu, A.K. Seminoma in hybrid catfish [*Clarias batrachus* (Linnaeus) ♀ × *Clarius gariepinus* (Burchell) ♂]. *Indian Journal of Experimental Biology* 2004;42:626–627.

103. Masahito, P., Ishkawa, T., Takayama, S. and Sugimura, H. Gonadal neoplasms in largemouth bass, *Micropterus salmoides* and Japanese dace (ugui), *Tribolodon hakonensis. Japanese Journal of Cancer Research* 1984;75(9): 776–783.

104. Burns, J.R. and Kallman, K.D. An ovarian regression syndrome in the platyfish, *Xiphophorus maculatus. Journal of Experimental Zoology* 1985;233:301–316.

105. Blazer, V.S. Histopathological assessment of gonadal tissue in wild fishes. *Fish Physiology and Biochemistry* 2002;26(1):85–101.

106. Smolowitz, R., Hanley, J. and Richmond, H. A three-year retrospective study of abdominal tumors in zebrafish maintained in an aquatic laboratory animal facility. *The Biological Bulletin* 2002;203:265–266.

107. Spitsbergen, J.M., Buhler, D.R. and Peterson, T.S. Neoplasia and neoplasm associated lesions in laboratory colonies of zebrafish emphasizing key influences of diet and aquaculture system design. *ILAR Journal* 2012;53(2):114–125.

108. Khoo, L., Camp, K.L., Leard, A.T. and Harshbarger, J.C. Granulosa cell tumor in a farm-reared channel catfish. *Journal of Aquatic Animal Health* 2000;12(3): 241–245.

109. Thomas, L. Les sarcomes fibrobastiques chez la morue. *Bulletin de l'Association Francaise pour l'Etude du Cancer* 1927;16:79–89.

110. Herman, R.L. and Landolt, M. A testicular leiomyoma in a largemouth bass, *Micropterus salmoides. Journal of Wildlife Diseases* 1975;11:128–129.

111. Budd, J., Schroder, J.D. and Dukes, K.D. Tumors of the yellow perch. In: *The Pathology of Fishes.* W.E. Ribelin and G. Migaki, eds. University of Wisconsin Press, Madison, WI, 1975; pp. 895–906.

112. Johnstone, J. Diseased and abnormal conditions of marine fishes. *Reports from Lancashire Sea-Fish Laboratory* 1914;23:18–56.

113. Haddow, A. and Blake, I. Neoplasms in fish. A report of six cases with a summary of the literature. *Journal of Pathological Bacteriology* 1933;36:41–47.

CHAPTER 15

NEUROLOGICAL DISEASES

SALVATORE FRASCA, JR.

STREPTOCOCCOSIS

Overview: Disease caused by bacteria of the genus *Streptococcus* or *Streptococcus*-like bacteria, such as enterococci and lactococci, is referred to as streptococcosis. Among the bacteria that have been identified as causing streptococcosis in fish, *Streptococcus iniae* is perhaps the most significant due to its virulence across a broad range of hosts, global distribution, economic impact and zoonotic risk.[1,2]

Etiology: *Streptococcus iniae* is a Gram-positive, encapsulated, beta-hemolytic coccus that is aerobic and facultatively anaerobic.[3] The bacterium has a global distribution with isolations in North America, the Middle East and the Asia-Pacific.[1]

Route of transmission: Experimental transmission of *S. iniae* has been achieved orally and by bath immersion, with and without skin abrasion, and by intraperitoneal injection.[1,4] Suspected other routes of transmission include ascension along the olfactory tract and direct contact.[1,4] Cannibalism of dead or dying infected fish may be a source of infection via the oral route.[1,4]

Host range: *Streptococcus iniae* has been reported from at least 27 species of fish, infecting feral and farmed populations of freshwater and marine fish from a wide range of genera including *Seriola*, *Anguilla*, *Oncorhynchus*, *Tilapia* and *Lates*.[1] The host range of *S. iniae* not only includes numerous species of fish, but also dolphins and humans, although the dolphin strain of *S. iniae* has not been associated with disease in fish.[1,5] *Streptococcus iniae* is a serious zoonotic pathogen with infections in humans handling raw fish being reported in North America and Asia.[2]

Clinical presentation: Disease caused by *S. iniae* varies with the virulence of the strain, fish host, route of infection, life stage of the fish, and environmental and water quality parameters.[1] In acute disease, sudden death may occur without premonitory signs, or signs may be limited to corneal opacification.[1,6] In subacute disease, a range of clinical signs, many nonspecific, can be seen and include unilateral or bilateral exophthalmos, corneal opacification, melanosis, lethargy, disorientation, erratic swimming behavior, anorexia, weight loss, and/or spinal rigidity or deviation (**Figures 15.1** through **15.3**).[1]

Pathology: Grossly apparent lesions include corneal opacification, exophthalmos and intracranial edema.[7] Principal histopathologic findings consist of septicemia in acute disease, and meningitis or meningoencephalitis and ophthalmitis in subacute disease.[4,7]

Differential diagnosis: Bacterial hemorrhagic septicemia, e.g., *Aeromonas* spp.; betanodaviral encephalitis; viral hemorrhagic septicemia.

Diagnosis: Diagnosis of streptococcosis requires correlation of clinical signs with histopathologic findings (e.g., meningitis, meningoencephalitis, pan- or endophthalmitis) and isolation of the bacterium.[1] The brain is the primary organ for culture isolation, although the bacterium may be isolated from other organs such as kidney and spleen, as well as from water.[1] It is worth noting that *S. iniae* has been isolated from fish that have survived outbreaks, as well as from apparently healthy barramundi and tilapia.[1,6,8]

Management/control: Antibiotic therapy is effective in treating fish during outbreaks, although efficacy varies with the drug, fish species, stocking density and morbidity of the population.[1] Vaccines against *S. iniae* have been developed; however, their efficacy has been limited and recrudescence of infection has occurred.[9,10] Identification of infected fish and implementation of biosecurity measures are

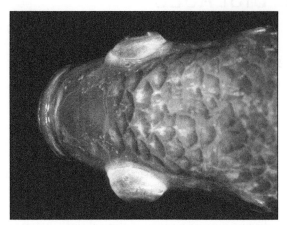

Figure 15.1 Bilateral exophthalmia in a Nile tilapia (*Oreochromis nilotica*) due to *Streptococcus iniae* infection. (Image courtesy of A. Camus.)

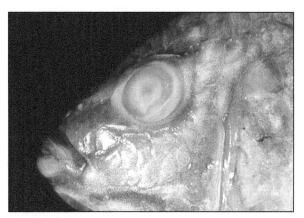

Figure 15.2 Corneal opacification in a Nile tilapia (*Oreochromis nilotica*) due to *S. iniae* infection. (Image courtesy of A. Camus.)

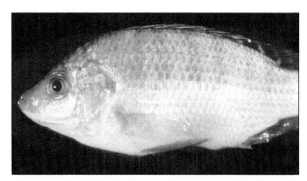

Figure 15.3 Weight loss and regional petechial hemorrhage of ventral abdomen near vent due to *S. iniae* infection in tilapia (*Oreochromis* sp.). (Image courtesy of S.A. Smith.)

critical to limiting the spread of disease within and between facilities.

ENTERIC SEPTICEMIA OF CATFISH

Overview: Enteric septicemia of catfish (ESC) and "hole-in-the-head disease" are different manifestations of disease caused by *Edwardsiella ictaluri* in channel catfish (*Ictalurus punctatus*) and other ictalurids, e.g., white catfish (*I. catus*) and brown bullhead (*I. nebulosus*). *Edwardsiella ictaluri* is an emergent pathogen to many non-ictalurid species of fish, in which the disease is referred to as edwardsiellosis.

Etiology: The causative agent of ESC is *Edwardsiella ictaluri*, a Gram-negative, rod-shaped, oxidase-negative, peritrichous, fermentative bacterium.[11]

Route of transmission: The bacterium has been shown to infect channel catfish via the intestine, nares and gill, as well as to invade skin at sites of abrasion in experimental immersion studies.[12]

Host range: Disease caused by *E. ictaluri* was originally documented in channel catfish but has been recognized in a broad range of cultured ictalurid species in the southeastern United States and Asia, e.g., walking catfish (*Clarias batrachus* L.) and hybrid catfish (*Clarias macrocephalus* × *Clarias gariepinus*) in Thailand; yellow catfish (*Pelteobagrus fulvidraco*) in China; and striped catfish (*Pangasius hypophthalmus*) in Vietnam.[13-15] Of significant epidemiologic concern is the fact that edwardsiellosis by *E. ictaluri* has been recognized in non-ictalurid fish in aquarium and laboratory settings, e.g., Bengal danio (*Danio devario*), Nile tilapia (*Oreochromis niloticus*), green knifefish (*Eigenmannia virescens*) and zebrafish (*Danio rerio*).[16-19]

Clinical presentation: Clinical signs of *E. ictaluri* infection in catfish include reduced feeding, listlessness and occasional rapid swimming at the water surface, and spiraling behavior. Gross external lesions reported in acute disease include petechial hemorrhages surrounding the mouth, along the ventrum and at the base of fins; gill pallor; slight exophthalmos; and numerous circular, white, slightly raised epithelial lesions.[20,21] In chronic disease there is characteristic ulceration of skin and muscle overlying the calvaria, exposing bone and occasionally brain, and resulting in the presentation that has

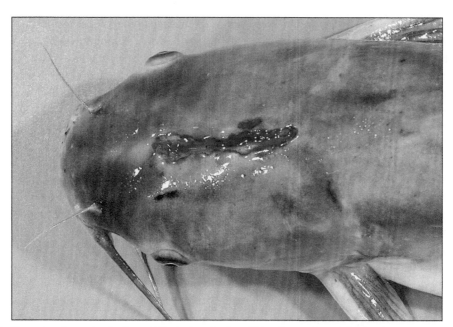

Figure 15.4 Chronic ulcerative lesion of "hole-in-the-head" in channel catfish (*Ictalurus punctatus*) infected with *Edwardsiella ictaluri*. (Image courtesy of L. Khoo.)

given rise to the name "hole-in-the-head disease" (**Figure 15.4**).[21]

Pathology: Internally, in acute disease, lesions are those of septicemia with petechial hemorrhages distributed throughout the liver, intestine, spleen, adipose tissue and mesenteries, together with a cloudy red coelomic effusion and gas-filled intestine.[20,21] In acute disease, histopathologic findings include acute granulocytic encephalitis localized to the medulla oblongata, whereas in chronic disease, there is granulomatous inflammation of the olfactory bulb and telencephalon.[21]

Differential diagnosis: Bacterial hemorrhagic septicemia, e.g., *Aeromonas* spp.

Diagnosis: Bacterial culture has been the conventional diagnostic modality with sampling including the brain. Real-time polymerase chain reaction (PCR) assays have been developed that provide rapid, sensitive, specific and accurate means of detecting and quantifying the presence of *E. ictaluri* in channel catfish and in pond water.[22,23]

Management/control: Key to management and control of edwardsiellosis in aquaculture settings is rapid and early detection of the bacterium. An avirulent live bacterin against *E. ictaluri*, available commercially under the name AQUAVAC-ESC™, has been used in aquaculture to protect channel catfish from ESC.[24]

MYCOBACTERIOSIS

Overview: Piscine mycobacteriosis is a collective term for the disease of fish caused by various species of *Mycobacterium*. The disease is a chronic, progressive, systemic infection that may take months, if not years, to manifest with clinical signs; it is often characterized by pronounced emaciation and has been referred to as "fish tuberculosis" or "wasting disease."[25]

Etiology: Collectively, the mycobacteria are pleomorphic, Gram-positive, acid-fast, nonmotile, aerobic rods that contain long-chain 3-hydroxy mycolic acids in their cell walls.[26] The species of *Mycobacterium* most frequently reported in cases of piscine mycobacteriosis are *M. marinum*, *M. fortuitum* and *M. chelonae*.[25,26] However, a growing number of experiences indicate that the assemblage of *Mycobacterium* species associated with disease in fish is much more diverse.

Route of transmission: Transmission of mycobacteria is considered to occur principally through ingestion of contaminated feed; consuming infected organic debris in the environment; or preying on, scavenging or cannibalizing infected fish.[27,28] Transovarian transmission has been reported in a viviparous fish, but it has not been documented in ovoviviparous fish.[25] Other vertebrates that share aquatic environments with fish, e.g., frogs, can serve as a source of mycobacteria to infect fish, as can certain aquatic invertebrates, e.g., snails.[25]

Host range: Mycobacteriosis affects an exceptionally broad range of fish, from freshwater to brackish to saltwater species, including both cold-water and warm-water species.[27,29] Piscine mycobacteriosis is a major concern in commercial aquaria and the aquaculture industry where recirculating water filtration systems are used. In addition, piscine mycobacteria, such as *M. marinum*, are capable of causing infections of the skin and deeper tissues of the extremities of humans, and therefore can be significant zoonotic pathogens.[30]

Clinical presentation: Clinical signs of mycobacteriosis in fish are often nonspecific and may include emaciation, lethargy, anorexia and listlessness. Fish may exhibit changes in their swimming behavior, such as slow swimming or aberrant swimming, changes in pigmentation, or clamping of their fins to their bodies. However, in many cases fish die of mycobacteriosis without exhibiting clinical signs.[25,31–34] Gross external lesions, if present, may include shallow, irregular, nonhealing, cutaneous ulcers (**Figure 15.5**).[31–33]

Pathology: Gross internal lesions consist of tan to white nodular granulomas located in the parenchyma of the coelomic viscera, particularly the head kidney, spleen and liver with varying degrees of renomegaly,

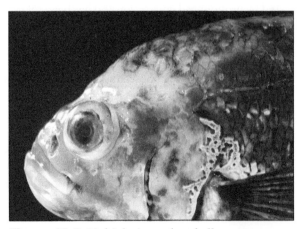

Figure 15.5 Multiple, irregular, shallow cutaneous ulcers of mycobacteriosis in an oscar (*Astronotus ocellatus*). (Image courtesy of L. Craig.)

splenomegaly and hepatomegaly.[29,31,33] However, the distribution of granulomas in mycobacteriosis is not strictly limited to the head kidney, spleen and liver; granulomas may be observed in other organs and tissues, e.g., gill, eye, brain, skeletal muscle, intestine, mesentery and pancreas.[35] Although granulomatous inflammation characterizes the response of all fish to mycobacterial infection, there is significant variation in the severity, distribution and cellular organization of the granulomatous response in different fishes.[26,33]

Differential diagnosis: Systemic granulomatous disease incited by *Nocardia* spp., or non-acid-fast bacteria, fungi or protists.

Diagnosis: Diagnosis of piscine mycobacteriosis traditionally has been based on histopathological assessment of granulomas and/or granulomatous inflammation for the presence of acid-fast bacteria; however, the relative scarcity of mycobacteria in some lesions coupled with the inability to provide species-level characterization of acid-fast bacteria in histologic section by microscopic examination alone has driven the development of additional methods of detection.[34] Mycobacteria may be distinguished by their *in vitro* growth characteristics (e.g., fast-growing vs. slow-growing, and photochromogenic vs. scotochromogenic), PCR amplification and sequencing of phylogenetically relevant genes, high-performance liquid chromatography, and capillary gas chromatography for fatty acid methyl ester analysis.[26,34] Because some piscine mycobacteria are slow growers, i.e., with results often not available in a clinically relevant timeframe, direct amplification from tissue with subsequent amplicon sequencing has become a prevalent means of detecting and characterizing mycobacterial infections.[34]

Management/control: There are no widely accepted treatments for piscine mycobacteriosis, and management in aquaria and aquaculture settings generally involves depopulation and disinfection.[26,34,36]

MENINGOENCEPHALITIS DUE TO *RENIBACTERIUM SALMONINARUM*

Granulomatous meningoencephalitis has been observed in salmonids with bacterial kidney disease due to *Renibacterium salmoninarum*. A range of encephalic lesions occurs in salmonids infected with

R. salmoninarum, with brain involvement occurring as part of multi-organ infections and in the absence of lesions in other organs. In some species of salmon, e.g., Atlantic salmon, encephalitis may occur with meningitis or absent meningitis, and encephalitis or meningitis occurs absent of systemic lesions.[37]

VIRAL NERVOUS NECROSIS

Overview: Disease of marine teleosts caused by betanodaviruses has been referred to as viral nervous necrosis, encephalomyelitis, and vacuolating encephalopathy and retinopathy.[38–40] The disease has been recognized on all continents where mariculture occurs, with the exception of the African continent, and it is the most serious viral infectious disease affecting marine farmed fish in the Mediterranean.[41]

Etiology: Viral nervous necrosis is caused by a clade of RNA viruses belonging to the family Nodaviridae, genus *Betanodavirus*, with four different genotypes currently recognized: red-spotted grouper nervous necrosis virus, striped jack nervous necrosis virus, tiger puffer nervous necrosis virus, and barfin flounder nervous necrosis virus.[41]

Route of transmission: The virus is transmitted horizontally, with vertical transmission also being a concern given that it has been achieved experimentally in European sea bass.[42]

Host range: This disease has emerged as a principal limiting factor to the culture of a number of marine fish, including sea bass and grouper (order Perciformes), flounder (order Pleuronectiformes), cod (order Gadiformes), eel (order Anguilliformes) and pufferfish (order Tetraodontiformes).[43]

Clinical presentation: Clinical signs of viral nervous necrosis include abnormal swimming behaviors (e.g. spiraling), swim bladder hyperinflation, and darkening of skin color.[43] Disease typically affects larval or juvenile life stages, and mortality rates can be extremely high, up to 100%.[43] In the case of sea bass and grouper, there has been an association between warmer water temperatures and disease in older, harvest-sized fish.[44,45]

Pathology: Histopathologic lesions consist of vacuole formation in the gray matter of the brain, accompanied by pyknosis, karyorrhexis, and shrinkage of affected neural cells and a mononuclear cell infiltrate, with basophilic intracytoplasmic inclusions of variable size.[38,39,43,46] Vacuole formation has also been reported in the cellular layers of the retina and in the rods and cones.[40,46] Subclinical nodaviral infections have been described in farmed juvenile Atlantic halibut and in farmed adult Atlantic cod.[47,48]

Differential diagnosis: Bacterial hemorrhagic septicemia, e.g., *Aeromonas* spp.; viral hemorrhagic septicemia.

Diagnosis: Diagnosis of betanodavirus can be accomplished by virus culture, reverse transcriptase PCR, indirect fluorescent antibody testing of tissue sections, or immunohistochemistry using an avidin–biotin–peroxidase technique. Isolation of virus by cell culture followed by characterization using immunostaining or reverse transcriptase PCR remains the "gold standard" for diagnostic purposes, with brain and eyes being the requisite diagnostic samples.[49]

Management/control: Control of nodaviral infection is centered on eliminating exposure to sources of infection. Incoming stock should be tested for the presence of betanodaviruses using an accepted diagnostic method, such as reverse transcriptase PCR, cognizant of the virus of interest and the detection limitations of the testing method.[43] Implementation of general hygiene practices, such as ultraviolet (UV) treatment of incoming water; adoption of sanitary barriers; regular fallowing of aquaculture sites; and disinfection of tanks, filters and equipment is recommended, along with approaches to control vertical transmission.[49] Vaccination using several different preparations, including recombinant viral coat protein and formalin-inactivated virus, has been shown to generate a protective immune response.[50–52]

VIRAL HEMORRHAGIC SEPTICEMIA

Overview: Viral hemorrhagic septicemia (VHS) is a viral disease of farmed and wild finfish that is of primary economic significance to salmonid aquaculture.[53]

Etiology: This disease is caused by a rhabdovirus of the genus *Novirhabdovirus* in the family Rhabdoviridae known as the Egtved virus, or viral hemorrhagic septicemia virus (VHSV).[54] Four genotypes of VHSV are currently recognized. Genetic differences between VHSV isolates appear more related to global geographic origin of the isolates than to year of isolation or host species or virulence.[53]

Route of transmission: Transmission of VHSV is horizontal and results from exposure to infected fish exhibiting clinical signs or seemingly healthy fish that contaminate water with virus, which is excreted in the urine and ovarian fluids of infected fish.[53,55] Incubation times and accumulated mortalities can vary with water temperature.[55]

Host range: The rainbow trout (*Oncorhynchus mykiss*) is considered the most susceptible salmonid species to VHS.[53] Natural infections of VHS have occurred in farmed turbot and Japanese flounder, as well as a wide range of freshwater and marine fish species.[53]

Clinical presentation: Clinical signs of VHS in rainbow trout are characterized by lethargy, slow swimming, darkening of the skin, hemorrhages of the skin at the base of fins and around the eyes and mouth, exophthalmos, and pallor of the gills, with occasional ascites (**Figure 15.6**).[53]

Pathology: Pathogenesis of VHS in rainbow trout includes viremia and systemic distribution of virus to multiple organs, including liver, brain, heart and gill, with tropism for endothelial cells. As the disease progresses, VHSV can be detected in neurons and neuroglia throughout the brain.[56] Mortality can be as high as 100% in fry, but ranges from 30% to 70% in older fish.[53] Chronically infected trout can develop dark skin discoloration and abnormal swimming behaviors.[53] Similar patterns of clinical signs have been demonstrated in other fish exposed to freshwater and marine VHSV isolates, including Pacific herring (*Clupea pallasii*) and freshwater drum (*Aplodinotus grunniens*), the latter also displaying

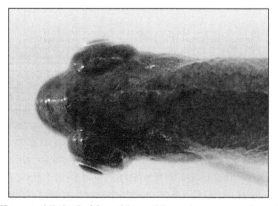

Figure 15.6 Golden shiner (*Notemigonus crysoleucas*) with cranial hemorrhage and exophthalmos as a result of VHSV infection. (Image courtesy of E. Cornwell.)

extensive iridal hemorrhage.[57,58] Virulent marine VHSV isolates have been shown to produce lesions in turbot (*Scophthalmus maximus* L.) comparable to those of freshwater VHSV isolates in rainbow trout.[59]

Differential diagnosis: Bacterial hemorrhagic septicemia, e.g., *Aeromonas* spp.; betanodaviral encephalitis.

Diagnosis: Diagnosis of VHS is dependent on identification of VHSV from tissues, with optimal sampling including the spleen, anterior kidney, heart, brain, and ovarian fluid or milt. The virus can be isolated in cell culture with subsequent identification by enzyme-linked immunosorbent assay, immunofluorescent staining or reverse-transcription PCR.[53]

Management/control: Management of VHS in aquaculture scenarios involves implementation of surveillance programs coupled with application of control and hygiene measures that reduce physiologic, metabolic and immunologic stress on fish. Water temperature, salinity and organic load are factors that affect the stability of VHSV in aquatic environments such that some VHSV isolates have been shown to be stable longer at colder temperatures and in freshwater as compared to seawater.[60]

CHANNEL CATFISH HERPESVIRUS

Channel catfish virus disease is a disease of cultured channel catfish (*Ictalurus punctatus*) fry and fingerlings caused by a highly pathogenic herpesvirus, i.e., channel catfish herpesvirus. The blue catfish, *Ictalurus furcatus*, has been experimentally infected, but other ictalurids appear resistant to infection.[61] The herpesvirus has been recognized as causing systemic mortalities of fry and fingerlings with hemorrhage, necrosis and edema of most tissues, as well as neuronal vacuolation and edema of the brain.[61,62] Disease occurrence is optimum at water temperatures above 25°C.[61] The channel catfish herpesvirus has been isolated from channel catfish brood stock, indicating that adults may serve as carriers.[63]

WHIRLING DISEASE OF SALMONIDS

Overview: Whirling disease is a parasitic disease of wild and cultured salmonid fish, particularly rainbow trout (*Oncorhynchus mykiss*) in North America and Europe.[64]

Etiology: The myxozoan *Myxobolus cerebralis* (phylum Myxozoa; class Myxosporea) is the causative agent of whirling disease of salmonids. The parasite has a complex life cycle characterized by alternation between an invertebrate and vertebrate host with sporogony in each, such that the myxosporean spore generated in the salmonid host is infective to *T. tubifex*, whereas the actinosporean triactinomyxon spore produced in *T. tubifex* is infective to the salmonid host.[64,65]

Route of transmission: Transmission of *M. cerebralis* to the susceptible salmonid host is dependent on contact with environments contaminated with the actinosporean triactinomyxon spore from *T. tubifex*, which previously must have been in contact with myxosporean spores from infected salmonids.[66]

Host range: Susceptibility to whirling disease among salmonids is variable. The rainbow trout (*Oncorhynchus mykiss*) is among the most susceptible species to whirling disease, as is the European Danube salmon (*Hucho hucho*), while the brown trout (*Salmo trutta*) and coho salmon (*Oncorhynchus kisutch*) are among the least susceptible.[64]

Clinical presentation: Clinical signs of whirling disease include darkening of the skin of the tail, referred to as "black tail," and radical tail-chasing swimming behavior (**Figure 15.7**). Gross lesions of whirling disease consist of caudal cutaneous melanosis; skeletal deformities manifest principally as lateral, dorsal or ventral curvatures of the spine; and foreshortening of the anterior portion of the head.[64,67,68] Disease commonly affects salmonid fry and fingerlings, as older fish become relatively resistant subsequent to the ossification of cranial and vertebral cartilages and acquired immunity.[69]

Pathology: The developmental stages of the parasite migrate through peripheral nerves, spinal cord and brain to invade vertebral and cranial cartilage.[64,69] Invasion and sporogonic development of the parasite in the cartilage results in chondrolysis and granulomatous chondritis of cranial, vestibular and vertebral cartilage, with subsequent deforming skeletal changes.[67–70] Lesions to the cranial cartilage result in the grossly recognized anterior cranial foreshortening, whereas deformation of semicircular canals and nerve impingement impairs vestibular function causing the observed whirling swimming behaviors. Vertebral instability due to lysis of vertebral cartilage contributes to spinal curvature, while collapse of vertebral foramina and compression on spinal nerves that control dermal melanocyte activity result in the caudal melanosis that is recognized as black tail.[67,68,70]

Differential diagnosis: Any viral, bacterial, fungal or protozoal agent causing central nervous system or vestibular lesions resulting in whirling behavior,[66] also vitamin C deficiency and vitamin A toxicity.[70]

Diagnosis: Diagnosis of whirling disease of salmonids requires detection of either the myxospore or the genomic DNA of *M. cerebralis*. Myxospores can be detected by histologic examination of tissue sections that include cranial and spinal cartilage, or by pepsin-trypsin digestion of cranial cartilage with subsequent microscopic examination of digestion preparations. DNA of *M. cerebralis* can be detected by PCR testing of cranial tissues.[71]

Management/control: Management strategies involve growing young fish in spore-free waters, using concrete raceways with high rates of water flow, employing routine disinfection protocols, and implementing surveillance practices for the presence of spores.[66] Inactivating triactinomyxon spores in source water is considered an essential control tactic in limiting or preventing infection with treatment largely focused on chemical or ultraviolet means of inactivating the myxosporean and actinosporean spores.[64] At the current time, no vaccine exists to prevent whirling disease in salmonids.

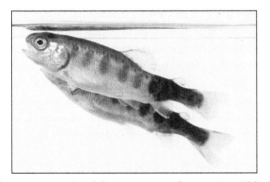

Figure 15.7 Caudal cutaneous melanosis, i.e., "black tail," in rainbow trout (*Oncorhynchus mykiss*) fingerlings due to infection with *Myxobolus cerebralis*. (Image courtesy of A. Mitchell.)

MYXOZOAN INFECTION OF YELLOW PERCH

Overview: Infection of the brain and spinal cord of wild and cultured yellow perch (*Perca flavescens*) by *Myxobolus neurophilus* results in disease with neurological clinical signs.[72,73] As demand for yellow perch is being met by a growing aquaculture industry using ponds or recirculating water systems or both, the significance of *M. neurophilus* as a potentially limiting infectious disease concern has also grown.[72]

Etiology: *Myxobolus neurophilus* is a neurotropic myxozoan that appears to infect only yellow perch.[72] Pathology is limited to the brain and spinal cord, and is manifest by the formation of pseudocysts containing myxospores, principally in the diencephalon and mesencephalon, with compression of the surrounding neuroparenchyma or protrusion into the lumen of the optic ventricle.[72]

Route of transmission: Transmission of *M. neurophilus* is presumed to occur by exposure of yellow perch to the actinospore released from the alternate invertebrate host (yet undetermined), which in turn must have been in contact with myxosporean spores from infected yellow perch. Myxospores of *M. neurophilus* are absent from organs other than the brain in yellow perch, and are presumed to be released when infected perch die and decompose or when they are eaten and their cranial tissues digested.[74]

Host range: This myxozoan is a parasite of wild and cultured yellow perch (*Perca flavescens*), though the parasite was originally identified in the johnny dater (*Etheostoma nigrum*).[73]

Clinical presentation: Infection with *M. neurophilus* results in expression of variable neurological clinical signs, principally abnormal swimming movements, although the lack of clinical signs has also been reported in infected fish.[72,73]

Pathology: Pseudocysts of myxospores are primarily observed in the diencephalon and mesencephalon where they cause compression of the surrounding neuroparenchyma or protrude into the lumen of the optic ventricle. A mild mononuclear meningoencephalitis was reported in regions of the brain where parasites were located free of pseudocysts.[72]

Differential diagnosis: Other neurotropic myxobolid myxozoans in perch (e.g., *Myxobolus*

aureatus), and bacterial or fungal causes of encephalomyelitis.

Diagnosis: Infection is diagnosed by microscopic examination of touch impressions, smears or homogenates of brain, or of histologic sections of brain and spinal cord. Molecular analyses of DNA extracted from homogenates of brain can be used to confirm the identity of *M. neurophilus*.[72,73]

Management/control: No treatment or vaccines are available. Control rests with implementation of biosecurity measures that identify and remove infected fish and prevent their introduction, and with chemical and ultraviolet disinfection of source water in a manner similar to that used to control *M. cerebralis*.

MISCELLANEOUS MYXOZOAN INFECTIONS OF THE CENTRAL NERVOUS SYSTEM

Scoliosis resulting from infection by *Myxobolus acanthogobii*, synonymous with *Myxobolus buri*, is a cause of significant economic losses in the aquaculture of yellowtail (*Seriola quinqueradiata*) particularly since disease is manifest in market-sized fish.[75–77] *Myxobolus acanthogobii* infects the brain of the yellowfin goby (*Acanthogobius flavimanus*), in which it causes slight exophthalmos and numerous white, bean-shaped pseudocysts distributed on the surfaces of the brain, olfactory nerve and vertebral column, but not the skeletal abnormalities it produces in yellowtail.[77] In contrast to infections by *Myxobolus neurophilus* and *Myxobolus acanthogobii* wherein lesions occur in association with spore-forming developmental stages, i.e., sporogonic plasmodia, several myxozoan-induced neurological conditions are incited by presporogonic or extrasporogonic plasmodia that invade the brain and spinal cord. Such is the case in the parasitic encephalitis associated with mass mortality of farmed Atlantic salmon known as nervous mortality syndrome and in the case of *Myxobolus spirosulcatus* infection in cultured yellowtail.[78–80]

ENCEPHALITIC MYCETOMA

Epizootic outbreaks of encephalitic mycetoma caused by a *Phialophora*-like melanized fungus, which was named *Exophiala salmonis*, have been reported in farmed cutthroat trout.[81] The primary lesion developed in the brain and spread outward to involve the eye and other tissues.[68]

ENCEPHALITIS DUE TO *EXOPHIALA PISCIPHILA* IN ATLANTIC SALMON

A cranial mycosis of low incidence but high mortality was described in Atlantic salmon caused by *Exophiala pisciphila*.[82] Fungal hyphae invaded cranial canals of the lateral line system and extended into cranial cartilage, retrobulbar tissues, brain and semicircular canals, inciting a granulomatous inflammatory reaction and necrosis of cartilage. Clinical signs included depression, darkening, exophthalmos and, in a few individuals, erratic swimming behavior, along with fistulae on the head and operculae.[82]

BRAIN AND SPINAL CORD INFECTION BY *PSEUDOLOMA NEUROPHILIA*

Overview: The most significant infection of neural tissues in laboratory fishes is that caused by *Pseudoloma neurophilia* in zebrafish (*Danio rerio*).[83] This parasite is considered by some to be the most common pathogen of zebrafish in research laboratories.[84]

Etiology: *Pseudoloma neurophilia* is a microsporidium that has a pronounced tropism for neural tissues, with clusters of developmental stages including spores forming within axons of the hindbrain, spinal cord and ventral nerve roots of the zebrafish.[81,85]

Route of transmission: The microsporidium has been shown to be transmissible directly by waterborne exposure, and spores have been identified in the ovary, suggesting vertical transmission.[83,86]

Host range: This microsporidium has predominantly been known as a pathogen of laboratory zebrafish, but has been shown to also infect other fish species such as *Betta splendens*, *Xiphophorus maculatus*, *Devario aequipinnatus*, *Pimephales promelas*, *Oryzias latipes*, *Carassius auratus* and *Paracheirodon innesi*.[87]

Clinical presentation: The most common clinical sign of infection in zebrafish is emaciation, while spinal curvatures, specifically lordosis and scoliosis, are also seen.[85]

Pathology: The parasite has a pronounced tropism for neural tissues, where clusters of developmental stages form in the axons of the hindbrain, spinal cord and ventral nerve roots.[84,85] Inflammation is typically not present when stages are seen in host axons and is minimal when spores are located in the neuroparenchyma.[84,85] Spores of *P. neurophilia* may also be seen in muscle tissue in association with myositis.[86]

Differential diagnosis: Other causes of emaciation, e.g., mycobacteriosis, or abnormal swimming behavior.

Diagnosis: Diagnosis is accomplished by microscopic examination of histologic sections for developing stages and spores, or by PCR assay.[84]

Management/control: No treatments or vaccines are available, and this microsporidium is resistant to chlorine disinfection at the levels commonly used to treat zebrafish eggs.[83,86,88] *Pseudoloma neurophilia* infections have the potential to alter the behavioral response of zebrafish given the regions of brain and spinal cord involvement, and as such may complicate experimental applications.[68,84]

MISCELLANEOUS CENTRAL AND PERIPHERAL INFECTIONS BY MICROSPORIDIA

Fish are hosts to a wide variety of microsporidia, belonging to a number of genera, several of which infect central and peripheral nervous tissues.[89] *Spraguea lophii* is a microsporidium that infects the brain and peripheral ganglia of black and white anglerfish in the North Atlantic and Mediterranean resulting in xenoma formation in spinal and cranial ganglia.[90] A microsporidium with genetic relatedness to members of the genus *Spraguea* has been identified in association with encephalomyelitis in farmed amberjack. Affected fish displayed spiraling swimming and had lesions that were most severe in the tegmentum, medulla oblongata and anterior spinal cord with spores in the perikaryon and axons of neurons.[91] An encephalitis of farmed Atlantic salmon in net pens due to a microsporidium, *Microsporidium cerebralis*, has been described.[92] The disease, "spinner disease," is characterized by an abnormal swimming behavior described as a slow spiraling ascent to the surface with loss of equilibrium; lesions occur in the myelencephalon of affected salmon and consist of degenerating and necrotic neurons, including the Mauthner cells, which contain microsporidial spores in the perikaryon and sometimes in the axon, and are accompanied by neuronophagic glial nodules.[68,92]

REFERENCES

1. Agnew, W. and Barnes, A.C. *Streptococcus iniae*: An aquatic pathogen of global veterinary significance and a challenging candidate for reliable vaccination. *Veterinary Microbiology* 2007;122:1–15.

2. Gauthier, D.T. Bacterial zoonoses of fishes: A review and appraisal of evidence for linkages between fish and human infections. *The Veterinary Journal* 2015;203:27–35.

3. Pier, G.B. and Madin, S.H. *Streptococcus iniae* sp. nov., a betahemolytic *Streptococcus* isolated from an Amazon freshwater dolphin, *Inia geoffrensis*. *International Journal of Systematic Bacteriology* 1976;26:545–553.

4. Bromage, E.S. and Owens, L. Infection of barramundi *Lates calcarifer* with *Streptococcus iniae*: Effects of different routes of exposure. *Diseases of Aquatic Organisms* 2002;52:199–205.

5. Buchanan, J.T., Colvin, K.M., Vicknair, M.R., Patel, S.K., Timmer, A.M. and Nizet, V. Strain-associated virulence factors of *Streptococcus iniae* in hybrid-striped bass. *Veterinary Microbiology* 2008;131:145–153.

6. Bromage, E.S., Thomas, A. and Owens, L. *Streptococcus iniae*, a bacterial infection in barramundi *Lates calcarifer*. *Diseases of Aquatic Organisms* 1999;36:177–181.

7. Eldar, A. and Ghittino, C. *Lactococcus garvieae* and *Streptococcus iniae* infections in rainbow trout *Oncorhynchus mykiss*: Similar, but different diseases. *Diseases of Aquatic Organisms* 1999;36:227–231.

8. Shoemaker, C.A., Klesius, P.H. and Evans, J.J. Prevalence of *Streptococcus iniae* in tilapia, hybrid striped bass, and channel catfish on commercial fish farms in the United States. *American Journal of Veterinary Research* 2001;62:174–177.

9. Eldar, A., Horovitcz, A. and Bercovier, H. Development and efficacy of a vaccine against *Streptococcus iniae* infection in farmed rainbow trout. *Veterinary Immunology and Immunopathology* 1997;56:175–183.

10. Bachrach, G., Zlotkin, A., Hurvitz, A., Evans, D.L. and Eldar, A. Recovery of *Streptococcus iniae* from diseased fish previously vaccinated with a streptococcus vaccine. *Applied Environmental Microbiology* 2001;67:3756–3758.

11. Hawke, J.P., McWhorter, A.C., Steigerwalt, A.G. and Brenner, D.J. *Edwardsiella ictaluri* sp. nov., the causative agent of enteric septicemia of catfish. *International Journal of Systematic Bacteriology* 1981;31:396–400.

12. Menanteau-Ledouble, S., Karsi, A. and Lawrence, M.L. Importance of skin abrasion as a primary site of adhesion for *Edwardsiella ictaluri* and impact on invasion and systematic infection in channel catfish *Ictalurus punctatus*. *Veterinary Microbiology* 2011;148:425–430.

13. Kasornchandra, J., Rogers, W.A. and Plumb, J.A. *Edwardsiella ictaluri* from walking catfish, *Clarias batrachus* L., in Thailand. *Journal of Fish Diseases* 1987;10:137–138.

14. Liu, J.Y., Li, A.H., Zhou, D.R., Wen, Z.R. and Ye, X.P. Isolation and characterization of *Edwardsiella ictaluri* strains as pathogens from diseased yellow catfish *Pelteobagrus fulvidraco* (Richardson) cultured in China. *Aquaculture Research* 2010;41:1835–1844.

15. Crumlish, M., Dung, T.T., Turnbull, J.F., Ngoc, N.T.N. and Ferguson, H.W. Identification of *Edwardsiella ictaluri* from diseased freshwater catfish, *Pangasius hypophthalmus* (Sauvage), cultured in the Mekong Delta, Vietnam. *Journal of Fish Diseases* 2002;25:733–736.

16. Waltman, W.D., Shotts, E.B. and Blazer, V.S. Recovery of *Edwardsiella ictaluri* from danio (*Danio devario*). *Aquaculture* 1985;46:63–66.

17. Soto, E., Griffin, M., Arauz, M., Riofrio, A., Martinez, A. and Cabrejos, M.E. *Edwardsiella ictaluri* as the causative agent of mortality in cultured Nile tilapia. *Journal of Aquatic Animal Health* 2012;24:81–90.

18. Kent, M.L. and Lyons, J.M. *Edwardsiella ictaluri* in the green knife fish, *Eigenmannia virescens*. *Fish Health News* 1982;11:1–2.

19. Hawke, J.P., Kent, M., Rogge, M.L., Baumgartner, W., Wiles, J., Shelley, J., Savolainen, L.C., Wagner, R., Murray, K. and Peterson, T.S. Edwardsiellosis caused by *Edwardsiella ictaluri* in laboratory populations of zebrafish *Danio rerio*. *Journal of Aquatic Animal Health* 2013;25:171–183.

20. Jarobe, H.H., Bowser, P.R. and Robinette, H.R. Pathology associated with a natural *Edwardsiella ictaluri* infection of channel catfish (*Ictalurus punctatus* Rafinesque). *Journal of Wildlife Diseases* 1984;20:352–354.

21. Blazer, V.S., Shotts, E.B. and Waltman, W.D. Pathology associated with *Edwardsiella ictaluri* in catfish, *Ictalurus punctatus* Rafinesque, and *Danio devario* (Hamilton-Buchanan 1822). *Journal of Fish Biology* 1985;27:167–175.

22. Bilodeau, A.L., Waldbieser, G.C., Terhune, J.S., Wise, D.J. and Wolters, W.R. A real-time polymerase chain reaction assay of the bacterium *Edwardsiella ictaluri* in channel catfish. *Journal of Aquatic Animal Health* 2003;15:80–86.

23. Griffin, M.J., Mauel, M.J., Greenway, T.E., Khoo, L.H. and Wise, D.J. A real-time polymerase chain reaction assay for quantification of *Edwardsiella ictaluri* in catfish pond water and genetic homogeneity of diagnostic case isolates from Mississippi. *Journal of Aquatic Animal Health* 2011;23:178–188.

24. Klesius, P.H. and Shoemaker, C.A. Development and use of modified live *Edwardsiella ictaluri* vaccine against enteric septicemia of catfish. *Advances in Veterinary Medicine* 1999;41:523–537.

25. Decostere, A., Hermans, K. and Haesebrouck, F. Piscine mycobacteriosis: A literature review covering the agent and the disease it causes in fish and humans. *Veterinary Microbiology* 2004;99:159–166.

26. Gauthier, D.T. and Rhodes, M.W. Mycobacteriosis in fishes: A review. *The Veterinary Journal* 2009;180:33–47.

27. Nigrelli, R.F. and Vogel, H. Spontaneous tuberculosis in fishes and other cold-blooded vertebrates with special reference to *Mycobacterium fortuitum* Cruz from fish and human lesions. *Zoologica* 1963;48:131–144.

28. Chinabut, S., Limsuwan, C. and Chanratchakool, P. Mycobacteriosis in the snakehead, *Channa striatus*. *Journal of Fish Diseases* 1990;13:531–535.

29. Chinabut, S. Mycobacteriosis and nocardiosis. In: *Fish Diseases and Disorders, Volume 3: Viral, Bacterial and Fungal Infections*. P.T.K. Woo and D.W. Bruno, eds. CAB International, New York, 1999; pp. 319–340.

30. Petrini, B. *Mycobacterium marinum*: Ubiquitous agent of waterborne granulomatous skin infections. *European Journal of Clinical Microbiology and Infectious Diseases* 2006;25:609–613.

31. Hedrick, R.P., McDowell, T. and Groff, J. Mycobacteriosis in cultured striped bass from California. *Journal of Wildlife Diseases* 1987;23:391–395.

32. Noga, E.J., Wright, J.F. and Pasarell, L. Some unusual features of mycobacteriosis in the cichlid fish *Oreochromis mossambicus*. *Journal of Comparative Pathology* 1990;102:335–344.

33. Wolf, J.C. and Smith, S.A. Comparative severity of experimentally induced mycobacteriosis in striped bass *Morone saxatilis* and hybrid tilapia *Oreochromis* spp. *Diseases of Aquatic Organisms* 1999;38:191–200.

34. Jacobs, J.M., Stine, C.B., Baya, A.M. and Kent, M.L. A review of mycobacteriosis in marine fish. *Journal of Fish Diseases* 2009;32:119–130.

35. Majeed, S.K., Gopinath, C. and Jolly, D.W. Pathology of spontaneous tuberculosis and pseudotuberculosis in fish. *Journal of Fish Diseases* 1981;4:507–512.

36. Mainous, M.E. and Smith, S.A. Evaluation of various disinfectants on *Mycobacterium marinum*. *Journal of Aquatic Animal Health* 2005;17:284–288.

37. Speare, D.J. Differences in patterns of meningoencephalitis due to bacterial kidney disease in farmed Atlantic and chinook salmon. *Research in Veterinary Science* 1997;62:79–80.

38. Yoshikoshi, K. and Inoue, K. Viral nervous necrosis in hatchery-reared larvae and juveniles of Japanese parrotfish, *Oplegnathus fasciatus* (Temminck & Schlegel). *Journal of Fish Diseases* 1990;13:69–77.

39. Bloch, B., Gravningen, K. and Larsen, J.L. Encephalomyelitis among turbot associated with a picornavirus-like agent. *Diseases of Aquatic Organisms* 1991;10:65–70.

40. Munday, B.L., Langdon, J.S., Hyatt, A. and Humphrey, J.D. Mass mortality associated with a viral-induced vacuolating encephalopathy and retinopathy of larval and juvenile barramundi, *Lates calcarifer* Bloch. *Aquaculture* 1992;103:197–211.

41. Vendramin, N., Toffan, A., Mancin, M., Cappellozza, E., Panzarin, V., Bovo, G., Cattoli, G., Capua, I. and Terregino, C. Comparative pathogenicity study of ten different betanodavirus strains in experimentally infected European sea bass, *Dicentrarchus labrax* (L.). *Journal of Fish Diseases* 2014;37:371–383.

42. Breuil, G., Pepin, J.F., Boscher, S. and Thiéry, R. Experimental vertical transmission of nodavirus from broodfish to eggs and larvae of the sea bass, *Dicentrarchus labrax* (L.). *Journal of Fish Diseases* 2002;25:697–702.

43. Munday, B.L., Kwang, J. and Moody, N. Betanodavirus infections of teleost fish: A review. *Journal of Fish Diseases* 2002;25:127–142.

44. Breton A. L., Grisez, L., Sweetman, J. and Ollevier, F. Viral nervous necrosis (VNN) associated with mass mortalities in cage-reared sea bass *Dicentrarchus labrax* L. *Journal of Fish Diseases* 1997;20:145–153.

45. Tanaka, A., Aoki, H. and Nakai, T. Pathogenicity of the nodavirus detected from diseased sevenband grouper *Epinephelus septemfasciatus*. *Fish Pathology* 1998;33:31–36.

46. Grotmol, S., Totland, G.K., Kvellestad, A., Fjell, K. and Olsen, A.B. Mass mortality of larval and juvenile hatchery-reared halibut (*Hippoglossus hippoglossus* L.) associated with the presence of virus-like particles in the central nervous system and retina. *Bulletin of the European Association of Fish Pathologists* 1995;15:176–180.

47. Johansen, R., Ranheim, T., Hansen, M.K., Taksdal, T. and Totland, G.K. Pathological changes in juvenile Atlantic halibut *Hippoglossus hippoglossus* persistently infected with nodavirus. *Diseases of Aquatic Organisms* 2002;50:161–169.

48. Gjessing, M.C., Kvellestad, A., Ottesen, K. and Falk, K. Nodavirus provokes subclinical encephalitis and retinochoroiditis in adult farmed Atlantic cod, *Gadus morhua* L. *Journal of Fish Diseases* 2009;32:421–431.

49. OIE. *Manual of Diagnostic Tests for Aquatic Animals*, 7th ed. OIE Organisation Mondiale de la Santé Animale, Paris, 2016.

50. Tanaka, S., Mori, K., Arimoto, M., Iwamo, T. and Nakai, T. Protective immunity of sevenband grouper, *Epinephelus septemfasciatus* Thunberg, against experimental viral nervous necrosis. *Journal of Fish Diseases* 2001;24:15–22.

51. Yamashita, Y., Fujita, Y., Kawakami, H. and Nakai, T. The efficacy of inactivated virus vaccine against viral nervous necrosis (VNN). *Fish Pathology* 2005;40:15–21.

52. Thiéry, R., Cozien, J., Cabon, J., Lamour, F., Baud, M. and Schneemann, A. Induction of a protective immune response against viral nervous necrosis in the European sea bass *Dicentrarchus labrax* by using betanodavirus virus-like particles. *Journal of Virology* 2006;80:10201–10207.

53. Skall, H.F., Olesen, N.J. and Mellergaard, S. Viral haemorrhagic septicaemia virus in marine fish and its implications for fish farming—A review. *Journal of Fish Diseases* 2005;28:509–529.

54. Walker, P.J., Benmansour, A., Dietzgen, R. et al. Family Rhabdoviridae. In: *Virus Taxonomy. Classification and Nomenclature of Viruses. Seventh Report of the International Committee on Taxonomy of Viruses*. M.H.V. Van Regenmortel, C.M. Fauquet, D.H.L. Bishop et al. eds. Academic Press, San Diego, 2000; pp. 563–583.

55. Smail, D.A. and Snow, M. Viral haemorrhagic septicaemia. In: *Fish Diseases and Disorders, Volume 3: Viral, Bacterial and Fungal Infections*, 2nd ed. P.T.K. Woo and D.W. Bruno, eds. CABI, Wallingford, 2011; pp. 110–142.

56. Brudeseth, B.E., Castric, J. and Evensen, Ø. Studies on pathogenesis following single and double infection with viral hemorrhagic septicemia virus and infectious hematopoietic necrosis virus in rainbow trout (*Oncorhynchus mykiss*). *Veterinary Pathology* 2002;39:180–189.

57. Lovy, J., Lewis, N.L., Hershberger, P.K., Bennett, W., Meyers, T.R. and Garver, K.A. Viral tropism and pathology associated with viral hemorrhagic septicemia in larval and juvenile Pacific herring. *Veterinary Microbiology* 2012;161:66–76.

58. Lumsden, J.S., Morrison, B., Yason, C., Russell, S., Young, K., Yazdanpanah, A., Huber, P., Al-Hussinee, L., Stone, D. and Way, K. Mortality event in freshwater drum *Aplodinotus grunniens* from Lake Ontario, Canada, associated with viral haemorrhagic septicemia virus, Type IV. *Diseases of Aquatic Organisms* 2007;76:99–111.

59. Brudeseth, B.E., Raynard, R.S., King, J.A. and Evensen, Ø. Sequential pathology after experimental infection with marine viral hemorrhagic septicemia virus isolates of low and high virulence in turbot (*Scophthalmus maximus* L.). *Veterinary Pathology* 2005;42:9–18.

60. Hawley, L.M. and Garver, K.A. Stability of viral hemorrhagic septicemia virus (VHSV) in freshwater and seawater at various temperatures. *Disease of Aquatic Organisms* 2008;82:171–178.

61. Plumb, J.A. Epizootiology of channel catfish virus disease. *Marine Fisheries Review* 1978;40:26–29.

62. Major, R.D., McCraren, J.P. and Smith, C.E. Histopathological changes in channel catfish (*Ictalurus punctatus*) experimentally and naturally infected with channel catfish virus disease. *Journal of the Fisheries Research Board of Canada* 1975;32:563–567.

63. Bowser, P.R., Munson, A.D., Jarboe, H.H., Francis-Floyd, R. and Waterstrate, P.R. Isolation of channel catfish virus from channel catfish, *Ictalurus punctatus* (Rafinesque), broodstock. *Journal of Fish Diseases* 1985;8:557–561.

64. Sarker, S., Kallert, D.M., Hedrick, R.P. and El-Matbouli, M. Whirling disease revisited: Pathogenesis, parasite biology and disease intervention. *Diseases of Aquatic Organisms* 2015;114:155–175.

65. Wolf, K. and Markiw, M.E. Biology contravenes taxonomy in the myxozoa: New discoveries show alternation of invertebrate and vertebrate hosts. *Science* 1984;225:1449–1452.

66. Hoffman, G.L. *Myxobolus cerebralis*, a worldwide cause of salmonid whirling disease. *Journal of Aquatic Animal Health* 1990;2:30–37.

67. Hedrick, R.P., McDowell, T.S., Gay, M., Marty, G.D., Georgiadis, M.P. and MacConnell, E. Comparative susceptibility of rainbow trout *Oncorhynchus mykiss* and brown trout *Salmo trutta* to *Myxobolus cerebralis*, the cause of salmonid whirling disease. *Diseases of Aquatic Organisms* 1999;37:173–183.

68. Speare, D.J. and Frasca, S. Jr. Nervous system. In: *Systemic Pathology of Fish, a Text and Atlas of Normal Tissues in Teleosts and Their Responses in Disease*, 2nd ed. H.W. Ferguson, ed. Scotian Press, London, 2006; pp. 218–243.

69. El-Matbouli, M., Hoffmann, R.W. and Mandok, C. Light and electron microscopic observations on the route of the triactinomyxon sporoplasm of *Myxobolus cerebralis* from epidermis into rainbow trout (*Oncorhynchus mykiss*) cartilage. *Journal of Fish Biology* 1995;46:919–935.

70. Turnbull, J. Musculoskeletal system. In: *Systemic Pathology of Fish, A Text and Atlas of Normal Tissues in Teleosts and their Responses in Disease*, 2nd ed. H.W. Ferguson, ed. Scotian Press, London, 2006; pp. 289–311.

71. Kelley, G.O., Zagmutt-Vergara, F.J., Leutenegger, C.M. et al. Evaluation of five diagnostic methods for the detection and quantification of *Myxobolus cerebralis*. *Journal of Veterinary Diagnostic Investigation* 2004;16:202–211.

72. Khoo, L., Rommel, F.A., Smith, S.A., Griffin, M.J. and Pote, L.M. *Myxobolus neurophilus*: Morphologic, histopathological and molecular characterization. *Diseases of Aquatic Organisms* 2010;89:51–61.

73. Scott, S.J., Griffin, M.J., Quiniou, S., Khoo, L. and Bollinger, T.K. *Myxobolus neurophilus* Guilford 1963 (Myxosporea: Myxobolidae): A common parasite infecting yellow perch *Perca flavescens* (Mitchell, 1814) in Saskatchewan, Canada. *Journal of Fish Diseases* 2015;38:355–364.

74. Dzulinksy, K., Cone, D., Faulkner, G.T. and Cusack, R. Development of *Myxobolus neurophilus* (Guilford, 1963) (Myxosporea) in the brain of yellow perch (*Perca flavescens*) in Vinegar Lake, Nova Scotia. *Canadian Journal of Zoology* 1994;72:1180–1185.

75. Egusa, S. *Myxobolus buri* sp. n. (Myxosporea: Bivalvulida) parasitic in the brain of *Seriola quinqueradiata* Temminck et Schlegel. *Fish Pathology* 1985;19:239–244.

76. Sakaguchi, S., Hara, T., Matsusato, T., Shibahara, T., Yamagata, Y., Kawai, H. and Maeno, Y. Scoliosis of cultured yellowtail caused by parasitic *Myxobolus buri*. *Bulletin of National Research Institute of Aquaculture* 1987;12:79–86.

77. Yokoyama, H., Freeman, M.A., Yoshinaga, T. and Ogawa, K. *Myxobolus buri*, the myxosporean parasite causing scoliosis of yellowtail, is synonymous with *Myxobolus acanthogobii* infecting the brain of the yellowfin goby. *Fisheries Science* 2004;70:1036–1042.

78. Rodger, H.D., Turnbull, T., Scullion, F.T., Sparrow, D. and Richards, R.H. Nervous mortality syndrome in farmed Atlantic salmon. *The Veterinary Record* 1995;137:616–617.

79. Frasca, Jr. S., Poynton, S.L., West, A.B. and Van Kruiningen, H.J. Epizootiology, pathology, and ultrastructure of the myxosporean associated with parasitic encephalitis of farmed Atlantic salmon *Salmo salar* in Ireland. *Diseases of Aquatic Organisms* 1998;32:211–225.

80. Yokoyama, H., Yanagida, T., Freeman, M.A., Katagiri, T., Hosokawa, A., Endo, M., Hirai, M. and Takagi, S. Molecular diagnosis of *Myxobolus spirosulcatus* associated with encephalomyelitis of cultured yellowtail, *Seriola quinqueradiata* Temminck & Schleg. *Journal of Fish Disease* 2010;33:939–946.

81. Carmichael, J.W. Cerebral mycetoma of trout due to a phialophora-like fungus. *Sabouraudia* 1966;2:120–123.

82. Langdon, J.S. and MacDonald, W.L. Cranial *Exophiala pisciphila* infection in *Salmo salar* in Australia. *Bulletin of the European Association of Fish Pathologists* 1987;35:117–119.

83. Kent, M.L., Buchner, C., Watral, V.G., Sanders, J.L., LaDu, J., Peterson, T.S. and Tanguay, R.L. Development and maintenance of a specific pathogen free (SPF) zebrafish research facility for *Pseudoloma neurophilia*. *Diseases of Aquatic Organisms* 2011;95:73–79.

84. Spagnoli, S.T., Xue, L., Murray, K.N., Chow, F. and Kent, M.L. *Pseudoloma neurophilia*: A retrospective and descriptive study of nervous system and muscle infections, with new implications for pathogenesis and behavioral phenotypes. *Zebrafish* 2015;12:189–201.

85. Matthews, J.L., Brown, A.M.V., Larison, K., Bishop-Stewart, J.K., Rogers, P. and Kent, M.L. *Pseudoloma neurophilia* n. g., n. sp., a new microsporidium from the central nervous system of the zebrafish (*Danio rerio*). *Journal of Eukaryotic Microbiology* 2001;48:227–233.

86. Kent, M.L. and Bishop-Stewart, J.K. Transmission and tissue distribution of *Pseudoloma neurophilia* (Microsporidia) of zebrafish, *Danio rerio* (Hamilton). *Journal of Fish Diseases* 2003;26:423–426.

87. Sanders, J.L., Watral, V., Stidworthy, M.F. and Kent, M.L. Expansion of the known host range of the microsporidium, *Pseudoloma neurophilia*. *Zebrafish* 2016;13:S102–S106.

88. Ferguson, J.A., Watral, V., Schwindt, A.R. and Kent, M.L. Spores of two fish Microsporidia (*Pseudoloma neurophilia* and *Glugea anomala*) are highly resistant to chlorine. *Diseases of Aquatic Organisms* 2007;76:205–214.

89. Lom, J. and Dyková, I. Microsporidia (Phylum Microspora Sprague, 1977). In: *Protozoan Parasites of Fishes*. Elsevier, Amsterdam, 1992; pp. 125–157.

90. Colmenero, A.I., Barría, C., Feist, S.W. and Tuset, V.M. Observations on the occurrence of *Spraguea lophii* in Mediterranean lophiids. *Parasitology Research* 2015;114:1977–1983.

91. Miwa, S., Kamaishi, T., Hirae, T., Murase, T. and Nishioka, T. Encephalomyelitis associated with microsporidian infection in farmed greater amberjack, *Seriola dumerili* (Risso). *Journal of Fish Diseases* 2011;34:901–910.

92. Brocklebank, J.R., Speare, D.J. and Kent, M.L. Microsporidian encephalitis of farmed Atlantic salmon (*Salmo salar*) in British Columbia. *Canadian Veterinary Journal* 1995;36:631–633.

CHAPTER 16

NUTRITIONAL DISEASES

*SIMON J. DAVIES, THARANGANI K. HERATH, AND
PETER BOWYER*

Overview: The relevance of fish nutrition has become increasingly important in the 21st century, largely due to the global increase in aquaculture production and the need for diets to meet growth at all stages of production from larvae to full grow-out and harvest. There are many established aquaculture species such as rainbow trout, carp, salmon and tilapia, but attention is now focused on a number of novel marine species such as cobia, mahi mahi and barramundi in the United States, and sea bass and sea bream in the Mediterranean as well as in Southeast Asia and the Indian subcontinent. Currently, the majority of farmed fish are freshwater or brackish with growth predominantly in China, Egypt, Vietnam and Thailand.[1]

Although temperate and warm water fish have been cultured commercially for several decades, diet formulations for many of these species are based on rather limited information of their nutrient requirements. Nutritional status is one of the most important factors governing the ability of fish to combat stress and enhance disease resistance. The onset of fish disease is often triggered when fish are stressed due to a variety of interplaying factors including poor diet management and suboptimal nutrition. The need for adequate diets to promote health and mitigate against diseases of farmed finfish is widely recognized.

In the most extreme situations, diets that are inadequate with respect to essential macro and micro nutrients (e.g., protein, amino acids, essential fatty acids, vitamins and minerals) can lead to gross malnutrition and increased disease susceptibility. However, in modern aquaculture, gross malnutrition scenarios are fortunately rare, as the industry has developed well-defined feed formulations based on years of practical experience especially with respect to salmonids (i.e., salmon and trout).

It is widely recognized that many issues contribute toward the viable production of farmed fish, especially during the hatchery phase when critical developmental stages of the juvenile fish occur including ontogeny of the digestive, immune and skeletal system. The latter has important implications for the overall conformation and health of the larval stage and resulting fry health, in addition to being a key factor in the survival and successive growth of the fish and feed efficiency at later stages of the production cycle. It is clear that early fish development is a complex interplay of numerous abiotic (e.g., environmental, such as temperature and water chemistry) and biotic, physiological, biochemical, and metabolic factors that can influence the different control mechanisms and expression of important biosynthesis routes at the organismal level, as well as locally for specific tissues and organs.

In the past two decades significant advances have been made in establishing the quantitative requirements of more than 50 essential nutrients for optimum growth and feed utilization, as well as to prevent deficiency diseases of single or multiple nutrients. However, significant gaps in our knowledge remain, particularly with regard to diets for new species, brood-stock nutrition and the effects of nutrition on the immune systems of fish. Economic and environmental sustainability pressures are also forcing changes in traditional formulations, producing challenges in satisfying nutritional requirements.[2]

The relationship between the correct nutritional status of fish and health is of paramount interest since previous attention was focused primarily on achieving fast growth rates and improved feed conversion efficiency. Since the advent of lower cost diets based on replacing fishmeal with an alternate protein, there is more flexibility in meeting the fundamental nutritional requirements of fish but also the potential for suboptimal nutrition when considering essential amino acids and more importantly vitamins and trace elements found in marine and terrestrial animal by-products.[3]

Nutritional diseases in fish must be viewed in a more generic manner as it is unlikely that one vitamin or mineral will be deficient as modern diets may be processed to include vitamin and mineral pre-mixes at variable levels, which may not always satisfy stringent nutritional demands of different species, at different life stages and culture conditions. As a consequence of changes in hatchery management strategies, use of new artificial diets to replace algae and live feeds present possibilities for dietary imbalance and deficiencies. The development of diets low in fishmeal and introduction of new protein and oil sources in extruded diets involving high temperatures and pressure pose further risks as these processes may affect thermolabile vitamins and nutrient bioavailability. Thus, fish nutrition is at a threshold or physiological "knife-edge" in some respects as the boundaries of fish nutrition are pushed in terms of feed formulations with novel ingredients, possibly limiting essential nutrients and growth-promoting factors at the critical stages of fish growth and development.

Etiologies: Feed and nutrient deprivation is usually the result of poor husbandry. For example, a poorly designed or maintained system is likely to develop water quality issues with related fish morbidity or mortality. In an effort to correct the water quality problems, the producer may reduce feed to the point where fish are in a negative energy and protein balance and begin to lose weight; or if the problem becomes chronic, starvation can result in loss of conformation and production losses.

The most likely cause of a nutritional deficiency in farmed fish will be a suboptimal level of an essential nutrient class such as one of the 10 essential amino acids, essential fatty acids or vitamins. Mineral deficiencies may be particularly specific and all relate to metabolic disturbances of major biochemical pathways associated with protein biosynthesis/catabolism and energy utilization or immune function in fish. Different strains and

types of fish such as use of triploid salmon and trout can exacerbate the situation.

CLINICAL PRESENTATIONS AND PATHOLOGY

Protein and essential amino acid imbalance

If protein is not supplied at the correct level in feeds, then the most likely outcome is suboptimal growth performance as opposed to any chronic pathologies, although very low protein intake may impede the long-term health of fish and skeletal and immune development. A well-balanced protein source is required to provide for the essential amino acids (EAAs) and an "ideal protein" is one where all 10 essential amino acids constitute the correct pattern matching the exact requirements of growing fish for muscle development, bone formation, and other vital structural and metabolic uses.[4]

Dietary imbalances of protein may also arise from the presence of disproportionate levels of specific amino acids such as leucine/isoleucine antagonisms, and to a lesser extent arginine/lysine and cysteine/methionine antagonisms. For example, blood meal is a rich source of valine, leucine and histidine, but is a poor source of methionine and isoleucine. Indeed, blood meal has been used in diets for salmon where it has been shown to be a very important source of histidine for the synthesis of a polypeptide with antioxidant function in the eye to prevent bilateral lenticular type cataract development (**Figure 16.1**).[5] However, in view of the antagonistic effect of excess leucine on isoleucine, animals fed high dietary levels of blood meal suffer from an isoleucine deficiency caused by an excess of dietary leucine. Although similar antagonisms have also been reported for cysteine/methionine and arginine/lysine in terrestrial farm animals, they have not been reported to occur in fish fed synthetic amino acid diet combinations. There is now a clear trend to greatly reduce or even remove the inclusion of fishmeal in diets for carnivorous fish, and formulate diets with alternative protein sources such as plant-based products such as soybean meal, pulses and grains that can be deficient in essential amino acids where methionine and lysine can be rate limiting to fish.

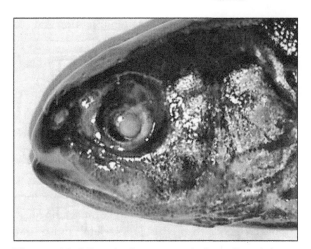

Figure 16.1 Lenticular cataract in juvenile rainbow trout (*Oncorhynchus mykiss*). Cataracts can result from an imbalance of amino acids in the ration.

Lipids and essential fatty acid imbalance and deficiencies

There is a delicate balance between the level of energy supplied by oils in fish diets to meet the optimum requirements of fish to achieve maximum protein utilization efficiency while ensuring a desired amount of lipid retention in tissues and the whole animal. An inappropriate protein-to-energy ratio caused by the overuse of oils in feeds can lead to excess lipid deposition in the carcass, especially in the visceral cavity around the intestine and vital organs such as the liver. Protein-to-energy (fat) ratio must therefore be carefully controlled throughout the production cycle to avoid excessive fat accumulation. This can be a serious problem for large trout approaching 1 kg in weight or hybrid striped bass reaching production size. Hepatic lipidosis is a common problem in captive fishes and can occur for multiple reasons, including starvation, a high percentage of carbohydrates in the diet, a high amount of lipids in the diet, and rancidity of feeds resulting in liver lipoid disease–type scenarios (**Figure 16.2**).[6,7] Modern high-energy salmon diets with oil levels exceeding 30% lead to changes in lipid accumulation in the flesh and retention in the visceral organs such as the intestinal tract. When the diet is properly balanced, the protein-to-energy ratio is optimized to prevent hepatic accumulation of fat; however, there is evidence that higher inclusions of

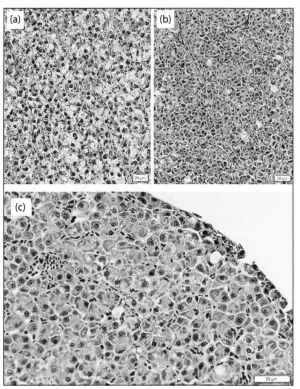

Figure 16.2 Light microscopy (H&E stained) of the liver of Atlantic salmon (*Salmo salar*) fry. (a) Healthy liver containing lipid. (b) Severely damaged hepatocytes with eosinophilic coagula (ceroid deposits). Ceroid deposition can result from a high level of antinutritive factors such as gossypol in the diet. (c) Fatty depletion and glycogen deposition in the liver in fish can result from dietary imbalances.

soy oil in salmonid diets can cause elevated hepatic and visceral fat (**Figure 16.3**).

Fish tissues contain relatively higher concentrations of highly unsaturated fatty acids (HUFAs) than terrestrial mammals. These are important constituents of all cell membranes, which makes fish tissue highly vulnerable to lipid peroxidation. Generally, essential fatty acids (EFAs) requirements of freshwater fish can be met by the supply of 18:3n-3 and 18:2n-6 fatty acids in diets, whereas the EFA requirement of marine fish can only be met by supplying long-chain HUFAs, 20:5n-3 and 22:6n-6.[8] Freshwater fish are able to elongate and desaturate 18:3n-3 to 22:6n-3, whereas marine fish, which lack or have a very low activity of 5-desaturase, require

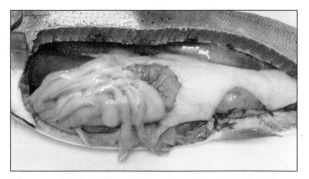

Figure 16.3 Adult rainbow trout (*O. mykiss*) with excess fat deposition around viceral organs.

the long-chain HUFA, eicosapentaenoic acid (20:5n-3; EPA), and docosahexaenoic acid (22:6n-3; DHA) in their diet.[9]

It is noteworthy that high dietary ratios of n-3 to n-6 fatty acids have been shown to reduce severity of cardiomyopathy, as well as the susceptibility of Atlantic salmon to stress.[10,11] Therefore, n-3 polyunsaturated fatty acids (PUFAs) are essential fatty acids in fish not only for optimal growth and feed efficiency, but also for cardiovascular function and immunological efficacy. Cardiomyopathy in salmon, which may present as cardiovascular breakdown and cardiac tamponade (i.e., hemopericardium) due to rupture of the atrium or sinus venosus, may be related to a fatty acid imbalance, vitamin E deficiency or selenium deficiency (**Figure 16.4**).[12,13]

Several biochemical abnormalities and disease syndromes are also associated with feeds that have become rancid where substantial loss of HUFAs and vitamin activity occurs due to lipid peroxidation. Some of the common epidermal lesions associated with fin erosion and skin inflammation problems in farmed fish have been linked to fatty acid imbalances

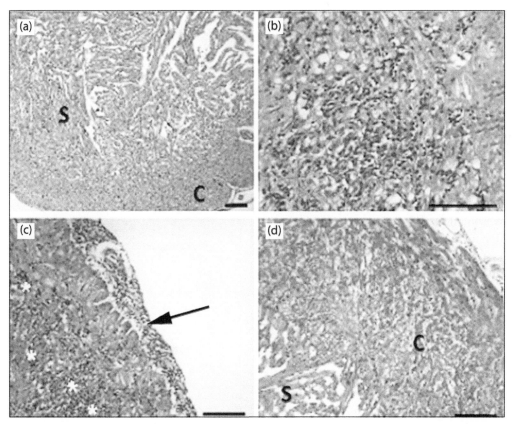

Figure 16.4 Light microscopy (H&E stained) of the heart from trout experimentally infected with salmonid alpha virus 1. (a) Control fish with healthy spongy (S) and compact (C) layers. (b) Severe inflammation of the compact layer. (c) Severe mononuclear infiltration of the compact layer and epicardium (arrow). (d) Severe vacuolation of the compact layer (C).

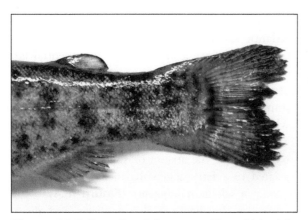

Figure 16.5 Juvenile rainbow trout (*O. mykiss*) with erosions on the pelvic and the caudal fins as a result of chronic zinc deficiency.

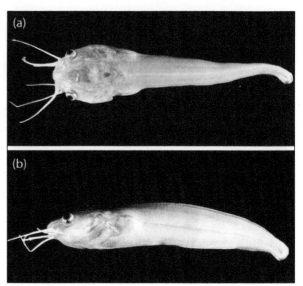

Figure 16.6 Cranial/skeletal abnormalities in African catfish (*Clarias gariepinus*) fingerling fed a diet deficient in vitamin C. (a) dorsal view, (b) lateral view.

(**Figure 16.5**). It is important to establish that the dietary lipid supply is not only at the correct level with the proper balance of EFAs for optimum growth and feed utilization, but can also maintain proper immune function and prevent infectious diseases in farmed fish.[9,14]

Carbohydrate excess in fish

Temperate carnivorous fish have a limited ability to utilize carbohydrate for energy purposes.[15] In general, excess dietary carbohydrates can lead to glycogen deposition in the liver and may produce irreversible pathological conditions in the liver. While reports on the detrimental effects of carbohydrates on fish health and immune function are not conclusive, an imbalance may also affect the normal gut microbial ecology leading to adverse effects on digestive physiology.

Micronutrient deficiencies
Vitamin C

Ascorbic acid (vitamin C) is essential for collagen formation, wound healing, hematopoiesis, detoxification of compounds as well as for several metabolic functions including being part of the antioxidant system in fish and other contaminants as well as toxins in diets.[16] One of the main effects of a vitamin C deficiency is skeletal malformations due to abnormal collagen synthesis. Skeletal deformities and malformations in farmed fish vary enormously in their severity and may include cranial abnormalities, vertebral column disorders, kyphosis, and

lordosis (**Figures 16.6** through **16.9**).[17] Skeletal and fin abnormalities of farmed fish cannot only hinder locomotion, which may lead to out-competition for food and exhaustion under intensive rearing conditions, but skeletal abnormalities are also problematic for processors by hampering filleting, reducing yield and causing poor fillet uniformity. The nutritional components affecting skeletal development in

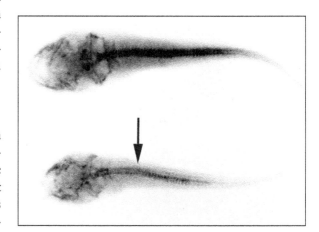

Figure 16.7 Radiograph (dorsal-ventral view) of African catfish (*Clarias gariepinus*) fingerling with normal axial skeleton (upper image) and skeletal deformity (lower image, arrow) due to a diet deficient in vitamin C.

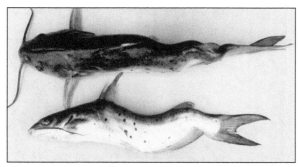

Figure 16.8 Pond raised channel catfish (*Ictalurus punctatus*) fed a diet deficient in vitamin C. (Image courtesy of A. Mitchell.)

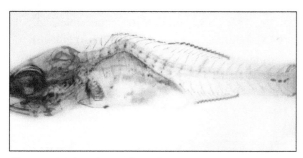

Figure 16.9 Alcian blue–alizarin red double stained first feeding sea bass fry showing skeletal lordosis due to a diet deficient in vitamin C.

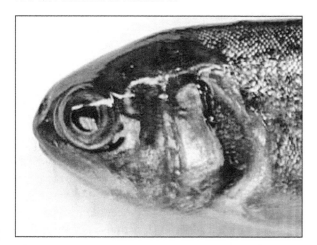

Figure 16.10 Juvenile rainbow trout (*O. mykiss*) with incomplete opercula exposing gill tissue typical of a diet deficient in vitamin C.

marine fish larvae has been reviewed.[18] Other related problems are incomplete opercula development, gill arch malformation and cataracts in sensitive species (**Figure 16.10**). Deformities of the opercula, can impinge on fish health by increasing exposure

of the delicate gill lamellae to suspended solids and pathogens, as well as reducing the value of whole fish products. Fin erosion and hemorrhages of the skin and internal organs may also be evident. Other vitamin C–related pathologies include exophthalmia, anemia and reduced egg hatchability. Vitamin C is a readily available, low-cost commercial product. Furthermore, dietary toxicity cannot occur in fish. Consequently, vitamin C presents a valuable option for supplementing (e.g., top dressing) feeds at particular strategic times in the rearing process, due to its multifaceted importance in maintaining fish health.

Vitamin E deficiencies

The vitamin E family of tocopherols are vital components of cell membranes in animals and play an important antioxidant function in combination with vitamin C and also selenium.[19] Vitamin E deficiency has been related to myopathy, including muscular deformities. Skeletal muscle abnormalities have been associated with selenium deficiency and rancid feeds.[20] Rancid feeds have also been linked to steatitis in a number of fish species. In addition, vitamin E and other antioxidant nutrients (e.g., ascorbic acid, carotene and selenium) are required for optimum function of the immune system in terrestrial and aquatic animals.[21,22]

Other vitamin deficiencies

The fat-soluble vitamin A and major water-soluble B vitamins are major cofactors and play vital roles in intermediate cellular metabolism in oxidation reactions and energy liberating pathways. Vitamin A deficiency has been associated with inferior growth and retinal atrophy, and more recently cranial and axial deformities in fish such as in salmon. Excess vitamin A has been linked to pathologies due to the metabolism of vitamin A into retinoic acid that can modulate gene expression and affect axial development.[23]

The B vitamins act as enzyme activators and play a key role in carbohydrate, protein, and lipid metabolism and function in a concerted synergistic manner. Several dietary factors and feed processing conditions may affect the stability and bioavailability of B vitamins in commercial fish diets. In addition, there may be varying bioavailability in different raw materials. Any reduction in B vitamin intake may also adversely impair the immune function in fish. Of the B vitamins, folic acid deficiency has been associated with poor growth and, in channel catfish, with anemia.[24,25] This disorder has been described as nutritional anemia of catfish and is caused by microbial contamination of feed that can result in folic acid depletion. The diagnosis is often based initially on history, with multiple production units developing similar signs at the same time. Acute thiamine deficiency has been associated with neurologic signs, including convulsions and death, whereas chronic deficiency has resulted in loss of equilibrium, edema and poor growth in fish.[26] Riboflavin deficiency has been associated with vascularization of the cornea of the eye, hyperpigmentation, clouding and hemorrhage of the eyes. Niacin, biotin and pyridoxine deficiencies have been associated with neurologic abnormalities, including spasms and convulsions.[27] Niacin deficiency has been associated with malpigmentation and caudal fin erosions in salmonid species. Choline and inositol deficiency have been linked to poor growth and feed efficiency in fish.

Nutritional gill disease has been described in a number of fish species and is primarily caused by a pantothenic acid deficiency.[28] The primary lamellae at the tips of the gill filaments of affected fish are fused, resulting in a very characteristic histologic lesion (**Figure 16.11**). Other effects are exophthalmia, edema (i.e., dropsy), pale liver, impaired energy metabolism and skin lesions (**Figure 16.12**).

Minerals and trace element imbalance and deficiency

The availability and utilization of dietary trace elements in fish is dependent upon the dietary source and form of the element ingested, the adequacy of stores within the body, interactions with other mineral elements present in the gastrointestinal tract and within the body tissues (i.e., antagonisms), and finally by element interactions with other dietary ingredients or their metabolites, such as vitamins, fiber and phytic acid found in soybean meal binding phosphorous.[29] There are at least 10 elements deemed to be essential in the diets of fish; these being calcium, phosphorous, magnesium,

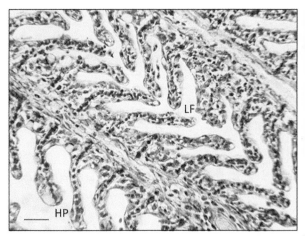

Figure 16.11 Light microscopy (periodic acid–Schiff [PAS] stain) of rainbow trout (*O. mykiss*) gill with morphology typical of pantothenic acid deficiency showing lamellar hyperplasia (HP) leading to necrosis and lamellar fusion (LF) due to "clubbed" lamellar tips. Bar = 50 um. (Image courtesy of R. Handy.)

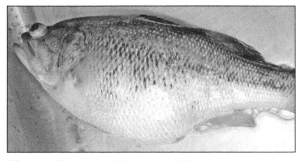

Figure 16.12 Adult largemouth bass (*Micropterus salmoides*) with dropsy and exophthalmia typical of a pantothenic acid deficiency.

potassium, iron, zinc, copper, iodine, selenium and manganese.[3] Other trace elements such as cobalt, vanadium, molybdenum and chromium may also be of significance in some fish.[30] Accurately quantifying dietary mineral requirements in fish is very difficult, most notably due to the water solubility of many elements. Indeed, many of the essential elements can be derived, to varying extents, from the surrounding water, such as calcium in marine fish. This has meant that specific requirements for elements in fish remain poorly defined and as a result a number of nutritional pathologies have arisen in intensive finfish farming as a consequence of improper provision of minerals and trace elements.

As previously discussed, specific vitamin deficiencies and imbalances can result in pronounced skeletal malformations due to the regulatory role they play in bone development. Similarly, dietary deficiencies and imbalances of the nutrients that are structural components of bone can influence skeletal dynamics and modeling during rapid phases of growth.[31] Minerals and trace elements are therefore key components in ensuring normal osteological development and ossification of the bone tissues of fish, particularly associated with water flow rate dynamics in aquaculture.[32] Phosphorous (P) deficiency in particular may promote significant increases in skeletal abnormalities and reduced bone mineralization in fish, which may impair growth potential and increase the number of fish routinely culled under intensive rearing conditions to maintain welfare. Calcium (Ca) is similarly vital in the growth and development of fish. However, dietary dependence is generally somewhat lower than P considering that most of the fish requirement can be met via absorption from the surrounding water especially in the marine environment. In freshwater, fish achieve this by uptake through the gills and skin, whereas in seawater, the ingestion of water becomes the primary mechanism of acquisition. Lordosis, scoliosis, jaw and cranial irregularities, as well as fin, rib and opercula abnormalities, can often be associated to improper provision of P and Ca (**Figures 16.13** through **16.15**). Adequate dietary provision of P and Ca, particularly during times of heightened environmental stress, can mitigate the risk of poor ossification. For example, enhanced Ca and P supplementation has been advocated as an effective feeding strategy during the early seawater transfer phase of Atlantic salmon smolts from freshwater to reduce the incidence of skeletal abnormalities much later when the fish reached harvest size. A deficiency or imbalance of magnesium (Mg), zinc (Zn) or manganese (Mn) can also cause skeletal abnormalities in fish, especially in diets low in fishmeal.

Deficiency of trace elements may cause other morphological effects, aside from those associated with bone material. Copper (Cu), Mn, Mg or Zn deficiencies have all been associated with specific or compounded clinical manifestations in numerous fish species. Examples include incidences of

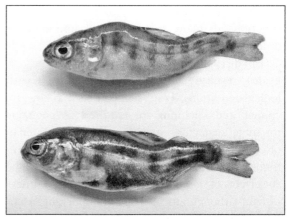

Figure 16.13 Skeletal lordosis and scoliosis in juvenile rainbow trout (*O. mykiss*). Amino acids (e.g., tryptophan, leucine, isoleucine, lysine, arginine and histidine) and mineral deficiencies are known to be responsible for skeletal deformities in fish.

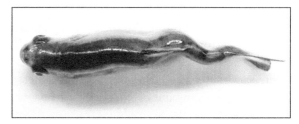

Figure 16.14 Dorsal view of skeletal scoliosis of rainbow trout in Figure 16.13.

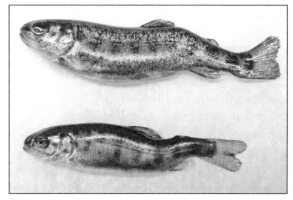

Figure 16.15 Skeletal lordosis and scoliosis in juvenile rainbow trout (*O. mykiss*).

cataracts, and Zn deficiency, in particular, has been reported to increase the onset of fin erosions and external bleeding at the base of fins, which is an important indicator of welfare conditions in intensively farmed fish.

Minerals and trace elements also have integral functions in many metabolic and immunological processes. For this reason, suboptimal dietary levels can disrupt normal physiological functioning and health, resulting in a plethora of different pathological conditions. Trace elements such as zinc, iron, copper and selenium are required as coenzymes for metalloenzymes, and are vital for maintenance of cellular functions and in the immune system of higher vertebrates. However, little is known about the effects of trace elements on the immune function of fish, although zinc is deemed important in many animal systems.

Iron (Fe) is an essential nutrient for fish as well as microorganisms, and the ability of pathogens to infect a host depends on its availability. Maintaining low concentrations of free Fe in mucus membranes and in other tissues is thought to be one of the primary nonspecific host defensive systems against bacterial insult. Levels of Fe in fish during bacterial infection decline rapidly in the spleen, liver and kidney, particularly in fish fed a diet with low Fe content. Low dietary Fe may protect against infection by limiting the amount of Fe available to bacteria, and Fe supplementation would increase susceptibility to infection.[33] On the other hand, iron deficiency has been reported to cause microcytic anemia in several fish species. Generally, Fe deficiency is not a problem in fish culture because water and feed ingredients in production diets tend to supply sufficient quantities of Fe to meet the metabolic physiological needs of fish. However, feed formulations containing high blood and fishmeal inclusions should be closely monitored because they supply large amounts of Fe, which may predispose fish to common bacterial pathogens.

Similar to higher vertebrates, an iodine deficiency can result in thyroid hyperplasia in teleost fish. The condition can occur as a consequence of a nutritional deficiency, but may also be associated with chronic nitrite and nitrate exposure and/or the application of ozone. Consequently, the potential for an iodine deficiency occurrence in a recirculating aquaculture system is heightened.

The form in which elements are provided in the diet is an important aspect of preventing mineral and trace element deficiencies in fish, as total dietary levels will seldom be actual bioavailable levels in practice and this must be a prime responsibility of the feed compounder and specialized fish nutritionist. In order to guarantee that nutritional requirements are met in compound fish diets, supplementation of minerals and trace elements, in freely available forms, is currently implemented during aquafeed formulation by using carefully designed trace element premixes that are often now co-mixed with vitamins into a single mixture designed for different fish species.

Anti-nutritional factors

The recent development of fish feeds with much lower fishmeal inclusion and an increased dependency on plant protein concentrates such as soybean meals and a range of other legume, pulses and grain-based proteins can introduce undesirable effects. The presence of anti-nutritional factors (ANFs) are well known in animal nutrition and fish can be sensitive to various protease inhibitors, saponins, tannins, hemagglutinins and non-starch polysaccharides (NSPs), of which some may negatively interact with the morphology and function of the gastrointestinal tract of fish. Specific oligosaccharides may interfere with digestion and together with saponins cause a degree of gut leakage leading to inflammation and impaired gut integrity. This may lead to potential secondary infection and an increased risk of systemic entry of pathogenic bacteria. Salmonid fish and carnivorous fish like sea bass and sea bream are sensitive to some standard grades of soybean included in fish feeds. The inclusion of soybean meal (SBM), especially in the diet of Atlantic salmon, induces an inflammatory response in the distal intestinal mucosa, known as SBM-induced enteritis (**Figure 16.16**).[34,35] The degree of processing of soybean meal and the removal of these deleterious ANFs can vastly alleviate this problem in diets containing high levels of such plant proteins.

Differential diagnosis: It is important to recognize that numerous factors may cause skeletal abnormalities in fish, including genetics, pathogens, trauma, environmental parameters and handling. This can complicate the diagnosis of skeletal defects caused by nutrition. Numerous pathogens and conditions can also mimic the gill pathology and exophthalmia

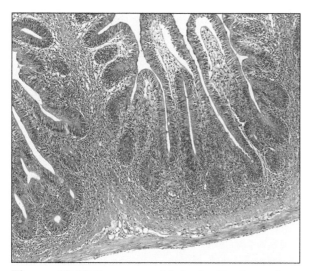

Figure 16.16 Severe enteritis in the distal gut of Atlantic salmon (*Salmo salar*) stained with periodic acid–Schiff (PAS). Carnivorous fish fed with soybean meal–based diet can develop enteritis (SBM-induced enteritis) characterized by severe infiltration of leukocytes and edema in the lamina propria. (Image courtesy of P. Silva.)

associated with a pantothenic acid deficiency, thus careful diagnostic examination for other conditions is paramount.

Diagnosis: The initial diagnosis of a nutritional disease in fish is generally based on a complete history. Specific nutritional diseases in fish are most often diagnosed after other causes of disease have been ruled out and the diet is more closely examined. However, it is of importance to consider that nutritional inadequacies may secondarily exacerbate other pathologies. Indeed, specific nutrient requirements are not constant throughout the life cycle of fish, being influenced by environmental stressors, pathogens and injury, as well as the animal's life stage.[8] It is therefore important for aquaculturists and aquarists to understand the nutritional requirements and signs of nutrient deficiencies and imbalances within their chosen cultured species.

Management/control: It is well known that nutritional deficiencies predispose fish to infectious diseases and conversely that modulation of nutritional supplements can improve disease resistance. The immune system of fish is constantly responding to true and opportunistic pathogens trying to invade body systems using the nonspecific or innate and specific or adaptive arm of the immune system similar to terrestrial animals. These responses occur via a cascade of events including pathogen recognition, antigen presentation and killing, and finally immune expansion and memory response. The initial events associated with pathogen recognition and antigen presentation drive fish into a hypermetabolic status, allowing them to activate cellular (e.g., phagocytes) and molecular (cytokines and chemokines) determinants of the innate immune system.[36] When challenged by an infection, metabolism shifts activating mobilization of protein and energy reserves in favor of immune defense to resolve disease establishment and to generate adaptive (i.e., memory) immunity.[37]

The interrelationship between nutrition and the immune system is complex, and is associated with numerous direct and indirect factors. Maintaining minimal levels of exogenous nutrients is therefore paramount to maintaining basal levels of immune competence and restoring collateral damage caused by pathogens. However, provision of some nutrients that are completely independent of sustaining basic physiological functions such as growth and reproduction were found to be helpful in improving immune competences in battling invading pathogens.

Functional feeds, which are defined as specially formulated diets containing essential or nonessential ingredients fed either singly or in combination, can influence immune function and fish health. Application of clinical nutrition strategies to improve stock health would benefit farmed organisms in many ways including fast growth, resistance to infections and the ability to cope with stress more efficiently. Functional feeds have been considered as an alternative measure for controlling infections, especially viral diseases (e.g., salmon pancreas disease [PD], heart and skeletal muscle inflammation [HSMI], cardiac myopathy syndrome [CMS]) and therefore health management through nutrient supplement is a new strategy to improve sustainability of the aquaculture industry.[38,39]

A plethora of feed additives, including vitamins, carotenoids, prebiotics, probiotics, and symbiotic and herbal remedies, have been tested as components in functional feeds. For example, inclusion of prebiotic mixes derived mainly from microbial and plants including mannan-oligosaccharide (MOS), beta-glucans, polysaccharides and nucleotides appear to improve nonspecific immune response translating into pro-inflammatory and chemotactic cytokines, such as interleukin (IL)-1β, IL-6, IL-8, tumor necrosis factor (TNF)-α, and γ-interferon (IFN), along with upregulation of important pattern recognition receptors (PRRs) such as toll-like receptor (TLR)3, TLR5, and TLR9 in different fish species.[40–42] Improving nutrient supplements, such as glutamine and arginine, that enhance phagocytes also appeared to be responsible for enhancing disease resistance status in fish. In addition, nutrients important to sustain membrane fluidity, such as n-3 or n-6 PUFAs, or antioxidant compounds, such as vitamin C and vitamin E, have been successful in improving immune competence of fish against pathogens. Further, these supplements also appeared to improve cell proliferation and maturation capacities, especially for lymphocytes that induce adaptive immune responses, producing pathogen-specific immunoglobulins and an enhanced immunological memory response.

In light of pressures to expand aquaculture in areas where water supply is limited, as well as provide production strategies with less environmental influence and ecological impact, the farming of aquatic livestock is increasingly adopting closed containment systems that recirculate or reuse water.[43] These recirculating aquaculture systems (RASs), typically indoors, minimize total water usage by removing waste products via continuous filtration. Recirculating aquaculture systems indispensably require mechanical filters to remove solid waste, as well as biofilters, where nitrifying bacteria oxidize excreted ammonia to nitrite, followed by oxidation of nitrite to nitrate, allowing a reduction in the buildup of toxic excretions and metabolites in the fish's rearing environment.

Feed utilized in an RAS can impact heavily upon the efficiency of its filtration systems and thus the overall efficiency of the operation and performance of its housed livestock. Consequently, it is increasingly being recognized that traditional diets may not be appropriate for these systems, such that RAS-specific feeds have become an emerging area in the growing aquafeed sector. These RAS feeds are somewhat unique in that they must ensure optimum performance of both the animals and the filtration systems. The aim of RAS feeds is to limit, as much as possible, nitrogen loading of the water while simultaneously allowing easy recovery of solid waste. Metabolic oxygen needs and carbon dioxide release by the fish is also of consideration, since these must similarly be managed within an RAS. These aims are approached through careful selection of highly digestible ingredients, optimized balancing of energy to protein ratios, and tailored amino-acid profiles, all of which depend upon the species being cultured. It will be of utmost importance that the process of designing diets that cater to filtration system capacity does not lose sight of possible nutrient imbalances and deficiencies.

In general, excellent progress has been made in designing specific feeds for fish that can sustain all stages of the production cycle. However, there are still issues relating to nutritional deficiencies in fish due to differences in formulations, choice of raw materials and processing methods used in the aquaculture feed industry. Increasingly, the diets for many fish species are subject to the pressure of raw material costs and availability leading to increasing variation in feed formulations and with reduction in fishmeal use with reliance on alternative ingredients. These include not only plant by-products but also novel ingredients such as algae, yeasts, bacteria and insect-based proteins, which can alter amino acid profile of diets as well as other nutrient components. New processing technologies and the effect of extrusion on feeds may affect the micronutrient balance warranting more attention to mineral and vitamin premixes in feeds designed for high performance, faster growth rates and superior feed conversion efficiencies. As an increasing volume of aquaculture production moves inland and indoors in coming years, traditional dietary formulations may require readjustment to suit filtration technologies. In addition, as a consequence of the complex interplay of the gut epithelium and its resident bacteria (microbiome), there is now increasing interest in how nutrition can influence the gut microbiome, immune-competence and improved disease resistance, and mucosal health in farmed fish. However, feed manufacturers and aquaculture producers should not lose sight of the key nutrient requirements and anti-nutrients that have been identified as contributors to fish nutritional health status.

REFERENCES

1. FAO. *The State of World Fisheries and Aquaculture 2016: Contributing to Food Security and Nutrition for all.* Rome, 2016.
2. Tacon, A.G.J. and Metian, M. Feed matters: Satisfying the feed demand of aquaculture. *Reviews in Fisheries Science & Aquaculture* 2015;23:1–10.
3. Watanabe, T., Kiron, V. and Satoh, S. Trace minerals in fish nutrition. *Aquaculture* 1997;151:185–207.
4. Wilson, R.P. and Halver, J. E. Protein and amino acid requirements of fishes. *Annual Review of Nutrition* 1986;6:225–244.
5. Remø, S.C., Hevrøy, E.M., Olsvik, P.A., Fontanillas, R., Breck, O. and Waagbø, R. Dietary histidine requirement to reduce the risk and severity of cataracts is higher than the requirement for growth in Atlantic salmon smolts, independently of the dietary lipid source. *British Journal of Nutrition* 2014;111(10):1759–1772.
6. Roald, S.O. An outbreak of lipoid liver degeneration (LLD) in Atlantic salmon (*Salmo salar*) in a fish farm and attempts to cure the disease (author's transl). *Nordisk Veterinaer Medicin* 1976;28(4–5):243–249.
7. Weisman, J.L. and Miller, D.l. Lipoid liver disease and steatitis in a captive sapphire damsel, *Pomacentrus pavo*. *Acta Ichthyologica et Piscatoria* 2006;36(2):9–104.
8. NRC. *Nutrient Requirements of Fish and Shrimp. Animal Nutrition Series, National Research Council of the National Academies*, The National Academies Press, Washington DC, 2011.
9. Bell, J.G., Ashton, I., Secombes, C.J., Weitzel, B.R., Dick, J.R. and Sargent, J.R. Dietary lipid affects phospholipid fatty acid compositions, eicosanoid production and immune function in Atlantic salmon (*Salmo salar*). *Prostaglandins, Leucotrienes and Eicosanoid Fatty Acids* 1996;54:173–182.
10. Martinez-Rubio, L., Morais, S., Evensen, Ø., Wadsworth, S., Ruohonen, K., Vecino, J. L. G., Bell, J. G. and Tocher, D. R. Functional feeds reduce heart inflammation and pathology in Atlantic salmon (*Salmo salar* L.) following experimental challenge with Atlantic salmon reovirus (ASRV). *PLoS ONE* 2012;7(11): e40266.
11. Thompson, K.D., Tatner, M.F. and Hendersoon, R.J. Effects of dietary (n-3) and (n-6) polyunsaturated fatty acid ratio on the immune response of Atlantic salmon, *Salmo salar* L. *Aquaculture Nutrition* 1996;2:21–31.
12. Bell, J.G., McVicar, A.H., Park, M.T. and Sargent, J.R. High dietary linoleic acid affects the fatty acid compositions of individual phospholipids from tissues of Atlantic salmon (*Salmo salar*): Association with stress susceptibility and cardiac lesion. *Journal of Nutrition* 1991;121:1163–1172.
13. Bell, J.G., Dick, J.R., McVicar, A.H., Sargent, J.R. and Thompson, K.D. Dietary sunflower, linseed and fish oils affect phospholipid fatty acid composition, development of cardiac lesions, phospholipase activity and eicosanoid production in Atlantic salmon (*Salmo salar*). *Prostaglandins, Leucotrienes and Eicosanoid Fatty Acids* 1993;49:665–673.
14. Fracalossi, D.M. and Lovell, R.T. Dietary lipid sources influence responses of channel catfish (*Ictalurus punctatus*) to challenge with the pathogen *Edwardsiella ictaluri*. *Aquaculture* 1994;119:287–298.
15. Polakof S., Panserat, S., Soengas, J.L. and Moon, T.W. Glucose metabolism in fish: A review. *Journal of Comparative Physiology B* 2012;182(8):1015–1045.
16. Sandnes, K. Vitamin C in fish nutrition—A review. *Fiskeridirektoratets skrifter. Serie Ernæring* 1991;4(1): 3–32.
17. Fjelldal, P. G., Hansen, T., Breck, O., Ørnsrud, R., Lock, E.-J., Waagbø, R., Wargeliusand, A. and Eckhard Witten, P. Vertebral deformities in farmed Atlantic salmon (*Salmo salar* L.)—Etiology and pathology. *Journal of Applied Ichthyology* 2012;28:433–440.
18. Cahua, C., Zambonino Infantea, J. and Takeuchib, T. Nutritional components affecting skeletal development in fish larvae. *Aquaculture* 2003;227(1–4):254–258.
19. Rider, S.A., Davies, S.J., Jha, N.A., Fisher, A.A., Knight, J. and Sweetman, J. Supra-nutritional dietary intake of selenite and selenium yeast in normal and stressed rainbow trout (*Oncorhynchus mykis*): Implications on selenium status and health responses. *Aquaculture* 2009;295:282–291.
20. Baker, R.T.M. and Davies, S.J. Modulation of tissue α-tocopherol in African catfish (*Clarias gariepinus*) fed oxidized oils, and the compensatory effect of supplemental dietary vitamin E. *Aquaculture Nutrition* 1997;3(2):91–97.
21. Hardie, L.J., Fletcher, T.C. and Secombes, C.J. The effect of dietary vitamin E on the immune response of the Atlantic salmon (*Salmo salar* L.). *Aquaculture* 1990;87:1–13.
22. Erdal, J.I., Evensen, O., Kaurstad, O.K., Lillehaug, A. Solbakken, R. and Thorud, K. Relationship between diet and immune response in Atlantic salmon (*Salmo salar* L.) feeding various levels of ascorbic acid and omega-3 fatty acids. *Aquaculture* 1991;98:363–379.
23. Lall, S.P. and Lewis-McCrea, L.M. Role of nutrients in skeletal metabolism and pathology in fish—An overview. *Aquaculture* 2007;267(1–4):3–19.
24. Cowey, C.B. and Woodward, B. The dietary requirement of young rainbow trout (*Oncorhynchus mykiss*) for folic acid. *J Nutr.* 1993;123(9):1594–600.
25. Cowey, C.B. and Woodward, B. Water-soluble vitamins in fish ontogeny. *Aquaculture* 2010;41(5):733–744.
26. Morito, C.L.H., Conrad, D.H. and Hilton, J.W. The thiamin deficiency signs and requirement of rainbow trout (*Salmo gairdneri*, Richardson). *Fish Physiology and Biochemistry* 1986;1(2):93–104.

27. Woodward, B. and Frigg, M. Dietary biotin requirements of young rainbow trout (*Salmo gairdneri*) determined by weight gain, hepatic biotin concentration and maximal biotin-dependent enzyme activities in liver and white muscle. *Journal of Nutrition* 1989;119(1):54–60.

28. Karges, R.G. and Woodward, B. Development of lamellar epithelial hyperplasia in gills of pantothenic acid-deficient rainbow trout, *Salmo gairdneri* Richardson. *Journal of Fish Biology* 1984;25(1):57–62.

29. Hilton, J.W. The interaction of vitamins, minerals and diet composition in the diet of fish. *Aquaculture* 1989;79:223–233.

30. Ahmed, A.R., Jha, A.N. and Davies, S.J. The efficacy of chromium as a growth enhancer for mirror carp (*Cyprinus carpio* L): An integrated study using biochemical, genetic and histological responses. *Biological Trace Elements Research* 2012;148(2):187–197.

31. Fox, S.W. and Davies, S.J. Corn-expressed dietary phytase augments vertebral and scale mineral content in juvenile rainbow trout (*Oncorhynchus mykiss*). *Aquaculture Nutrition* 2011;17(4):840–852.

32. Owen, M.A.G., Eynon B., Woodgate S., Davies S.J. and Fox S. Increased water current induces microarchitectural changes to the vertebral bone of juvenile rainbow trout (*Oncorhynchus mykiss*). *Aquaculture* 2012;344–349:141–146.

33. Rigos, G., Samartzis, A., Henry, M., Fountoulaki, E., Cotou, E., Sweetman, J., Davies, S. and Nengas, I. Effects of additive iron on growth, tissue distribution, hematology and immunology of gilthead sea bream, *Sparus aurata*. *Aquaculture International*, 2010;18:1093.

34. Baeverfjord, G.T. and Krogdahl, A. Development and regression of soybean meal induced enteritis in Atlantic salmon, *Salmo salar* L., distal intestine: A comparison with the intestines of fasted fish. *Journal of Fish Diseases* 1996;19(5):375–387.

35. Ruytera, B., Moya-Falcóna, C., Rosenlundb, G. and Vegusdala, A. Fat content and morphology of liver and intestine of Atlantic salmon (*Salmo salar*): Effects of temperature and dietary soybean oil. *Aquaculture* 2006;252(2–4):441–452.

36. Blazer, V.S. Piscine macrophages function and nutritional influences: A review. *Journal of Aquatic Animal Health* 1991;3:77–86.

37. Blazer, V.S. Nutrition and disease resistance in fish. *Annual Review of Fish Diseases* 1992;1:309–323.

38. Tacchia, L., Bickerdike, R., Douglasa, A., Secombes, C.J. and Martia, S.A.M. Transcriptomic responses to functional feeds in Atlantic salmon (*Salmo salar*). *Fish & Shellfish Immunology* 2011;31(5):704–715.

39. Luckstadt, C. The use of acidifiers in fish nutrition. *CAB Reviews: Perspectives in Agriculture, Veterinary Science, Nutrition and Natural Resources* 2008;3(044).

40. Hoseinifar, S.H., Esteban, M.A. Cuesta, A. and Sun, Y. Prebiotics and fish immune response: A review of current knowledge and future perspectives. *Reviews in Fisheries Science & Aquaculture* 2015;23(4):315–328.

41. Dimitroglou, A., Merrifield, D.L., Carnevali, O., Picchietti, S., Avella, M., Daniels, C.L., Güroy, D. and Davies, S.J. Microbial manipulations to improve fish health and production—A Mediterranean perspective. *Fish & Shellfish Immunology* 2011;30:1–16.

42. Merrifield, D.L., Bradley, G., Harper, G., Baker, R.T.M., Munn, C.B. and Davies, S.J. Assessment of the effects of vegetative and lyophilised *Pediococcus acidilactici* on growth, feed utilisation, intestinal colonisation and health parameters of rainbow trout (*Oncorhynchus mykiss* Walbaum). *Aquaculture Nutrition* 2010;17:73–79.

43. Piedrahita, R.H. Management of aquaculture effluents: Reducing the potential environmental impact of tank aquaculture effluents through intensification and recirculation. *Aquaculture* 2003;226(1–4):35–44.

SEDATION, ANESTHESIA, ANALGESIA AND EUTHANASIA

LYSA PAM POSNER, CRAIG A. HARMS, AND STEPHEN A. SMITH

Fish of all types are routinely sedated or anesthetized for transport, husbandry, diagnostics, medical and therapeutic procedures, or prior to euthanasia. As with mammals, reptiles or avian species, anesthesia in fish should produce unconsciousness in a way that causes minimal stress or discomfort to the animal and maintains physiologic parameters as close to normal range as possible. In addition to the physiologic effects, other considerations in choosing an anesthetic include access to agents, ease of administration, risks with human exposure, cost and environmental impact.

To date, more than 33,000 different species of fish have been described. Fish are generally divided into one of three groups: aquatic vertebrates (e.g., bony fishes, such as salmonids, carp and catfishes) exclusive of tetrapods, cartilaginous fishes (e.g., sharks, rays and chimaeras) or jawless aquatic craniates (e.g., lampreys and hagfishes). Further, differences exist in each group by habitat, as there are marine, brackish and freshwater species, and cold-, cool- and warm-water species. This variability of animals between and even within each group makes extrapolation of drug doses or effects from different species questionable.

BASIC CONSIDERATIONS FOR ANESTHESIA IN FISH

Fish scheduled for anesthesia should be granted similar pre-anesthetic considerations as with any other animal. In general, a health exam should be performed to assess overall health, gill health and appropriateness of anesthesia. Withholding food before anesthesia may be prudent as regurgitation of food while sedated or anesthetized can occur and could result in food particles in the gills (sestonosis), which would hinder exchange of gases and electrolytes. Most fish can easily accommodate a short fasting period (12–24 hr) without any adverse sequelae. While there is little reported evidence that sick fish have greater mortality when anesthetized, it is likely that, similar to other animals, sick fish may have greater mortality in the peri-anesthetic period.

Care should also be taken to match water quality of the anesthesia water as closely as possible with that of the culture or holding water (e.g., temperature, pH, salinity, hardness), ideally using the same water. All equipment and supplies for the procedures to be performed should be prepared beforehand, and a source of recovery water should be available before initiating anesthesia in order to minimize anesthesia time and time out of water. Anesthesia equipment should be cleaned and disinfected between uses with a suitable disinfectant such as dilute chlorhexidine, and rinsed well prior to each use. Thorough drying of equipment between uses also provides an additional degree of disinfection.

Once anesthetized, fish should be handled gently and with care to avoid damaging their protective mucous layer and thin skin epithelium (**Figures 17.1** and **17.2**). It is important to avoid having fish contact dry surfaces, including dry human hands. Moistened latex or nitrile gloves are preferable to bare hands, and all surfaces the fish contacts directly should ideally be smooth and moist. During anesthesia, the gills of fish must be supplied with adequately oxygenated water for gas exchange and the exposed skin must be kept moist. In prolonged procedures or when fish are held in very deep planes of anesthesia that reduce opercular effort, it may be necessary to artificially supply the needed volumes of oxygenated water to the gills to maintain the fish's physiology. Water flow rate should be sufficient to irrigate gill arches bilaterally, without engorging the gastrointestinal tract. A flow rate of ~1 L/kg/min

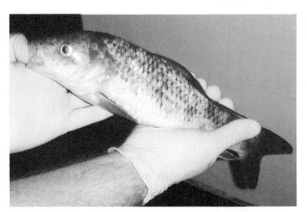

Figure 17.1 Holding a koi (*Cyprinus carpio*) with a gloved finger in the mouth to prevent damage to the skin and restrain the fish during transport or physical examination.

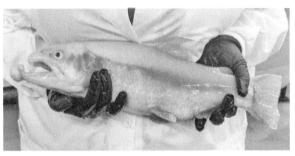

Figure 17.2 Restraining a large "golden" rainbow trout (*Oncorhynchus mykiss*) after sedation to minimize damage to the skin and fins during transport or examination. Note the large kype, or hook-like protuberance on the lower jaw, which is a normal secondary sexual characteristic of some mature male salmonids. (Image courtesy of B. Reed-Grimmett.)

is suitable in most cases.[1,2] Though anesthetized fish can survive removal from water and exposure of their gills to air for short periods of time sufficient for minor procedures (e.g., gill biopsy), care should be taken to prevent desiccation of skin, eyes, and gills, and the physiologic derangements of not exchanging oxygen and carbon dioxide at the gill–water interface.

ANESTHESIA

Routes of administration

Fish exchange oxygen and carbon dioxide via the gills. The movement of these gases requires a

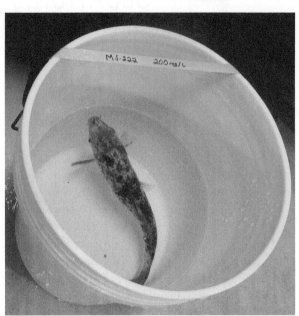

Figure 17.3 Anesthesia induction of a koi (*C. carpio*) immersed in 200 mg/L MS-222. An air diffuser stone was removed to make the fish more readily visible, but aeration is recommended as a standard procedure for immersion anesthesia.

thin, permeable membrane in close proximity to a capillary. This makes administration of drugs by immersion, via gill uptake, unique and useful in fish species. The proximity of the gill capillary results in rapid uptake of drugs with similarities to both inhalation and intravenous injection in other species (i.e., very close to a central compartment). The vast majority of fish are sedated or anesthetized by drug absorption across the gills using an immersion route of administration (**Figure 17.3**). Alternatively, anesthetic drugs can be administered parenterally, that is, intravenously (IV) or intramuscularly (IM), or orally. Physical restraint is always required for IV injections and usually required for IM injections. Intramuscular injections may be administered via handheld syringe caudal to a pectoral or pelvic fin (especially in koi to avoid any potential marring of the dorsal color pattern) or caudal to the dorsal fin where scales are often less developed and there is interstitial space where muscle bundles come together that can accommodate the injection volume (**Figures 17.4** and **17.5**). Intramuscular injections may also be administered by handheld syringe or

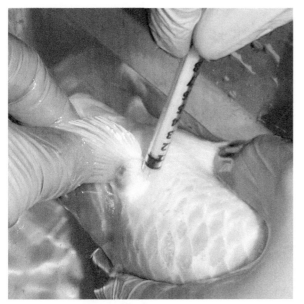

Figure 17.4 Intramuscular (IM) injection site in the pectoral muscle behind the pectoral fin of a koi (*C. carpio*). This ventral location is preferred for IM injections in order to prevent marring the dorsal color pattern in case of an injection site complication.

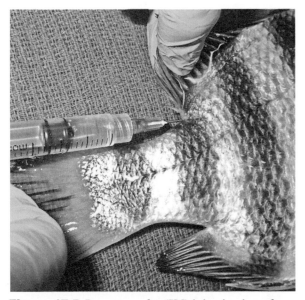

Figure 17.5 Intramuscular (IM) injection into the dorsal musculature of a fish, immediately caudal to the dorsal fin. In many teleost species, this location has minimal scales making needle insertion easier, and leakage of injected drug out of muscle bundles may be retained within the midline interstitial space between muscle bundles rather than leaking out of the fish.

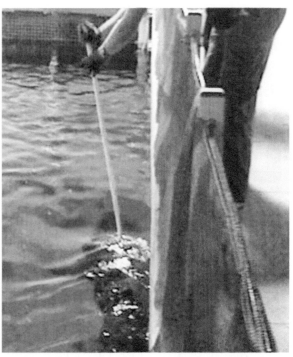

Figure 17.6 Pole syringe intramuscular (IM) injection into the dorsal musculature of a sand tiger shark (*Carcharias taurus*). Pole syringes allow injections into unrestrained large fish.

pole syringe (for unrestrained fish) directly into the epaxial muscle bellies in the dorsal half of larger fish (**Figure 17.6**). Epaxial muscles provide a large target area, but injections in this area are more likely to have leakage through the needle track than when administered behind a fin. If IM injections are administered forcefully, as with a "jab stick" pole syringe, local muscle damage may ensue (**Figure 17.7**). Interestingly, some drugs (e.g., alfaxalone) that are effective by immersion or IV administration in fish are not reliably effective when administered IM.[3,4] Oral administration of sedative and anesthetic drugs is less commonly used in fish, because precise dosing is difficult and there is uncertainty regarding rate and degree of absorption.

Duration of anesthesia

Fish are commonly anesthetized for brief procedures for which induction doses of anesthetic drugs are usually sufficient. However, some fish require prolonged anesthetic times in order to facilitate the procedures needed (e.g., extended surgery or imaging). In those

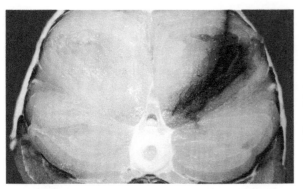

Figure 17.7 Hemorrhage and dorsal muscle damage from high-pressure "jab stick" pole syringe injection of dexamethasone sodium phosphate into a sand tiger shark (*C. taurus*). Although injections by this method may be the only option for getting drugs into the patient, resulting tissue damage may suggest that the technique should not be used repeatedly for a sustained period.

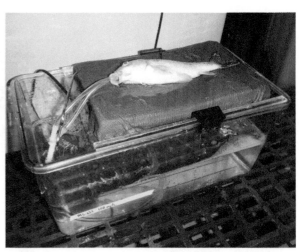

Figure 17.8 Recirculating anesthesia machine with a koi resting on moistened platform while anesthesia water is pumped across the gills before draining back into the reservoir tank. The reservoir tank in this image is a plastic rodent cage, and the recirculating pump is in the left corner of the reservoir tank.

cases, consideration must be taken for the concentration of anesthetic drug used and the ability to provide well-oxygenated water to the gills for gas exchange. For fish that need to be removed from water, care should be taken to provide a continuous flow of anesthetic water over the gills and keep the skin moist to prevent disruption of the slime coat. This can be accomplished by the use of a recirculating anesthetic system utilizing a pump, flexible plastic tubing, clamps, an open cell foam platform cut to fit the patient, and a support fitted to an aquarium or plastic container of suitable size to serve as a reservoir (**Figure 17.8**).[5] One places the fish on the water-soaked foam platform and pumps water containing anesthesia over the gills; the water then percolates through the foam and trickles back into the reservoir tank for recirculation (**Figure 17.9**). The trickling helps to maintain aeration of the water, but this can be further supplemented using a diffuser stone (i.e., air stone) in the reservoir water. Either air or oxygen can be pumped through the diffuser stone. A recirculating system of varying complexity, portability and cost can be designed to fit the needs of the clinicians and the fish to be anesthetized.

Monitoring anesthesia

As with most other animals that are anesthetized, it is important to monitor fish for both anesthetic depth as well as physiologic stability. Opercular rate can be

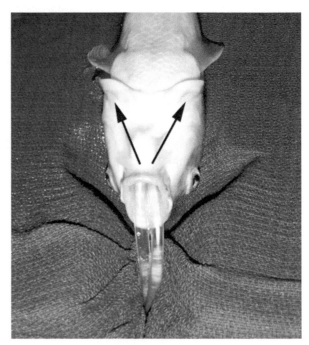

Figure 17.9 Dual flow of anesthetic water into the oral cavity of a koi (*C. carpio*) showing direction of water flow (arrows) over the gills and exiting the branchial cavity.

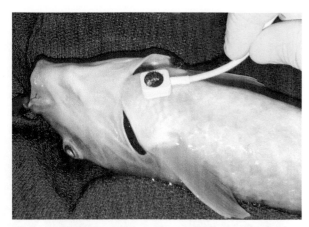

Figure 17.10 Doppler probe positioned over the heart of a koi (*C. carpio*) to detect blood flow, confirm cardiac activity and measure heart rate. Temporarily suspending water flow over the gills may be necessary to detect blood flow using a Doppler probe.

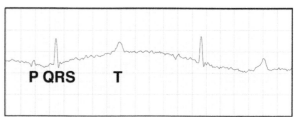

Figure 17.11 Modified lead I ECG recording from an anesthetized weakfish (*Cynoscion regalis*) in dorsal recumbency using broad clip-on leads attached to the pelvic fins, left pectoral fin and opercular isthmus. Recording shows normal sinus rhythm with a heart rate of 30/min. Recording speed is 50 mm/s, gain is 40 mm/mV, small squares = 1 mm, large squares = 5 mm, interbeat interval = 2 sec (100 mm).

assessed visually and is inversely related to anesthetic depth (i.e., the slower the opercular rate the deeper the plane of anesthesia). Heart rate can be monitored by Doppler with the probe being placed directly over the heart, although water flow over the gills may have to be paused briefly to avoid interference (**Figure 17.10**). Jaw tone and response to stimuli, particularly surgical stimuli, can also be monitored. In larger fish, blood samples can be obtained to assess oxygen (pO$_2$) and carbon dioxide (pCO$_2$) tensions, pH, and lactate levels. Although it is possible in some species to sample blood from the sinus venosus (i.e., pure venous blood) through the opercular membrane or intra-oral dorsal aorta (i.e., pure arterial blood), mixed venous and arterial blood is commonly obtained from the caudal hemal arch of the tail region. However, interpretation of results of mixed venous blood can still be useful for physiological monitoring, as pO$_2$ is the only blood gas value that varies markedly between venous and arterial samples to any extent clinically significant. Furthermore, the pO2 from mixed venous blood is useful as a broad indication of oxygenation status.

Whereas blood pressure and ECG monitoring are routinely measured in mammals, they are rarely measured in a clinical setting in fish. Blood pressure can be determined by cannulating the dorsal aorta, and ECG tracings can be acquired by attaching leads to needles or wire probes inserted into lateral muscles to measure electrical vectors generated by cardiac cells.

Although the two-chambered heart of fish is quite different from mammals, the acquired ECG tracing is remarkably similar with respect to generation of a characteristic sinus rhythm (**Figure 17.11**).[6,7] Electrocardiographic tracings can be acquired using standard ECG machines, but caution must be exercised with electrical equipment and water. Anesthetized fish that are removed from water for procedures are good candidates for ECG acquisition. Electrocardiograms can be generated from electrodes in or on the skin that record the electrical activity of the heart. The waveforms are a summation of the vectors of those electrical changes (depolarization and repolarization and the direction). In mammals, there are standardized placements for the electrodes and body position to produce consistent waveforms that can be further analyzed. While there are no reported standards for the placement in fish, it is logical to place the leads in a triangular or box pattern around the heart. Thus, the "arm" leads (i.e., black and white leads in the American color-coding system; or red and yellow leads in the European color-coding system) of an ECG machine can be attached either directly with alligator clips or attached to needles placed near each pectoral fin and the "leg" lead (i.e., red and green leads in the American system; or green and black leads in the European system) placed near the caudal end of the fish (**Figures 17.12** and **17.13**). The sensitivity of the equipment, the shape and attachment of the leads, and the size and shape of the fish can affect the quality of ECG acquisition.

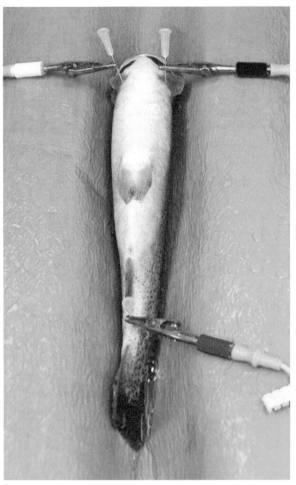

Figure 17.12 Placement of ECG needle electrodes (American color system) in a rainbow trout (*O. mykiss*).

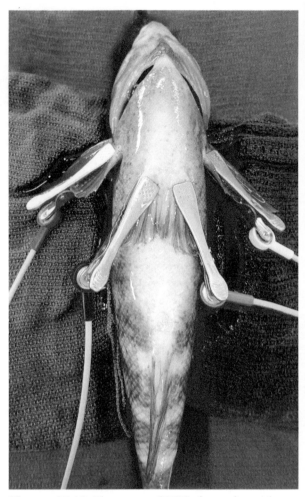

Figure 17.13 Placement of ECG clamp electrodes (European color system) in tautog (*Tautoga onitis*).

Depth and stages of anesthesia

Anesthetized fish undergo behavioral and physiologic changes associated with increasing depth similar to other animals (**Table 17.1**).[8] A surgical plane of anesthesia should occur in stage III anesthesia. Remember that not all anesthetic compounds discussed in this chapter produce surgical planes of anesthesia.

Induction and maintenance of anesthesia

Induction of anesthesia with immersion agents is generally accomplished by placing an individual fish into a container containing anesthetic agent (**Figures 17.14** through **17.17**). Even with pH balancing, fish often react to being placed into water

with a novel chemical. Fish should be left unstimulated in the container, but observed for any adverse reactions (e.g., termination of opercular activity) or attempt to escape the container. Fish are considered in stage I of anesthesia when they voluntarily react to the effects of the agent (analogous to feeling the effects of alcohol), which may appear anxious or uncoordinated. Stage II includes involuntary excitement where fish are generally active but uncoordinated. Stage III is generally considered true anesthesia where the fish should have little or no response to stimuli. Heart rate and opercular rate of the fish should decrease. At the deepest planes of stage III, fish should be nonresponsive to invasive procedures or surgery. Stage IV follows and is characterized as the beginning of medullary death. Fish

Table 17.1 Stages of anesthesia in fish

STAGE	PLANE	LEVEL OF ANESTHESIA	GENERAL DEMEANOR	ACTIVITY	EQUILIBRIUM	GILL VENTILATION RATE	REACTIVITY	HEART RATE	MUSCLE TONE	EXAMPLES OF PROCEDURES
0		None	Normal	Normal	Normal	Normal	Normal	Normal	Normal	
I		Voluntary excitement	Normal to agitated	Normal to increased	Normal	Normal to increased	Normal to increased	Normal	Normal	
II		Involuntary excitation	Agitated	Increased	Altered	Increased	Increased	Increased	Normal	
III	1	Deep sedation	Poorly responsive	Little	Grossly affected	Decreased	Decreased response to stimuli	Normal to decreased	Decreased	Physical inspection; weighing
	2	Light anesthesia	Lack of response	None	Absent	Decreased	Responds only to painful stimuli	Decreased	Decreased	External tags (skin, fin and opercular); gill, skin and fin biopsies; blood draws
	3	Surgical	Anesthetized	None	Absent	Shallow to none	None	Decreased	Decreased	Internal tags (intracoelomic); surgery
IV		Medullary collapse	Overanesthetized	None	Absent	None	None	Decreased to irregular	Lost	Near death

Source: Modified from Sneddon, L.U., *Journal of Exotic Pet Medicine* 2012;21(1):32–43.

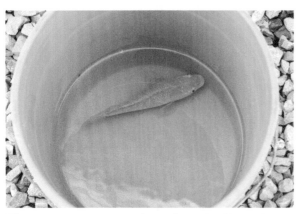

Figure 17.14 Stage 0 of anesthesia in tilapia (*Oreochromis* sp.). Fish should present normal equilibrium and normal ventilation rate.

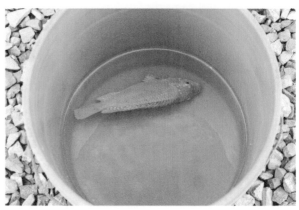

Figure 17.15 Stage II of anesthesia in tilapia. Fish commonly exhibit excitement, an increased ventilation rate, and an altered equilibrium where the fish continues to try to right itself.

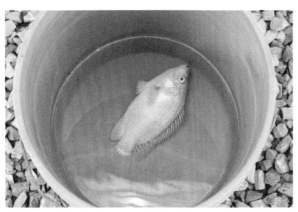

Figure 17.16 Stage III (plane 1) of anesthesia in tilapia. Fish commonly display very little response to stimuli, a decreased ventilation rate and severely affected equilibrium where the fish no longer tries to right itself.

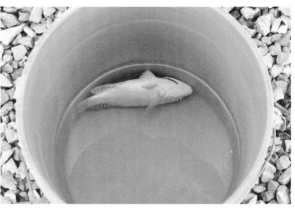

Figure 17.17 Stage III (plane 3) of anesthesia in tilapia. Fish commonly demonstrate no response to stimuli, an extremely reduced ventilation rate and a complete lack of equilibrium.

in stage IV are very deeply anesthetized and close to dying.

Following induction of anesthesia, the clinician will need to determine whether the procedure can be accomplished quickly and the fish placed in water without anesthetic for recovery, or if the fish needs to be maintained under anesthesia for longer duration. Anesthesia can be maintained by removing the fish from the induction chamber, and running anesthetic containing water over the gills to both keep the fish asleep, as well as provide a changing interface for oxygen and carbon dioxide exchange. Maintenance of anesthesia this way is easily accomplished by way of a recirculating water pump that delivers the water through the mouth over the gills and then collects the water for redistribution. Fish may be kept anesthetized this way for minutes to hours (**Figure 17.8**). Concentration of anesthetic required during the maintenance phase is generally less than the induction doses (25%–60%), but will need to be adjusted based on the needs of each individual fish, the duration of anesthesia, and procedure being performed. By monitoring the depth of anesthesia, fish can be maintained successfully on recirculating anesthesia systems for procedures lasting over 3 hr.

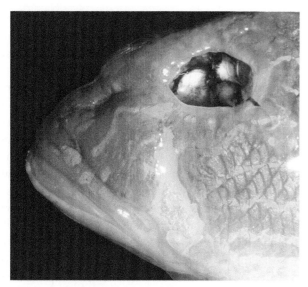

Figure 17.18 Sand perch (*Diplecrum formosum*) that was anesthetized for a minor procedure and returned to its multispecies tank before fully recovered, resulting in bilateral exenteration by aggressive tank mates taking advantage of the fish's compromised state.

Recovery

Recovery from anesthesia should occur when the fish is removed from exposure to the chemical agent in the water, or given time to metabolize parenterally administered drugs. Time to recovery is based on the agent, concentrations and duration of exposure. Most immersion agents are cleared from the body via the gills, so active gilling or assisted exposure to anesthesia-free water is required. Fish that are not operculating autonomously will have delayed recoveries from immersion agents. Fish are considered recovered from anesthesia when they can right themselves, maintain buoyancy, have normal opercular rates and can swim normally. It is essential to ensure complete recovery prior to returning a fish to water with aggressive tank mates (**Figure 17.18**).

ANESTHETIC AGENTS

Tricaine methanesulfonate (MS-222, TMS, Tricaine-S®, Fiquel®)
Chemistry

Tricaine (3-aminobenzoic acid ethyl ester methanesulfonate) is a white crystalline power that has a water solubility of 1.25 g/mL at 20°C. Depending on the buffering capacity of the water, the addition of tricaine to water at clinically relevant doses likely will cause the water to become acidic. At 100 mg/L, the pH of a poorly buffered solution can be a pH of 5 or lower. Therefore, most solutions should be buffered with sodium bicarbonate. Short of monitoring the anesthetic water with a pH meter, sodium bicarbonate at a 1:1 ratio by weight with tricaine provides a reasonably close approximation to the original pH, or at least moderates the reduction without overcompensating to a more basic solution.[9] Although saltwater is sometimes presumed to have adequate buffering capacity to moderate pH shifts caused by tricaine, this is not necessarily the case, at least with some artificial seawater mixes, and buffering tricaine with sodium bicarbonate is recommended for seawater as well as freshwater.[9] A stock solution of tricaine may be prepared at a concentration of 10 g/L, which allows easy calculation for working in 100 mg/L dilutions. Stock solutions should be stored in an airtight, darkened container at room temperature. Old stock solutions or those exposed to light will turn brown in color and lose potency. Duration of potency is poorly defined, with reports of efficacy lasting 1–3 months if protected from light and stored in a cool location, but if in doubt, starting with a fresh stock solution is recommended.[10]

Mechanism of action

Tricaine is a water-soluble chemical in the local anesthetic family. Local anesthetics function by blocking conduction of sodium channels in neurons, which prevents transmission of ascending neural information. However, the mechanism of central action of tricaine as a general anesthetic is unknown, and it is reasonable to consider whether the lack of movement seen in fish anesthetized with tricaine is at least partially associated with blocked conduction of muscle as opposed to true central nervous system (CNS) depression. While there is evidence that tricaine administered by immersion does decrease peripheral neural conduction in the oyster toadfish, *Opsanus tau*, there is also evidence that local anesthetics like tricaine likely have CNS effects.[11,12] Lidocaine, a structurally related drug, is an analgesic and functions as a CNS depressant when given centrally in humans and domestic mammals.[13–15] Furthermore, higher concentrations of tricaine in the blood and CNS tissue is associated with deeper anesthesia in snapper, *Pagrus auratus*, indicating that its use as a general anesthetic in fish likely has merit.[12]

Anesthetic effects

Tricaine is rapidly absorbed via diffusion across the gill tissue and provides a fairly rapid induction and recovery. The early stages of anesthesia can show some excitatory effects as fish pass through stage II anesthesia before becoming immobile. Once the fish is immobile, tricaine can completely abolish further muscle movement. Tricaine causes physiologic changes in fish, including increased cortisol, glucose, hematocrit and lactate concentrations.[16] In salmon anesthetized with 100 mg/L of tricaine, cardiovascular changes include a steady decrease in blood pressure (i.e., dorsal aortic), but with minimal changes to cardiac output.[17]

The half-life of tricaine in teleost fish is estimated to be 1.4–4.0 hr.[18] The majority of tricaine is eliminated unchanged by excretion via gills, although a minor portion of tricaine and its polar metabolites are excreted via the kidney.[10,18] Repeated exposure of different fish species to tricaine produces differing anesthetic requirements. Tilapia exposed weekly to tricaine at 200 mg/L were anesthetized more quickly following repeated exposure, whereas daily exposure to tricaine anesthesia in goldfish resulted in increased anesthetic requirements to achieve an equivalent plane of anesthesia.[19,20] The cause of the increased anesthetic requirement in goldfish remains unknown, but was not associated with any gill pathology.[21] Historically, the use of old stock solutions have been blamed for increasing drug needs with repeated exposure. While this may be a factor, goldfish do indeed appear to require increased concentrations of freshly prepared tricaine with repeated anesthetic events.

Tricaine is likely the most commonly used agent for the anesthesia of fish in the United States. It is the only anesthetic approved by the United States Food and Drug Administration (FDA) for cold-blooded aquatic animals and for fish intended as food.[22] The FDA requires a 21-day withdrawal period for fish used for food or released into the wild.[22] Despite suggestions that tricaine could be carcinogenic, mutagenic or teratogenic, references cited to support the suggestion do not in fact provide primary evidence for the claim nor does the material safety data sheet (MSDS).[16,23–25] In addition, the FDA "is not aware of any peer reviewed reference that documents that MS-222 is a known carcinogen/teratogen" (FDA Center for Veterinary Medicine Compliance, personal communication). The powder, however, is a respiratory and mucous membrane irritant, so mixing stock solutions under adequate ventilation control to minimize exposure to airborne powder is recommended. A single report of chronic occupational exposure to tricaine has been associated with reversible retinal toxicity in an ichthyologist presumably by interference with normal rhodopsin regeneration.[26] However, daily exposure of koi carp to tricaine for 2 weeks did not result in any electroretinography (ERG) changes.[27] This indicates that clinical exposure of tricaine to aquatic patients is unlikely to produce adverse visual effects in fish but does not suggest that people should be cavalier with their own exposure.

Dose

The dose of tricaine varies widely based on species, size and age of the fish, as well as type of water (marine vs. freshwater, soft vs. hard). Additionally, the dose will be dependent on the depth of CNS depression required and speed desired for induction of anesthesia. In general, lower doses should be used with physiologically compromised or diseased fish.

- Tricaine sedation dose: 20–50 mg/L
- Tricaine anesthesia dose: 50–150 mg/L
- Tricaine long-term anesthesia via recirculating system: ~2/3 of induction dose, adjusted as required to maintain anesthetic depth

Eugenol (clove oil; eugenol, AQUI-SE® [2-methoxy-4-(2-propenyl) phenol], isoeugenol, AQUI-S® [2-methoxy-4 propenylphenol])

Chemistry

Eugenol is the primary active ingredient in clove oil, which is distilled from various parts of the clove tree, *Syzygium aromaticum*, also known as *Eugenia aromatica*. Eugenol is a pale yellow liquid that is poorly water soluble and must be dissolved in ethanol (1:9) before dilution into water. AQUI-SE® and AQUI-S® are proprietary formulations of eugenol and isoeugenol, respectively, which are sufficiently soluble to allow direct addition to induction water. Clove oil and eugenol are classified by the FDA as GRAS (i.e., "generally regarded as safe") for human use, but their use for sedation and anesthesia of food fishes is prohibited by the FDA in the United States (http://www.fda.gov/downloads/AnimalVeterinary/GuidanceComplianceEnforcement/Guidancefor Industry/ucm052520.pdf).

Clove oil

Clove oil is a natural analgesic and antiseptic that historically has been used to treat dental pain. Eugenol is the main ingredient of clove oil, but since it is primarily sold over the counter in pharmacies and health food stores, the concentration of eugenol can vary greatly (60%–90%).[28] Although eugenol has been shown to produce immobility in fish, the variation in concentration of active drug in clove oil makes sedation and anesthesia less predictable from a clinical standpoint.

Isoeugenol and eugenol

Isoeugenol is chemically similar to eugenol, but it is not present in clove oil. Specific gravity of eugenol and isoeugenol are 1.06 and 1.08, respectively, so for practical purposes of calculating doses, 1 mL of a pure product can be taken to be 1 g. Effects of these products marketed for fish are likely to be more predictable than the mixture of chemicals in clove oil. AQUI-S is a 50% isoeugenol solution that is approved for sedation and anesthesia in finfish, crustacea and abalone in Australia, New Zealand, Chile and Korea.[29] In those countries it has no withdrawal time for fish destined for human consumption or release to the wild. Attempts to gain approval of AQUI-S in the United States were discontinued following studies indicating carcinogenicity in male laboratory mice and efforts shifted to AQUI-SE.[30] Since 2015, AQUI-SE (50%, or 500 mg/mL eugenol solution) and AQUI-S 20E (10%, or 100 mg/mL eugenol solution) can be used in the United States under an FDA INAD (Investigational New Animal Drug) exemption for research purposes. Under this INAD exemption, AQUI-SE and AQUI-S 20E can be used in 10–100 mg/L solutions for up to 15 min in duration as a single treatment. As of September 2016 under an expanded INAD, freshwater and marine finfish administered AQUI-S 20E at 10–100 mg/L, for field-based fishery management activities, may be released immediately. Following use in hatcheries, freshwater and marine fish have a 72 hr withdrawal period; however, fish that are illegal for harvest may be released immediately.

Mechanism of action

The mechanism of action of eugenol as an analgesic is likely due to blocking voltage gated Na^+ channels (as in local anesthetics) and possibly through interaction with transient receptor potential channels. These receptors are also known as vanilloid or capsaicin binding site receptors and have been shown to attenuate ascending pain pathways, particularly c-fiber neurons. Similar to tricaine, the mechanism of central action of eugenol as a general anesthetic is unknown.

Anesthetic effects

Eugenol produces immobility in fish, but recovery time is dose and time related.[28] Compared with tricaine, eugenol (e.g., red pacu dosed at 50, 100 and 200 mg/L) produces faster induction of anesthesia but slower recovery and the fish remained more reactive to noxious stimuli.[31] Physiologic effects of anesthetic doses of eugenol (e.g., Chinook salmon dosed at 60 mg/L) decreased cardiac output by decreasing heart rate, cardiac output, and dorsal aortic pressure, while also decreasing PaO_2 by 75%.[17] Metabolic effects following eugenol anesthesia have shown mixed responses; in salmon there were increased catecholamines, glucose and hematocrit values, whereas catfish did not show any rise in cortisol.[16,17,31,32] As a sedative, isoeugenol is reported to have a good safety margin, but compared with tricaine anesthesia, eugenol (e.g., red pacu) had a smaller therapeutic index (therapeutic dose/lethal dose).[28,31] The combination of hypoxemia, decreased cardiac output, plus increased sympathetic demand may result in adverse physiological derangements.

Dose

Accurate dosing for clove oil is difficult, as the percentage of eugenol (active ingredient) varies as does the requirements for various species. Concentrations of active ingredients in AQUI-S and AQUI-SE are known, so their effects on various species can be more accurately assessed.

- Reported doses of clove oil range from 2–120 mg/L[28]
- Clove oil sedation dose for transportation: 2–5 mg/L
- Clove oil anesthesia dose: 20–60 mg/L

Dosing for AQUI-S 20E and AQUI-S (based on percentage of active ingredient)

- AQUI-S 20E and AQUI-S sedation dose: 15–20 mg/L
- AQUI-S 20E and AQUI-S anesthesia dose: 20–60 mg/L

Metomidate (metomidate hydrochloride, Aquacalm™)

Chemistry

Metomidate is an imidazole anesthetic and is marketed as Aquacalm™ (metomidate hydrochloride) for immersion use in ornamental finfish only. It is not sold for use in fish intended for human or animal consumption. It is supplied as a white powder consisting solely of metomidate hydrochloride. It is not formally approved for fish by the FDA, but is legally marketed as an FDA indexed product under MIF 900–002. Therefore, the product is available in the United States for use in minor species but has not undergone the extensive review process necessary for an approved animal drug.

Mechanism of action

Imidazole anesthetics work by enhancing the effects of gamma amino butyric acid (GABA), a primary inhibitory neurotransmitter, on the GABA receptor. GABA agonists work by binding to GABA receptors, increasing chloride conduction, which hyperpolarizes the nerve and decreases neural conduction. Both GABA and GABA receptors are present in fish species.[33] Imidazole anesthetics (e.g., etomidate) are commonly used in mammalian anesthesia and also produce anesthesia in fish species. Imidazole anesthetics generally are poor muscle relaxants and provide no analgesia.[34]

Anesthetic effects

Imidazoles anesthetics are often incorrectly referred to as "stress-free" anesthetics because following administrations, patients do not experience an increase in plasma cortisol concentration. The lack of increased cortisol is due to reversible inhibition of the enzyme 11β hydroxylase in the pathway for the production of cortisol from cholesterol. Salmon anesthetized with metomidate did not show a rise in cortisol, but did have a clinically relevant lactate increase, which implies that the lack of increased plasma cortisol is not due to lack of stress.[35] Therefore, users of metomidate should be cautious regarding interpreting interrenal parameters, and should be cautioned not to rely on cortisol values to help determine stress response in fish. Additionally, short-circuiting the normal homeostatic interrenal stress response could even be detrimental in some circumstances.

Imidazole anesthetics generally have a wide safety margin in fish and produce a rapid induction with a more prolonged recovery. Metomidate has been shown to be effective in many fish species but was ineffective with increased mortality in larval goldfish.[36–39] One of the authors (LPP) has also noted that goldfish require higher than recommended doses and often do not achieve a surgical plane of anesthesia (unpublished observation). Induction and recovery times for metomidate are dose dependent, with high doses (16 mg/L) resulting in mortality in catfish.[38] Metomidate at anesthetic concentrations in salmon produced minimal changes to heart rate or cardiac output.[17] This is similar to the lack of cardiovascular changes seen with other imidazole anesthetics in mammalian species where there is no change in cardiac contractility.[8]

Fish and other aquatic species (e.g., frogs) exposed to metomidate can have darkened skin coloration after exposure. Since cortisol inhibits the release of ACTH, and ACTH stimulates melanocyte stimulating hormone (MSH), it has been hypothesized that the decrease in cortisol production that occurs with the use of these drugs results in an increase in MSH.[40] Normal color returns after recovery from the anesthetic. Metomidate has been successfully used as an immersion agent in fish, and has also been successfully used intravenously and orally to anesthetize turbot and halibut.[41] However, the manufacturer of metomidate advises caution with (1) larval fish species, which may be more sensitive to sedation than

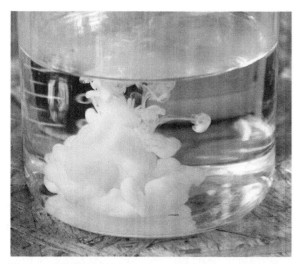

Figure 17.19 Addition of propofol to water in preparation for sedating a fish. Note that the propofol will normally turn the water cloudy as opposed to MS-222 that does not change the clarity of the water.

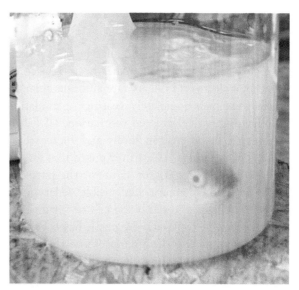

Figure 17.20 Initial placement of fish in propofol anesthetic water. Note that the propofol may make observing the various stages of anesthesia difficult.

older fish of the same species; (2) fish species such as knifefish and gouramis; and (3) any fish species for extended periods (e.g., >24 hr) during transportation.

Dose

- Metomidate sedation dose: 0.1–1.0 mg/L
- Metomidate anesthesia dose: 1.0–10.0 mg/L
- Metomidate anesthesia IV dose: 3.0 mg/kg IV[41]
- Metomidate anesthesia oral dose: 7.0 mg/kg oral[41]

Propofol (Diprivan®)
Chemistry
Propofol is an alkyl-phenol compound commercially available as an emulsion. Various formulations are available with varying types and concentrations of preservative (e.g., benzyl alcohol, EDTA), though most fish immersion studies have primarily been performed with formulations containing EDTA.[42,43] The pH of propofol is 7.5–8.5, so additional buffering of the water is not necessary when used as an immersion agent. It should be noted that propofol turns the anesthetic water a cloudy white color unlike the other immersion anesthetics, which do not change the clarity of the water (**Figures 17.19 through 17.21**).

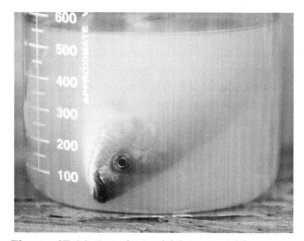

Figure 17.21 Anesthetized fish in propofol anesthetic water.

Mechanism of action
Propofol produces anesthesia by enhancing the effects of GABA, similar to the mechanism of action for metomidate.[33] Propofol is used extensively as a sedative and anesthetic in human and veterinary medicine where it provides good muscle relaxation but no analgesia. In mammals, propofol must be administered intravenously to produce sedation or anesthesia. While IV administration is effective in fish species, propofol is absorbed quickly via immersion presumably across the gills.[42–45]

Anesthetic effects

Propofol by immersion produces dose- and duration-dependent sedation and anesthesia in goldfish, koi carp and catfish.[42,43,46] Anesthesia is accompanied by a decrease in heart rate and opercular rate, with some fish completely ceasing operculation.[43] Coinciding with decreased ventilation, all fish had decreased blood oxygen levels and increased lactate concentrations.[43] Catfish exposed to a low dose of propofol (0.4 mg/L) for 12 hr for the purpose of transportation demonstrated visible sedation with minimal changes to red blood cell or serum chemistry values.[47] Propofol at 3.0 mg/L has been evaluated for use during 20 minutes of anesthesia in koi carp via a recirculating system. Although the propofol was successful in keeping the fish asleep, 1 of 9 fish had a prolonged recovery and 1 of 9 fish died.[43] Anecdotal reports to one of the authors (LPP) has indicated that some clinicians switch to anesthetic-free water while on the recirculating system, which has prevented complications and long recoveries. In sturgeon, *Acipenser oxyrinchus*, given IV propofol produced light anesthesia accompanied with respiratory depression and bradycardia.[44] However, in bamboo sharks, *Chylloscyllium plagiosum*, anesthetic effects were more pronounced and lasted over 1 hr in most animals.[45]

Dose

- Propofol anesthesia dose: 5.0 mg/L[43]
- Propofol sedation dose: 0.4 mg/L[47]
- Propofol long-term immersion anesthesia via recirculating system: $\sim 1/2$ of induction dose, adjusted as required to maintain anesthetic depth
- Propofol anesthesia IV dose: 2.5–7.5 mg/kg IV[44,45]

Alfaxalone (Alfaxan®)
Chemistry

Alfaxalone is a neurosteroid anesthetic. It is available in the veterinary preparation Alfaxan®, which is licensed for intravenous use in dogs and cats in the United States. Alfaxalone has limited water solubility, but in the Alfaxan formulation, alfaxalone is encased in a cyclodextrin shell that is water soluble.

After administration, the cyclodextrin is metabolized releasing the active agent. The pH of alfaxalone is 6.5–7.0, so buffering of water is not necessary for immersion administration.

Mechanism of action

Alfaxalone produces anesthesia by enhancing the effects of GABA, similar to the mechanism of action of metomidate.[33]

Anesthetic effects

Alfaxalone by immersion produces dose- and duration-dependent sedation and anesthesia in koi carp and goldfish.[4,48] Anesthesia was accompanied by a decrease in heart rate and opercular rate with higher doses stopping operculation.[4] Coincident with the decrease in heart rate and operculation, blood oxygen partial pressure decreased and lactate levels increased.[4]

Alfaxalone administered to koi carp by intramuscular (IM) route produced highly variable results, with 33% of the fish never becoming anesthetized, 33% having prolonged effects (>10 hr) and 33% dying.[3] Although IM administration is documented only in koi carp, such administration in other fish species should be considered with caution.

Dose

- Alfaxalone sedation dose: 2.5–7.0 mg/L
- Alfaxalone anesthesia dose: 10.0 mg/L
- Alfaxalone long-term immersion anesthesia via recirculating system: $\sim 1/4$ of induction dose, adjusted as required to maintain anesthetic depth

2-Phenoxyethanol (2-PE)
Chemistry

Phenoxyethanol is a clear, oily, organic compound that is fairly water soluble. It has been used as a topical anesthetic in humans and is considered bacteriocidal and fungicidal.[25,49] It has also been used as a tissue fixative, as it preserves many cell biochemical properties.[49] Although phenoxyethanol is used in dermatological and cosmetic products, the compound has been reported as an allergen and topical irritant.[28,50,51]

Mechanism of action

The mechanism of action of phenoxyethanol as a general anesthetic in fish is unknown. Its use as a topical anesthetic implies that it might interrupt neural transmission via blocking Na^+ channels, similar to tricaine or lidocaine.

Anesthetic action

Phenoxyethanol produces sedation and immobility in many fish species.[36,52–54] Induction and recovery from anesthesia are generally considered rapid, but some authors report difficulty reaching stages of complete surgical anesthesia.[28,53] Increased water temperature requires higher dosing of the drug.[28,52] In trout, phenoxyethanol produces dose-dependent heart rate depression as well as a decrease in dorsal aortic pressure.[54]

Dose

- 2-Phenoxyethanol anesthesia dose: 0.2–0.5 mL/L

Carbon dioxide (CO_2)

Carbon dioxide has a long history of use for sedation and anesthesia of fish. It is inexpensive, readily available, safe for humans with proper ventilation and leaves no tissue residues of regulatory concern when used in food fish. Acidification of water and patient, adverse physiologic effects, and difficulty regulating and monitoring concentrations make CO_2 a less desirable agent in most cases.

Chemistry

Carbon dioxide (CO_2) is an odorless, colorless gas that is soluble in water. High levels of CO_2 produce a dose-dependent CNS depression, ranging from somnolence to complete anesthesia in fish and mammals.[55] Carbon dioxide is a normal by-product of aerobic metabolism of all animals and is generally easy to remove from the body as it diffuses 15 times faster than oxygen. Based on the carbonic acid equation, increased plasma concentrations of CO_2 result in an acidemia that has physiologic consequences such as cerebral vasodilation, cell receptor deactivation and changes to coagulation in mammals. The physiological effects of acidemia have not been well investigated in fish.

Mechanism of action

The CNS depression associated with high CO_2 levels are associated with H^+ levels in the CNS, although the mechanism by which those protons produce sedation is unknown.

Anesthetic effects

Carbon dioxide produces sedation and anesthesia in a variety of fish species.[56–58] In general, anesthetic induction (~12 min) and recovery times (~22 min) are longer compared with other anesthetic agents, and some fish will show distress likely associated with either the low pH or low oxygen content of the water.[28,56] Although sedative doses are generally considered safe (i.e., no mortality), anesthetic doses (>150 mm Hg) have been associated with increased mortality in koi carp.[56] Therefore, it is not surprising then that CO_2 is used in the aquaculture industry as a sedative for transportation and non-surgical procedures, but not for prolonged surgical procedures.[28]

High concentrations of CO_2 (150–200 mm Hg) are required to produce anesthesia. At these doses, there is concern for lowered pH of the water and the reduced amount of O_2 available for the fish (O_2 will be displaced by the high concentration of CO_2). Buffering the water with sodium bicarbonate decreases the excitability reaction in trout to water with CO_2.[28] Supplemental oxygen is also recommended.[56]

Dose

Carbon dioxide can be administered directly by bubbling CO_2 gas into water through a diffuser stone, placing a block of dry ice in the water, or can be generated by administration of sodium bicarbonate in the water. Use of a diffuser stone is preferred for efficient delivery. The generation of CO_2 following bicarbonate administration in water is fairly slow and hard to estimate, but is increased in acidic water. Carbon dioxide has been generated by the addition of Alka-Seltzer® Original tablets to water, but actual CO_2 concentrations in those situations are difficult to estimate and the product also contains aspirin and citric acid, so is not recommended. Carbon dioxide has also been used as an adjunct for anesthesia and euthanasia by providing sedation before an alternative method/drug is administered (see later section on euthanasia). Accurate dosing requires specific monitoring equipment, but it is more commonly dosed to effect.

- CO_2 sedation dose: 50–125 mmHg
- CO_2 anesthesia dose: 150–200 mmHg
- $NaHCO_3$ anesthesia dose: 200–600 mg/L

Benzocaine (ethyl aminobenzoate, Anesthesin®, Anesthone®, Orthesin®, Parathesin®, Benzoak®)

Chemistry

Benzocaine is commonly used as a local anesthetic in humans (e.g., cough drops, sunburn aid). Benzocaine occurs in two forms: a crystalline salt (benzocaine HCl) that is soluble in water at 0.4 g/L and a non-water-soluble basic form that must be dissolved in ethyl alcohol before it is sufficiently soluble in water. Benzocaine is often prepared as a stock solution of 100 g/L and should be stored in a dark container protected from light. Clinically relevant solutions are acidic and should be buffered with sodium bicarbonate to raise the pH to between 7.0 and 7.5. Chemically similar to tricaine, benzocaine has a long history of use in research settings as a more economical anesthetic alternative, but is less convenient and less easily accessible for use in clinical practice.

Mechanism of action

Benzocaine is a local anesthetic that blocks neuronal sodium channel conduction. As with tricaine, the mechanism of central action as a general anesthetic is unknown.

Anesthetic effects

Benzocaine produces sedation and anesthesia in a wide range of fish species. Likely due to similar mechanisms of action, induction and recovery times are similar to tricaine. Heart rate and opercular rate show dose-dependent depression.

Dose

- Benzocaine anesthetic dose: 25–200 mg/L

Ketamine (Ketaject®, Ketaset®, Vetalar®)

Chemistry

Ketamine is a white crystalline powder that is supplied in a water-soluble solution. The various formulations of ketamine are approved by the FDA for use in cats, non-human primates and humans. Commercially prepared ketamine is acidic with a pH of 3.5–5.5, which can sting at the site of intramuscular administration.

Mechanism of action

Ketamine is a N-methyl-D-aspartate (NMDA) receptor antagonist that produces dissociative anesthesia by blocking binding of the excitatory neurotransmitter glutamate and dissociating the thalamocortical and limbic systems. Additionally, NMDA antagonists interrupt pain transmission in the dorsal horn of the spinal cord, mediating somatic, visceral, neuropathic and orthopedic pain, often at subanesthetic doses.[59] Glutamate-binding NMDA receptors are present in fish species.[60]

Anesthetic effects

Ketamine has been evaluated both by IV and IM routes in multiple fish species. Intravenous injections produce more reliable effects, but have been associated with prolonged effects and ventilatory depression in trout and salmon.[61] Administration of ketamine is more commonly accomplished with an intramuscular injection, although the anesthetic effects are less reliable. As in mammals, IM ketamine is often used in combination with alpha-2 agonists to provide additional CNS depression and better muscle relaxation. The combination of ketamine and alpha-2 agonists (e.g., dexmedetomidine, medetomidine) has been effective for immobilization and deep sedation but not surgical anesthesia in varying fish species, such as sturgeon, bonitos, mackerel, and black sea bass. However, it was not effective in red porgy.[44,62,63] Behavioral effects such as excitement, loss of shoaling behavior and apparent incoordination can also be seen.[64]

Dose

- Ketamine anesthesia IV dose: 30 mg/kg IV
- Ketamine anesthesia IM dose: 20–80 mg/kg IM

Alpha-2 receptor agonists (xylazine, dexmedetomidine, medetomidine)

Chemistry

Alpha-2 agonists are lipophilic, crystalline substances that are water soluble. The pH of commercial preparations varies between 5.5 and 7.0.

Mechanism of action

Alpha-2 agonists bind and activate alpha-2 adrenergic receptors. Activation of the receptors causes a decrease in systemic norepinephrine, as well as a decrease in neural transmission, resulting in sedation and analgesia. At least five alpha-2 receptors have been identified in zebrafish.[65]

Anesthetic effects

Alpha-2 agonists have sedative effects in fish with zebrafish showing a dose-dependent decrease in locomotion following dexmedetomidine.[65] However, anesthetic doses of xylazine are associated with a complete cessation of operculation, seizure-like activity and death in trout.[66] Xylazine, medetomidine and dexmedetomidine have been used successfully as adjuncts with other sedatives/anesthetics such as ketamine to provide sedation and likely analgesia.

Alpha-2 antagonists (e.g., yohimbine, atipamezole) are effective reversal agents in fish species.[62,63] Atipamezole has been administered at 5 times the medetomidine dose and 10 times the dexmedetomidine dose.[62,63]

Dose

- Medetomidine anesthesia IM dose: 0.06–4.0 mg/kg IM (with ketamine 1–4 mg/kg)
- Dexmedetomidine anesthesia IM dose: 0.05–0.1 mg/kg IM (with ketamine 1–4 mg/kg)
- Dexmedetomidine (0.05–1.0 mg/kg) + midazolam (0.2 mg/kg) + ketamine 2–4 mg/kg IM (black sea bass and cobia), however similar dosing of dexmedetomidine, midazolam, and ketamine was not recommended for red porgy[63]

ANALGESIA

There is mounting evidence that fish have the neuroanatomic pathways and higher brain centers to perceive pain as well as a descending modulatory pathway to attenuate pain.[67] Readers are directed to an entire *ILAR Journal* issue (2009; volume 50, issue 4) where anatomy, physiology and behavioral responses are reviewed in relation to pain and distress in fish.[68] If one accepts that fish can perceive pain, then providing appropriate analgesia becomes obligatory. Even if one does not accept the evidence for pain perception in fish, physiologic and behavioral consequences of unrelieved nociception can compromise outcomes in both clinical and research settings.

Analgesia is defined as the moderation or blocking of the perception of pain without the loss of consciousness. Immersion anesthetics are unlikely to provide any post-anesthetic analgesia. In general there are five primary ways to attenuate the pain pathway in animal species: opioid agonists, alpha-2 agonists, local anesthetics, NMDA antagonists and NSAIDs. Opioid, alpha-2 and NMDA receptors are all present in fish. Local anesthetics block Na^+ channels in fish as they do in other animals, and fish have an inflammatory cascade that is blocked by NSAIDs. Although repeated doses of analgesics could extend the duration of effect following a surgical procedure, oral administration of analgesics and multiple-dose pharmacokinetics of NSAIDs have not been evaluated in fish, and the adverse consequences of multiple capture and restraint episodes for injections must be considered. Therefore, single doses of analgesics administered at the time of anesthesia are typically employed in fish medicine.

Opioids

Morphine

Morphine, a mu (μ) opioid agonist, is likely the most researched opioid for use in fish. It is analgesic in many fish species including trout, goldfish and koi carp.[20,69,70] Although the effective dosage appears similar between species, the pharmacokinetics of morphine in fish is species dependent. For example, morphine in flounder had a $T_{1/2}$ of ~34 hr, whereas trout had a $T_{1/2}$ of ~14 hr, which would make predicting dosing intervals difficult to extrapolate.[71] Morphine dose: 5–10 mg/kg IM.

Butorphanol

Butorphanol, a kappa opioid agonist, has been shown to be analgesic in koi carp, but at high doses

(10 mg/kg) produced problems with equilibrium where fish maintained a head down posture until the effects of the drug dissipated.[70,72] In a model that looked at anesthetic sparing effects, butorphanol only decreased anesthetic needs in goldfish at the lowest doses (0.1 mg/kg); but at higher doses increased anesthetic needs.[20] Butorphanol dose: 0.1–0.4 mg/kg IM.

Buprenorphine

Buprenorphine is a partial mu (μ) opioid agonist, and did not produce analgesia at any of three doses (i.e., 0.01, 0.05 and 0.10 mg/kg) evaluated in rainbow trout.[73]

NSAID

Fish are able to mount an inflammatory response that is attenuated by the use of NSAIDs.[74] Therefore it is logical to assume that blocking inflammation will decrease pain in fish species, which has been shown in koi carp, goldfish and rainbow trout.[20,72,73] Supporting this conclusion is the finding that ketoprofen produced analgesia in a MAC reduction model in goldfish.[20] Ketoprofen dose: 0.5–2.0 mg/kg IM; carprofen dose: 1.0–5.0 mg/kg IM.

Local anesthetics

Lidocaine stops neuronal Na^+ channel propagation in fish and has been shown to decrease pain when injected peripherally in trout.[74] Lidocaine dose: 1.0 mg/100 g trout (10 mg/kg).[73]

EUTHANASIA

The word *euthanasia* comes from the Greek words meaning "good death." The issue of euthanasia in fish is complicated as it must balance humanness to each animal (euthanasia) with the needs of aquaculture (slaughter) and occasional non-euthanasia research needs (humane killing). The issue is further complicated by the fact that many fish species are resistant to the effects of hypoxemia and are likely to be able to survive without oxygen for extended periods of time. The most recent American Veterinary Medical Association (AVMA) guidelines provide guidance for the euthanasia of fish.[75] Unfortunately, many inappropriate methods for euthanasia have been suggested for fish. The following methods do not meet the criteria for humane euthanasia: flushing of finfish into sewer, septic, or other types of outflow systems; placing fish in a freezer with or without water; or direct immersion in fixative or preservative.[62]

Euthanasia by immersion

Overdose of immersion anesthetic is a common method for fish euthanasia. Since fish progressively pass through the stages of sedation and anesthesia prior to euthanasia, the immersion solution still needs to be buffered for humane reasons depending on the euthanasia compound used. Recommendations generally include using approximately 3 to 5 times the anesthetic dose and leaving the fish in the solution for 10 min following the loss of operculation.[75] One of the authors (LPP) has personal experience with goldfish being exposed to various anesthetics at 5 times the anesthetic dose for 1 hr without operculation that fully recovered after being placed in anesthesia-free water (without any assisted ventilation). Likewise, another author (SAS) has observed koi carp recover from a 20 min exposure of MS-222 at 250 μg/L after being left on a table for examination. Recent evaluation of euthanasia by immersion demonstrated that exposure of goldfish to MS-222 up to 1000 mg/L did not consistently kill fish (i.e., 94% survived).[53] It is therefore likely that presumed overdoses with immersion anesthetics in many fish species are resulting in a deep plane of anesthesia rather than causing death, and should be followed by a second step, such as decapitation, cervical separation, pithing or freezing to ensure death.

Tricaine methanesulfonate

Tricaine will acidify the water and should be buffered appropriately to prevent discomfort before anesthesia. Tricaine dose for euthanasia: 250 to 500 mg/L (note that dose of 400 mg/L has been shown to be ineffective for a few species, e.g., Gulf of Mexico sturgeon).

Clove oil, eugenol and isoeugenol

Clove oil, AQUI-SE and AQUI-S doses for euthanasia: 100–300 mg/L.

Benzocaine

Benzocaine dose for euthanasia: 250 mg/L.

Carbon dioxide

Carbon dioxide can cause death at high doses or can be used as a sedative/anesthetic before a secondary means of euthanasia. Only CO_2 from a source that allows for careful regulation of concentration, such as from compressed gas cylinders, is acceptable.[75] Administration must be conducted in well-ventilated areas so that CO_2 gas that escapes out of the water does not affect personnel.

Propofol and alfaxalone

Both propofol and alfaxalone can produce anesthesia in fish. Therefore, they can be used as part of a two-step method for euthanasia: anesthesia by immersion, followed by a mechanical final form of death (decapitation, pithing, etc.). Propofol dose for euthanasia: 25 mg/L; alfaxalone dose for euthanasia: 50 mg/L.

Ethanol

Ethanol is considered a conditionally acceptable euthanasia method, however, immersing live, unanesthetized finfish directly into preservative concentrations of ethanol (>70%) is not acceptable.[65,75] Appropriate dilution of ethanol for euthanasia should be 1%–3% or 10–30 mL of 95% ethanol per L of water.

Quinaldine sulfate

Quinaldine sulfate will acidify water, therefore, buffering is required to prevent distress from an acute drop in pH. Quinaldine sulfate dose for euthanasia: 100 mg/L.

2-Phenoxyethanol

2-Phenoxyethanol dose for euthanasia: 0.5–0.6 mL/L or 0.3–0.4 mg/L. It is similarly suggested that this immersion dose be followed by a mechanical form (decapitation, pithing, etc.) of euthanasia.

Euthanasia by injection

Injectable agents have been administered via IV, IP, IM, and intracardiac routes (IC should only be performed after anesthesia). Any drug that would produce anesthesia followed by a second lethal method (decapitation, pithing, IC drugs) would be appropriate.

Pentobarbital

Sodium pentobarbital dose for euthanasia: 60–100 mg/kg IV, IP or IC following anesthesia by another secondary means.

Euthanasia by physical methods

Mechanical or physical methods of euthanasia are acceptable if they quickly produce unconsciousness. These methods should only be used by personnel properly trained in the techniques.

Decapitation followed by pithing

Decapitation and pithing cause rapid death and unconsciousness. Decapitation alone is not considered a humane approach to euthanasia, especially for species that may be particularly tolerant of low O_2 concentrations.[75]

Cranial concussion

Both blunt force trauma and captive bolts (for larger fish species) can produce quick unconsciousness. Both methods should be followed by a second lethal step to ensure death.

Maceration

Death is nearly instantaneous when appropriate equipment is used with appropriate-size fish. The AVMA guidelines warn that the process is aesthetically unpleasant for some operators and observers.[75]

Rapid cooling

Rapid cooling to 2°C–4°C without direct contact with ice is appropriate for euthanasia of zebrafish, and conditionally appropriate for other small-bodied (<3.8 cm total length), temperate and subtropical stenothermic species.[75] Whether this method meets the criteria for rapid, stress-free unconsciousness and death remains a matter of some debate, and it does not apply to larger-bodied, or cold- or cool-water fish.

REFERENCES

1. Klide, A.M. Questions depth of anesthesia and adequacy of ventilation in fish article. Letters to the editor. *Journal of the American Veterinary Medical Association* 2011;238(11):1402.

2. Harms, C., Bakal, R., Khoo, L., Spaulding, K. and Lewbart, G. Microsurgical excision of an abdominal mass in a gourami. *Journal of the American Veterinary Medical Association* 1995;207(9):1215–1217.

3. Bailey, K.M., Minter, L.J., Lewbart, G.A., Harms, C.A., Griffith, E.H. and Posner, L.P. Alfaxalone as an intramuscular injectable anesthetic in koi carp (*Cyprinus carpio*). *Journal of Zoo and Wildlife Medicine* 2014;45(4):852–858.

4. Minter, L.J., Bailey, K.M., Harms, C.A., Lewbart, G.A. and Posner, L.P. The efficacy of alfaxalone for immersion anesthesia in koi carp (*Cyprinus carpio*). *Veterinary Anaesthesia and Analgesia* 2014;41(4):398–405.

5. Lewbart, G.A. and Harms, C. Building a fish anesthesia delivery system. *Exotic DVM* 1999;1(2):25–28.

6. Sundeep, S.D., Dóró, E, Magyary, I., Egginton, S., Sík, A. and Müller, F. Optimisation of embryonic and larval ECG measurement in Zebrafish for quantifying the effect of QT prolonging drugs. *PLOS ONE* 2013;8(4):e60552. http://journals.plos.org/plosone/article/asset?id=10.1371/journal.pone.0060552.PDF.

7. Sherrill, J., Weber III, E.S., Marty, G.D. and Hernandez-Divers, S. 2008. Fish cardiovascular physiology and disease. *Veterinary Clinics of North America: Exotic Animal Practice* 2009;12:11–38.

8. Tranquilli, W.J., Thurmon, J.C. and Grimm, K.A. *Lumb and Jones' Veterinary Anesthesia and Analgesia*. John Wiley & Sons, 2013.

9. Christiansen, E.F. and Stoskopf, M.K. pH dynamics of tricaine methanesulfonate (MS-222) in fresh and artificial seawater. *North American Journal of Aquaculture* 2013;75(3):356–360.

10. Carter, K.M., Woodley, C.M. and Brown, R.S. A review of tricaine methanesulfonate for anesthesia of fish. *Reviews in Fish Biology and Fisheries* 2011;21(1):51–59.

11. Palmer, L.M. and Mensinger, A.F. Effect of the anesthetic tricaine (MS-222) on nerve activity in the anterior lateral line of the oyster toadfish, *Opsanus tau*. *Journal of Neurophysiology* 2004;92(2):1034–1041.

12. Ryan, S. The dynamics of MS-222 anaesthesia in a marine teleost (*Pagrus auratus*: Sparidae). *Comparative Biochemistry and Physiology Part C: Comparative Pharmacology* 1992;101(3):593–600.

13. Doherty, T.J. and Frazier, D.L. Effect of intravenous lidocaine on halothane minimum alveolar concentration in ponies. *Equine Veterinary Journal* 1998;30(4):300–303.

14. Valverde, A., Doherty, T.J., Hernandez, J. and Davies, W. Effect of lidocaine on the minimum alveolar concentration of isoflurane in dogs. *Veterinary Anaesthesia and Analgesia* 2004;31(4):264–271.

15. Gaughen, C.M. and Durieux, M. The effect of too much intravenous lidocaine on bispectral index. *Anesthesia & Analgesia* 2006;103(6):1464–1465.

16. Cho, G.K. and Heath, D.D. Comparison of tricaine methanesulphonate (MS222) and clove oil anaesthesia effects on the physiology of juvenile chinook salmon *Oncorhynchus tshawytscha* (Walbaum). *Aquaculture Research* 2000;31:537–546.

17. Hill, J.V. and Forster, M.E. Cardiovascular responses of Chinook salmon (*Oncorhynchus tshawytscha*) during rapid anaesthetic induction and recovery. *Comparative Biochemistry and Physiology: Toxicology & Pharmacology* 2004;137(2):167–177.

18. Hunn, J.B. and Allen, J.L. Movement of drugs across the gills of fishes. *Annual Review of Pharmacology* 1974;14(1):47–54.

19. Smith, D., Smith, S. and Holladay, S. Effect of previous exposure to tricaine methanesulfonate on time to anesthesia in hybrid tilapias. *Journal of Aquatic Animal Health* 1999;11(2):183–186.

20. Ward, J.L., McCartney, S.P., Chinnadurai, S.K. and Posner, L.P. Development of a minimum-anesthetic-concentration depression model to study the effects of various analgesics in goldfish (*Carassius auratus*). *Journal of Zoo and Wildlife Medicine* 2012;43(2):214–222.

21. Posner, L.P., Scott, G.N. and Law, J.M. Repeated exposure of goldfish (*Carassius auratus*) to tricaine methanesulfonate (MS-222). *Journal of Zoo and Wildlife Medicine* 2013;44(2):340–347.

22. FDA. *Tricaine-S in FDA GreenBook*. US Department of Health and Human Services, 2015, http://www.accessdata.fda.gov/scripts/AnimalDrugsAtFDA/details.cfm?dn=200–226.

23. Detar, J.E. and Mattingly, H.T. Response of southern redbelly dace to clove oil and MS-222: Effects of anesthetic concentration and water temperature. *Proceedings of the Annual Conference of the South-eastern Association of Fish Wildlife Agencies* 2004;58:219–227.

24. Summerfelt, R.C., Smith, L., Schreck, C. and Moyle, P. Anesthesia, surgery, and related techniques. In: *Methods for Fish Biology*. American Fisheries Society, Bethesda, MD 1990;8(9.6):2.

25. Yoshimura, H., Naamura, M. and Koeda, T. Mutagenicity screening of anesthetics for fishes. *Mutation Research: Genetic Toxicology and Environmental Mutagenesis* 1981;90(2):119–124.

26. Bernstein, P.S., Digre, K.B. and Creel, D.J. Retinal toxicity associated with occupational exposure to the fish anesthetic MS-222. *American Journal of Ophthalmology* 1997;124(6):843–844.

27. Bailey, K.M., Hempstead, J.E., Tobias, J.R., Borst, L.B., Clode, A.B. and Posner, L.P. Evaluation of the effects of tricaine methanesulfonate on retinal structure and function in koi carp (*Cyprinus carpio*). *Journal of the American Veterinary Medical Association* 2013;242(11):1578–1582.

28. Ross, L.G., Ross, B. and Ross, B. *Anesthetic and Sedative Techniques for Aquatic Animals*, 3rd ed. Blackwell, Oxford, 2008.

29. AQUI-S New Zealand Ltd. AQUI-S products. 2015; http://www.aqui-s.com/.

30. National Toxicology Program. Toxicology and carcinogenesis studies of isoeugenol in F344/N rats and

B63F1 mice. 2010; https://ntp.niehs.nih.gov/ntp/htdocs/lt_rpts/tr551.pdf.

31. Sladky, K.K., Swanson, C.R., Stoskopf, M.K., Loomis, M.R. and Lewbart, G.A. Comparative efficacy of tricaine methanesulfonate and clove oil for use as anesthetics in red pacu (*Piaractus brachypomus*). *American Journal of Veterinary Research* 2001;62(3):337–342.

32. Wagner, G.N., Singer, T.D. and Scott McKinley, R. The ability of clove oil and MS-222 to minimize handling stress in rainbow trout (*Oncorhynchus mykiss* Walbaum). *Aquaculture Research* 2003;34(13):1139–1146.

33. Kim, Y.-J., Nam, R.-H., Yoo, Y.M. and Lee, C.-J. Identification and functional evidence of GABAergic neurons in parts of the brain of adult zebrafish (*Danio rerio*). *Neuroscience Letters* 2004;355(1):29–32.

34. Stoelting, R. *Pharmacolgy and Physiology in Anesthetic Practice*, 3rd ed. Lippincott-Raven, Philadelphia, 1999.

35. Olsen, Y.A., Einarsdottir, I.E. and Nilssen, K.J. Metomidate anaesthesia in Atlantic salmon, *Salmo salar*, prevents plasma cortisol increase during stress. *Aquaculture* 1995;134(1–2):155–168.

36. Mattson, N. and Riple, T. Metomidate, a better anesthetic for cod (*Gadus morhua*) in comparison with benzocaine, MS-222, chlorobutanol, and phenoxyethanol. *Aquaculture* 1989;83(1):89–94.

37. Hill, J., Davison, W. and Forster, M. The effects of fish anaesthetics (MS222, metomidate and AQUI-S) on heart ventricle, the cardiac vagus and branchial vessels from Chinook salmon (*Oncorhynchus tshawytscha*). *Fish Physiology and Biochemistry* 2002;27(1–2):19–28.

38. Small, B.C. Anesthetic efficacy of metomidate and comparison of plasma cortisol responses to tricaine methanesulfonate, quinaldine and clove oil anesthetized channel catfish *Ictalurus punctatus*. *Aquaculture* 2003;218(1):177–185.

39. Massee, K.C., Rust, M.B., Hardy, R.W. and Stickney, R.R. The effectiveness of tricaine, quinaldine sulfate and metomidate as anesthetics for larval fish. *Aquaculture* 1995;134(3):351–359.

40. Harms, C.A. Anesthesia in fish. In: *Zoo and Wildlife Animal Medicine, Current Therapy, vol. 4*. M.E. Fowler and R. Miller, eds. WB Saunders, Philadelphia, 1999; pp. 158–163.

41. Hansen, M.K., Nymoen, U. and Horsberg, T.E. Pharmacokinetic and pharmacodynamic properties of metomidate in turbot (*Scophthalmus maximus*) and halibut (*Hippoglossus hippoglossus*). *Journal of Veterinary Pharmacology and Therapeutics* 2003;26(2):95–103.

42. J. Balko, S.K. Wilson, G. Lewbart, B.R. Gaines and L.P. Posner. Propofol as an immersion anesthetic and in a minimum anesthetic concentration (MAC) reduction model in goldfish (*Carassius auratus*). *ACVAA Scientifc Meeting*, Washington DC, 2015.

43. Oda, A., Bailey, K.M., Lewbart, G.A., Griffith, E.H. and Posner, L.P. Physiologic and biochemical assessments of koi (*Cyprinus carpio*) following immersion in propofol. *Journal of the American Veterinary Medical Association* 2014;245(11):1286–1291.

44. Fleming, G.J., Heard, D.J., Francis Floyd, R. and Riggs, A. Evaluation of propofol and medetomidine-ketamine for short-term immobilization of Gulf of Mexico sturgeon (*Acipenser oxyrinchus desoti*). *Journal of Zoo and Wildlife Medicine* 2003;34(2):153–158.

45. Miller, S., Mitchell, M., Heatley, J., Wolf, T., Lapuz, F., Lafortune, M. and Smith, J.A. Clinical and cardiorespiratory effects of propofol in the spotted bamboo shark (*Chylloscyllium plagiosum*). *Journal of Zoo and Wildlife Medicine* 2005;36(4):673–676.

46. Gressler, L., Parodi, T., Riffel, A., DaCosta, S. and Baldisserotto, B. Immersion anaesthesia with tricaine methanesulphonate or propofol on different sizes and strains of silver catfish *Rhamdia quelen*. *Journal of Fish Biology* 2012;81(4):1436–1445.

47. Gressler, L.T., Sutili, F.J., da Costa, S.T., Parodi, T.V., Pes Tda, S., Koakoski, G., Barcellos, L.J. and Baldisserotto, B. Hematological, morphological, biochemical and hydromineral responses in *Rhamdia quelen* sedated with propofol. *Fish Physiology and Biochemistry* 2015;41(2):463–472.

48. Bauquier, S., Greenwood, J. and Whittem, T. Evaluation of the sedative and anaesthetic effects of five different concentrations of alfaxalone in goldfish, *Carassius auratus*. *Aquaculture* 2013;396:119–123.

49. Nakanishi, M., Wilson, A.C., Nolan, R.A., Gorman, G.C. and Bailey, G.S. Phenoxyethanol: Protein preservative for taxonomists. *Science* 1969;163(3868):681–683.

50. Hausen, B.M. The sensitizing potency of Euxyl® K 400 and its components 1,2–dibromo-2,4–dicyanobutane and 2–phenoxyethanol. *Contact Dermatitis* 1993;28(3):149–153.

51. Stoskopf, M. and Posner, L. Anesthesia and restraint of laboratory fish. In: *Anesthesia and Analgesia in Laboratory Animals*, 2nd ed. R. Fish, P. Danneman, M. Brown and A. Karas, eds. Elsevier, San Diego, 2008; pp. 519–534.

52. Weyl, O., Kaiser, H. and Hecht, T. On the efficacy and mode of action of 2–phenoxyethanol as an anaesthetic for goldfish, *Carassius auratus* (L.), at different temperatures and concentrations. *Aquaculture Research* 1996;27(10):757–764.

53. Balko, J.A., Oda, A., Posner, L.P. Immersion euthanasia of goldfish (*Carassius auratus*). *47th Annual Conference of the IAAAM*, Virginia Beach, VA. May 21–26, 2016.

54. Fredricks, K.T., Gingerich, W.H. and Fater, D.C. Comparative cardiovascular effects of four fishery anesthetics in spinally transected rainbow trout, *Oncorhynchus mykiss*. *Comparative Biochemistry and Physiology Part C: Comparative Pharmacology* 1993;104(3):477–483.

55. Eisele, J., Eger 2nd, E. and Muallem, M. Narcotic properties of carbon dioxide in the dog. *Anesthesiology* 1966;28(5):856–865.

56. Yoshikawa, H., Ishida, Y., Ueno, S. and Mitsuda, H. Changes in depth of anesthesia of the carp anesthetized with a constant level of CO2. *Nippon Suisan Gakkaishi* 1988;54(3):457–462.

57. Trushenski, J.T., Bowker, J.D., Gause, B.R. and Mulligan, B.L. Chemical and electrical approaches to sedation of hybrid striped bass: induction, recovery, and physiological responses to sedation. *Transactions of the American Fisheries Society* 2012;141(2):455–467.

58. Iwama, G.K., McGeer, J.C. and Pawluk, M.P. The effects of five fish anaesthetics on acid–base balance, hematocrit, blood gases, cortisol, and adrenaline in rainbow trout. *Canadian Journal of Zoology* 1989;67(8):2065–2073.

59. Visser, E. and Schug, S.A. The role of ketamine in pain management. *Biomedicine & Pharmacotherapy* 2006;60(7):341–348.

60. Chen, J., Patel, R., Friedman, T.C. and Jones, K.S. The behavioral and pharmacological actions of NMDA receptor antagonism are conserved in zebrafish larvae. *International Journal of Comparative Psychology* 2010;23(1):82–90.

61. Graham, M.S. and Iwama, G.K. The physiologic effects of the anesthetic ketamine hydrochloride on two salmonid species. *Aquaculture* 1990;90(3):323–331.

62. Williams, T.D., Rollins, M. and Block, B.A. Intramuscular anesthesia of bonito and Pacific mackerel with ketamine and medetomidine and reversal of anesthesia with atipamezole. *Journal of the American Veterinary Medical Association* 2004;225(3):417–421.

63. Christiansen, E., Mitchell, J., Harms, C.A. and Stoskopf, M. Sedation of red porgy (*Pagrus pagrus*) and black sea bass (*Centroprisfis striata*) using ketamine, dexmedetomidine and midazolam delivered via intramuscular injection. *Journal of Zoo and Aquarium Research* 2014;2(3):62–68.

64. Riehl, R., Kyzar, E., Allain, A. et al. Behavioral and physiological effects of acute ketamine exposure in adult zebrafish. *Neurotoxicology and Teratology* 2011;33(6):658–667.

65. Ruuskanen, J.O., Peitsaro, N., Kaslin, J.V., Panula, P. and Scheinin, M. Expression and function of alpha-adrenoceptors in zebrafish: drug effects, mRNA and receptor distributions. *Journal of Neurochemistry* 2005;94(6):1559–1569.

66. Oswald, R. Injection anaesthesia for experimental studies in fish. *Comparative Biochemistry and Physiology Part C: Comparative Pharmacology* 1978;60(1):19–26.

67. Sneddon, L.U. Clinical anesthesia and analgesia in fish. *Journal of Exotic Pet Medicine* 2012;21(1):32–43.

68. Posner, L.P. Pain and distress in fish: A review of the evidence. *ILAR Journal* 2009;50(4):327–328.

69. Sneddon, L.U. The evidence for pain in fish: the use of morphine as an analgesic. *Applied Animal Behaviour Science* 2003;83(2):153–162.

70. Baker, T.R., Baker, B.B., Johnson, S.M. and Sladky, K.K. Comparative analgesic efficacy of morphine sulfate and butorphanol tartrate in koi (*Cyprinus carpio*) undergoing unilateral gonadectomy. *Journal of the American Veterinary Medical Association* 2013;243(6):882–890.

71. Newby, N.C., Mendonça, P.C., Gamperl, K. and Stevens, E.D. Pharmacokinetics of morphine in fish: Winter flounder (*Pseudopleuronectes americanus*) and seawater-acclimated rainbow trout (*Oncorhynchus mykiss*). *Comparative Biochemistry and Physiology Part C: Toxicology & Pharmacology* 2006;143(3):275–283.

72. Harms, C.A., Lewbart, G.A., Swanson, C.R., Kishimori, J.M. and Boylan, S.M. Behavioral and clinical pathology changes in koi carp (*Cyprinus carpio*) subjected to anesthesia and surgery with and without intra-operative analgesics. *Comparative Medicine* 2005;55(3):221–226.

73. Mettam, J.J., Oulton, L.J., McCrohan, C.R. and Sneddon, L.U. The efficacy of three types of analgesic drugs in reducing pain in the rainbow trout, *Oncorhynchus mykiss*. *Applied Animal Behaviour Science* 2011;133(3–4):265–274.

74. Frantz, S. Fishing for COX inhibitors. *Nature Reviews: Drug Discovery* 2002;1(7):486.

75. Leary, S., Underwood, W., Anthony, R. et al. *AVMA Guidelines for the Euthanasia of Animals*. 2013.

CHAPTER 18

SURGERY

SHANE M. BOYLAN

ANESTHESIA

Anesthesia is covered in detail in Chapter 17 but will be briefly mentioned here. Immersion anesthetics most commonly used for fish anesthesia are tricaine methanesulfonate/MS-222, eugenol (clove oil), 2-phenoxyethanol, isoflurane, aflaxalone, metomidate and propofol.[1,2] Isoeugenol (AQUI-S®) may become approved for use in the United States in the future as it has several benefits including a potential for no withdrawal time. Currently, only MS-222 is approved for food fish in the United States with a withdrawal period of 21 days.

As a general rule, induction baths of MS-222 start at 150–250 ppm, with maintenance doses varying from 25 to 120 ppm. The wide range is due to the diversity of fishes, gender, reproductive status and health status. An important guideline is that slow-moving (benthic) fish generally require greater concentrations of MS-222 for induction. Koi (*Cyprinus carpio*) and lined seahorses (*Hippocampus erectus*) are very different fish, but they may both require up to 200 ppm MS-222 for induction and 100–120 ppm for maintenance. Ram ventilators or constantly swimming pelagic fish often need less MS-222 for induction as a rule. Both mahi mahi (*Coryphaena hippurus*), which are stenohaline marine teleosts, and bonnethead sharks (*Sphyrna tiburo*), which are euryhaline elasmobranchs, are sensitive to MS-222 and often need only 50 ppm for induction and half that for maintenance. The gill physiology and oxygenation style of each fish species should be considered before anesthetizing a patient for surgery. Of the variety of fish immersion anesthetics available, MS-222 is recommended as the immersion anesthetic of choice due to its long history of safe use and scientific evaluation.

Injectable anesthetics are not as commonly used as immersion drugs in private practice, but alpha-2 agonists (dexmedetomidine), ketamine, opioids, and benzodiazepenes (midazolam) have extensive use among public aquarium veterinarians (Appendices A and B). Although safety concerns are rare, the diversity of fish species does potentially create opportunities for rare, negative reactions to the aforementioned injectable anesthetics.[3]

Ideally, oxygen supplementation should start before induction. Dissolved oxygen (DO) should be supersaturated from 115% to 150% (6–10 ppm depending on salinity and temperature) as gilling may be reduced or absent in long anesthetic procedures. Excessive saturation of >200% occurs routinely during shipping, which can cause mild to moderate sedation that resolves over several days. There are likely no benefits of DO saturation >150%, and oxidation of tissues (gills) and oxygen toxicity to the central nervous system (CNS) are possible although data is lacking.

ANALGESIA

Surgery cannot be discussed without mention of pain management. The controversy of whether fish feel pain has been documented in the literature.[4–7] Pain and analgesia have been experimentally documented with mild acetic acid dermal and thermal exposures.[8–11] From the veterinary perspective, fish experience pain as analgesics mask the symptoms of pain allowing for the expression of normal behaviors.

Symptoms of pain in teleosts include clamped fins, decreased swimming, decreased appetite, increased gilling rate and abnormal position in the water column (i.e., fish often near the bottom).[12,13] Benthic, slow-moving fish may only show decreased appetite and increased respiration. However, some fish normally only eat once weekly making appetite a poor indicator of pain. Similarly, increased gilling could be caused by pain, low dissolved oxygen or decreased gill function (parasites, chloramine damage, etc.). Knowing normal fish behavior and environmental parameters is critical in assessing pain. Social behaviors are also sensitive to the effects of pain. With social groups, individuals with decreased health are often pushed to the edges of populations where predation risks are greater. Fish in pain will be unable to maintain the same swim speeds and corrections in orientation compared to healthier specimens, especially in schooling fish. In captivity, healthy fish often become aggressive to compromised fish that cannot escape due to the confinements of their environment. Pain relief can help patients reintroduce themselves into the tank social structure with less chance of tank-mate aggression.

The classical definition of nociception of whether a drug provides true pain relief compared to sedation is a nuance for most fish clinicians. The benefits of analgesia are often mixed with sedation. Fish in pain may swim erratically and further injure themselves against tank walls/tank structures or elicit aggression/predation from other fishes. Whether a drug reduces this behavior by sedation or true analgesia is clinically irrelevant in a practical situation.

As a generalization, teleosts respond to nearly all classes of anesthetics and analgesics like the other vertebrate classes. Dosages may be much higher to achieve desired effects and environmental influences like water temperature, age, reproductive status, salinity and health may be more significant. In no other vertebrate class does reproductive state play such a significant role in physiology. Reproductive female fish may see their roe-filled ovaries comprise 25% or more of their total mass compared to <1% during nonreproductive times (S. Boylan, per observation). Fat and protein content of fish change drastically depending on their diet and reproductive status, which can have huge effects on protein- or lipid-bound drugs. Similarly, temperature and salinity may significantly alter drug metabolism. Very few studies have examined the effects of varying environmental parameters on the pharmacokinetics and pharmacodynamics of drugs in fish.

Elasmobranch analgesics represent a black box. Hole punches used to mark the dorsal fin elicit no pain response in bonnethead sharks (*S. tiburo*) and sandtiger sharks/gray nurse sharks (*O. taurus*), which suggests elasmobranch nociception may be dramatically different (Boylan, per observation). Opioid drugs that target mu and kappa opioid receptors appear to have limited effects in elasmobranchs.[14] Anecdotally, alpha 2 agonists, ketamine, and benzodiazepenes do affect elasmobranchs and produce sedation for capture (Boylan, per observation).[15] Propofol works well given via intrasinus/intravenous routes in a variety of elasmobranchs, whereas immersion propofol produces rapid but prolonged anesthesia in the chain dogfish (*Scyliorhinus retifer*) (Boylan, per observation).[15]

Just as with warm-blooded vertebrates, systemic and local analgesics are recommended with major surgery. Minor surgical procedures like gill clips, skin scrapes, fin clips, and minor cryotherapy may not need analgesia beyond the anesthetic procedure. Intracoelomic surgery, extensive external debridement, or orthopedic surgery warrant local anesthetics and perhaps continued oral or injectable analgesia for days to weeks. With little pharmacokinetic data available, injectable analgesics with the longest half-lives should be chosen to avoid repeat handling. Pain medications should be given based on the accessibility and stress level of the fish. For example, koi may tolerate and benefit from injections of a pain medication every other day, whereas a tarpon (*Megalops atlanticus*) may only receive one dose of an analgesic during recovery because recapture is more likely to injure the fish. Sick or painful fish often refuse to eat making oral analgesic therapy difficult. Dose intervals for injections are not provided here because stress/capture effects determine the frequency of administration.

Although not thoroughly studied, it is very plausible that immersion anesthetics provide no pain relief once a fish has recovered. Fish are considered "recovered" from immersion anesthetics when their control of buoyancy, behavior and activity require no more support. In zebrafish, fish recovered from anesthesia were behaviorally identical to controls suggesting no lingering effect.[16] Like gas anesthesia in mammals, recovery occurs when the effects

Table 18.1 **Analgesics for fish surgery**
Hydromorphone 0.5–2 mg/kg IM
Butorphanol 1–10 mg/kg IM (considered a weak analgesic in fish)
Buprenorphine 0.1–0.5 mg/kg IM
Tramadol 5–10 mg/kg PO

NSAIDS:
    Ketoprofen 2 mg/kg with loading dose of 5 mg/kg IM or PO
    Meloxicam 0.2–1.5 mg/kg IM (not useful in tilapia)[20]

Ketamine 1–20 mg/kg IM (lower doses are used in conjunction with other analgesics for pain, higher doses are used for capture/surgical anesthesia)
Propofol 2.5–5 mg/kg IV
Benzodiazepenes, Midazolam 0.5–2 mg/kg IM

of immersion anesthetics are gone. Tricaine methanesulfonate, eugenol/isoeugenol, 2-phenoxyethanol, and propofol should be treated like isoflurane or sevoflurane in that they may not provide adequate pain relief post-surgery.

Opioids, alpha-2 agonists, ketamine (NMDA antagonists), NSAIDS (meloxicam), and benzodiazepenes have research and anecdotal use among fish veterinarians as analgesics (**Table 18.1**).[17–21] Although a benzodiazepine may not be considered a true analgesic in mammals, the sedative effects post-surgery may keep a fish from causing further injury to itself and is therefore included as a post-surgical treatment.

LOCAL ANESTHETICS

Lidocaine and/or bupivacaine are routinely administered for local analgesia. Either drug can be mixed with sodium bicarbonate immediately before administration in equal amounts when injecting an awake fish to reduce the pain associated with pH.[22] Lidocaine and bupivacaine are often mixed in equal volume, combining the benefit of lidocaine's rapid onset and the prolonged activity of bupivacaine. As it may improve analgesic longevity, the addition of an opioid to a local block mixture should be considered in those fish which are unlikely to receive more analgesia due to recapture considerations.[23] Lidocaine with epinephrine is commonly used to provide pain relief and reduce bleeding in the initial skin incision.

SURGERY

Pre-surgical examination

Pre-surgical evaluation usually involves taking a history, observing the fish in its environment, gill clip/gill endoscopic exam, fin clip, skin scrape, water quality evaluation, and a thorough physical exam under anesthesia. Observing the fish in its environment should not be overlooked. Capturing the patient can often cause severe trauma, and every effort should be made to understand the fish's normal activity to facilitate its safe and smooth immobilization and assess its post-surgical recovery. During observation, flashing, increased gilling, abnormal buoyancy, and other clinical signs may guide further diagnostics or alter surgical plans. Packed cell volume (PCV) and total solids are recommended minimal database values with a complete biochemistry profile being preferred for major surgery. Formalin-fixed blood can be submitted for complete blood counts to clinical pathology labs, or an in-house evaluation of a blood smear may be sufficient.[24] Severe anemia/hypoproteinemia may force a surgery to be postponed to start supportive therapy (e.g., antibiotics, IV colloids, balanced fluids therapy, blood transfusions, iron therapy, tube feeding, vitamins). Radiography should be performed on the anesthetized fish, as it provides valuable information concerning the anatomy for surgery, and ultrasound may also be instrumental for certain surgeries like mass removal or ovariectomy.[25] Contrast radiography should be conducted 24 hours before any foreign body surgery is attempted. Iodine compounds (e.g., diatrizoate meglumine) are preferred due to their safety with gastric ulcerations and decreased likelihood to accrete with the foreign body compared to barium compounds. The location and size of the foreign body will guide the surgical approach, and contrast may reveal gastrointestinal (GI) ruptures/torsion that could require small suture for resection and anastomosis. Oral/rectal endoscopy (rigid or flexible) may also be useful as a pre-surgical diagnostic depending on the location of foreign bodies. Frayed fins, ulcers or severe scale loss may necessitate systemic antibiotic therapy prior to surgery. A history of prolonged inappetence may suggest vitamin therapy and nutritional support (e.g., force feeding, partial parenteral nutrition, isotonic fluids) may need to occur for several days to weeks before surgery, as decreased fat and protein will change drug distribution and metabolism during anesthesia. Gills should be bright red and the gill surfaces free of parasites and excessive mucous/damage. Fish are often fasted for 24–48 hours prior to surgery to avoid water fouling during surgery. If a rigid endoscope is available, the gills should be examined for parasites, telangiectasia, pallor, and excessive mucous (see Chapter 3 on diagnostics).

Surgical prep

Skin represents a major portion of both the innate and acquired immune response in teleost. Antibodies, white blood cells, alarm cells, and antimicrobial molecules are abundant in the mucous skin layer, which is often compared to the mucosal immunity of the mammalian gastrointestinal system. Preparation of teleost surgical sites usually involves removing only the mucous and scales in the surgical area to make an incision. Povidone-iodine compounds (1:10 to 1:50 dilutions) are the recommended topical disinfectant due to their broad spectrum of activity and reduced desiccating effects. Alcohol-containing products should be avoided if possible in teleosts and are contraindicated in elasmobranchs. Many teleost incision sites are never treated with disinfectants. Elasmobranch surgical sites are often flushed with sterile saline or sterile water to osmotically shock and/or mechanically remove surface microorganisms, but elasmobranch skin should never be treated with any chemical if possible. Clear surgical drapes allow visual monitoring of the patient while providing a sterile surgical field. Drapes are usually held in place with an adhesive or clamp on the sponge/surgical table as attaching the drape to a fish is difficult and damaging. Petroleum jelly can also help drapes adhere to the fish skin without removing valuable mucous.[26]

Induction, maintenance and surgery

Fish anesthesia devices have been documented in several articles.[26–33] They may be as simple as a foam surgical bed on top of a 10-gallon tank sump, whereas more complicated systems may have multiple sumps with varying concentrations

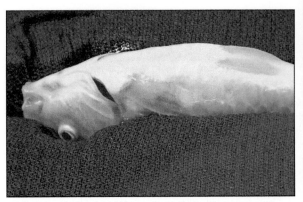

Figure 18.1 Foam surface modified for holding a fish during anesthesia and surgery. Note surface is widened at head area to avoid contact with eyes. (Image courtesy of C. Harms.)

of anesthetics. The simplest setup generally has an open cell foam block with a V shape cut as a surgery table that rests on top of a tank/sump (see Figure 17.8 in Chapter 17).[27,32] The foam area around the head is usually widened to avoid foam contact with eyes (**Figure 18.1**). Clear, plastic film (Saran wrap) is often placed on the foam to prevent contact mucous loss between the foam and patient. Maintenance anesthetic water is pumped from the sump through tubing into the fish's mouth. Water should cover the gills equally without causing gill damage or filling the stomach with excessive water pressure. Water exits the operculum and drains back into the sump through a perforated lid or table that supports the foam. Small towels or other barriers can be placed between the gill opercula and surgical site to prevent anesthetic water entering the surgical incision. Water flow rate can be modified by changing pump strength, restricting water flow through valves, or reducing tubing diameter either by clamps or choosing smaller tubing. All tissues not directly in the surgical field should be kept wet, especially the eyes. Irrigating the fish with water from a syringe or adding a second, low-pressure water line from the pump to frequently moisten the fish are the most commonly used methods.

Surgical events of one hour or more typically have increasing depths of anesthesia requiring the maintenance solution to be diluted. In simple systems, this involves adding fresh water to the sump for dilution of the anesthetic water. A sump with a known volume and anesthetic concentration allows accurate measurement. Prior to surgery, marks on the sump may be made with tape or markers that indicate what amount of clean, anesthetic-free water should be added to reduce the immersion anesthetic concentration to a particular concentration. In complex systems, different sumps with less concentrated solutions would be switched into the anesthetic circuit. Access to the pump, tubing and water is therefore necessary throughout a surgery. Monitoring the heart rate and/or opercular rate generally determines the effective depth of anesthesia.

Standard companion animal spay packs usually have the necessary surgical tools for fish surgery. A variety of forceps, blade handles, blade sizes and clamp types are useful. Tissue retractors (e.g., Army-Navy, Gelpi, and ophthalmic speculums) are very helpful to keep surgical sites open (**Figure 18.2**). Intracoelomic surgery may benefit from magnification (ocular loops, endoscopes) and supplemental lighting in small fish.

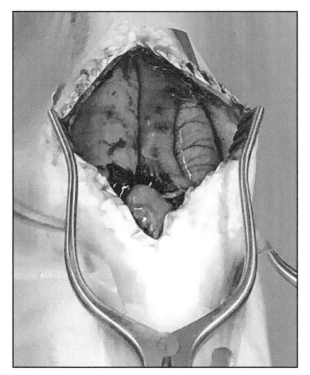

Figure 18.2 Gelpi style retractors being used for exposing coelomic organs during ovariectomy in a striped bass (*Morone saxatalis*).

Synthetic monofilament suture is the preferred suture in fish, as it usually produces the least amount of tissue reaction in most ectotherms.[30,34–37] Braided suture is often described as "wicking" bacteria and water into the wound. Braided sutures may also cut the skin in areas under mechanical stress.[38] Cat gut, silk and other natural suture materials may provoke significant inflammation causing the incision to dehisce.[36,39] Due to the difference in leukocyte enzymes, even absorbable suture may remain in fish for years.[40] Cutting needles are preferred in most situations as fish skin/scales can quickly dull tapered surgical needles.

Hemostasis can occur in a variety of ways. Lidocaine with epinephrine usually controls superficial skin bleeding when used as a local anesthetic for the initial incision. When sterility is less of a concern (i.e., skin bleeding), silver nitrate sticks are very effective and inexpensive. Single-use electrocautery (e.g., low and high temperature single use pens) or unipolar and bipolar electrocautery units should be considered with fish >3 kg. While pressure with sterile gauze and/or hemostat clamps alleviates most internal bleeding, ligation of visible blood vessels can be done with ophthalmic suture or hemoclips. Products like Gelfoam® and Surgicel® can be useful for complicated internal bleeds that cannot be controlled with the aforementioned methods. The small/thin nature of fish blood vessels and lower blood pressure make excessive bleeding rare compared to mammalian species.

Surgical closure is often completed with a one suture closure layer in fish skin, although two layer closures (i.e., muscle and skin) are preferred when anatomically possible (fish >5 kg). Simple interrupted, horizontal mattress, Ford interlocking, cruciate and simple continuous patterns are the most commonly used skin suture patterns. Both marine and freshwater fish can heal large coelomic ulcerations, even with organs exposed to the environment, without intervention when otherwise healthy. The failure of one simple interrupted suture is often not significant, and interrupted suture patterns are preferred to the continuous patterns for this reason. Simple interrupted sutures should be placed 2–3 mm from each other (**Figure 18.3**). Most fish form an everting skin reaction to simple interrupted knots, but the horizontal mattress may be preferred

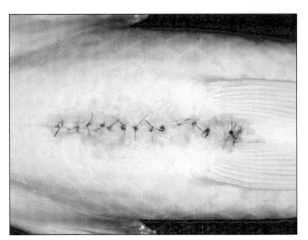

Figure 18.3 **Exploratory coeliotomy in a koi closed with a simple interrupted pattern of 4-0 PDS®II, thirteen days post-surgery. (Image courtesy of L.S. Christian.)**

when the skin does not naturally evert with the simple interrupted pattern. Fish skin generally heals quickly with close apposition. Fortunately for the clinician, fish skin usually heals without obvious scar tissue in 3 to 6 weeks when not complicated by infection. The lytic enzymes of fish white blood cells do not degrade absorbable suture and most sutures are actually extruded by the skin as a foreign body if left in place. Manual removal of suture is often necessary when sutures are not extruded naturally. Once immersed in water, most topical antimicrobials and skin adhesives do not adhere well to incision sites. Staples are not efficacious in fish, and tissue adhesives can cause irritation.[41] Skin glue can be placed on suture knots when necessary. Different topical creams with antimicrobial and wound healing properties have been tried with varying successes: silver sulfadiazine, triple antibiotic ointment, medical grade honey, silver collasate, phenytoin/misoprostol combination creams, etc.[42,43]

Misoprostol/phenytoin and silver collasate appear to have the best adherence to fish skin. Misoprostol/phenytoin combinations are available at compounding pharmacies as either powders or creams. Post-surgical cold laser wound therapy is appropriate if the tissues are kept moist to avoid thermal/dehydration injury. Collagen patches can also be sutured to wounds to facilitate healing.[44] Keeping dissolved oxygen elevated to 115%–150% over days to weeks may facilitate wound healing using the principles of hyperbaric wound treatment.

Anesthesia water should be clean and match all the critical parameters of the patient's environment: pH, temperature, salinity, hardness (see Chapter 2 on water quality). Although using tank water for surgical maintenance reduces the risk of water quality parameter differences, tank water is often rich in opportunistic organisms that may pose a risk to wound healing. As most fish surgeries are considered clean but not sterile, it is up to the clinician to determine what sources to use. Atypical mycobacteria, *Aeromonas* spp., *Vibrio* spp., fungi, protozoa, and other pathogens will likely be more abundant in tank water compared to recently prepared salt water or dechlorinated freshwater. Anesthetic induction should be conducted in tank water, and maintenance water can be made specifically for surgery, or use treated tank water to remove opportunistic pathogens. If maintenance water looks rich in organic debris, treating the water with hydrogen peroxide several hours prior to use may reduce contamination risks. Hydrogen peroxide breaks down to water and oxygen as it oxidizes bacteria and protozoa. A DO meter can be used to monitor hydrogen peroxide activity, which should return to pretreatment levels before being used for surgery to avoid oxidation damage to wounds/gills. Fish are often fasted for 24 hours prior to surgery to avoid defecation and regurgitation during surgery. Fasting also reduces the risk of pain-induced, decreased gastrointestinal motility that can lead to infection through colic. Salinity and temperature should not be overlooked during surgery or recovery. Adding salt (i.e., 3–6 ppt) for many freshwater fish reduces both opportunistic pathogens and osmotic gradients, thereby assisting wound healing. Similarly, reducing salinity in euryhaline fish to 20–25 ppt may reduce wound dehydration. Temperature is a major factor in wound healing and immune function in fish. Although many surgeons prefer to keep their operating rooms cooler for their comfort, a chilled fish will have decreased wound healing and poor immune function that may take weeks to recover even in ideal conditions given the stresses of surgery. As mentioned earlier, DO should minimally be 100% oxygen saturation or preferably slightly supersaturated (110%–150%) to facilitate healing and reduce stress.

Fluid therapy (e.g., IV, intracoelomic, or subcutaneous) is a typical supportive therapy in companion animal medicine surgery that is often overlooked in fish medicine (Appendix C). The majority of mammal surgeries have an IV line placed to administer fluids, and equivalent supportive care should be considered for fish. Continuous IV fluid therapy is rare in fish, but intracoelomic fluid therapy is relatively easy to administer. The osmolarity of the fluid should match the selected patient. Freshwater teleosts can receive normal replacement crystalloid fluids like lactate ringers (LRS) or Normosol-M® either IV or intracoelomically. Marine teleosts have much greater concentrations of ions (e.g., Na, Cl, and Mg) compared to freshwater teleosts and air breathing vertebrates. When generating a replacement fluid for a marine teleost, measured osmolarity is preferred to calculated osmolarity. Calculated osmolarity may miss important fluid components like trimethylamine oxide (TMAO) in elasmobranchs. Formulations for elasmobranch ringers and green moray eel ringers solutions have been published.[45–47] Sterile crystalloid fluids should be injected intracoelomically or intravenously (when blood loss is significant) at the end of surgery before closure. Intravenous colloids (Hetastarch®, Vetstarch®) should be given when significant blood loss occurs or ultrasound/Doppler findings suggest cardiac insufficiency.

Monitoring

Capillary refill time is a simple clinical indicator of perfusion of which all veterinarians are familiar. Its approximate analog in fish is the visual examination of the gills. Gills should normally be bright red, whereas pallor usually suggests anemia. MS-222 causes vasodilation and fin rays (particularly the tail fin) will become pale pink in fish that are not heavily pigmented. If a sedated fish does not exhibit pink vasodilation in the fins, the gills should be immediately examined for normal coloration.

Besides its normal diagnostic imaging value, ultrasound is useful to monitor heart rate and gill perfusion. Water is a superb conductor of sound. Submerging the patient's head facilitates gas exchange and provides access to the cranially located heart to ultrasonography. Placing an ultrasound probe directly on the gills with color Doppler

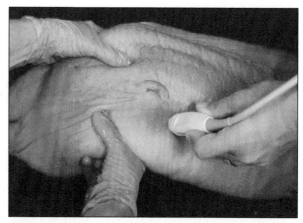

Figure 18.4 Ultrasound detection of the caudal location of heart in a green moray eel (*Gymnothorax funebris*).

mode can evaluate cardiopulmonary function rapidly when the heart cannot be found. If an ultrasound is not available, portable Doppler probes are just as effective in monitoring heart rate. It is important to find the heart prior to surgery, as Doppler probes may need to be placed in unique positions such as inside the opercular cavity to detect a heart rate (**Figure 18.4**). ECG monitors have been used effectively to monitor fish cardiovascular activity, and pulse oximetry has met with limited success. ECG probes are placed at the base of each pectoral and the anal fin or attached to similar locations.[48]

Gilling/opercular movement in fish is the equivalent to respiratory rate in terrestrial mammals. Many sedated procedures occur with the fish ventilating, but most surgical procedures of >15 minutes experience a cessation or severe reduction of autonomic opercular/spiracle movement. For surgery, fish should be placed in water with an increased dissolved oxygen concentration (i.e., 115%–150%) for several minutes before induction. Increasing dissolved oxygen in water is as simple as connecting an air stone to an oxygen tank. DO can be measured through various probes and kits (e.g., YSI, Hach, Chemetrics). Increased oxygenation should continue throughout surgery and recovery. To date, no negative effect has been shown on DO levels >115% for hours, and fish have been kept at 200+% DO for 24 or more hours during shipping without permanent side effects. Oxidation damage to the gills and mild oxygen narcolization are possible, particularly in elasmobranchs exposed to >200% DO for greater than 24 hours. Although many fish surgeries are successful with using room air, the use of supplemental oxygen is recommended, as blood gas analysis (e.g., I-STAT®) has shown respiratory acidosis and anoxia can occur during long surgeries without the use of supplemental oxygen.

Rapid blood gas analysis is usually accomplished with portable devices like the I-STAT®. Considerable research is available on blood gases, electrolytes, and lactate levels associated with the stress of capture or anesthetic monitoring in elasmobranchs and teleost game fish.[49–52] Blood collected during surgery may show trends that demand changes in oxygenation, electrolyte administration or sodium bicarbonate therapy for metabolic acidosis. Blood gas analysis is recommended when dealing with elasmobranch surgery, as there are numerous therapies that can support elasmobranchs.

Common surgical procedures in fish

Fin repair: The large pectoral and tail fins of butterfly koi often split. The show quality of these fish is partially dependent on the fins, and a veterinarian may be asked if they can assist. Once sedated, the edges of fins at the split should be gently scraped with a scalpel blade or mildly debrided to create fresh edges. The roughened edges of the fin are juxtaposed and held in place with simple interrupted, monofilament sutures. Skin adhesives have met with poor success in fish and are generally avoided.[26,41] Sutures should be removed after a few weeks depending on healing. This procedure may need to be repeated several times until split fins heal.

Superficial/integument mass removal: Cryosurgery is a quick, relatively painless and safe method of removing external masses less than 3 cm. Liquid nitrogen (LN) and over-the-counter (OTC) wart removers have both been documented in fish literature.[53,54] Cryotherapy removes superficial, unwanted tissue without the bleeding associated with surgical steel removal. The OTC applicators are suitable for small dermal masses (<2 cm), while LN can treat a range of lesions from millimeters to several centimeters (**Figure 18.5**). "Sumi" or black spots are sometimes unwanted areas of pigmentation on koi

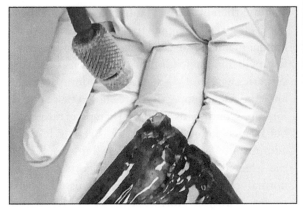

Figure 18.5 Liquid nitrogen cryotherapy in a southern flounder (*Paralichthys lethostigma*) to remove a rostral mass.

that can be quickly removed with a cryogun during any handling procedure. Repeat application may be necessary depending on the type of tissue that replaces the surgically frozen area. Koi pox, caused by cyprinid herpesvirus 1 (CyHV-1), produces melting waxlike lesions that can also be treated with cryotherapy if they do not resolve satisfactorily for the client.

Large masses/tumors (>2 cm) may need standard surgical debulking before LN cryotherapy is applied to the base of the lesion. Cryotherapy improves the chance of removing all atypical cells without the excessive debulking necessary with surgical steel surgery. LN cryotherapy often acts as a form of chemical cautery, although other forms of hemostasis should always be available.

Wen surgery: The wen is a proliferation of tissue on the cranial aspect of several breeds of fancy goldfish. Excessive proliferation may alter buoyancy or cover the eyes and nares, which reduces normal feeding behaviors.[55] Cryotherapy or surgical debridement can be done quickly under anesthesia. Although hemorrhage is rare, pressure or silver nitrate can quickly stop bleeding. Sharp scissors are often used to "trim" the wen (**Figure 18.6**). If the wen is suspected in altering buoyancy, a note of caution needs to be mentioned. An anesthetized fish's natural buoyancy is usually dorsal recumbency (i.e., belly up) with the head being more buoyant than the tail. This may not be true of fancy goldfish, which have atypical swim bladders. Once a radiograph has

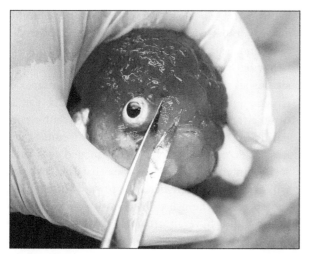

Figure 18.6 Wen trimming in a sedated goldfish to remove excessive proliferation of tissue around the eyes. (Image courtesy of S.A. Smith.)

ruled out coelomic or gastrointestinal gas, the wen should be superficially trimmed and the fish completely recovered from sedation. Only when the fish is fully awake with conscious control over its orientation should the buoyancy be evaluated. Removing too much of the wen at first can make it difficult for the fish to readjust its buoyancy. It may take a few days for the fish to correct itself before another wen trimming is recommended. Only after the wen is considered normal, vestibular/CNS disease ruled out, and the buoyancy remains atypical, should aspirations of the swim bladder be conducted.

Coelomotomy: Opening the coelom surgically is usually done to collect biopsies, identify reproductive state or remove internal masses (tumors, reproductive tissues, foreign bodies). With the anesthetized fish in dorsal recumbency, the ventral midline of a fish is given a local block that is allowed to take effect (minimum 5 minutes). Scale removal is limited to the incision site, and a stab incision is made cranial to vent where the skin is loose and tented by forceps. The forceps are placed in the incision and used to raise the skin, while the scalpel blade (blade facing "up" or ventral) is placed between the points of the forceps, which lift the skin away from organs and guide the scalpel incision while avoiding coelomic organs. Incisions may extend through the pelvic fins, typically accomplished using scissors instead of a scalpel blade to cut through the cartilage or bone of the pelvic girdle.

In larger fish, a subcuticular/muscle and superficial skin layer closure is possible with this incision reducing the risks of dehiscence. Despite large incisions, fish heal quickly, even in the areas of the pelvic/pectoral fins, which are hard to close.

Removal of internal masses is surgically identical to that of mammals, and standard veterinary surgical processes apply. Masses/organs should have their blood supplies ligated with suture, clamps or hemoclips.[56] Incisions are made near the mass, usually with the fish in dorsal recumbency.[57] Potential neoplasias and granulomas should be examined by histopathology, and cultures should be taken when signs of infection are present.[48] The biggest difference with fish tumor removal compared to mammals is that there can be a change in buoyancy. Fish need time to adjust to buoyancy changes. This author uses volume-filling crystalloid fluids during large tissue resection for a variety of reasons. Intracoelomic fluids also help dislodge atmospheric gas that can become trapped during surgery. Intracoelomic gas bubbles alter buoyancy and absorb slowly. Bolus intracoelomic fluid therapy may also offset some of the changes in weight distribution and support the cardiovascular system provided the fluids are isotonic (surgical blood loss).

Ovariectomy is common among older teleosts and elasmobranchs in captivity. Teleost ovariectomy uses a ventral, midline or slightly, off midline approach (**Figure 18.7**). Older koi (*Cyprinus carpio*) and brook

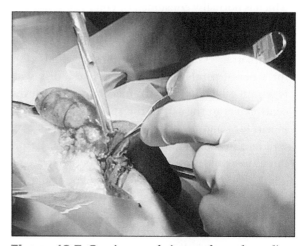

Figure 18.7 Ovariectomy being performed to relieve dystocia in a koi.

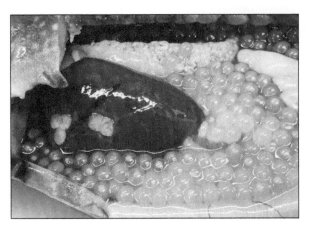

Figure 18.8 Brook trout (*Salvelinus fontinalis*) with old intracoelomic eggs adhered to the liver.

trout (*Salvelinus fontinalis*) commonly present with retained eggs that require ovariectomy.[56] Roe-filled ovaries are delicate and require careful handling to avoid rupture. Stay sutures should not be placed in a reproductively active ovary. Ligating the ovaries at their communication with the cloaca requires careful observation, as there can be retained ovarian tissue or eggs. Intracoelomic eggs often lead to inflammation/yolk peritonitis or create desiccated, flat foreign bodies (**Figure 18.8**). Manual debridement, flushing and suction, and cautery may be used to make sure all ovarian remnants/eggs are properly removed. In certain batoid species like Southern stingrays (*Dasyatis americana*) females continually fill their uterus with histotroph (i.e., nutritive material derived from maternal tissues other than blood), which is normally consumed by embryos. If not bred, the female still continues to produce histotroph, which eventually distends the uterus leading to mucometra.[58] The unique anatomy of batoids allows for a dorsal paralumbar approach if the disk width is within 50 and 60 cm. An incision is made several centimeters to the left of the spine to approach the uterus for removal.[33,58]

The clinician should remember that fish have protandranous and protogynous reproductive strategies. Thus, exploratory surgeries may be confusing with hermaphroditic states possible, especially in polluted waters where estrogenic compounds abound.

Ophthalmic surgery: Fish eyes suffer from a variety of problems including but not limited to infectious disease, gas exophthalmia, cataracts, trauma and lipid keratopathy. Enucleation/exenteration is a common surgery in petfish.[59] In passive species like koi/goldfish, enucleation generally causes little change in behavior, whereas in tanks/ponds with more aggressive fishes, enucleation can result in behavioral detriments and increased stress. Fish with one eye are often attacked by tank-mates and have trouble competing for food and habitat. In many circumstances, it is preferred to let a nonvisual, damaged eye heal by second intention with the hopes that the other fish will not change their behavior toward the patient if they perceive the fish to have both eyes even if one eye is blind. Several attempts at placing false eyes in fish have met with short-term success.[60] Fish with a false eye show improvement regarding tank-mate behaviors, but false eyes invariably dislodge (suture or adhesive failures over time) and have to be replaced. Enucleation should occur with ocular neoplasia, but second intention healing of damaged eyes is preferred when possible.

Removal of a fish eye is similar to enucleation in companion animals except for the lack of functional eyelids/palpebral. Adipose lids, which occur in certain species, are the equivalent to palpebra and may need to be resected prior to enucleation in some teleosts.[53] Local analgesics should be provided to the eye periphery where ocular muscles need to be cut while avoiding injections near the optic nerve due to its close proximity to the brain. Lidocaine with epinephrine can be used to reduce potential bleeding. A scalpel blade or small, curved scissors can carefully dissect the sclera from ocular muscles and attachments. If not already collapsed, the contents of the eye can be aspirated prior to surgical removal to facilitate enucleation. The optic nerve should not be stretched or otherwise irritated if possible. The surgery site is left to heal by second intention, and the globe generally fills with scar tissue in a few months unless there are complications. It is recommended that the fish be isolated or kept with gentle tank-mates during the recovery period. Systemic antibiotics are recommended and analgesics are generally not needed beyond a few days, as most fish begin to feed quickly if kept in quiet tanks.

Cataracts are common in public aquariums where fish live beyond normal life expectancy and trauma is common. If the retina remains functional,

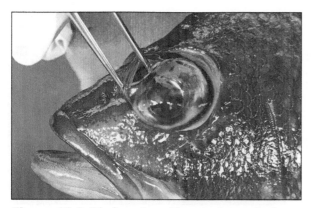

Figure 18.9 Black sea bass (*Centropristis striata*) with recurrent exophthalmia having lens surgically removed.

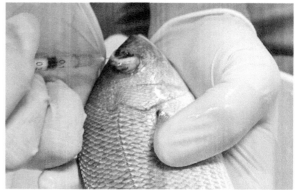

Figure 18.10 Fine needle aspirate of gas accumulation in the eye of a scup (*Stenotomus chrysops*).

phacoemulsification or lens extraction is recommended to provide improved vision.[61] The lens often completely luxates in chronic exophthalmia cases and can be removed with forceps after making an incision into the cornea (**Figure 18.9**). Eyes can be restored to normal size with isotonic fluids in freshwater fish, and in this case of marine fishes with marine teleost ringers.[62] Closing the cornea can be accomplished with suture and sometimes skin glue. Without the lens, the brain will need time to adjust to inverted image processing, but companion animals adjust to changes in image processing from unilateral phacoemulsification within a short time (i.e., week). Lipid keratopathy is a condition common in captive moray eels. Surgical and dietary management of the condition is well described.[63–65]

Unilateral pseudobranchectomy is a simple surgical procedure used to treat gas exophthalmia caused by gas supersaturation. Small cracks in plumbing with powerful pumps can create venturi like effects that result in gas super saturation (typically nitrogen). The pseudobranch (see Chapter 1, Figure 1.10) is a gill-like structure attached to the medial surface of the operculum within the gill chamber. It exchanges gas with water to deliver oxygen to the eyes. When the water is gas supersaturated, the pseudobranch delivers gas-rich blood to the ocular tissues where gas emboli form. Radiography can help guide gas aspiration, which is only palliative if the source of gas saturation is not corrected (see Chapter 3, Figure 3.53). The affected eye(s) are usually treated with ophthalmic antibiotics before a

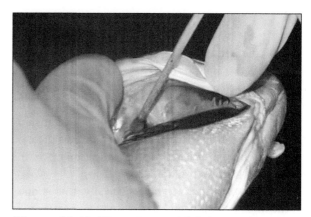

Figure 18.11 Silver nitrate stick being used to burn the pseudobranch in a vermillion snapper (*Rhomboplites aurorubens*).

small gauge needle aspirates the gas (**Figure 18.10**). Anti-inflammatory agents (ophthalmic prednisone or ophthalmic NSAIDS like flurbiprofen) are often applied topically post-aspiration. Unilateral pseudobranchectomy helps reduce gas delivery to prevent recurrence and should be conducted on the most affected side. Bilateral pseudobranchectomy is contraindicated, as it may cause blindness. The gill chamber is carefully opened during sedation, and a silver nitrate stick is used to burn the pseudobranch gill tissue by contact (**Figure 18.11**). Unilateral pseudobranchectomy can be done in stages (e.g., 25%, 50%, 75% and 100%) until the clinician is familiar with the response to treatment. Usually, it takes >50% reduction in pseudobranch tissue to reduce recurrence. The theory behind pseudobranchectomy is

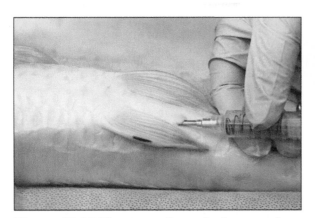

Figure 18.12 Placement of a passive integrated transponder (PIT) tag in the coelomic cavity of koi using a large gauge needle device. (Image courtesy of S.A. Smith.)

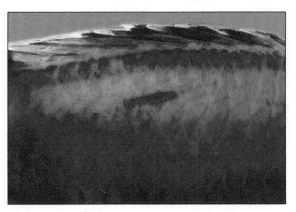

Figure 18.13 PIT tag placement in dorsal musculature of a tilapia highlighted by transillumination. (Image courtesy of S.A. Smith.)

that the reduction in pseudobranch surface area reduces the amount of gas absorbed from the water and released into ocular tissues. Carbonic anhydrase inhibitors (e.g., acetazolamide, 2–3 mg/kg intradermally or intramuscularly every 5 to 7 days for up to three treatments) may also assist in certain cases, although their efficacy for gas saturation or trauma-induced gas exophthalmia is unknown.

Transmitter placement: Historically, this is one of the most common surgical procedures performed in fish. The fish literature is rich in papers that describe a variety of transmitters and methods of placement.[38,66] In recent years, a number of papers have highlighted the need for veterinary guidance in this area, as sterility has been ignored or considered a low priority in previous decades.[38,67] However, antenna and transmitters need to be made as sterile as possible without affecting their function.[66] Most types of intracoelomic transmitters are placed into the caudal coelom using a small ventral-lateral incision. Pressure necrosis or changes in buoyancy should be evaluated in controlled pilot studies before large studies are conducted to ensure fish behavior, buoyancy, reproduction and viability are not significantly altered.[68] Many intracoelomic transmitters may be shed through the gastrointestinal tract or the body wall.[69,70] Swim bladders may need increased gas volumes to offset the weight of transmitters, and the time to accommodation may require holding animals in captivity for days to weeks before release.[71] There

may be a mandatory withdrawal period if MS-222 is used to sedate the fish, so this is an excellent time to evaluate changes in buoyancy, behavior and transmitter retention. PIT (passive integrated transponders) tags are also used to identify individual fish. These are small enough to be implanted intracoelomically or intramuscularly using large bore needles (**Figures 18.12** and **18.13**).

Orthopedic surgery: Orthopedic repairs in fish are rare. Smaller external fixation kits (avian/exotic products) are available that can be used to correct certain orthopedic fractures. Aquatic environments promote biofilms that rapidly colonize external pins that direct infection into the bone. Internal fixation devices show more promise in the aquatic environment.[72] Cerclage wire was successful to repair mandibular factures, a common occurrence in aggressive feeding fish, in arowana.[73] If antimicrobials can be placed on external fixation devices that are neutrally buoyant enough to allow normal activity, external fixation may be possible. Spinal trauma is a common occurrence in fish due to collisions with tank walls, lightning strikes in koi ponds, capture/handling trauma, or metabolic disorders.[74–76] Spinal surgery to correct scoliosis or traumatic spinal fractures have occurred in koi.[77] Vertebroplasty is the process of injecting bone cement into vertebral bodies to provide support and stop progressive lesions. This technique shows promise in stabilizing spines in large fish patients (sandtiger sharks) in public aquariums or larger koi before the lesions progress beyond unsuitable quality of life. Bone morphogenetic protein should also be considered in difficult-to-repair orthopedic fractures.

Pneumocystectomy: Swim bladder surgery or ligation of the physostomous duct are often surgeries of last resort.[78] Pneumocystectomy was successful in ameliorating buoyancy issues in a goldfish with fungal pneumocystitis.[79] Ligation of the physostomous duct has been tried in koi, cichlids, goldfish and catfish to prevent recurrent water entry into the swim bladder. With the fish in dorsal recumbency, gentle traction of the liver and stomach can expose the physostomous duct's connection to the cranial swim bladder where hemoclips or suture can be used to seal the physostomous duct. Before surgical ligation is attempted, blocking the physostomous duct may be achievable by injecting blood (blood patch) or tissue adhesive into the duct's opening, which is usually located on the dorsal surface of the caudal pharynx. This nonsurgical method has been found to have a greater safety margin.

REFERENCES

1. Beckman, M.S., Spooner, T.M., Meyer, A.C., Waltenburg, M.A. and Mitchell, M.A. Immersion anesthetics in freshwater stingrays: Comparing the effects of MS-222 and alfaxalone on *Potamotrygon* sp. *47th IAAAM Conference*, Virginia Beach, Virginia, May 21–26, 2016.
2. Vaughan, D.B., Penning, M.R. and Christison, K.W. 2-Phenoxyethanol as anaesthetic in removing and relocating 102 species of fishes representing 30 families from Sea World to uShaka Marine World, South Africa. *Onderstepoort Journal of Veterinary Research* 2008;75(3):189–198.
3. Christiansen, E.F., Mitchell, J.M., Harms, C.A. and Stoskopf, M.K. Sedation of red porgy (*Pagrus pagrus*) and black sea bass (*Centroprisfis striata*) using ketamine, dexmedetomidine and midazolam delivered via intramuscular injection. *Journal of Zoo and Aquarium Research* 2014;2(3):62.
4. Weber, E.S. Fish analgesia: Pain, stress, fear aversion, or nociception? *Veterinary Clinics of North America: Exotic Animal Practice* 2011;14(1):21–32.
5. Rose, J.D., Arlinghaus, R., Cooke, S.J., Diggles, B.K., Sawynok, W., Stevens, E.D. and Wynne, C.D. Can fish really feel pain? *Fish and Fisheries* 2014;15(1):97–133.
6. Sneddon, L.U., Braithwaite, V.A. and Gentle, M.J. Do fishes have nociceptors? Evidence for the evolution of a vertebrate sensory system. *Proceedings of the Royal Society of London B: Biological Sciences* 2003;270(1520):1115–1121.

7. Sneddon, L.U. Evolution of nociception in vertebrates: Comparative analysis of lower vertebrates. *Brain Research Reviews* 2004;46(2):123–130.
8. Sneddon, L.U. The evidence for pain in fish: The use of morphine as an analgesic. *Applied Animal Behaviour Science* 2003;83(2):153–162.
9. Sneddon, L.U., Braithwaite, V.A. and Gentle, M.J. Novel object test: Examining nociception and fear in the rainbow trout. *The Journal of Pain* 2003;4(8):431–440.
10. Sneddon, L.U. Pain perception in fish: Indicators and endpoints. *ILAR Journal* 2009;50(4):338–342.
11. Nordgreen, J., Kolsrud, H.H., Ranheim, B. and Horsberg, T.E. Pharmacokinetics of morphine after intramuscular injection in common goldfish *Carassius auratus* and Atlantic salmon *Salmo salar*. *Diseases of Aquatic Organisms* 2009;88(1):55–63.
12. Harms, C.A., Lewbart, G.A., Swanson, C.R., Kishimori, J.M. and Boylan, S.M. Behavioral and clinical pathology changes in koi carp (*Cyprinus carpio*) subjected to anesthesia and surgery with and without intra-operative analgesics. *Comparative Medicine* 2005;55(3):221–226.
13. Baker, T.R., Baker, B.B., Johnson, S.M. and Sladky, K.K. Comparative analgesic efficacy of morphine sulfate and butorphanol tartrate in koi (*Cyprinus carpio*) undergoing unilateral gonadectomy. *Journal of the American Veterinary Medical Association* 2013;243(6):882–890.
14. Davis, M.R., Mylniczenko, N., Storms, T., Raymond, F. and Dunn, J.L. Evaluation of intramuscular ketoprofen and butorphanol as analgesics in chain dogfish (*Scyliorhinus retifer*). *Zoo Biology* 2006;25(6):491–500.
15. Pening, M.R., Vaughan, D.B., Fivaz, K. and McEwan, T. Chemical immobilization of elasmobranchs at uShaka Sea World, Durban South Africa. In: *Elasmobranch Husbandry Manual II*. M. Smith, D. Warmolts, D. Thoney, R. Hueter, M. Murray and J. Ezcurra, eds. Ohio Biological Survey Inc., 2017; chap. 32.
16. Nordgreen, J., Tahamtani, F.M., Janczak, A.M. and Horsberg, T.E. Behavioural effects of the commonly used fish anaesthetic tricaine methanesulfonate (MS-222) on zebrafish (*Danio rerio*) and its relevance for the acetic acid pain test. *PLOS ONE* 2014;9(3):e92116.
17. Mettam, J.J., Oulton, L.J., McCrohan, C.R. and Sneddon, L.U. The efficacy of three types of analgesic drugs in reducing pain in the rainbow trout, *Oncorhynchus mykiss*. *Applied Animal Behaviour Science* 2011;133(3):265–274.
18. Nordgreen, J., Garner, J.P., Janczak, A.M., Ranheim, B., Muir, W.M. and Horsberg, T.E. Thermonociception in fish: Effects of two different doses of morphine on thermal threshold and post-test behaviour in goldfish (*Carassius auratus*). *Applied Animal Behaviour Science* 2009;119(1):101–107.
19. Nordgreen, J., Bjørge, M.H., Janczak, A.M., Poppe, T., Koppang, E.O., Ranheim, B. and Horsberg, T.E. The effect of morphine on changes in behaviour and physiology in intraperitoneally vaccinated Atlantic

salmon (*Salmo salar*). *Applied Animal Behaviour Science* 2013;145(3):129–137.

20. Fredholm, D.V., Mylniczenko, N.D. and KuKanich, B. Pharmacokinetic evaluation of meloxicam after intravenous and intramuscular administration in Nile tilapia (*Oreochromis niloticus*). *Journal of Zoo and Wildlife Medicine* 2016;47(3):736–742.

21. Alvarez, F.A., Rodriguez-Martin, I., Gonzalez-Nuñez, V., de Velasco, E.M., Sarmiento, R.G. and Rodríguez, R.E. New kappa opioid receptor from zebrafish *Danio rerio*. *Neuroscience Letters* 2006;405(1):94–99.

22. Bartfield, J.M., Gennis, P., Barbera, J., Breuer, B. and Gallagher, E.J. Buffered versus plain lidocaine as a local anesthetic for simple laceration repair. *Annals of Emergency Medicine* 1990;19(12):1387–1389.

23. Bazin, J.E., Massoni, C., Bruelle, P., Fenies, V., Groslier, D. and Schoeffler, P. The addition of opioids to local anaesthetics in brachial plexus block: The comparative effects of morphine, buprenorphine and sufentanil. *Anaesthesia* 1997;52(9):858–862.

24. Arnold, J.E., Matsche, M.A. and Rosemary, K. Preserving whole blood in formalin extends the specimen stability period for manual cell counts for fish. *Veterinary Clinical Pathology* 2014;43(4):613–620.

25. Harms, C.A., Bakal, R.S., Khoo, L.H., Spaulding, K.A. and Lewbart, G.A. Microsurgical excision of an abdominal mass in a gourami. *Journal of the American Veterinary Medical Association* 1995;207(9):1215.

26. Murray M.J. Fish surgery. *Seminars in Avian and Exotic Pet Medicine*. 2002;11(4):246–257.

27. Lewbart, G.A. and Harms, C.A. Building a fish anesthesia delivery system. *Exotic DVM* 1999;1(2):25–28.

28. Harms, C.A. and Lewbart, G.A. Surgery in fish. *Veterinary Clinics of North America: Exotic Animal Practice* 2000;3(3):759–774.

29. Wildgoose, W.H. Fish surgery: An overview. *Fish Veterinary Journal* 2000;5:22–36.

30. Harms, C.A. Surgery in fish research: Common procedures and postoperative care. *Lab Animal* 2005;34(1):28–34.

31. Weber, E.P., Weisse, C., Schwarz, T., Innis, C. and Kilde, A. Anesthesia, diagnostic imaging, and surgery of fish. *Compendium on Continuing Education for the Practicing Veterinarian* 2009;31(2):E1–E9.

32. Roberts, H.E. Surgery and wound management in fish. In: *Fundamentals of Ornamental Fish Health*. H.E. Roberts, ed. Wiley-Blackwell, Ames, 2010; pp. 185–196.

33. Sladky, K.K. and Clarke, E.O. Fish surgery: Presurgical preparation and common surgical procedures. *Veterinary Clinics of North America: Exotic Animal Practice* 2016;19(1):55–76.

34. Nematollahi, A., Bigham, A.S., Karimi, I. and Abbasi, F. Reactions of goldfish (*Carassius auratus*) to three suture patterns following full thickness skin incisions. *Research in Veterinary Science* 2010;89(3):451–454.

35. Govett, P.D., Harms, C.A., Daczm, K.E., Marsh, J.C. and Mem, J.W. Effect of four different suture materials on the surgical wound healing of loggerhead sea turtles, *Caretta caretta*. *Journal of Herpetological Medicine and Surgery Volume* 2004;14(4).

36. Anderson, E.T., Davis, A.S., Law, J.M., Lewbart, G.A., Christian, L.S. and Harms, C.A. Gross and histologic evaluation of 5 suture materials in the skin and subcutaneous tissue of the California sea hare (Aplysia californica). *Journal of the American Association for Laboratory Animal Science* 2010;49:64.

37. Hurty, C.A., Brazik, D.C., Law, J.M., Sakamoto, K. and Lewbart, G.A. Evaluation of the tissue reactions in the skin and body wall of koi (*Cyprinus carpio*) to five suture materials. *The Veterinary Record* 2002;151(11):324–328.

38. Harms, C.A. and Lewbart, G.A. The veterinarian's role in surgical implantation of electronic tags in fish. *Reviews in Fish Biology and Fisheries* 2011;21(1):25–33.

39. Jepsen, N., Koed, A., Thorstad, E.B. and Baras, E. Surgical implantation of telemetry transmitters in fish: How much have we learned? In: *Aquatic Telemetry*. E.B. Thorstad, I.A. Fleming and T.F. Naesje, eds. Springer, Netherlands, 2002; pp. 239–248.

40. Cavin, J. Seventeen month suture retention with severe tissue response in a sea raven (*Hemitripterus americanus*). *Proceedings of the IAAAM*, 2011.

41. Baras, E. and Jeandrain, D. Evaluation of surgery procedures for tagging eel Anguilla anguilla (L.) with biotelemetry transmitters. *Advances in Invertebrates and Fish Telemetry*. Springer, Netherlands, 1998; pp. 107–111.

42. Clarke, E.O. Topical application of misoprostol and phenytoin gel for treatment of dermal ulceration in teleosts. *47th IAAAM Conference*, Virginia Beach, Virginia, May 21–26, 2016.

43. Fontenot, D.K. and Neiffer, D.L. Wound management in teleost fish: Biology of the healing process, evaluation, and treatment. *Veterinary Clinics of North America: Exotic Animal Practice* 2004;7(1):57–86.

44. Mylniczenko, N.D. and Travis, E.K. Techniques using BioSISt in aquatic animals. *AAZV Conference*, San Diego, California, 2004; pp. 104–107.

45. Stamper, M.A. Immobilization of elasmobranchs. In: *The Elasmobranch Husbandry Manual*. M. Smith, D. Warmolts, D. Thoney and R. Hueter, eds. Ohio Biological Survey, Columbus, OH, 2004; p. 293.

46. Boylan, S.M., Camus, A., Gaskins, J., Oliverio, J., Parks, M., Davis, A. and Cassel, J. Spondylosis in a green moray eel, *Gymnothorax funebris* (Ranzani 1839), with swim bladder hyperinflation. *Journal of Fish Diseases* 2016;40:963–969.

47. Mylniczenko, N.D. and Clauss, T. Pharmacology of elasmobranchs: Updates and techniques. In: *Elasmobranch Husbandry Manual II*. M. Smith, D. Warmolts, D. Thoney, R. Hueter, M. Murray and J. Ezcurra, eds. Ohio Biological Survey, Columbus, OH, 2017; p. 298.

48. Weisse, C., Weber, E.S., Matzkin, Z. and Klide, A. Surgical removal of a seminoma from a black sea bass. *Journal of the American Veterinary Medical Association* 2002;221(2):280–283.

49. Mandelman, J.W. and Skomal, G.B. Differential sensitivity to capture stress assessed by blood acid–base status in five carcharhinid sharks. *Journal of Comparative Physiology B* 2009;179(3):267.

50. Hyatt, M.W., Anderson, P.A., O'Donnell, P.M. and Berzins, I.K. Assessment of acid–base derangements among bonnethead (*Sphyrna tiburo*), bull (*Carcharhinus leucas*), and lemon (*Negaprion brevirostris*) sharks from gillnet and longline capture and handling methods. *Comparative Biochemistry and Physiology Part A: Molecular & Integrative Physiology* 2012;162(2):113–120.

51. Harter, T.S., Morrison, P.R., Mandelman, J.W., Rummer, J.L., Farrell, A.P., Brill, R.W. and Brauner, C.J. Validation of the i-STAT system for the analysis of blood gases and acid–base status in juvenile sandbar shark (*Carcharhinus plumbeus*). *Conservation Physiology* 2015;3(1):002.

52. Naples, L.M., Mylniczenko, N.D., Zachariah, T.T., Wilborn, R.E. and Young, F.A. Evaluation of critical care blood analytes assessed with a point-of-care portable blood analyzer in wild and aquarium-housed elasmobranchs and the influence of phlebotomy site on results. *Journal of the American Veterinary Medical Association* 2012;241(1):117–125.

53. Boylan, S.M., Harms, C.A., Waltzek, T., Law, J.M., Garner, M., Cassell, J., Fatzinger, M.H. and Govett, P. Clinical report: Hyperplastic adipose lids in mackerel scad, *Decapterus macarellus* (Cuvier). *Journal of Fish Diseases* 2011;34(12):921–925.

54. Harms, C.A., Christian, L.S., Burrus, O., Hopkins, W.B., Pandiri, A.K., Law, J.M., Wolf, K.N., Butler, C.M. and Lewbart, G.A. Cryotherapy for removal of a premaxillary mass from a chain pickerel using an over-the-counter wart remover. *Exotic DVM* 2008;10:15–17.

55. Angelidis, P., Vatsos, N.I. and Karagiannis, D. Surgical excision of skin folds from the head of a goldfish *Carassius auratus* (Linnaeus 1758). *Companion Animal Practice* 2009;19:49.

56. Stamper, M.A. and Norton, T. Ovariectomy in a brook trout (*Salvelinus fontinalis*). *Journal of Zoo and Wildlife Medicine* 2002;33(2):172–175.

57. Raidal, S.R., Shearer, P.L., Stephens, F. and Richardson, J. Surgical removal of an ovarian tumour in a koi carp (*Cyprinus carpio*). *Australian Veterinary Journal* 2006;84(5):178–181.

58. George, R.H., Gangler, R., Steeil, J. and Baine, K. Ovariectomy of sub-adult southern rays (*Dasyatis americana*) as a tool for managing an exhibit population. *Drum and Croaker* 2014;19.

59. Wildgoose, W.H. Exenteration in fish. *Exotic DVM* 2007;9:25–29.

60. Nadelstein, B., Bakal, R. and Lewbart, G.A. Orbital exenteration and placement of a prosthesis in fish. *Journal of the American Veterinary Medical Association* 1997;211(5):603–606.

61. Adamovicz, L., Lewbart, G. and Gilger, B. Phacoemulsification and aspiration for cataract management in a dollar sunfish, *Lepomis marginatus* (Holbrook)—A case report. *Journal of Fish Diseases* 2015;38:1089–1092.

62. Boylan, S.M., Camus, A., Gaskins, J., Oliverio, J., Parks, M., Davis, A. and Cassel, J. Spondylosis in a green moray eel, *Gymnothorax funebris* (Ranzani 1839), with swim bladder hyperinflation. *Journal of Fish Diseases* 2017;40:963–969.

63. Clode, A.B., Harms, C., Fatzinger, M.H., Young, F., Colitz, C. and Wert, D. Identification and management of ocular lipid deposition in association with hyperlipidaemia in captive moray eels, *Gymnothorax funebris* (Ranzani), *Gymnothorax moringa* (Cuvier) and *Muraena retifera* (Goode and Bean). *Journal of Fish Diseases* 2012;35(9):683–693.

64. Colitz, C.M., Manire, C.A., Clode, A. and Harms, C. Surgical management of lipid keratopathy in green moray eels (*Gymnothorax funebris*) under human care. *Veterinary Ophthalmology* 2011;14(6):422.

65. Greenwell, M.G. and Vainisi, S.J. Surgical management of lipid keratopathy in green moray eels (*Gymnothorax funebris*). *Proceedings of the Association of Reptilian and Amphibian Veterinarians* 1994;155–157.

66. Helm, W.T. and Tyus, H.M. Influence of coating type on retention of dummy transmitters implanted in rainbow trout. *North American Journal of Fisheries Management* 1992;12(1):257–259.

67. Mulcahy, D.M. Surgical implantation of transmitters into fish. *ILAR Journal* 2003;44(4):295–306.

68. Martin, S.W., Long, J.A. and Pearsons, T.N. Comparison of survival, gonad development, and growth between rainbow trout with and without surgically implanted dummy radio transmitters. *North American Journal of Fisheries Management* 1995;15(2):494–498.

69. Jepsen, N., Mikkelsen, J.S. and Koed, A. Effects of tag and suture type on survival and growth of brown trout with surgically implanted telemetry tags in the wild. *Journal of Fish Biology* 2008;72(3):594–602.

70. Groocock, G.H. Pathologic changes associated with coelomic radio-transmitter expulsion and a modified surgical technique for implantation. *New York Chapter of the American Fisheries Society Annual Meeting*, Lake Placid, NY, February 1–3, 2012.

71. Perry, R.W., Adams, N.S. and Rondorf, D.W. Buoyancy compensation of juvenile Chinook salmon implanted with two different size dummy transmitters. *Transactions of the American Fisheries Society* 2001;130(1):46–52.

72. Royal, L.W., Grafinger, M.S., Lascelles, B.D., Lewbart, G.A. and Christian, L.S. Internal fixation of a femur fracture in an American bullfrog. *Journal of the American Veterinary Medical Association* 2007;230(8):1201–1204.

73. Lloyd, R. and Sham, N. Surgical repair of mandibular symphyseal fractures in three Silver Arowana (*Osteoglossum bicirrhosum*) using interfragmentary wire. *Journal of Zoo and Wildlife Medicine* 2014;45(4):926–930.

74. Preziosi, R., Gridelli, S., Borghetti, P., Diana, A., Parmeggiani, A., Fioravanti, M.L., Marcer, F., Bianchi, I., Walsh, M. and Berzins, I. Spinal deformity in a sandtiger shark, *Carcharias taurus* Rafinesque: A clinical–pathological study. *Journal of Fish Diseases* 2006;29(1):49–60.

75. Anderson, P.A., Huber, D.R. and Berzins, I.K. Correlations of capture, transport, and nutrition with spinal deformities in sandtiger sharks, *Carcharias taurus*, in public aquaria. *Journal of Zoo and Wildlife Medicine* 2012;43(4):750–758.

76. Tate, E.E., Anderson, P.A., Huber, D.R. and Berzins, I.K. Correlations of swimming patterns with spinal deformities in the sand tiger shark, *Carcharias taurus*. *International Journal of Comparative Psychology* 2013;26:75–82.

77. Lewbart, G. Stabilization of scoliosis in two koi. *Immunity* 1993;61:5309–5314.

78. Lewbart, G.A., Stone, E.A. and Love, N.E. Pneumocystectomy in a Midas cichlid. *Journal of the American Veterinary Medical Association* 1995;207(3):319–321.

79. Zoller, G., Santamaria-Bouvier, A., De Lasalle, J., Cluzel, C., Duhamelle, A., Larrat, S. and Maccolini, E. Total pneumocystectomy in a telescope Goldfish (*Carassius auratus*) with fungal pneumocystitis. *Journal of Exotic Pet Medicine* 2017;26:19–28.

THERAPEUTANTS FOR FISH

GRACE A. KARREMAN*, PATRICIA S. GAUNT†,
RICHARD G. ENDRIS‡, AND NICK SAINT-ERNE§

Aquatic animal practice by veterinarians ranges from the individual pet to public aquarium displays, to wildlife/fisheries, to large-scale commercial aquaculture. Aquatic veterinary medicine shares fundamental principles with terrestrial animal practice, including basic principles of veterinary medicine and legal requirements for practice. However, the aquatic veterinarian's pharmaceutical tool kit contains only a fraction of the drugs approved for terrestrial species. Developing drugs for minor species ("minor use/minor species," or "MUMS"), especially food-fish species, is particularly challenging due to very small markets and stringent drug approval requirements. Having fewer tools at hand, aquatic food-fish veterinarians must be aware of their legal responsibilities and have a working knowledge of the pharmaceutical products legally marketed for aquatic species.

The purpose of this chapter is to give the aquatic animal veterinarian information and context to make decisions about pharmaceutical treatments for fish species. Legally marketed products for food fish in the United States under the U.S. Food and Drug Administration (FDA) Center for Veterinary Medicine (CVM) are discussed in the first section, and the second section addresses drugs and regulations in the European Union (EU), Norway and Canada, with an appendix at the end of the book for other countries in which the information was publicly available but not complete. The third section of this chapter will discuss treatments in ornamental and tropical fish species. This chapter will cover

drugs and treatment methods for these drugs, but will not cover pesticides and other compounds.

THERAPEUTANTS FOR AQUATIC SPECIES IN THE UNITED STATES

The FDA definitions for drugs and associated terms can be found on its website along with a document titled "FDA Answers Your Questions About Fish Drugs" that provides a good overview.[1] This website lists all drugs and medicated articles, grouped by method of administration (immersion, injectable, in medicated feed). The U.S. Fish and Wildlife Service's Aquatic Animal Drug Approval Partnership (AADAP) Program's "Guide to Using Drugs, Biologics and Other Chemicals in Aquaculture" provides practical information for drug treatments.[2]

Veterinarians can also contact the individual drug sponsors, extension agents and various veterinary and nonveterinary websites for further information.

The FDA's "Letter to Aquaculture Professionals" details the benefits of FDA approvals for drugs and medicated articles for food fish.[3] New animal drug applications (NADAs) for aquatic species, as for terrestrial species, have undergone rigorous scrutiny and scientific testing to prove they are safe and effective, including establishing tissue residues and withdrawal times.

Approved drugs

Under the Food, Drug, and Cosmetic Act (FDCA), a new animal drug is a drug that is not recognized as safe

---

* Food fish, United States and Canada

† Food fish, United States

‡ Food fish, Europe, Norway and Canada

§ Ornamental fish

and effective for use in animals, and can only be legally marketed if it is approved, conditionally approved, or indexed.[4] Drugs and/or medicated articles have been approved to treat aquatic species for bacterial gill disease, columnaris disease, saprolegniasis (i.e., fungus on fish eggs), bacterial hemorrhagic septicemia, furunculosis, ulcer disease, gaffkemia in lobsters and various parasites.[5] **Table 19.1** lists the current NADAs and medicated articles grouped by treatment indication. The table also includes one approved drug for anesthesia, six for marking fish and one as an aid to spawning.

Conditional approval

Although none are currently listed for aquatic species, drugs for minor species may be marketed under "conditional approval."[6] The drug sponsor must have already met all safety requirements for the drug approval and have shown "substantial evidence of effectiveness." The sponsor is given one year to accumulate data and demonstrate substantial evidence of efficacy.

Investigational new animal drugs (INADs)

An investigational new animal drug (INAD) exemption is a process by which the FDA authorizes and controls the use of unapproved drugs by qualified researchers to investigate safety and effectiveness. In turn, data generated through studies is expected to lead to a new animal drug approval.[7,8] Compassionate INADs for aquatic species may be obtained through the U.S. Fish and Wildlife Service's AADAP program, which administers the National INAD Program (NIP).[9,10] The program allows both public and private agencies in all 50 states exemptions to use INADs for health and maintenance of aquatic species. In turn, all data generated by INAD users is submitted by AADAP to the FDA in support of new animal drug approvals. INADs currently available through the AADAP program are listed in **Table 19.2**. Other public partners include UMESC (Upper Midwest Environmental Sciences Center) and NRSP-7 (National Research Support Program No. 7).[11,12]

Low regulatory priority drugs

The FDA has deemed certain compounds classified as new animal drugs for use in aquaculture species to be of "low regulatory priority" (LRP) under its enforcement discretion, e.g., povidone-iodine used to disinfect eggs (Ovadine®) and salt (sodium chloride).[13] These substances must only be used (1) for the stated indications; (2) at the stated levels; (3) in accordance with best management practices (BMPs); (4) so as not to result in an adverse effect on the environment, e.g., must comply with applicable environmental requirements such as National Pollution Discharge Elimination System (NPDES) permits; and (5) be of an appropriate grade for use in food animals. **Table 19.3** lists all LRP compounds.

Deferred regulatory status drugs

Copper sulfate and potassium permanganate have been given "deferred regulatory status," pending further evaluation by CVM. Both can be used to treat external protozoan or metazoan infestations as well as external bacterial or fungal infections on fish.[13]

Veterinary Feed Directive

The Veterinary Feed Directive (VFD) applies to animal drugs approved by the FDA that are to be used in feeds under the supervision of a veterinarian.[14] Citing antimicrobial resistance, the FDA finalized a guidance document in 2012 outlining its policy regarding judicious use of antimicrobial drugs medically important in human medicine and used in food-producing animals.[15] Medically important antimicrobial drugs (MIADs) could only be used to ensure animal health and could only be administered with veterinary oversight. With the institution of the Second (revised) VFD Rule in 2015, the FDA changed the marketing status of all feeds containing MIADs from over-the-counter (OTC) to VFD. Beginning in January 2017, this changed the status of several animal antimicrobials from OTC to VFD drugs for medicated feed products and from OTC to prescription drugs for medications administered in water.[14,16] For aquaculture medicated feeds, this rule affected Terramycin® (oxytetracycline dihydrate) and Romet® (sulfadimethoxine/ormetoprim). Aquaflor® (florfenicol) was already a VFD drug under the First VFD Rule when it was initially marketed in 2005.

The Second VFD Rule specified the roles and responsibilities of the veterinarian, client and distributor of the VFD feed. As part of the responsibilities, the veterinarian must be licensed in the

Table 19.1 FDA-approved drugs and medicated feed articles by treatment indication

INDICATION[a]	DRUG	APPROVED SPECIES	WITHDRAWAL PERIOD	DOSE
Infectious disease or parasites				
Bacterial gill disease	Chloramine-T Powder for Immersion HALAMID AQUA® NADA 141-423	Immersion—For the control of mortality in freshwater-reared salmonids due to bacterial gill disease associated with *Flavobacterium* spp.	0 days	12–20 mg/L
	35% PEROX-AID® for Immersion (Hydrogen peroxide) NADA 141-255	Immersion—For control of mortality in freshwater-reared salmonids due to bacterial gill disease associated with *Flavobacterium branchiophilum*	0 days	50–100 mg/L
Bacterial hemorrhagic septicemia	Terramycin® 200 for Fish (Oxytetracycline dihydrate) NADA 038-439	Oral via feed—For the control of bacterial hemorrhagic septicemia caused by *Aeromonas liquefaciens* in salmonids as well as catfish	21 days	2.5–3.75 g/100 lb of fish/10 days
Cold water disease	Aquaflor® Type A Medicated Article (florfenicol) NADA 141-246	Oral via feed—For the control of mortality in freshwater-reared salmonids due to cold water disease associated with *Flavobacterium psychrophilum*	15 days	10–15 mg/kg of fish/day for 10 consecutive days
	Terramycin® 200 for Fish (Oxytetracycline dihydrate) NADA 038-439	Oral via feed—For the control of mortality in freshwater-reared salmonids due to cold water disease associated with *Flavobacterium psychrophilum*	21 days	2.5–3.75 g/100 lb of fish for 10 days
Columnaris disease	Chloramine-T Powder for Immersion HALAMID AQUA® NADA 141-423	Immersion—For the control of mortality in Walleye and freshwater-reared warm water finfish due to external columnaris disease associated with *Flavobacterium columnare*	0 days	12–20 mg/L
	35% PEROX-AID® for Immersion (Hydrogen peroxide) NADA 141-255	Immersion—For control of mortality in freshwater-reared cold water finfish and channel catfish due to external columnaris disease associated with *Flavobacterium columnare (Flexibacter columnaris)*	0 days	50–100 mg/L
	Aquaflor® Type A Medicated Article (florfenicol) NADA 141-246	Oral via feed—For the control of mortality in freshwater-reared finfish due to columnaris disease associated with *Flavobacterium columnare*	15 days	10–15 mg/kg/day for 10 days
	Terramycin® 200 for Fish (Oxytetracycline dihydrate) NADA 038-439	Oral via feed—For control of mortality in freshwater-reared *Oncorhynchus mykiss* due to columnaris disease associated with *Flavobacterium columnare*	21 days	3.75 g/100 lb of fish/10 days

(Continued)

Table 19.1 (*Continued*) **FDA-approved drugs and medicated feed articles by treatment indication**

INDICATION[a]	DRUG	APPROVED SPECIES	WITHDRAWAL PERIOD	DOSE
Enteric septicemia	Aquaflor® Type A Medicated Article (florfenicol) NADA 141-246	Oral via feed—For the control of mortality in catfish due to enteric septicemia associated with *Edwardsiella ictaluri*	15 days	10 mg/kg of body weight for 10 days
	Romet-30® and Romet TC NADA 125-933	Oral via feed—For the control of mortality in catfish due to enteric septicemia associated with *Edwardsiella ictaluri* susceptible to the sulfadimethoxine and ormetoprim combination	3 days	50 mg/kg of body weight for 5 days
Furunculosis and ulcer disease	Terramycin® 200 for Fish (Oxytetracycline dihydrate) NADA 038-439	Oral via feed—For the control of ulcer disease in salmonids caused by *Haemophilus piscium* and furunculosis caused by *Aeromonas salmonicida*	21 days	2.5–3.75 g/100 lb of fish/10 days
	Aquaflor® Type A Medicated Article (florfenicol) NADA 141-246	Oral via feed—For the control of mortality in freshwater-reared salmonids due to furunculosis associated with *Aeromonas salmonicida*	15 days	10–15 mg/kg of fish/day for 10 days
	Romet-30® and Romet TC NADA 125-933	Oral via feed—For the control of mortality in salmonids (trout and salmon) due to furunculosis associated with *Aeromonas salmonicida*	42 days	50 mg/kg body weight for 5 days
Gaffkemia	Terramycin® 200 for Fish (Oxytetracycline dihydrate) NADA 038-439	Oral via feed—For the control of gaffkemia in lobsters caused by *Aerococcus viridans*	30 days	1 g/lb of med feed for 5 days
Parasiticides (various)	Formalin-F™ (formalin: approximately 37% by weight of formaldehyde gas) NADA 137-687	Immersion—For the control of external protozoa (*Chilodonella* spp., *Costia* spp., *Epistylis* spp., *Ichthyophthirius* spp. *Scyphidia* spp. and *Trichodina* spp.) and the monogenetic trematode parasites (*Cleidodiscus* spp., *Dactylogyrus* spp., and *Gyrodactylus* spp.) on all finfish and for the control of protozoan parasites (*Bodo* spp., *Epistylis* spp., and *Zoothamnium* spp.) on penaeid shrimp	0 days	Up to 170 μL/L (above 50°F); below 50°F, up to 250 μL/L
	Formacide-B (formalin) Aqueous solution ANADA 200-414	Immersion—For the control of external protozoa (*Chilodonella* spp., *Costia* spp., *Epistylis* spp., *Ichthyophthirius* spp., *Scyphidia* spp., and *Trichodina* spp.), and the monogenetic trematode parasites (*Cleidodiscus* spp., *Dactylogyrus* spp., and *Gyrodactylus* spp.) on cultured finfish and for the control of external protozoan parasites (*Bodo* spp., *Epistylis* spp., and *Zoothamnium* spp.) on penaeid shrimp	0 days	Up to 170 μL/L (above 50°F); below 50°F, up to 250 μL/L 50–100 μL/L for penaeid shrimp
	PARASITE-S® (formalin) NADA 140-989	Immersion—All finfish and penaeid shrimp. Finfish external protozoa: *Chilodnella* spp., *Costia* spp., *Epistylis* spp., *Ichthyophthirius* spp., *Scyphidia* spp., *Trichodina* spp. Finfish monogenetic trematode parasites: *Cleidodiscus* spp., *Dactylogyrus* spp., and *Gyrodactylus* spp. Penaeid shrimp external protozoan parasites: *Bodo* spp., *Epistylis* spp. and *Zoothamnium* spp.	0 days	Up to 170 μL/L (above 50°F); below 50°F, up to 250 μL/L 50–100 μL/L for penaeid shrimp

(*Continued*)

Table 19.1 (Continued) FDA-approved drugs and medicated feed articles by treatment indication

INDICATION[a]	DRUG	APPROVED SPECIES	WITHDRAWAL PERIOD	DOSE
Pseudomonas disease	Terramycin® 200 for Fish (Oxytetracycline dihydrate) NADA 038-439	Oral via feed—For the control of pseudomonas disease in salmonids and catfish	21 days	2.5–3.75 g/100 lb of fish/10 days
Saprolegnia (fungus on fish eggs)	Formalin-F™ (formalin: approximately 37% by weight of formaldehyde gas) NADA 137-687	Immersion—For the control of fungi of the family Saprolegniaceae on all finfish eggs	0 days	1000–2000 µL/L for 15 minutes
	35% PEROX-AID® for Immersion (Hydrogen peroxide) NADA 141-255	Immersion—For the control of mortality in freshwater-reared finfish eggs due to saprolegniasis	0 days	50–100 mg/L
	Formacide-B (formalin) Aqueous solution ANADA 200-414	Immersion—For the control of fungi of the family Saprolegniaceae in finfish eggs	0 days	1000–2000 µL/L for 15 minutes
	PARASITE-S® (formalin) NADA 140-989	Immersion—For the control of fungi of family Saprolegniaceae on all finfish eggs	0 days	1000–2000 µL/L for 15 minutes
Streptococcal septicemia	Aquaflor® Type A Medicated Article (florfenicol) NADA 141-246	Oral via feed—For the control of mortality in freshwater-reared warm water finfish due to streptococcal septicemia associated with *Streptococcus inaie*	15 days	2.5–3.75 g/100 lb of fish for 10 days
Treatment type				
Anesthetics	Tricaine-S (Tricaine methane sulfonate) ANADA 200-226	Immersion—Temporary immobilization of fish, amphibians and other aquatic cold-blooded animals (i.e., manual spawning, fish stripping, weighing, measuring, marking, surgical operations, transport, photography, research)	21 days	10–1000 mg/L; species-dependent

(Continued)

Table 19.1 (*Continued*) **FDA-approved drugs and medicated feed articles by treatment indication**

INDICATION[a]	DRUG	APPROVED SPECIES	WITHDRAWAL PERIOD	DOSE
Marking fish	Oxymarine™ (Oxytetracycline hydrochloride) NADA 130-435	Immersion—To mark skeletal tissues, most often otoliths, of all finfish fry and fingerlings for identification	0 days[b]	200–700 mg/L (buffered) for 2–6 hours
	Oxytetracycline HCL Soluble Powder - 343 (Oxytetracycline hydrochloride) NADA 200-247	Immersion—For marking of skeletal tissue of finfish fry and fingerlings for identification	0 days[b]	200–700 mg/L (buffered) for 2–6 hours
	PENNOX 343(Oxytetracycline hydrochloride) ANADA 200-026	Immersion—For marking of skeletal tissue of finfish fry and fingerlings for identification	0 days[b]	200–700 mg/L (buffered) for 2–6 hours
	Terramycin-343 (Oxytetracycline HCl) Soluble Powder NADA 008-622	Immersion—For marking of skeletal tissue of finfish fry and fingerlings for identification	0 days[b]	200–700 mg/L (buffered) for 2–6 hours
	TETROXY Aquatic (Oxytetracycline hydrochloride) ANADA 200-460	Immersion—To mark skeletal tissues, most often otoliths, of all finfish fry and fingerlings for identification	0 days[b]	200–700 mg/L (buffered) for 2–6 hours
	Terramycin® 200 for Fish (Oxytetracycline dihydrate) NADA 038-439	Oral via feed—For marking of skeletal tissue in Pacific salmon	21 days	2.5–3.75 g/100 lb of fish/10 days
Spawning aid	Chorulon® (Chorionic gonadotropin) NADA 140-927	Injectable—Indicated as an aid in improving spawning function in male and female brood finfish	0 days (broodfish treated per label directions)	50–510 I.U/lb/BW (male); 67–1816 I.U./lb/ BW (female)

[a] From http://www.fda.gov/AnimalVeterinary/DevelopmentApprovalProcess/Aquaculture/ucm132954.htm.

[b] For all oxytetracycline HCl approved uses 0-day withdrawal times.

Table 19.2 **Publicly available INADs through the AADAP program**

DELIVERY METHOD	TARGET PATHOGENS/INDICATIONS/OBJECTIVES
Medicated feeds	
Aquaflor® (active ingredient: 50% florfenicol)	Bacterial pathogens susceptible to florfenicol, exclusive of already approved claims Control mortality caused by certain bacterial diseases in lobsters
Terramycin® 200 for Fish (active ingredient: oxytetracycline dihydrate)	Bacterial pathogens susceptible to oxytetracycline, exclusive of already approved claims Bacterial shrimp pathogens susceptible to oxytetracycline
SLICE® (active ingredient: emamectin benzoate)	Parasitic copepods
17α-methyl testosterone	Feed additive to larval tilapia to produce populations comprising over 90% male fish
Immersion	
35% PEROX-AID® (active ingredient: 35% hydrogen peroxide)	Ectoparasites of the genera *Ambiphrya, Chilodonella, Dactylogyrus, Epistylis, Gyrodactylus, Ichthyobodo, Ichthyophthirius, Trichodina, Trichophrya, Argulus, Salmincola, Lernaea*, and *Ergasilus* in freshwater fish species; and of the genera *Neobenedenia, Amyloodinium, Cryptocaryon*, and *Uronema* in marine fish species
HALAMID® (active ingredient: chloramine-T) Actamide® (active ingredient: chloramine-T)	External flavobacteriosis
PENNOX® 343 (active ingredient: oxytetracycline hydrochloride)	Bacterial pathogens susceptible to oxytetracycline
Reward® (active ingredient: diquat)	External flavobacteriosis (e.g., bacteria responsible for bacterial gill disease and external columnaris)
Sedatives	
AQUI-S®20E (active ingredient: eugenol)	To establish the effectiveness and safety of AQUI-S® 20E as an anesthetic/sedative in a variety of fish species under a variety of environmental conditions
Spawning aids	
Common carp pituitary	To establish the effectiveness of Common Carp Pituitary to induce gamete maturation in a variety of fish species
Catfish pituitary	To establish the efficacy of Channel Catfish Pituitary on gamete maturation in a variety of catfish species
Luteinizing hormone-releasing hormone analog (LHRHa)	To establish the effectiveness of LHRHa to induce gamete maturation in a variety of fish species
Ovaplant® (active ingredient: salmon gonadotropin-releasing hormone analogue (sGnRHa))	To establish the effectiveness of sGnRHa/Ovaplant® to induce gamete maturation in a variety of fish species
OvaRH®	To determine the efficacy of OvaRH® (sGnRHa) injection to induce gamete maturation (ovulation and spermiation) in a variety of fish species
Marking	
SE-MARK® (active ingredient: calcein)	To establish the effectiveness of calcein to mark fin rays, scales, otoliths, and other calcified fish or selected mussel tissues via immersion baths
Injectables	
Erymicin 200 Injectable (active ingredient: erythromycin)	Bacterial kidney disease (BKD; *Renibacterium salmoninarum*)

Source: https://www.fws.gov/fisheries/aadap/inads.html.

Table 19.3 **Drugs of low regulatory priority**

COMPOUND	DOSE/INDICATION
Parasiticides/protozoacides	
Acetic acid	Parasiticide for fish
Calcium oxide	Used as an external protozoacide for fish
Garlic (whole form)	Used for control of helminth and sea lice infestations of marine salmonids
Magnesium sulfate	Used to treat external monogenean infestations and external crustacean infestations in fish
Onion (whole form)	Used to treat external crustacean parasites and to deter sea lice from infesting external surface of salmonids at all life stages
Sodium chloride	Used as a parasiticide
Osmotic regulation/transport	
Calcium chloride	Used to increase the hardness of water for holding and transporting fish
Ice	Used to reduce metabolic rate of fish during transport
Potassium chloride	Used as an aid in osmoregulation; relieves stress and prevents shock
Sodium chloride	Used as an osmoregulatory aid for the relief of stress and prevention of shock
Anesthetics	
Carbon dioxide gas	Used as an anesthetic for fish
Sodium bicarbonate	Used to introduce carbon dioxide into the water to anesthetize fish
Egg treatments	
Calcium chloride	Used to increase water calcium concentration to ensure proper egg hardening
Fuller's earth	Used to reduce the adhesiveness of fish eggs
Papain	Used to remove the gelatinous matrix of fish egg masses
Povidone-iodine	Egg surface disinfectant
Sodium sulfite	Used to improve egg hatchability
Urea and tannic acid	Used to denature the adhesive component of fish eggs
Thiamine deficiency	
Thiamine hydrochloride	Used to prevent or treat thiamine deficiency in salmonids

Source: http://www.fda.gov/downloads/AnimalVeterinary/GuidanceComplianceEnforcement/PoliciesProceduresManual/UCM046931.pdf
Note: The compounds have undergone review by the Food and Drug Administration and have been determined to be new animal drugs of low regulatory priority.

state where he/she is practicing and have a valid veterinary–client–patient relationship (VCPR). The VCPR is defined by either state or federal requirements.[17] If the state veterinary licensing board VCPR guidelines meet or exceed the federal guidelines, the state licensing board's criteria determine the VCPR in that state. For those state boards that do not meet the basic federal guidelines for a VCPR, the federal guidelines are in effect. A federal VCPR requires that the veterinarian has recently examined or has

knowledge of the history of the fish in question and that appropriate clinical judgment is applied to determine treatment of the fish. The veterinarian must use appropriate medication with prompt initiation of the treatment using the correct regime and be available for emergency or follow-up treatment of the fish.

In addition to the VCPR responsibilities, a veterinarian must maintain appropriate records that include either a written hard copy or electronic version of the VFD order and issue a copy of the written order either in paper or electronic form to both the client and the distributor. All VFD orders must be retained by the veterinarian, the client, and distributor, and be available for FDA inspection for 2 years after issuance. Electronic submission of VFD orders must be compliant with the requirements of 21 CFR Part 11. Although electronic VFD submission programs decrease paperwork, monthly access and account maintenance fees are charged. E-mailing a portable document format (PDF) or sending a facsimile (fax) of a VFD order to a distributor is not considered an electronic copy of a VFD order because hard-written originals are associated with each of these.

In compliance with the VCPR agreement, the client must agree to cooperate with the veterinarian and follow the dose rate, duration, expiration date and withdrawal times of the VFD drug. As part of the distributor's responsibilities, he or she must notify the FDA of the intent to distribute VFD medicated feed prior to distribution. A distributor must have a signed VFD order prior to the delivery of the VFD feed to a client.

A VFD order issued by a veterinarian must contain the following information:[18]

1. Name of the VFD drug.
2. Name and address of the client and veterinarian.
3. Identification of the animals to be treated, including the species, production class, approximate number, and location.
4. Disease being treated.
5. Amount of drug to be mixed in the feed.
6. Duration of use and feeding directions according to the label.
7. Warning or cautionary statements such as residue warning.
8. Date of ordering the drug and veterinarian's signature.
9. Expiration date of the VFD order.
10. Number of refills (not currently permitted for fish).
11. Affirmation of intent for combination VFD drugs.
12. Statement "Extra-label use of VFD drugs is prohibited."

The expiration of a VFD order is up to 6 months at the discretion of the veterinarian, even though the maximum duration of use for the currently approved VFD drugs is 10 consecutive days. An expiration date of up to 6 months offers an advantage to aquaculture facilities where medicated feed availability is limited, and it can take several weeks to obtain medicated feed during an outbreak. If a veterinarian is allowed to order and a producer is allowed to retain a VFD drug for this extended period, it might provide a potential advantage in fighting future bacterial outbreaks in areas where there are limited feed mills producing VFD feeds. If the VFD order expires prior to completing the antimicrobial's duration of use, the veterinarian must issue a new order for the client to be able to finish feeding the medicated feed. Currently, there are no refills allowed for aquaculture VFD medicated feeds. If the same pond of fish that was treated with a VFD drug breaks again with the bacterial disease post-treatment, a new order must be issued by a veterinarian for the client to use additional VFD feed.

The information required under "affirmation of intent" (no. 11 of the VFD order) applies to whether the veterinarian will allow additional drugs combined with the VFD drug in the feed. Because there are no combination drugs approved for aquaculture at this time, regulations require a veterinarian to state under "affirmation of intent" that no other animal drugs are allowed in the VFD feed.

The statement "extra-label use of VFD drugs is strictly prohibited" (no. 12 of the VFD order) is required on the aquaculture VFD order form. However, the FDA recently issued a revision to the "Extra-label Use of Medicated Feeds for Minor Species" Compliance Policy Guide (CPG Section 615.115) that will allow extra-label use of VFD medicated feeds for minor species including fish if the animal's health is threatened or death may result from lack of treatment.[19] The FDA has indicated it will use enforcement discretion for extra-label use of VFD medicated feeds in minor species because delivery of medication to fish through feed is the most practical method of administration. The extra-label use of medicated feeds is limited to farmed or confined fishes. No regulatory action will be taken against the veterinarian, client or feed distributor for this extra-label use if the guidelines of CPG 615.115 are followed. Some of the stipulations are that there must be a VCPR in place and the medicated feeds used are only those approved for use in aquatic species.

Prepopulated VFD forms issued by drug sponsors facilitate the VFD order process for veterinarians and allow them to quickly complete the remaining information. Veterinarians can also create their own VFD forms as long as all required information is included. Generic versions of the VFD form can be downloaded from the FDA's website and from the members' section of the American Veterinary Medical Association's website.[20,21] Alternatively, private companies such as GlobalVetLink (https://www.globalvetlink.com) or RxExpress (www.dvm-rxexpress.com) offer electronic submission of VFD orders that comply with federal regulations.

VFD drugs supplied by pharmaceutical companies are Type A medicated articles. These are the most concentrated forms of the drugs and cannot be fed undiluted. The currently marketed VFD Type A medicated articles for aquaculture are florfenicol, oxytetracycline and sulfadimethoxine/ormetoprim. Type B medicated feeds contain concentrates of the drug in feed and also cannot be fed undiluted. Type C medicated feed is manufactured by diluting the Type A medicated article or Type B or C medicated feed with feed to the final concentration that is fed to fish. For clarification, drugs are categorized according to their potential to create unsafe drug residues in edible tissues of major species (e.g., cattle, pigs), with Category I having the lowest potential and Category II having the highest. Category I drugs do not require a preslaughter withdrawal period in major species at the lowest dose rate that they are approved. Category II drugs either do require a withdrawal period in major species at the lowest dose rate that they are approved, or are regulated on a "no-residue" basis or with zero tolerance.

Under the new VFD rules, oxytetracycline dihydrate (Terramycin®) remains a Category I medicated article (even though a preslaughter withdrawal time is required in fish), and florfenicol (Aquaflor®) and sulfadimethoxine/ormetoprim (Romet®) remain Category II medicated articles. According to 21 CFR Sec. 558.4(b)(1), a medicated feed mill license is not required to manufacture Type B or C (finished) medicated feed from the Category I Type A medicated article.[22] Oxytetracycline dihydrate (Terramycin®) medicated feed can be blended on farms and in unlicensed and licensed feed fills. For florfenicol (Aquaflor®) and sulfadimethoxine/ormetoprim (Romet®), only a licensed feed mill can manufacture medicated feed with the Category II Type A medicated article. However, Romet® TC is a Category II Type B medicated feed and does not require a medicated feed mill license to manufacture Type B or Type C medicated feed.[22] Romet® TC can be blended on farms, and in unlicensed and licensed feed fills.

Extra-label use of approved drugs in food fish

Extra-label drug use (ELDU) refers to use in another species, for another disease or condition, at different frequencies, at different dose rates, or deviation from the withdrawal times listed on the label. Prior to 1994 the FDCA did not allow ELDU of animal drugs. The Animal Medicinal Drug Use Clarification Act (AMDUCA) of 1994 amended the FDCA to allow the ELDU of animal drugs under certain circumstances when there were no approved treatment options available. It did not permit the extra-label use of medicated feeds. However, with minor species such as fish, medicated feed was the most practical route of drug administration. Subsequently, in its compliance policy guide (CPG 615.115, 2016), the FDA stated that it would use enforcement discretion for ELDU of medicated feed for minor species.[19] Under the terms of this CPG, if a veterinarian determined that the health of the fish was at risk, the fish were suffering or death could ensue from failure to treat, the veterinarian could prescribe medicated feeds in an extra-label manner, with the following certain conditions.

- The ELDU of medicated feed must be used only under the written authorization of a licensed veterinarian in a VCPR. Under the federal VCPR, the client must agree to comply with the veterinarian's instructions.
- The extra-label use of medicated feed for aquaculture is limited to only those that are FDA-approved for use in aquatic species.
- The feed must be manufactured and labeled according to approved methods.
- Extra-label use of medicated feeds is for use only in fish confined to enclosures such as ponds, tanks, and aquariums, and not for treatment of fish in the wild.

- It may be used only to treat conditions threatening the health of the fish and may not be used for weight gain or for production purposes.
- Adverse events (AEs) must be reported to the FDA within 10 days of occurrence.

For ELDU of a VFD medicated feed, the veterinarian must complete a written recommendation (separate from the VFD order) for the medical rationale for extra-label use including the diagnosis, drug selection, dose rate, duration and withdrawal period.[19] This must be dated within 6 months of the date of issuance of the VFD order. The veterinarian must keep a paper or electronic copy of the recommendation and provide a copy to the client. The VFD order must be completed with the following information noted in the space allotted for "Special instructions" for ELDU.

- "This VFD is issued in accordance with CPG 615.115."
- The actual species and indication for which the medicated feed is being used, if different than on the VFD form. If it is the same species or indication listed on the VFD prepopulated form, this should be circled.
- If the withdrawal time for a species of fish is different from the withdrawal time listed on the VFD order form, it should be extended beyond that of the approved use based on scientific information.

Both the ELDU written recommendation and VFD order must be signed and dated by the veterinarian within 6 months prior to use.[19] Paper or electronic copies of both must be available for FDA inspection for 2 years. Some states require retention of medical records for longer than 2 years. Thus, veterinarians should check with their state licensing boards for the period of time they are required to maintain records. The veterinarian must issue a copy of the VFD order and written recommendation to the producer and only a copy of the VFD order to the distributor of the feed.

The producer should keep complete records of medicated feeds received including labels, invoices and dates fed. The identity of the fish receiving medicated feeds should be traceable. The withdrawal times for the use of the medications must be met to avoid unsafe residues in edible tissues. The producer should use the feed in accordance with federal, state and local laws and have permits from the NPDES if required. These records must be maintained for 2 years from the date of delivery of the feed and be available for FDA inspection. The distributor of the VFD medicated feeds used for ELDU must observe regulations discussed under VFD drugs, i.e., delivery of the VFD feed to a client after receipt of the VFD order and record retention for 2 years, subject to FDA inspection. Manufacturers of VFD feeds for ELDU must manufacture according to Good Manufacturing Practices and retain manufacturing records for 1 year for FDA inspection.

When VFD orders are inspected by FDA field personnel, enforcement action can be taken against the veterinarian, client, distributor, and/or manufacturer of the medicated feed for extra-label use in which there is use or manufacture that is inconsistent with the policies. For example, during a course of inspection, if VFD records indicated that a producer inadvertently observed a shortened withdrawal time of 10 days for florfenicol medicated feed (instead of the 15 days as per the approved label), enforcement action may be taken. A warning letter from the FDA may be followed by seizure of products, misdemeanor fines, or criminal prosecution for more serious offenses.

Compounding

Compounding in veterinary medicine is the customized preparation of a drug or therapeutant for an animal patient.[23] This is done when there is no FDA-approved product that can meet the animal's medicinal needs. One class of compounded drugs is formulated from FDA-approved products but used in an extra-label manner, e.g., the use of praziquantel (approved for the treatment of tapeworms in dogs) for tapeworm treatment in ornamental fish. Under the Food, Drug, and Cosmetic Act (FDCA) and AMDUCA, veterinarians are allowed the ELDU of approved drugs for compounding. The second class of compounded drugs, those formulated from "bulk substances," which are raw (non-FDA-approved) active pharmaceutical ingredients, is currently illegal for animal drugs under FDCA.[23,24] Individual state licensing boards regulate how the compounded product is administered and dispensed by veterinarians.

Veterinarians should check with their state licensing boards to ensure they are in compliance.

Record keeping

Veterinarians must maintain written and/or electronic medical records on their patients' medical diagnoses, treatments and progress. As discussed under VFD drugs, the federal law requires that VFD orders be retained for 2 years subject to FDA inspection. However, most states require veterinarians to retain all medical records for a period of 3–5 years after the last patient examination or treatment.[25] Veterinarians must also consider statutes of limitation that are applicable in malpractice lawsuits and retain records accordingly. State veterinary practice acts are interpreted and enforced by each state's veterinary medical board. Veterinarians with legal questions pertaining to practice and record keeping should contact the veterinary medical board in the state(s) in which they are licensed.

Adverse event reporting

Veterinarians must report adverse events in aquatic species, including side effects and issues with efficacy or safety.[26] Veterinarians should report to the drug company directly (contact information is usually found on the product label) and may report to the FDA as well.[27] If the adverse event involves ELDU of a VFD medicated feed, the veterinarian is obligated to report this to the FDA within 10 days of occurrence.[19] The report to the FDA includes a standardized form submitted through the FDA's electronic gateway.[28] The report should include information about the aquatic animals, a description of the event(s) and the veterinarian's evaluation. Drug companies are required to report all adverse events to the FDA.

Tissue residues

Following the stated withdrawal times on the label minimizes the possibility of detecting violative residues in edible tissues of aquatic species. The veterinarian who writes an ELDU VFD or prescription is responsible for setting the withdrawal time. Useful resources for determining residue depletion of medications and withdrawal times in fishes include the Phish-Pharm database, the Food Animal Residue Avoidance Databank (FARAD), and Chapter 11 of the HACCP Guidelines.[29–31]

High enforcement priority drugs

Drugs that have a high enforcement priority in food animals and those that are forbidden from extra-label use are listed in **Table 19.4**. This may be due to a combination of safety concerns including safety to the target animal, the environment, or humans who may come in contact with the drug either directly (e.g., during the administration of the drug) or indirectly (e.g., via consumption of an animal with drug residues or exposure to effluent water containing the drug).[13]

Antimicrobial stewardship

With few approved antimicrobials that have a limited number of indications in aquatic veterinary medicine practice, it behooves veterinarians and their clients to be judicious in their use and to ensure that they remain efficacious for treatment of bacterial diseases. On January 1, 2017, changes to CVM regulations mandated that the veterinarian be involved with all in-feed medicated articles (i.e., drugs) including those that had previously been over-the-counter (OTC). With so much responsibility on veterinarians to safeguard antibiotic efficacy, the American Veterinary Medical Association (AVMA), American Fisheries Society (AFS) Fish Culture Section, and other veterinary and fish health organizations issued guidelines to ensure judicious use of antibiotics.[2,32] These include but are not limited to:

1. Perform a necropsy and bacterial culture with antimicrobial susceptibility testing on isolates for clinically ill and freshly dead fish. Document and maintain all findings related to a more specific diagnosis. This will improve efficacy of antibiotics for treatment of diseased fish by ensuring appropriate use, while supplying information for aquatic animal bacteria susceptibility databanks.
2. Use FDA-approved antibiotics for fish species and bacterial diseases for which the drug is approved, if available, in accordance with the label. This should be used at the lowest approved dose rate, for the full duration of use, with the approved withdrawal times. Antibiotics with Gram-negative activity should be rotated periodically to help decrease resistance.

Table 19.4 **Drugs forbidden for use in food animals in the United States**
Drugs the FDA considers to be of high enforcement priority
Chloramphenicol
Fluoroquinolones and Quinolones
Malachite green
Nitrofurans
Steroid hormones
Drugs prohibited by the FDA from being used in an extra-label manner in food animals
Chloramphenicol
Clenbuterol
Diethylstilbestrol (DES)
Dimetridazole
Fluoroquinolones
Furazolidone
Glycopeptides
Ipronidazole
Nitrofurazone
Other nitroimidazoles
Phenylbutazone in female dairy cattle 20 months of age or older
Sulfonamide drugs in lactating dairy cattle (except approved use of sulfadimethoxine, sulfabromomethazine, and sulfaethoxypyridazine)

Source: http://www.fda.gov/downloads/AnimalVeterinary/GuidanceComplianceEnforcement/PoliciesProceduresManual/UCM046931.pdf

3. Re-evaluate diseased fish if clinical signs continue following the complete duration of treatment. If it is determined that additional VFD medicated feed is needed, the veterinarian must issue a new order.[14] There are no allowed refills for VFD aquaculture drugs, and once fish have been treated for the full duration of use, these fish cannot receive additional VFD medicated feed unless a new order is written.

4. Under the Second VFD rule, veterinarians are allowed to write VFD orders for medicated feeds with an expiration date of up to 6 months. Veterinarians should exercise good clinical judgment to ensure the expiration date of the order is reasonable. When choosing the expiration date, the veterinarian should consider the species of fish, the bacterial disease, the time of year, the duration of the disease outbreaks, the infrastructure of the local fish industry, and whether medicated feed is readily available. For example, if a catfish farmer located in the southern United States has outdoor ponds that break with enteric septicemia of catfish (ESC) in September, and he requests a VFD order for medicated feed with a 6-month expiration date, the veterinarian should consider that within 3 months, the pond temperatures will be too cold for bacterial disease outbreaks and for the fish to feed at the commonly blended medicated feeding rates of 3%. The veterinarian should be familiar with the availability of medicated feed within his/her locale. If the infrastructure is such that medicated feed is readily available, long expiration dates are unnecessary.

5. Use drugs in an extra-label fashion only under a VCPR in compliance with AMDUCA and CPG 615.115.[33,34] When ELDU is used for food fish not listed on the label, a prolonged preslaughter withdrawal time should be observed based on scientific information as available. Resources for withdrawal times can be found through Phish-Pharm, FARAD and the FDA.[19,30,35]

6. Ensure that facility personnel comply with the proper use of VFD medicated feeds, other antibiotics and medications.[32]

7. Ensure that the client is engaged in BMPs to prevent bacterial outbreaks. Preventative practices include use of available bacterial vaccines; maintenance of optimal water quality; good fish nutrition; and good pond husbandry, such as weed control, parasite control, vector control, low stocking density, and biosecurity.[2]

8. Ensure that the facility complies with local, state and federal environmental regulations for water discharge, including antibiotic concentration limits.

9. Educate veterinarians about bacterial susceptibility to antibiotics used in aquatic animals. Resources include the Clinical & Laboratory Standards Institute (CLSI), CVM, AVMA, Phish-Pharm, World Aquatic Veterinary Medical Association (WAVMA), and fisheries journals.[35–39]

Administration of treatment

Treatment of aquatic species includes proper diagnostic workup, a treatment plan, and knowledge of the pharmacology of the intended therapeutant and key water quality parameters. Technical support and/or information is available from the drug sponsors as well as extension agents, feed company veterinarians, and academic and field veterinarians and nonveterinary fish health professionals. The U.S. Fish and Wildlife Service AADAP program and the AFS Fish Culture Section have practical publications including their "Guide to Using Drugs, Biologics and Other Chemicals in Aquaculture."[2] The AADAP guide includes a treatment calculator to expedite dose and administration calculations. Good practices include but are not limited to the following.

Before treating:[2,40]

1. Accurately determine the water volume, flow rate and temperature.

2. Accurately determine the number and total weight of fish to be treated.

3. Confirm the identity, expiration date and active ingredient concentration of the regulated product to be applied.

4. Double-check treatment calculations. Beware of confusion from mixing metric and English units.

5. Have aeration devices ready for use if needed.

6. If treated water is to be discharged, make sure all appropriate permits are in place and regulatory authorities have been notified.

7. If unfamiliar with the fish species, the therapeutant in that particular fish species, or water conditions, should conduct a bioassay on a small group of fish before treating the population of fish to be treated.

When treating:

1. Dilute the regulated product with rearing water before applying it (or follow product directions).

2. Ensure the regulated product is well mixed and evenly applied to the population of fish to be treated.

3. Observe fish closely and frequently during treatment for signs of distress.

4. Monitor temperature and dissolved oxygen levels in the water during treatment.

5. Except for oral treatments, discontinue feeding during treatment. Fish are unlikely to feed during treatment, and uneaten feed will pollute the system and may reduce the efficacy of some treatments.

6. Discontinue treatment and restore normal culture conditions if fish become distressed.

After treating:

1. Observe fish frequently for at least 24 hours following treatment.

2. Do not stress treated fish for at least 48 hours.

3. Recheck fish to determine efficacy of treatment.

The following are examples of immersion, injectable, and in-feed treatments.

Immersion treatments

Tricaine-S (Syndel USA, Ferndale, Washington) is a short-acting anesthetic encompassing a variety of uses and a wide dose range to accommodate various species and desired levels of anesthesia. Tricaine-S is a powder that is dissolved in water with a dose-dependent fish response. Directions for use and the package insert are detailed on several websites.[41] The volume of the container, tank or pond must be calculated prior to treatment.[2] The drug sponsor's website provides a treatment calculator.[42] Generally, fish are dipped or netted out of their holding vessel and treated in a container outside of their normal environment. The premeasured anesthetic powder is added to the container of water prior to the fish being added. Fish may also be treated in a static bath *in situ* in their original container. The drug is strongly acidic, and in water with poor buffering capacity, it is wise to use a buffer such as sodium bicarbonate. The fish are placed in fresh, clean water to reverse anesthetic properties of the drug. A comprehensive discussion of sedation and anesthesia in fishes can be found in Chapter 17, and a presentation on anesthesia and tranquillization of aquatic animals can be found on the World Aquatic Veterinary Medical Association's website.[43] AADAP's "Quick Desk Reference Guide to Approved Drugs for Use in Aquaculture" also provides an example of treatment calculations.[44]

Injection treatments

Chorulon (Merck Animal Health, Madison, New Jersey) is a freeze-dried preparation of human chorionic gonadotropin approved for use as an aid in improving spawning function in fishes. When reconstituted with the accompanying sterile diluent, each 10 mL vial contains 10,000 IU chorionic gonadotropin.[45] Chorulon should be administered as an intramuscular injection. Any single injection should be administered, depending on the fish species, at a dose of 110–1122 IU/kg body weight (bw) for males and 147–3995 IU/kg bw for females.[45,46] Fish should be sedated or restrained manually while injecting to decrease trauma.[47] Intramuscular injections are administered in the epaxial muscles along the back of a fish with a 22–25 gauge needle inserted along one side of the dorsal fin between scales while angling the needle toward the head. The needle should be inserted forward from the injection site during administration so that the injected material does not leak from under the skin. Intramuscular injections can also be given in epaxial muscles by inserting the needle on the dorsal midline behind the dorsal fin, and angling it forward to either side in the muscles. Because skin in this area does not have scales, it is easier to insert the needle without accidently piercing or removing a scale by the needle.

In-feed treatments

Aquaflor® (Merck Animal Health, Madison, New Jersey) is a Type A medicated article that contains 50% florfenicol. The drug florfenicol (FFC) is fed by diluting it in fish feed to produce a Type C medicated feed. Florfenicol dose rates and the amount of drug to be mixed in the feed can be found on the sponsor's prepopulated VFD order forms.

Scenario: Fingerling catfish located in two 10-acre earthen ponds are diagnosed with enteric septicemia of catfish (ESC) by a licensed veterinarian based on clinical signs and lesions. The bacterial isolate *Edwardsiella ictaluri* is found to be susceptible to the antibiotic florfenicol. The fish are approximately 6 inches in length, weigh 58.8 pounds/1000 fish, and feed at a rate of 3% body weight. The farmer estimates there are a total of 2,100,000 fish in the two ponds, and he requests a VFD from his veterinarian to use florfenicol medicated feed. If the veterinarian agrees this is the best treatment, the veterinarian must then complete a VFD order and provide a copy to the client and distributor of the feed.

Below are explanations for calculations required on the VFD order form that the veterinarian must complete.

1. Calculate an approximate total weight of the fish in the ponds:

    Multiply the number of fish times the weight of 1000 fish = 123,480,000 then divide by 1000 = 123,480 pounds of catfish.

2. Calculate the total quantity of Aquaflor® medicated feed needed*:

---

* Under the Second VFD Rule, the veterinarian does not need to calculate the quantity of feed. The veterinarian only has to list the production class and approximate number of fish. The client and distributor calculate the actual quantity of feed for each VFD order. This section is supplied as optional information that the veterinarian may enter on the order form at the client's request.

If fish are feeding at a 3% body weight, then the amount of feed they are eating is 3% × 123,480 pounds = 3704 pounds of feed/day. The duration of use for Aquaflor is 10 days so the fish will need a total of 37,040 pounds (or 18.52 tons) of medicated feed for the complete treatment.

3. Calculate the amount of Aquaflor needed for medicated feed:

A dose rate of 10 mg florfenicol/kg bw is the dose rate that is sufficient to treat most ESC-diseased catfish. To calculate the ppm of florfenicol in feed, the following formula is used:

PPM (mg/kg) in feed = Dose rate ÷ % Feeding rate[48]

$$PPM = 10 \text{ mg/kg} \div 0.03$$

The medicated feed should contain 333 mg FFC/kg feed, which is equivalent to 300 grams of FFC/ton of feed. This number must be entered by the veterinarian in "g/ton" on the VFD form under "Drug level" (see following chart). Since Aquaflor is a 50% premix, this requires 666 mg (or 0.67 g) Aquaflor/kg feed. To prepare a ton of feed medicated at this dose rate, 0.67 g of Aquaflor is multiplied by 907.18 kg feed (number of kg in a ton) = 607.81 g/ton, which is equivalent to 1.32 lb of Aquaflor/ton of feed.

The drug sponsor of florfenicol (and other VFD drug sponsors) supplies this information on its prepopulated forms, but if such forms are not available, the veterinarian can calculate this number based on the aforementioned formula. Following is a portion of a prepopulated form excerpted from an Aquaflor VFD form provided by Merck Animal Health, Inc.

If a farmer's feed bin or storage area does not hold the entire quantity of medicated feed ordered, he/she can have the distributor deliver it in several shipments. The VFD feed must be fed for the entire duration of use, which is 10 consecutive days. A 15-day preslaughter withdrawal time must be observed for food-sized fish. If fish in this pond break again with ESC post-florfenicol treatment and the farmer wishes to treat again with medicated feed, a new VFD order must be issued by the veterinarian since there are no refills for VFD medicated feeds used in aquaculture. The VFD medicated feed treating fish from other ponds on the farm may also not be used to retreat the fish in the previously treated pond.

THERAPEUTANTS FOR AQUATIC SPECIES IN THE EU, NORWAY AND CANADA

Internationally, few drugs used in aquatic food species (i.e., aquaculture) have undergone a full review and approval process by government authorities. The role of veterinarians with regard to aquaculture drugs varies greatly between countries, from legislative requirements for veterinary prescriptions to no veterinary involvement. Drugs not specifically approved for use in fish are frequently available through off-label (extra-label) use. Off-label use may include restrictions that vary within regions and between countries.

Information regarding approved drugs for aquaculture species and the role of veterinarians will be presented for the European Union (EU), Norway and Canada in this section. References for additional countries in which information is available are listed at the end of this chapter. General principles regarding veterinary responsibilities discussed earlier in the chapter apply, as do those discussed for therapeutant administration.

FEEDING RATE % BIOMASS	FFC CONCENTRATION IN FEED GRAMS/TON		AMOUNT OF AQUAFLOR® PER TON OF FEED POUNDS		BIOMASS OF FISH MEDICATED/ TON OF FEED/10-DAY TREATMENT POUNDS
	Dose: 10 mg/kg	Dose: 15 mg/kg	Dose: 10 mg/kg	Dose: 15 mg/kg	
1%	908	1,362	4.0	6.00	20,000
2%	454	681	2.0	3.00	10,000
3%	300	450	1.32	1.98	6,666

Europe

Volume 5 of "The Rules Governing Medicinal Products in the European Union" contains the legislation for veterinary medicinal products in the EU.[49] Drugs may be approved by a member state (i.e., country), mutual recognition between states, by a centralized route including all EU member states, or a decentralized route. As a result, approvals and market authorizations vary among member states. Most countries in the EU require a veterinary prescription for approved aquaculture drugs. However, only salmon are classified as a "major species" for which a maximum residue limit (MRL) for drug residues in flesh have been established. All other fish species are considered "minor species."[50] Presently there are 19 drugs licensed in the EU for finfish (including Salmonidae). **Table 19.5** lists these drugs.[51,52] There are 23 other drugs approved for "all food-producing animals" in the EU that could be prescribed for use in fish via the "cascade system."

Table 19.5 **Drugs available for use in aquaculture in Europe[a]**

	REGULATORY APPROVAL		
DRUG	**FINFISH OR SALMONIDAE**	**ALL FOOD-PRODUCING ANIMALS**	**MAXIMUM RESIDUE LIMIT (MRL) (μG/KG)**
Amoxicillin		X	50
Ampicillin		X	50
Azagly-nafarelin	X		None
Azamethiphos	X		None
Benzocaine	X		None
Benzylpenicillin		X	50
Bronopol	X		None
Chlortetracycline		X	100
Cloxacillin		X	300
Colistin		X	150
Cypermethrin	X		50
Danofloxacin		X	100
Deltamethrin	X		10
Difloxacin		X	300
Diflubenzuron	X		1000
Doxycycline		X	100
Emamectin	X		100
Enrofloxacin		X	100
Erythromycin		X	200
Florfenicol	X		100
Flumequine	X		600
Gentamicin	X		50
Hexaflumuron	X		500
Isoeugenol	X		6000
Lufenuron	X		1350
Neomycin		X	500

(Continued)

Table 19.5 (Continued) Drugs available for use in aquaculture in Europe[a]

| | REGULATORY APPROVAL | | |
DRUG	FINFISH OR SALMONIDAE	ALL FOOD-PRODUCING ANIMALS	MAXIMUM RESIDUE LIMIT (MRL) (μG/KG)
Oxacillin		X	300
Oxolinic acid		X	100
Oxytetracycline		X	100
Paromomycin		X	500
Sarafloxacin	X		30
Somatosalm	X		None
Spectinomycin		X	300
Sulfonamides		X	100
Teflubenzuron	X		500
Tetracycline		X	100
Thiamphenicol		X	50
Tilmicosin		X	50
Tosylchloramide sodium	X		None
Tricaine mesylate	X		None
Trimethoprim		X	50
Tylosin		X	100

Source: http://ec.europa.eu/health//sites/health/files/files/eudralex/vol-5/reg_2010_37/reg_2010_37_en.pdf; http://www.ema.europa.eu/ema/index.jsp?curl=pages/regulation/document_listing/document_listing_000165.jsp.
[a] Exclusive of dietary supplements.

Veterinarians in the EU may prescribe off-label use under the cascade system under the following conditions: (1) no veterinary medicine is authorized for the indication or fish species in that member state; (2) the prescribing veterinarian takes direct responsibility for the animals (i.e., fish) under his/her care; and (3) treatment will avoid unacceptable suffering in those animals (fish). A minimum withdrawal period of 500 degree days (number days withdrawal = 500 × water temperature °C) applies to all "off-label use" and/or compounded (extemporaneously prepared) substances under this system.[53]

Figure 19.1 diagrams the cascade procedure (decision tree) of the EU, while Appendix D provides a detailed example of the cascade system in the United Kingdom.[50]

Medicated feed containing a premix of veterinary medicines requires a veterinary prescription. Directive 90/167/EEC of the EU governs the conditions for mixing veterinary medicine into feed, its marketing and use across the EU.[54]

Norway

Legislation concerning medicinal products for animals and humans is similar in Norway and the EU, due to the extended EEA (European Economic Association) agreement between the EU and EFTA (European Free Trade Association) countries (except Switzerland) in the field of medicinal products. All veterinary medicinal products (VMPs) used for fish treatment in Norway must be prescribed by an authorized veterinarian/fish health biologist. **Table 19.6** lists the approved drugs for aquaculture in Norway.[55,56]

EU Cascade Procedure

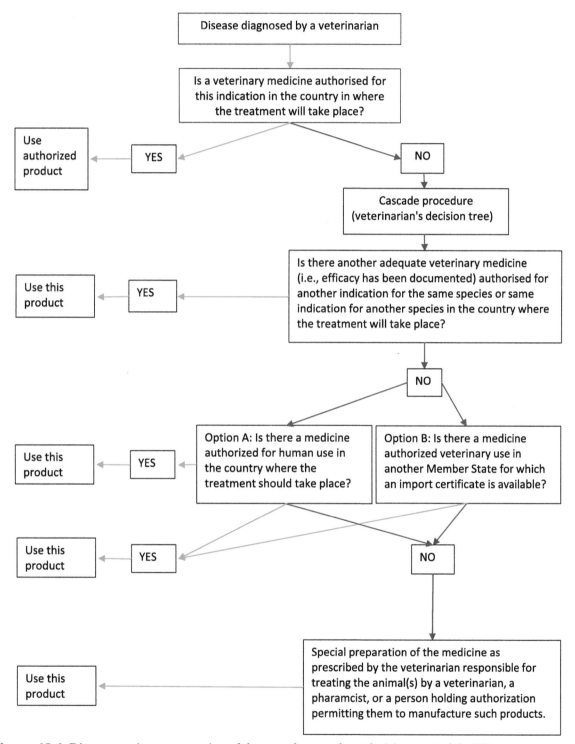

Figure 19.1 Diagrammatic representation of the cascade procedure (decision tree) of the EU.

Table 19.6 **Drugs approved for aquaculture in Norway**

PRODUCT NAME/PHARMACEUTICAL FORM	ACTIVE INGREDIENT	FISH SPECIES
Antibacterials		
Aquaflor vet premix 50% for medicated feed	Florfenicol	Salmon
Floraqpharma vet medicated pellets 2 g/kg	Florfenicol	Salmon
Oxolinsyre vet medicated pellets 5 g/kg	Oxolinic acid	Salmonidae
Tribrissen powder for medicated feed	Sulfadiazine/trimethoprim	Finfish
Sea Lice Treatment		
Alpha Max vet solution 10 mg/mL	Deltamethrin	Salmon
Azasure vet 500 mg/g powder for suspension	Azamethiphos	Atlantic salmon
Betamax vet solution 50 mg/mL	Cypermethrin	Salmon
Ektobann vet medicated pellets 2 g/kg	Teflubenzuron	Salmon
Hydrogen peroxide concentrate for bath solution 49.5% w/w	Hydrogen peroxide	Atlantic salmon
Paramove concentrate for bath solution 49.5% w/w	Hydrogen peroxide	Salmon
Releeze (former Lepsidon) vet medicated pellets 0.6 g/kg	Diflubenzuron	Salmon
Salmosan vet 500 mg/g powder for suspension	Azamethiphos	Atlantic salmon
SLICE vet premix 0.2% for medicated feed	Emamectin	Salmon and rainbow trout
Anesthetics		
AQUI-S vet concentrate for bath solution 540 mg/mL	Isoeugenol	Salmon and rainbow trout
Benzoak vet concentrate for bath solution 200 mg/mL	Benzocaine	Salmon and trout
Finquel vet powder for bath solution 1000 mg/g	Tricaine	Salmon, rainbow trout and cod
Tricaine Pharmaq vet powder for bath solution 1000 mg/g	Tricaine	Finfish
Antifungal		
Pyceze concentrate for bath solution 500 mg/mL	Bronopol	Salmon and rainbow trout

Source: List of approved aquaculture drugs in Norway, https://legemiddelverket.no/Documents/Veterin%C3%A6rmedisin/Fisk%20og%20legemidler/Pharmaceuticals-fish-MA-2017-09-22.pdf; Pharmaceuticals for fish holding marketing authorization in Norway (not all products may actually be marketed) are listed in the Norwegian regulations, under Fish Medicine https://legemiddelverket.no/Documents/Veterin%C3%A6rmedisin/Fisk%20og%20legemidler/General%20information-%20medicines%20for%20fish-2016-07-06.pdf.

All medicinal products for fish are prescription-only medicines (POMs) in Norway, regardless of the legal status of the medicinal product.

- *Marketing authorization (MA)*: Following an application from the manufacturer or his authorized representative, the product is approved by the Norwegian Medicines Agency (NoMA) to be put on the market after an assessment of quality, safety and efficacy according to the national requirements.
- *Special exemption (SE)*: Permission given to individual authorized veterinarians/fish health biologists to use proprietary

medicinal products without an MA in Norway. Veterinarians/fish health biologists must apply for an SE to NoMA.

- *Exemption from marketing authorization (MA) under exceptional circumstances*: Following an application from the manufacturer or his authorized representative, NoMA may under exceptional circumstances grant a special permit for a product to be put on the market without an MA. Such permits may be given on the condition that the manufacturer agrees to certain commitments. The permits are only valid for a specified time period, but may be renewed.

- *Veterinary medicinal product extemporaneously prepared*: Prepared in a pharmacy according to a prescription from an authorized veterinarian/fish health biologist.
- *Medicated feed*: Medicated feed must be manufactured by a feed mill authorized by NoMA. Good manufacturing practices (GMPs) are required.

All prescribers must report prescriptions to the Norwegian Food Safety Authority, the competent authority responsible for quality control of fish products, including the residue control and monitoring program.[57] The Norwegian legislation concerning residues of VMPs in food intended for human consumption is similar to the EU legislation. Withdrawal periods are based on EU-approved maximum residue limits (MRLs). All pharmacologically active substances administered to fish intended for human consumption must be listed in Commission Regulation (EU) No 37/2010 (Replacing Annex I, II or III of Council Regulation 2377/90) for at least one food-producing species.[58] According to EU and Norwegian legislation, veterinarians/fish health biologists may use medicinal products holding MA for other species for the treatment of fish, and also veterinary medicinal products prepared extemporaneously, in accordance with the cascade principle of Article 11 in Directive 2001/82/EC, as amended by Directive 2004/28/EC.[59]

This provision is implemented in Norway in Volume 4 and Volume 5 of the Regulation on Use of Medicinal Products in Animals of 2007-01-16.[60] Use of products approved in other EEA (European Economic Area) countries in accordance with the cascade system requires permission from NoMA as a special exemption. The NoMA is responsible for setting withdrawal periods for VMPs holding a Norwegian marketing authorization (MA). When products not holding MA in Norway are used, the veterinarian/fish health biologist is responsible for setting adequate withdrawal periods. As in the EU's cascade principle, the withdrawal period when using medicines off label for fish must be greater than 500 degree days (e.g., greater than 50 days at water temperature 10°C).[51] The MRL requirement must be met.

Canada

Approved drugs for aquatic food species

Canada's Food and Drugs Act and Regulations (FDAR), administered by Health Canada, governs the approval of drugs in Canada including aquaculture drugs. Twelve drugs are currently approved for immersion or in-feed treatments for various indications in aquatic food fish including anesthesia, antibacterials, fungicides and parasiticides.[61] **Table 19.7** lists the drugs available for aquatic food fish in Canada by use.[62,63]

Veterinarians are licensed by the provinces in Canada. They must maintain a valid VCPR as defined by Health Canada. Veterinary prescriptions are required for application of certain approved drugs to aquaculture species in Canada, i.e., the anesthetic MS-222 (tricaine methanesulfonate) as well as antibiotics applied in-feed. In accordance with recent Health Canada policies on antimicrobial use, antibiotics previously on the Medicated Ingredient Brochure (MIB) (e.g., oxytetracycline hydrochloride [oxytetracycline dehydrate] 75 mg/kg fish/day) now require veterinary prescription.[64]

Fewer options are available to the veterinarian in Canada than in the United States for accessing drugs not approved for aquaculture. There is no minor use/minor species legislation, and although an investigational new drug (IND) category is part of the drug approval process, there is no public program analogous to the U.S. Fish and Wildlife Service's AADAP program and no alternate avenues such as conditional approval or low regulatory priority drugs. However, the veterinarian may request Health Canada approval to import drugs not available in Canada under the Emergency Drug Release (EDR) program.[65] Nonveterinary researchers may also apply for Health Canada approval under the Experimental Studies Certificate (ESCert).[66]

The veterinarian may also prescribe extra-label use (ELDU). The veterinarian must have a valid VCPR. Veterinary extra-label use of drugs is defined by Health Canada as the "use or intended use of a drug approved by Health Canada in an animal in a manner not in accordance with the label or package insert. It also includes the use of all unapproved drugs, including unapproved bulk active pharmaceutical ingredients (APIs) and compounded drugs." The major concerns with ELDU are violative tissue

Table 19.7 Drugs approved for aquaculture in Canada

TREATMENT TYPE	PRODUCT NAME/ PHARMACEUTICAL FORM	ACTIVE INGREDIENT	FISH SPECIES	INDICATION	WITHDRAWAL TIME (DAYS)
Anesthetics					
	Aqualife TMS DIN 02168510	Tricaine methanesulfonate	Salmonids	Anesthesia or sedation	5
Infectious Diseases					
Fungicide (*Saprolegnia* spp.)	PARASITE-S DIN 02118114	Formalin	Salmonids—eggs	Fungi (Saprolegniaceae)	None
	PEROX-AID DIN 02238749	Hydrogen peroxide	Salmonids—eggs	Fungal infections	None
	Pyceze DIN 02298880	Bronopol	Salmonids—eggs	Fungi (Saprolegniaceae)	None
	Pyceze DIN 02298880	Bronopol	Salmonids—Atlantic salmon and rainbow trout (fry and smolts/fingerlings)	Fungal infections (*Saprolegnia* spp.)	None
Fish egg disinfectant (various organisms)	Ovadine DIN 02305712	Povidone-iodine	Salmonids (genera *Salmo* and *Oncorhynchus*)—eggs	Fish egg disinfectant; *Aeromonas salmonicida*, *Chondrococcus columnaris*, *Cytophaga psychrophila*, *Renibacterium salmonicida*, *Vibrio anguillarum*, *Yersinia ruckeri*, infectious hematopoietic necrosis virus, infectious pancreatic necrosis virus, infectious salmon anemia virus and viral hemorrhagic septicemia virus associated with fish egg surfaces	None
Furunculosis	Aquaflor DIN 02233742	Florfenicol	Salmon	Furunculosis (*Aeromonas salmonicida*)	12
	Romet 30 DIN 02242954	Sulfadimethoxine and Ormetoprim	Salmonids (trout and salmon)	Furunculosis (*Aeromonas salmonicida*)	42
	Terramycin-Aqua DIN 00607657	Oxytetracycline hydrochloride	Salmonids (salmon and trout)	Furunculosis (*Aeromonas salmonicida*)	40

(Continued)

Table 19.7 (*Continued*) Drugs approved for aquaculture in Canada

TREATMENT TYPE	PRODUCT NAME/ PHARMACEUTICAL FORM	ACTIVE INGREDIENT	FISH SPECIES	INDICATION	WITHDRAWAL TIME (DAYS)
Bacterial diseases (various)	Terramycin-Aqua DIN 00607657	Oxytetracycline hydrochloride	Salmonids (salmon and trout)	Ulcer disease (*Haemophilus piscium*), columnaris disease (*Chondrococcus [Flexibacter] columnaris*), cold water disease (*Cytophaga psychrophila*) and enteric redmouth disease (*Yersinia ruckeri*)	40
Vibriosis	Tribrissen 40% powder DIN 02146037	Trimethoprim and Sulfadiazine	Salmon	Disease caused by *Vibrio anguillarum*	80
Gaffkemia (in lobsters)	Oxysol-220 DIN 02223902	Oxytetracycline hydrochloride	Lobsters	Gaffkemia (red tail disease) caused by *Aerococcus viridans*	30
	Oxysol-440 DIN 00685224	Oxytetracycline hydrochloride	Lobsters	Gaffkemia (red tail disease) caused by *Aerococcus viridans*	30
	Terramycin-Aqua DIN 00607657	Oxytetracycline hydrochloride	Lobsters	Gaffkemia (red tail disease) caused by *Aerococcus viridans*	30
Parasiticide (various)	PARASITE-S DIN 02118114	Formalin	Salmonids	External protozoan parasites, *Ichthyophthirius* spp. (*Ich*), *Chilodonella* spp., *Costia* spp., *Epistylis* spp., *Scyphidia* spp., and *Trichodina* spp.; and for the monogeneans, *Cleidodiscus* spp., *Gyrodactylus* spp., and *Dactylogyrus* spp.	None
Parasiticide, sea lice	SLICE DIN 02328216	Emamectin benzoate	Atlantic salmon	Parasitic infestations caused by all parasitic stages (chalimus I- IV and adult) of the sea louse (*Lepeophtheirus salmonis*)	0

Source: Fish, https://www.canada.ca/en/health-canada/services/drugs-health-products/veterinary-drugs/legislation-guidelines/policies/list-veterinary-drugs-that-authorized-sale-health-canada-use-food-producing-aquatic-animals.html; and eggs, https://www.canada.ca/en/health-canada/services/drugs-health-products/veterinary-drugs/legislation-guidelines/policies/list-veterinary-drugs-that-authorized-sale-health-canada-use-hatchery-eggs-aquaculture.html.

residues and development or dissemination of anti-microbial resistance. However, Health Canada issued a policy that recognized that ELDU within a valid VCPR is a necessary tool for the practice of veterinary medicine to access certain drugs for the treatment of animals.[67] The practice should be done by the veterinarian or under the supervision of a veterinarian, may not include use of banned substances (FDAR section C.01.610.1) and/or result in violative residues. A veterinarian may prescribe a medicated feed under an ELDU for therapeutic purposes only (C.08.012). The drug or drugs used as the medicating ingredient of the medicated feed must have an assigned drug identification number (DIN) pursuant to section C.01.014.2 or be permitted under section C.08.005 (Investigational New Drug), C.08.011 (Emergency Drug Release) or C.08.013 (Experimental Study Certificate). The medicated feed must be for the treatment of animals under the direct care of that veterinary practitioner and the written prescription must contain the following information:

- Name and address of the person named on the prescription as the person for whom the medicated feed is to be mixed.
- Species, production type and age or weight of the animals to be treated with the medicated feed.
- Type and amount of medicated feed to be mixed.
- Proper name, or the common name if there is no proper name, of the drug or each of the drugs as the case may be, to be used as medicating ingredients in the preparation of the medicated feed, and the dosage levels of those medicating ingredients.
- Any special mixing instructions.
- Labeling instructions including:
  o Feeding instructions.
  o A warning statement respecting the withdrawal period to be observed following the use of the medicated feed.
  o Where applicable, cautions with respect to animal health or to the handling or storage of the medicated feed.

The Canadian Veterinary Medical Association (CVMA) recently published "Veterinary Oversight of Antimicrobial Use—A Pan-Canadian Framework of Professional Standards for Veterinarians."[68] The document makes recommendations for prescribing, dispensing, high importance antimicrobial drugs, off-label drug use, and active pharmaceutical ingredients and compounding, and advocates for a decision cascade for antimicrobial use.[69]

Other countries

Information from government sources on approved drugs for aquaculture for countries in Asia, Latin America, the Near East and Africa is not as readily available as it is for the EU, Canada and the United States. Consequently, the information presented in Appendix E comes from a number of sources that include both government and published journal articles. It is recognized that aquaculture drug use rapidly evolves in response to the needs of the aquaculture industry, and as a result the list for countries may not reflect current use patterns. The information presented is grouped by geographic area—Southeast Asia (ASEAN countries, Bangladesh and India); Northeast Asia (China, Japan, Korea); Australia and New Zealand; and Latin/South America (Chile)—and may include both drugs and chemicals used in aquaculture.

THERAPEUTICS IN ORNAMENTAL FISH

Ornamental fish include tropical freshwater and saltwater fish kept in aquariums, and cool-water fish species such as goldfish and koi that are often maintained in backyard ponds. Fish farms, primarily in Asia and the southeastern United States, produce over 90% of the freshwater fish sold in tropical fish stores in the United States. Wild fish collected from around the world, mostly from South America and Africa, make up less than 10% of the freshwater fish sold in the United States. Most saltwater fish sold commercially in the United States are still collected from the wild, though the number of saltwater species now being produced by aquaculture production techniques is increasing. Ornamental fish are the third most popular pet in the United States, according to the American Pet Products Association survey (2017–2018). The survey found that in the United states there were 60.2 million dog owners, 47.1 million cat owners, and 12.5 million freshwater fish plus 2.5 million saltwater fish-keeping households.[70] However, the total number of these animals in U.S. households was 139.3 million freshwater fish plus another 18.8 million saltwater fish, 94.2 million cats and 89.7 million dogs.[70]

Ornamental fish, like aquaculture species, can succumb to a variety of viral, bacterial, fungal and parasitic diseases, as well as from poor water quality, toxins, predation, interspecies aggression, neoplasia, trauma, and metabolic diseases. It is important to assess all of these factors and perform good diagnostic testing to ensure that correct treatments are being recommended. Also, there can often be more than one problem occurring at the same time. For example, an obvious bacterial lesion might actually be secondary to damage of the epithelium caused by external parasites. Thus, both pathogens must be treated to ultimately provide relief for the fish.

Medications used for treating ornamental fish are often the same as those used in other veterinary patients, but some are unique to treating fish and not available through the normal pharmacy distribution network. There are a few FDA-approved medications used in aquaculture species (i.e., food fish), and some of these have application for treatment of ornamental fish diseases. Treating aquarium and pond fish has also utilized many chemicals that are not approved by the FDA for veterinary use. Historically these unapproved compounds have been marketed through pet stores and pond supply companies. It deserves repeating that unapproved drugs do not qualify for extra-label drug use. The reader should refer to previous sections of this chapter for a definition and legal requirements for the use of indexed drugs in fish. For ornamental fish this includes Ovaprim® (i.e., injectable sGnRHa + domperidone; Syndel USA) for use as a spawning aid in ornamental brood stock, and Aquacalm™ (i.e., metomidate hydrochloride soluble powder; Syndel USA) for the sedation and anesthesia of ornamental finfish.

When administering therapeutics to ornamental fish, it is important to assess the quality of the water in which they live. It is difficult to control or prevent infectious diseases or noninfectious problems of fish when the water quality is less than optimal. By improving the water quality, stress on the fish is reduced and the immune system of the fish can keep many diseases in check. It may be possible to separate diseased fish into an isolation tank for treatment versus treating the whole aquarium or pond. The isolation tank can be of a known volume of water and smaller than the main habitat, which makes dosing of medications for a water bath easier to calculate and requires less medication. However, if treating for an infectious pathogen, even fish that are not currently showing clinical signs of infection may need to be treated. It is important that the effects of medications on the biological filter in an aquarium or pond should also be considered. If the drug affects the nitrifying bacteria, then daily water testing and water changes may be required.

Aeromonas sp. and other bacterial species are commonly present in water and even on the fish itself. Most of these bacteria are often opportunistic pathogens that proliferate when the fish is weakened (i.e., stressed) or injured. Maintaining the water temperature in the treatment tank at the fish's optimum temperature (e.g., 20°C–3°C for koi and goldfish; 24°C–26°C for tropical fish) can increase the fish's immune response and aid healing. Some fish diseases, such as cyprinid herpesvirus-3 and *Ichthyophthirius multifiliis*, are best treated at even higher water temperatures. Osmotic stress due to skin lesions can often be decreased by adding salt to the water (0.1%–0.3% solution) for freshwater fish species.

Maintaining good nutrition during treatment of fish is also critical to proper treatment. Some fish, however, when severely affected will stop eating and may need to be force fed or tube fed. Feeding frozen brine shrimp or freeze-dried tubifex worms may entice reluctant eaters more than the standard flake or pelleted fish food. Frozen brine shrimp are also good to mix into a medicated diet for feeding tropical fish. Nutritional deficiencies, especially of amino acids, fatty acids, and vitamins C, A and E, have been shown to reduce the amount of globulin and antibody an animal can produce in response to an infection. This would ultimately reduce the animal's resistance to a pathogen. Therefore, proper nutrition, with adequate vitamin, mineral and fatty acid supplementation, is essential in maintaining optimum fish health.[71]

Therapeutics are administered to ornamental fish by a variety of routes. The most common route is by adding the therapeutic directly to the aquarium or pond water. Treating fish by prolonged immersion in a medication added to the aquarium or pond water is often termed a "bath." Alternatively, removing the fish from their original aquarium or pond and exposing them for a short immersion in a concentrated medicated solution, followed by returning the fish to the aquarium water is termed a "dip." This latter method allows more accurate measurement of the water volume to ensure the correct dose is administered and reduces the amount of medication used per dose. Medication can also be topically applied directly to the skin of the fish while the fish is briefly held out of the water. Additionally, some medications can be incorporated into or on the food, and fed or administered orally using a rubber feeding tube placed through the mouth into the stomach or intestines. Larger-sized fish can be injected with medications intramuscularly, intracoelomically and rarely intravenously. With any treatment method, water quality must be considered, as even with the best medication, fish in poor quality water are less likely to recover.

For bath treatments, mixing a measured dose of a powdered medication into a small volume of warm water and shaking vigorously in a tightly closed container followed by pouring the solution into the water allows for better distribution of medication in the aquarium or pond water. For liquid medications, measuring the required dose into a syringe and injecting the medication through a needle under the water surface allows better dispersal into the aquarium or pond water. Water changes may need to be completed between doses of medications given via bath application. Medications commonly added to aquarium or pond water in a bath application include formalin, hydrogen peroxide, and salt (i.e., sodium chloride).

Topical medications can be used for skin lesions in fish when it is deemed not too stressful to handle the fish. It is often helpful to debride open wounds and then gently swab or spray the lesion with Betadine or similar skin disinfectant before applying an antibiotic ointment (**Figure 19.2a**). This will help remove necrotic tissue and reduce bacterial and fungal growth. Care should be taken to avoid damaging new epithelial skin growth on subsequent days of topical treatment. Topical medications commonly used for skin lesions of fish include antibiotic ointments (ophthalmic preparations work well), Betadine solutions and hydrogen peroxide.

Intramuscular injections are generally given in the epaxial muscles along the back next to or immediately

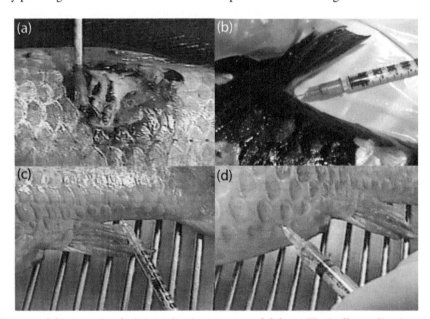

Figure 19.2 Routes of therapeutic administration in ornamental fish. (a) Topically medicating an ulcer in a koi using Betadine solution. (b) Intramuscular injection with needle inserted into the epaxial muscles behind the dorsal fin. (c) Intramuscular injection into the caudal peduncle with needle inserted between the pelvic fin and tail. (d) Intracoelomic injection with the needle inserted into the ventral coelomic cavity of the fish.

behind the dorsal fin, or in the caudal peduncle, i.e., the area posterior to the vent and anterior to the tail fin (**Figures 19.2b and c**). The needle is pointed anteriorly at a shallow angle and is advanced forward along the surface of the scale, and under the anterior scale. In many species of fish there is an area immediately behind the dorsal fin where the skin does not have scales so the needle can be inserted without penetrating or damaging any scales. Fish skin is not elastic so some medication may flow out the injection site if large volumes are injected in one area. Digital pressure can be applied over the injection site to help diffuse the medication and to seal the puncture.

Intraperitoneal (i.e., intracoelomic) injections are given in the abdomen, above and behind the pelvic fin (**Figure 19.2d**). It is often helpful to hold the fish upside down to facilitate movement of the internal organs away from the body wall. In some fish species there may be an area caudal to the pelvic fin devoid of scales that facilitates needle entry into the coelom. The hypodermic needle is inserted anteriorly at a shallow angle to avoid deep penetration and entry into the intestines or other organs. The drug is then injected just inside the internal body wall into the space between the body wall and the internal organs. Medications given by the intramuscular injection route commonly include antibiotics, analgesics, anti-inflammatory drugs and vitamins.

Intravenous injections are difficult to accomplish in fish, but can be given in the caudal vein below the spine in the caudal peduncle. In larger fish species, there may be veins in the oral cavity or inside the operculum that are large enough to use for IV injections.

Medicated food for ornamental fish (i.e., not food fish) can be made by mixing the medication with the appropriate amount of fish food pellets or flakes, and adding some egg whites, cod liver oil or vegetable oil as a binding agent. The mixture is then stirred together and spread out in a pan to dry. The medicated food can be fed in place of the regular diet or at regular intervals along with the regular diet depending on the medication and the dosing regimen. Tube-feeding the medicated food can also be an option for larger fish. Medicated food should be stored in an air-tight container in the refrigerator. Medications commonly incorporated into fish food include antibiotics, parasiticides and vitamin supplements.

REFERENCES

1. https://www.fda.gov/Drugs/InformationOnDrugs/ucm079436.htm
2. https://drive.google.com/file/d/0B43dblZIJqD3Q2NqQkhfeV84emc/view
3. http://www.fda.gov/animalveterinary/safetyhealth/productsafetyinformation/ucm324048.htm
4. http://www.fda.gov/AnimalVeterinary/DevelopmentApprovalProcess/NewAnimalDrugApplications/default.htm
5. https://www.fda.gov/AnimalVeterinary/DevelopmentApprovalProcess/Aquaculture/ucm132954.htm
6. https://www.fda.gov/AnimalVeterinary/ResourcesforYou/ucm413948.htm#drugs
7. http://www.fda.gov/AnimalVeterinary/GuidanceComplianceEnforcement/GuidanceforIndustry/ucm123818.htm
8. https://srac.tamu.edu/serveFactSheet/242
9. https://www.fws.gov/fisheries/aadap/about_background.html
10. https://www.fws.gov/fisheries/aadap/inads.html
11. https://www.umesc.usgs.gov/
12. http://www.nrsp-7.org/
13. http://www.fda.gov/downloads/AnimalVeterinary/GuidanceComplianceEnforcement/PoliciesProceduresManual/UCM046931.pdf
14. http://www.fda.gov/downloads/AnimalVeterinary/GuidanceComplianceEnforcement/GuidanceforIndustry/UCM052660.pdf
15. http://www.fda.gov/downloads/AnimalVeterinary/GuidanceComplianceEnforcement/GuidanceforIndustry/UCM216936.pdf
16. https://www.aasv.org/documents/DraftFDAGFI213.pdf
17. http://www.fda.gov/AnimalVeterinary/DevelopmentApprovalProcess/ucm460406.htm
18. http://www.fda.gov/downloads/AnimalVeterinary/GuidanceComplianceEnforcement/GuidanceforIndustry/UCM474640.pdf
19. http://www.fda.gov/ucm/groups/fdagov-public/@fda-gov-afda-ice/documents/webcontent/ucm074659.pdf
20. https://www.fda.gov/downloads/animalveterinary/guidancecomplianceenforcement/guidanceforindustry/ucm474640.pdf
21. https://www.avma.org/Pages/home.aspx
22. https://www.gpo.gov/fdsys/pkg/CFR-2012-title21-vol6/pdf/CFR-2012-title21-vol6-sec558-4.pdf
23. https://www.avma.org/KB/Resources/Reference/Pages/Compounding.aspx
24. https://www.avma.org/KB/Policies/Pages/Compounding-from-Unapproved-Bulk-Substances-in-Food-Animals.aspx
25. https://www.avma.org/Advocacy/StateAndLocal/Pages/sr-records-retention.aspx
26. http://www.fda.gov/downloads/AnimalVeterinary/GuidanceComplianceEnforcement/GuidanceforIndustry/UCM213153.pdf

27. http://www.fda.gov/AnimalVeterinary/SafetyHealth/ReportaProblem/ucm055305.htm
28. http://www.fda.gov/downloads/AboutFDA/ReportsManualsForms/Forms/AnimalDrugForms/UCM048810.pdf
29. https://www.fda.gov/AnimalVeterinary/ScienceResearch/ToolsResources/Phish-Pharm/default.htm
30. http://www.farad.org/
31. http://www.fda.gov/downloads/food/guidanceregulation/ucm251970.pdf
32. https://www.avma.org/KB/Policies/Pages/Judicious-Use-of-Antimicrobials-for-Treatment-of-Aquatic-Animals-by-Veterinarians.aspx?PF=1
33. http://www.fda.gov/AnimalVeterinary/GuidanceComplianceEnforcement/ActsRulesRegulations/ucm085377.htm
34. http://www.fda.gov/AnimalVeterinary/NewsEvents/CVMUpdates/ucm529164.htm?linksOrder=Sorter_link_name&linksDir=ASC
35. http://www.fda.gov/AnimalVeterinary/ScienceResearch/ToolsResources/Phish-Pharm/default.htm
36. Clinical and Laboratory Standards Institute. Performance Standards for Antimicrobial Susceptibility Testing of Bacteria Isolated from Aquatic Animals; Second Informational Supplement. CLSI document VET03/VET04-S2. 2014.
37. https://www.avma.org/
38. http://www.fda.gov/animalveterinary/default.htm
39. https://www.wavma.org/
40. https://www.fws.gov/fisheries/AADAP/PDF/GUIDE_June_2014b.pdf
41. https://dailymed.nlm.nih.gov/dailymed/drugInfo.cfm?setid=315d9bc7-24b3-4e2b-9777-33878d46f1df
42. http://www.syndel.com/downloads/dl/file/id/111/
43. https://www.wavma.org/Webinars/B-1007-Tranquillisation-Anaesthesia-and-Euthanasia-in-Pet-Fish
44. https://www.fws.gov/fisheries/AADAP/PDF/deskreference.pdf
45. https://www.fws.gov/fisheries/aadap/PDF/2nd-Edition-FINAL.pdf
46. http://www.merckvetmanual.com/exotic-and-laboratory-animals/aquarium-fishes/management-of-fish
47. Saint-Erne, N. Clinical procedures. In: *Advanced Koi Care*. N. Saint-Erne, ed. Erne Enterprises, Glendale, AZ; 2002, pp. 39–61.
48. http://avmajournals.avma.org/doi/full/10.2460/javma.229.3.362
49. https://ec.europa.eu/health/documents/eudralex/vol-5_en
50. http://web.oie.int/RR-Europe/eng/events/docs/11.10__FEAPchallenges%20in%20AM%20use.pdf
51. http://ec.europa.eu/health//sites/health/files/files/eudralex/vol-5/reg_2010_37/reg_2010_37_en.pdf
52. http://www.ema.europa.eu/ema/index.jsp?curl=pages/regulation/document_listing/document_listing_000165.jsp
53. https://assets.publishing.service.gov.uk/government/uploads/system/uploads/attachment_data/file/424668/VMGNote13.PDF
54. http://eur-lex.europa.eu/legal-content/en/ALL/?uri=CELEX:31990L0167
55. https://legemiddelverket.no/Documents/Veterin%C3%A6rmedisin/Fisk%20og%20legemidler/Pharmaceuticals-fish-MA-2016-06-15.pdf
56. https://legemiddelverket.no/Documents/Veterin%C3%A6rmedisin/Fisk%20og%20legemidler/General%20information-%20medicines%20for%20fish-2016-07-06.pdf
57. www.mattilsynet.no
58. https://ec.europa.eu/health/sites/health/files/files/eudralex/vol-5/reg_2010_37/reg_2010_37_en.pdf
59. https://ec.europa.eu/health/sites/health/files/files/eudralex/vol-5/dir_2004_28/dir_2004_28_en.pdf
60. https://ec.europa.eu/health/documents/eudralex/vol-5_en
61. https://www.canada.ca/en/health-canada/services/consumer-product-safety/reports-publications/pesticides-pest-management/decisions-updates/registration-decision/2017/azamethiphos-2017-13.html
62. Fish: https://www.canada.ca/en/health-canada/services/drugs-health-products/veterinary-drugs/legislation-guidelines/policies/list-veterinary-drugs-that-authorized-sale-health-canada-use-food-producing-aquatic-animals.html
63. Eggs: https://www.canada.ca/en/health-canada/services/drugs-health-products/veterinary-drugs/legislation-guidelines/policies/list-veterinary-drugs-that-authorized-sale-health-canada-use-hatchery-eggs-aquaculture.html
64. http://www.inspection.gc.ca/animals/feeds/medicating-ingredients/mib/mib-35a/eng/1330987515269/1330987584088
65. https://www.canada.ca/en/health-canada/services/drugs-health-products/veterinary-drugs/emergency-drug-release-veterinary-drugs.html
66. https://www.canada.ca/content/dam/hc-sc/documents/services/drugs-health-products/veterinary-drugs/applications-submissions/ESC-Form_Final_CPAB-eng.pdf
67. https://www.canada.ca/en/health-canada/services/drugs-health-products/veterinary-drugs/extra-label-drug-use.html
68. https://www.canadianveterinarians.net/documents/pan-canadian-framework
69. https://www.canada.ca/en/public-health/services/antibiotic-antimicrobial-resistance/animals/actions/responsible-use-antimicrobials.html
70. http://www.americanpetproducts.org/press_industry-trends.asp
71. Saint-Erne, N. Nutrition. In: *Advanced Koi Care*. N. Saint-Erne, ed. Erne Enterprises, Glendale, AZ; 2002, pp. 89–93.

THERAPEUTICS FOR ORNAMENTAL, TROPICAL, BAIT AND OTHER NON-FOOD FISH: ANTIMICROBIAL AND ANTIFUNGAL AGENTS

JESSICA GASKINS AND SHANE M. BOYLAN

Statement: None of these therapeutic compounds are approved or available for extra-label use in food fish.

MEDICATION	DRUG CLASS	DOSE AND ROUTE	SPECIES	COMMENTS
Acriflavine	Slow-acting topical antiseptic	10 mg/L IV every 4 hours[48]	Channel catfish	Clinical Note: Also known as Euflavin
Amikacin	Aminoglycoside antibiotic	5 mg/kg IM every 12 hours[63]		Caution: Use with care in any animal with suspected renal impairment
		5 mg/kg IM every 72 hours for 3 treatments[71]		Clinical Note: Aminoglycosides can be nephrotoxic in certain species
		5 mg/kg ICe every 24 hours for 3 days then every 48 hours for 2 treatments (PD)[30]	Koi	
Amoxicillin	Beta-lactam antibiotic	25 mg/kg PO every 12 hours[64]		Clinical Note: Medication has primarily Gram-positive coverage so may not be indicated for ornamental fish
		40 mg/kg IV every 24 hours[8]	Sea bream	
		80 mg/kg PO every 24 hours for 10 days[8]	Sea bream	
		40 mg/kg IV or 80 mg/kg PO every 24 hours for 10 days[8]	Sea bream	
		110 mg/kg PO in feed every 24 hours[2]	Channel catfish	
Ampicillin	Beta-lactam antibiotic	10 mg/kg IM every 24 hours[68]	Atlantic salmon	Clinical Note: Medication has primarily Gram-positive coverage so may not be indicated for ornamental fish
		10 mg/kg IV every 24 hours[46]	Striped bass	
		50–80 mg/kg PO every 24 hours in feed for 10 days[43]		
Azithromycin	Macrolide antibiotic	30 mg/kg PO every 24 hours for 14 days[15]	Chinook salmon	
		40 mg/kg ICe[16]	Chinook salmon	
Aztreonam	Monocyclic beta-lactam antibiotic (aka Monobactam)	100 mg/kg IM or ICe every 48 hours for 7 doses[53]		
Benzalkonium chloride	Topical Category III antiseptic	0.5 mg/L in tank water long term[68]		Counseling Point: Unlike many other topical antiseptics this product does not cause irritation
		10 mg/L for 10 minute bath[68]		Clinical Note: Often a preservative in many pharmacologic preparations (i.e., eye drops)

(Continued)

MEDICATION	DRUG CLASS	DOSE AND ROUTE	SPECIES	COMMENTS
Bronopol	Standardized chemical allergen by increasing histamine release and cell-mediated immunity and antifungal activity	15–50 mg/L×30–60 minute bath/immersion[43]		
Ceftazidime	Third-generation cephalosporin antibiotic	22 mg/kg IM, ICe every 72–96 hours for 3–5 treatments[53]		
Ceftiofur	Third-generation cephalosporin antibiotic	8 mg/kg IM (may see up to 40 mg/kg)[11]	Representatives from following families: Anabantidae, Callichthyidae, Cichlidae, and Cyprinidae	Caution: Volume can be irritating (aseptic granulomatous reactions) and may want to divide into two doses on either side of animal
		20 mg/kg IM once, 60 mg/kg IM once or 30 mg/kg ICe once, 60 mg/kg ICe once[23]	Koi	Clinical Note: Dosing in koi found to be ineffective
Chloramine-T	Chlorinated sulfonamide derivative biocide disinfectant	2.5–20 mg/L prolonged immersion[68]		Clinical Note: Dose and duration vary widely with species and water quality

Clinical Note: Used in aquaculture to prevent external flavobacterial diseases and fluke infections in koi and goldfish[43] |
| Chloramphenicol | Highly lipophilic, bacteriostatic antimicrobial similar to a macrolide antibiotic | 50 mg/kg PO or IM once then 25 mg/kg every 24 hours[64]

50 mg/kg PO every 24 hours[6] | Trout | Caution: Long-term exposure leads to bone marrow suppression

Caution: Prohibited for use in food animals |
| Ciprofloxacin | Fluoroquinolone antibiotic | 15 mg/kg IM, IV[44] | Carp, African catfish, rainbow trout | Clinical Note: Binds to magnesium, calcium, and aluminum, rendering the medication ineffective

Counseling Point: Medication has decreased uptake in hard water and will need to increase dose for marine patients |

(Continued)

MEDICATION	DRUG CLASS	DOSE AND ROUTE	SPECIES	COMMENTS
Difloxacin	Second-generation synthetic fluoroquinolone antibiotic	10 mg/kg PO every 24 hours[14]	Atlantic salmon	Clinical Note: Levels were higher in marine species versus freshwater species
		10 mg/kg PO and IV once at 14°C and 22°C[66]	Olive flounder	Clinical Note: Study with temperature demonstrated lower temperature with lower elimination rates[51,66]
		20 mg/kg PO every 24 hours for 3 days[10]	Crucian carp	Counseling Point: Medication has decreased uptake in hard water and will need to increase dose for marine patients
				Clinical Note: Binds to magnesium, calcium, and aluminum, rendering the medication ineffective
Enrofloxacin	Fluoroquinolone antibiotic	2.5 mg/kg IV every 24 hours[9]	Sea bream	Clinical Note: To examine the use of quinolones from a review perspective please see reference to Samuelsen[59]
		5 mg/kg PO, IM, ICe every 24 hours[64]		
		5–10 mg/kg PO every 24 hours[68]		Counseling Point: Medication has decreased uptake in hard water and will need to increase dose for marine patients
		5–10 mg/kg IM, ICe every 48 hours for 7 treatments[37]	Red pacu	Clinical Note: On average 10%–40% will be metabolized into ciprofloxacin in most species (humans, dogs, cats, horses, cattle, turtles, and snakes),[49] however only about 5% observed in fish[17]
		10 mg/kg PO every 24 hours[9,35,59]	Sea bream, common carp, rainbow trout	
		10 mg/kg PO or IV[17,33,34]	Brown trout, Korean catfish, allogynogenetic silver crucian carp	Clinical Note: Binds to magnesium, calcium, and aluminum, rendering the medication ineffective; therefore, when tube feeding do not mix with high-calcium foods
		10 mg/kg PO in feed every 24 hours[36,43]	Tra catfish	
		20 mg/kg PO in feed for 7 days[7]	Nile tilapia	
		50 mg/kg PO every 24 hours for 7 days[74]	Red pacu	
		2.5–5 mg/L for 5 hour immersion every 24 hours for 5–7 days[37]		

MEDICATION	DRUG CLASS	DOSE AND ROUTE	SPECIES	COMMENTS
Erythromycin	Macrolide class of antibiotics	100 mg/kg PO every 24 hours for 10 days[16]	Chinook salmon	Counseling Point: Found in many over-the-counter drugs for treating full tanks but not recommended as they are harmful to nitrifying bacteria of tank
		100 mg/kg PO or IM every 24 hours for 7–21 days[64,68]		
		100–200 mg/kg PO every 24 hours for 21 days[42]	Chinook salmon	Clinical Note: Study with rainbow trout did reveal anorexia in treated fish
		110 mg/kg PO in feed once daily for 2 weeks[26]	Rainbow trout	
Florfenicol	Broad spectrum antibiotic (synthetic fluorinated analog of thiamphenicol)	5–20 mg/kg PO every 24 hours[28]	Atlantic salmon	Clinical Note: Variety of doses in a variety of species but many are pharmacokinetic and not actual clinical situations; adjust doses accordingly[19]
		10 mg/kg PO once daily in medicated feed pellet for 10 days[20]	Channel catfish	
		10 mg/kg IM every 24 hours[76]	Koi, carp, 3-spot gourami	
		10–20 mg/kg PO every 24 hours for 10 days[57]	Atlantic salmon	
		10 mg/kg IV once and 20 mg/kg IM once[40]	Olive flounder	
		10–24 mg/kg in oral slurry once[18,27]	Orange-spotted grouper, Atlantic salmon	
		25–50 mg/kg PO every 24 hours[57]	Atlantic salmon	
		40 mg/kg once IM[45]	White spotted bamboo shark	
		40–50 mg/kg PO, IM, ICe every 12–24 hours[39,64]	Red pacu	
		100 mg/kg IM every 24 hours[57]	Atlantic salmon	

(Continued)

MEDICATION	DRUG CLASS	DOSE AND ROUTE	SPECIES	COMMENTS
Flumequine	First-generation fluoroquinolone antibiotic	10 mg/kg PO every 48 hours[24]	Goldsinny wrasse and cod	Counseling Point: Medication has decreased uptake in hard water and will need to increase dose for marine patients
		12–25 mg/kg PO, ICe, or IV every 24 hours[55]	Atlantic halibut	
		25–50 mg/kg IM every 24 hours[54]	Atlantic salmon	Clinical Note: Binds to magnesium, calcium, and aluminum, rendering the medication ineffective
		30 mg/kg IM, ICe[4,43]	Atlantic salmon	
		50–100 mg/L for 3–5 hour immersion[4,43]	Brown trout and Atlantic salmon	
		10 mg/kg PO every 24 hours in feed for 10 days[43]		
Formalin	Highly reactive aldehyde gas formed by oxidation of hydrocarbons	0.23 mL/L bath for up to 60 minutes[43]		Note: All doses based on 100% formalin, which is 37% formaldehyde
	In solution, it has a wide range of uses such as a disinfectant and as a laboratory fixative or preservative	1mL in 38 L as 12–24 hour bath followed by 30%–70% water change, may be repeated[71]		Caution: Hazardous and carcinogenic, toxic to plants as well
		1–2 mL/L for 15 minute bath[43]		Clinical Note: Some species more sensitive than others so monitor closely for signs of respiratory distress (pale color, increased opercular movement, gasping)
		25 mg/L immersion for up to 144 hours (equal to 9.3 mg/L formaldehyde)[73]	Striped bass	
		300 ppm for 30 minute bath[62]	Guilthead sea bass	
		400 ppm for 1 hour bath[32]	Red porgy	
		250–400 ppm bath for 1 hour followed by a 5 minute freshwater dip[61]	Yellowtail kingfish	Clinical Note: Keep water well oxygenated as each 5 mg/L of formalin chemically removes 1 mg/L oxygen[43]
Furazolidone	Antibacterial and antiprotozoal nitrofuran	1 mg/kg PO, IV every 24 hours[47]	Channel catfish	Caution: Prohibited for use in food animals
		30 mg/kg once PO[74]	Nile tilapia	Clinical Note: Increased efficacy when 2 ppm furazolidone added with 0.2 ppm methylene blue (Shane Matthew Boylan, DVM, personal communication. South Carolina Aquarium. June 2018.)
		25–35 mg/kg PO every 24 hours in feed for 20 days[25]	Rainbow trout, brown trout, brook trout, and cutthroat trout	
		50–100 mg/kg PO every 24 hours in feed for 10–15 days[43]		
		1–10 mg/L in tank water for $\geq$ 24 hours[43]		

MEDICATION	DRUG CLASS	DOSE AND ROUTE	SPECIES	COMMENTS
Gentamicin	Aminoglycoside antibiotic	1 mg/kg IM or ICe every 24 hours[60]	Channel catfish	Clinical Note: Aminoglycosides can be nephrotoxic in certain species
		2 mg/kg IM then 1 mg/kg IM at 8 and 72 hours[65]	Brown shark	
		2.5 mg/kg IM every 72 hours[38]	Koi	
		3.5 mg/kg IM every 24 hours[31]	Toadfish and goldfish	
Iodine	Antiseptic that is bactericidal with fungicidal and sporicidal properties	20–100 mg/L bath for 10 minutes for egg disinfection[43]		Counseling Point: Avoid topical products that have detergent combined with the active drug (i.e., Betadine scrub)
	Often used as skin cleaner and antiseptic, but can be used for its drying effects	Topical application to wound, rinse immediately[68]		Counseling Point: Tends to stain skin, hair, and fabric.
				Caution: Avoid contact with eyes
Itraconazole	Synthetic triazole antifungal	1–5 mg/kg PO every 24 hours in feed for up to 7 days[64]		Clinical Note: Most often used to treat systemic mycoses (aspergillosis, cryptococcal meningitis, blastomycosis, and histoplasmosis)[49]
Kanamycin	Aminoglycoside antibiotic	20 mg/kg ICe once every 3 days for 5 treatments[43]		Clinical Note: Aminoglycosides can be nephrotoxic in certain species
		50 mg/kg PO every 24 hours in feed[43]		
		50–100 mg/L in tank water every 72 hours for 3 treatments[43]		
Ketoconazole	Imidazole antifungal	2.5–10 mg/kg PO, IM or ICe for 10 days[64]	Rainbow trout	Clinical Note: Most often used to treat systemic mycoses (aspergillosis, cryptococcal meningitis, blastomycosis, and histoplasmosis)[49]

(Continued)

MEDICATION	DRUG CLASS	DOSE AND ROUTE	SPECIES	COMMENTS
Malachite green	Organic compound that is a triarylmethane dye	0.1 mg/L in tank water every 3 days for 3 total treatments[43]		Caution: Mutagenic, teratogenic and toxic to certain fish species such as Centrarchids
		0.25 mg/L for 15 minute immersion every 24 hours[72]		Caution: Increased toxicity at higher temperatures and lower pH
		0.5 mg/L for 1 hour bath[43]		Caution: Histopathogical observations of livers and gills of rainbow trout exposed to series of exposures of 1–6 ppm 40 minute baths of malachite green at weekly intervals revealed sinusoidal congestion, focal necrosis on livers and necrosis and separation of epithelial lining from lamellar and interlamellar regions of gills; however hepatic changes not severe enough to be reflected in protein changes. Gills of treated fish showed separation of epithelial lining from both lameller and interlamellar regions.[21]
		1 mg/L for a 30–60 minute bath[43]		
		1 mg/L for 1 hour immersion for fungal control on fish eggs[68]		
		2 mg/L for 15 minute bath for fungal control on fish eggs[68]		
		1.6 mg/L 40 minute bath at 7, 14, and 21 days[1]		
		3.2 mg/L as dip for 7, 14, and 21 days[1]		
		10 mg/L for 10–30 minute bath for fungal control on freshwater fish eggs[43]		Counseling Point: Stains most objects, especially plastic aquarium decor or filtration equipment
		50–60 mg/L for 10–30 second bath[43]		
		100 mg/L topically to skin lesions[43]		
Marbofloxacin	Third-generation fluoroquinolone antibiotic	10 mg/kg once every 24 hours for 3 days at 15°C and 25°C[79]	Crucian carp	Clinical Note: Half-life of medication was longer at 10°C than at 25°C as expected
				Counseling Point: Medication has decreased uptake in hard water and will need to increase dose for marine patients
				Clinical Note: Binds to magnesium, calcium, and aluminum, rendering the medication ineffective

(Continued)

MEDICATION	DRUG CLASS	DOSE AND ROUTE	SPECIES	COMMENTS
Methylene blue	Thiazine dye	2 mg/L tank water treatment for 48 hours up to 3 treatments for freshwater egg infection prevention[43]		Caution: Toxic to nitrifying bacteria and plants Caution: Stains most objects, including aquarium decor and filtration equipment
Metronidazole	Antibiotic for anaerobes and antiprotozoal agent	25 mg/kg PO every 24 hours in feed for 5–10 days[43]	Angelfish	Counseling Point: Does not dissolve well in water so best to dissolve using properties of geometric dilution in small portions rather than adding directly into treatment tank
		50 mg/kg PO every 24 hours for 5 days[69]	Angelfish	
		100 mg/kg PO in feed every 24 hours for 3 days[43]		
		6.6 mg/L in tank water every 24 hours for 3 days[43]		
		25 mg/L in tank water every 48 hours for 3 treatments[43]	Koi	
		6.25–18 mg/g PO in feed for 5 days[70] Medicated feed of brine shrimp (625 mg per 100 mL for 15–20 minutes prior to feed) given daily for 5 treatments[30]		
Miconazole	Imidazole antifungal	10–20 mg/kg PO, IM, or ICe every 24 hours[63]		
Nalidixic acid	Synthetic quinolone antibiotic, though technically by structure it is a naphthyridone	5 mg/kg PO or IM every 24 hours[64]		
		20 mg/kg PO every 24 hours[68]		
		13 mg/L for 1–4 hour bath and repeat as needed[43]		
Neomycin	Aminoglycoside antibiotic	66 mg/L in tank water every 3 days for 3 treatments[43]		Caution: Tends to be more nephrotoxic and less effective against several bacterial species than either gentamicin or amikacin and is generally limited to topical formulations[49]

(Continued)

MEDICATION	DRUG CLASS	DOSE AND ROUTE	SPECIES	COMMENTS
Nifurpirinol	Nitrofuran derivative	0.45–0.9 mg/kg PO every 24 hours for 5 days[43]		Caution: Carcinogenic
		4–10 mg/kg PO in feed every 12 hours for 5 days[43]	Striped bass, palmetto bass	Caution: Toxic to scaleless fish
		0.1 mg/L of tank water every 24 hours for 3–5 days[43]		Counseling Point: Medication is inactivated in bright light
		1–2 mg/L as bath or immersion (5 minutes up to 6 hours)[43]		Counseling Point: Medication is absorbed from water, change 50%–75% of water between treatments
Nitrofurazone	Bactericidal chemical	2–5 mg/L in tank water every 24 hours for 5–10 days[71]		Caution: Carcinogenic
		50 mg/L for 3 hour immersion[5]	Gilt-head bream, Mozambique tilapia	Caution: Toxic to scaleless fish
		100 mg/L for 30 minute bath[43]		Counseling Point: Medication is inactivated in bright light
		100 mg/L for 6 hour immersion[5]	Gilt-head bream, Mozambique tilapia	Counseling Point: Medication is absorbed from water, change 50%–75% of water between treatments
Norfloxacin	Fluoroquinolone antibiotic	10 mg/kg PO given once[75]	Common carp, Crucian carp	Counseling Point: Medication has decreased uptake in hard water and will need to increase dose for marine patients
				Clinical Note: Binds to magnesium, calcium, and aluminum, rendering the medication ineffective
Oxolinic acid	Quinolone antibiotic	5–25 mg/kg PO every 24 hours[64]		Counseling Point: Medication has decreased uptake in hard water and will need to increase dose for marine patients
		10 mg/kg PO every 24 hours[68]		
		25 mg/kg ICe every 24 hours[56]	Corkwing wrasse	Clinical Note: Binds to magnesium, calcium, and aluminum, rendering the medication ineffective
		25–50 mg/kg PO every 24 hours[54,68]	Atlantic salmon	
		10 mg/kg PO in feed every 24 hours for 10 days[43]		
		3–10 mg/L in tank water for 24 hours[43]		
		25 mg/L for 15 minute bath every 12 hours for 3 days[43]		

(Continued)

MEDICATION	DRUG CLASS	DOSE AND ROUTE	SPECIES	COMMENTS
Oxytetracycline	Tetracycline antibiotic	3 mg/kg IV every 24 hours[12]	Red pacu	Counseling Point: Medication is light-sensitive and will degrade if not kept light-protected
		7 mg/kg IM every 24 hours[12]	Red pacu	Counseling Point: Medication may be decreased by binding to ions in saltwater[41,49]
		10 mg/kg IM every 24 hours[63]		
		20 mg/kg once ICe[68]	Salmonids	
		20 mg/kg PO every 8 hours[64]		
		25–50 mg/kg IM or ICe[43]		
		60 mg/kg IM every 7 days[22]	Carp	
		70 mg/kg PO every 24 hours for 10–14 days[70]		
		100 mg/kg IM every 24 hours[52]	Doctor fish (tench)	
		10–100 mg/L in tank water (hard water will require higher doses)[43]		
		7 mg/kg PO in feed every 24 hours for 10 days[70]		
		55–83 mg/kg PO every 24 hours in feed for 10 days[43]		
		75 mg/kg PO in feed every 24 hours for 10 days[68]		
		100 mg/kg PO every 24 hours for 5 days[77]	Yellow catfish	
		100 mg/kg PO every 24 hours for 7 days[78]	Grass carp	
		10–50 mg/L for 1 hour bath[43]		

(Continued)

MEDICATION	DRUG CLASS	DOSE AND ROUTE	SPECIES	COMMENTS
Potassium permanganate	Highly oxidative, water-soluble potassium salt compound with purple crystals	2 mg/L as indefinite bath[71]		Caution: Toxicity increases with increased pH
		5 mg/L bath for 30–60 minutes[43]		Caution: Never mix with formalin
		1000 mg/L bath for 10–40 seconds[43]		Counseling: May prove toxic to goldish species
				Counseling Point: Systems with high organic load will require higher doses
				Testing: Add KMnO4 to small sample of system water and red color should remain for at least 4 hours; continue adding KMnO4 until 4 hour test is adequate[13]
Sarafloxacin	Fluoroquinolone antibiotic	10–14 mg/kg PO every 24 hours for 10 days[64]		Counseling Point: Medication has decreased uptake in hard water and will need to increase dose for marine patients
		10 mg/kg PO every 24 hours[68]		
		10 mg/kg PO every 24 hours (6–14 mg/kg range) for 5–10 days[50,67]	Channel catfish	Clinical Note: Binds to magnesium, calcium, and aluminum, rendering the medication ineffective
Silver sulfadiazine	Topical antimicrobial targeting Gram-negative and Gram-positive bacteria as well as yeast	Topical use every 12 hours for external infection[38]	Koi	Counseling Point: Keep lesion out of water for 30–60 seconds after application (with gills submerged)

(Continued)

MEDICATION	DRUG CLASS	DOSE AND ROUTE	SPECIES	COMMENTS
Sulfadimethoxine/ ormetoprim	Sulfonamide antimicrobial	50 mg/kg PO in feed for 5 days[43] Medicated feed of brine shrimp (3 mg/L saltwater for 4 hours, rinse, then feed immediately)[43]		Counseling Point: May be possible to use with other forms of live food
Sulfamethoxazole/ trimethoprim	Potentiated sulfonamide antimicrobial	30 mg/kg PO every 24 hours for 10–14 days[43] 20 mg/L in 5–12 hour immersion every 24 hours for 5–7 days[3,43] 0.2% PO in feed every 24 hours for 10–14 days[43] 200 mcg m^{-1} bath for 72 hours[58]	Rainbow trout Atlantic halibut	Counseling Point: Change 50%–75% of water between treatments
Thiamphenicol	Methyl-sulfonyl analog of antibiotic chloramphenicol	15–30 mg/kg PO every 24 hours for 5 days[29]	Sea bass	
Tobramycin	Aminoglycoside antibiotic	2.5 mg/kg IM once then 1 mg/kg IM every 4 days[64]		Caution: Nephrotoxicity and ototoxicity
Triple antibiotic ointment (polymyxin B, bacitracin, neomycin)	Combination antibiotic topical ointment: Neomycin is an aminoglycoside antibiotic, polymyxin B interferes with tetrahydrofolic acid production and bacitracin is a polypeptide antibiotic	Topical use every 12 hours for external bacterial infection[38]	Koi	Counseling Point: Keep lesion out of water for 30–60 seconds after application (with gills submerged) Caution: Keep away from eyes as can be irritating

REFERENCES

1. Alderman, D.J. Malachite green: A pharmacokinetic study in rainbow trout, *Oncorhynchus mykiss* (Walbaum). *Journal of Fish Diseases* 1993;16:297–311.

2. Ang, C.Y., Liu, F.F., Lay, J.O. et al. Liquid chromatographic analysis of incurred amoxicillin residues in catfish muscle following oral administration of the drug. *Journal of Agricultural and Food Chemistry* 2000;48:1673–1677.

3. Bergjso, T. and Bergjso, H.T. Absorption from water as an alternative method for the administration of sulfonamides to rainbow trout, *Salmo gairdneri*. *Acta Veterinaria Scandinavica* 1978;19:102–109.

4. Bowser, P.R. and Babish, J.G. Clinical pharmacology and efficacy of fluoroquinolones in fish. *Annual Review of Fish Diseases* 1991;1:63–66.

5. Colorni, A. and Paperna, I. Evlauation of nitrofurazone baths in the treatment of bacterial infections of *Sparus aurata* and *Oreochromis mossambicus*. *Aquaculture* 1983;245:208–219.

6. Cravedi, J.P., Heuillet, G., Peleran, J.C. et al. Disposition and metabolism of chloramphenicol in trout. *Xenobiotica* 1985;15:115–121.

7. Danyi, S., Widart, J., Douny, C. et al. Determination and kinetics of enrofloxacin and ciprofloxacin in Tra catfish (*Pangasianodon hypophthalmus*) and giant freshwater prawn (*Macrobrachium rosenbergii*) using a liquid chromatography/mass spectrometry method. *Journal of Veterinary Pharmacology and Therapeutics* 2010;34:142–152.

8. Della Rocca, G., Zaghini, A., Zanoni, R. et al. Seabream (*Sparus aurata* L.): Disposition of amoxicillin after single intravenous or oral administration and multiple dose depletion studies. *Aquaculture* 2004;232:1–10.

9. Della Rocca, G., Di Salvo, A., Malvisi, J. et al. The disposition of enrofloxacin in seabream (*Sparus aurata*) after single intravenous injection or from medicated feed administration. *Aquaculture* 2004;232:53–62.

10. Ding, F., Cao, J., Ma, L. et al. Pharmacokinetics and tissue residues of difloxacin in crucian carp (*Carassius auratus*) after oral administration. *Aquaculture* 2006;256:121–128.

11. Dixon, B.A. and Issvoran, G.S. The activity of ceftiofur sodium for *Aeromonas* spp. isolated from ornamental fish. *Journal of Wildlife Diseases* 1992;28(3):453–456.

12. Doi, A.M., Stoskopf, M.K., Lewbart, G.A. et al. Pharmacokinetics of oxytetracycline in the red pacu (*Colossoma brachypomum*) following different routes of administration. *Journal of Veterinary Pharmacology and Therapeutics* 1998;21:364–368.

13. Duncan, T.O. A review of literature on the use of potassium permanganate (KMnO4) in fisheries. United States Fish and Wildlife Service, Report FWS - LR - 74 - 14, p. 61. 1974.

14. Elston, R.A., Drum, A.S., Schweitzer, M.G. et al. Comparative uptake of orally administered difloxacin in Atlantic salmon in freshwater and seawater. *Journal of Aquatic Animal Health* 1994;6:341–348.

15. Fairgrieve, W.T., Masada, C.L., McAuley, W.C. et al. Accumulation and clearance of orally administered erythromycin and its derivative, azithromycin, in juvenile fall Chinook salmon *Oncorhynchus tshawytscha*. *Diseases of Aquatic Organisms* 2005;64:99–106.

16. Fairgrieve, W.T., Masasda, C.L., Peterson, M.E. et al. Concentrations of erythromycin and azithromycin in mature Chinook salmon *Oncoryhynchus tshawytscha* after intraperitoneal injection, and in their progeny. *Diseases of Aquatic Organisms* 2006;68:227–234.

17. Fang, X., Liu, X., Liu, W. et al. Pharmacokinetics of enrofloxacin in allogynogenetic silver crucian carp, *Carassius auratus gibelio*. *Journal of Veterinary Pharmacology and Therapeutics* 2012;35:397–401.

18. Fend, J.B., Huang, D.R., Zhong, M. et al. Pharmacokinetics of florfenicol and behaviour of its metabolite florfenicol amine in orange-spotted grouper (*Epinephelus coioides*) after oral administration. *Journal of Fish Diseases* 2016;39:833–843.

19. Gaikowskiet, M.P., Whitsel, M.K., Charles, S. et al. Depletion of florfenicol amine in tilapia. *Aquaculture Research* 2015;46:1842–1857.

20. Gaunt, P.S. Multidose pharmacokinetics of orally administered florfenicol in the channel catfish (*Ictalurus punctatus*). *Journal of Veterinary Pharmacology and Therapeutics* 2012;36:502–506.

21. Gerundo, N., Alderman, D.J., Clifton-Hadley, R.S. et al. Pathological effects of repeated doses of malachite green: A preliminary study. *Journal of Fish Diseases* 1991;14:521–532.

22. Grondel, J.L., Nouws, J.F.M., De Jon, M. et al. Pharmacokinetics and tissue distribution of oxytetracycline in carp, *Cyprinus carpio* L., following different routes of administration. *Journal of Fish Diseases* 1987;10:153–163.

23. Grosset, C., Weber, E.S., Gehring, R. et al. Evaluation of an extended-release formulation of ceftiofur crystalline-free acid in koi (*Cyprinus carpio*). *Journal of Veterinary Pharmacology and Therapeutics* 2015;38:606–615.

24. Hansen, M.K. and Horseberg, T.E. Single dose pharmacokinetics of flumequine in cod (*Gadus morhua*) and goldsinny wrasse (*Ctenolabrus rupestris*). *Journal of Veterinary Pharmacology and Therapeutics* 2000;23:163–168.

25. Heaton, L.H. and Post, G. Tissue residue and oral safety of furazolidone in four species of trout. *The Progressive Fish-Culturist* 1968;30(4):208–215.

26. Hicks, B.D. and Geraci, J.R. A histological assessment of damage in rainbow trout, *Salmo gairdneri Richardson*, fed rations containing erythromycin. *Journal of Fish Diseases* 1984;7:457–465.

27. Horsberg, T.E., Hoff, K.A. and Nordmo, R. Pharmacokinetics of florfenicol and its metabolite florfenicol amine in Atlantic salmon. *Journal of Aquatic Animal Health* 1996;8:292–301.

28. Inglis, V., Richards, R.H., Varma, K.J. et al. Florfenicol in Atlantic salmon, *Salmo salar* L., parr: Tolerance and assessment of efficacy against furunculosis. *Journal of Fish Diseases* 1991;14:343–351.

29. Intorre, L., Castells, G., Cristofol, C. et al. Residue depletion of thiamphenicol in the sea-bass. *Journal of Veterinary Pharmacology and Therapeutics* 2002;25:59–63.

30. Johnson, E.L. *Koi Health and Disease. Johnson Veterinary Services*. Reade Printers, Athens, 2006.

31. Jones, J., Kinnel, M., Christenson, R. et al. Communications: Gentamicin concentrations in toadfish and goldfish serum. *The AAPS Journal* 2005;7(2), Article 30.

32. Katharios, P., Papandroulakis, N., Divanach, P. et al. Treatment of *Microcotyle* sp. (Monogenea) on the gills of cage-cultured red porgy, *Pagrus pagrus* following baths with formalin and mebendazole. *Aquaculture* 2006;251:167–171.

33. Kim, M.S., Lim, J.H., Park, B.K. et al. Pharmacokinetics of enrofloxacin in Korean catfish (*Silurus asotus*). *Journal of Veterinary Pharmacology and Therapeutics* 2006;29:397–402.

34. Koc, F., Uney, K., Atamanalp, M. et al. Pharmacokinetic disposition of enrofloxacin in brown trout (*Salmo trutta fario*) after oral and intravenous administrations. *Aquaculture* 2009;295:142–144.

35. Kyuchukova, R., Milanova, A., Pavlov, A. et al. Comparison of plasma and tissue disposition of enrofloxacin in rainbow trout (*Oncorhynchus mykiss*) and common carp (*Cyprinus carpio*) after a single oral administration. *Food Additives and Contaminants: Part A* 2015; 32(1):35–39.

36. Lewbart, G.A. Emergency pet fish medicine. In: *Current Veterinary Therapy XII: Small Animal Practice*. J.D. Bonagura and R.W. Kirk, eds. WB Saunders, Philadelphia, 1995; pp. 1369–1374.

37. Lewbart, G., Vaden, S., Deen, J. et al. Pharmacokinetics of enrofloxacin in the red pacu (*Colossoma brachypomum*) after intramuscular, oral, and bath administration. *Journal of Veterinary Pharmacology and Therapeutics* 1997;20:124–128.

38. Lewbart, G.A. Koi medicine and management. *Compendium on Continuing Education for the Practicing Veterinarian* 1998;20(3A Suppl):5–12.

39. Lewbart, G.A., Papich, M.G., Whitt-Smith, D. et al. Pharmacokinetics of florfenicol in the red pacu (*Piaractus brachypomus*) after single dose intramuscular administration. *Journal of Veterinary Pharmacology and Therapeutics* 2005;28:317–319.

40. Lim, J.H., Kim, M.S., Hwang, Y.H. et al. Pharmacokinetics of florfenicol following intramuscular and intravenous administration in olive flounder (*Paralichthys olivaceus*). *Journal of Veterinary Pharmacology and Therapeutics* 2010;34:206–208.

41. Lunestad, B.T. and Goksoyr, J. Reduction in the antibacterial effect of oxytetracycline in seawater by complex formation with magnesium and calcium. *Diseases of Aquatic Organisms* 1992;9:67–72.

42. Moffitt, C.M. Survival of juvenile Chinook salmon challenged with *Renibacterium salmoninarum* and administered oral doses of erythromycin thiocyanate for different durations. *Journal of Aquatic Animal Health* 1992;4:119–125.

43. Noga, E.J. *Fish Disease: Diagnosis and Treatment*, 2nd ed. Wiley-Blackwell, Ames, IA, 2010; p. 340.

44. Nouws, J.F.M., Grondel, J.L., Schutte, A.R. et al. Pharmacokinetics of ciprofloxacin in carp, African catfish, and rainbow trout. *Veterinary Quarterly* 1988;10: 211–216.

45. Zimmerman, D.M., Armstrong, D.L., Curro, T.G. et al. Pharmacokinetics of florfenicol after a single intramuscular dose in white-spotted bamboo sharks (*Chiloscyllium plagiosum*). *Journal of Zoo and Wildlife Medicine* 2006;37:165–173.

46. Plakas, S.M., DePaola, A. and Moxey, M.B. *Bacillus stearothermophilus* disk assay for determining ampicillin residues in fish muscle. *Journal Association of Official Analytical Chemists International* 1991;74:910–912.

47. Plakas, S.M., El Said, K.R. and Stehly, G.R. Furazolidone disposition after intravascular and oral dosing in the channel catfish. *Xenobiotica* 1994;24:1095–1105.

48. Plakas, S.M., El Said, K.R., Bencsath, F.A. et al. Pharmacokinetics, tissue distribution, and metabolism of acriflavine and proflavine in the channel catfish (*Ictalurus punctatus*). *Xenobiotica* 1998;28:605–616.

49. Plumb, D.C. *Plumb's Veterinary Drug Handbook*, 6th ed. Pharma Vet Inc., Stockholm, WI, 2008; pp. 457–462.

50. Plumb, J.A. and Vinitnantharat, S. Dose titration of sarafloxacin (A-56620) against *Edwardsiella ictaluri* infection in channel catfish. *Journal of Aquatic Animal Health* 1990;2:194–197.

51. Reimscheussel, R., Stewart, L., Squibb, E. et al. Fish Drug Analysis—Phish-Pharm: A searchable database of pharmacokinetics data in fish. *The AAPS Journal* 2005;7(2):Article 30.

52. Reja, A., Moreno, L., Serrano, J.M. et al. Concentration-time profiles of oxytetracycline in blood, kidney, and liver of tench (*Tinca tinca* L.) after intramuscular administration. *Veterinary and Human Toxicology* 1996;38:344–347.

53. Roberts, H.E., Palmeiro, B., Weber, E.S. III. Bacterial and parasitic diseases of pet fish. *Veterinary Clinics of North America: Exotic Animal Practice* 2009;12:609–638.

54. Rogstad, A., Ellingsen, O.F. and Syversten, C. Pharmacokinetics and bioavailability of flumequine and oxolinic acid after various routes of administration to Atlantic salmon in seawater. *Aquaculture* 1993;110: 207–229.

55. Samuelsen, O.B. and Ervik, A. Absorption, tissue distribution, and excretion of flumequine after intravenous, intraperitoneal and oral administration to Atlantic halibut (*Hippoglossus hippoglossus*) held in seawater at 9C. *Aquaculture* 1997;158:215–227.

56. Samuelson, O.B. and Ervik, A. Absorption, tissue distribution, and excretion of flumequine and oxolinic acid

in corkwing wrasse (*Symphodus melops*) following a single intraperitonial injection or bath treatment. *Journal of Veterinary Pharmacology and Therapeutics* 2001;23: 111–116.

57. Samuelsen, O.B., Hjeltnes, B., Glette, J. et al. Efficacy of orally administered florfenicol in the treatment of furunculosis in Atlantic salmon. *Journal of Aquatic Animal Health* 1998;10:56–61.

58. Samuelsen, O.B., Lunestad, B.T. and Jelmert, A. Pharmacokinetic and efficacy studies on bath - administering potentiated sulfonamides in Atlantic halibut, *Hippoglossus hippoglossiodes* L. *Journal of Fish Diseases* 1997;20:287–296.

59. Samuelsen, O.B. Pharmacokinetics of quinolones in fish: A review. *Aquaculture* 2006;255:55–75.

60. Setser, M.D. Pharmacokinetics of gentamicin in channel catfish (*Ictalurus punctatus*). *American Journal of Veterinary Research* 1998;46:2558–2561.

61. Sharp, N.J., Diggles, B.K., Poortenaar, C.W. et al. Efficacy of Aqui-S, formalin and praziquantel against the monogeneans, *Benedenia seriolae* and *Zeuxapta seriolae*, infecting yellowtail kingfish *Seriola lalandi lalandi* in New Zealand. *Aquaculture* 2004;236:67–83.

62. Sitjà-Bobadilla, A., de Felipe, M.C., Alvarez-Pellitero, P. et al. *In vivo* and *in vitro* treatments against *Sparicotyle chrysophrii* (Monogenea: Microcotylidae) parasitizing the gills of gilthead sea bream (*Sparus aurata* L.). *Aquaculture* 2006;261:856–864.

63. Stoskopf, M.K. Appendix V: Chemotherapeutics. In: *Fish Medicine*. M.K. Stoskopf, ed. WB Saunders, Philadelphia, 1993; pp. 832–839.

64. Stoskopf, M.K. Fish Pharmacotherapeutics. In: *Zoo and Wild Animal Medicine: Current Therapy 4*. M.E. Fowler and R.E Miller, eds. WB Saunders, Philadelphia, 1999; pp. 182–189.

65. Stoskopf, M.K., Kennedy-Stoskopf, S., Arnold, J. et al. Therapeutic aminoglycoside antibiotic levels in brown shark, *Carcharhinus plumbeus* (Nard). *Journal of Fish Diseases* 1986;9:303–311.

66. Sun, M., Li, J., Gai, C.L. et al. Pharmacokinetics of difloxacin in olive flounder *Paralichthys olivaceus* at two water temperatures. *Journal of Veterinary Pharmacology and Therapeutics* 2014;37:186–191.

67. Thune, R.L. and Johnson, M.C. Effect of oral sarafloxacin dose and dose duration on *Edwardsiella ictaluri*-infected channel Catfish. *Journal of Aquatic Animal Health* 1992;4:252–256.

68. Treves-Brown, K.M. *Applied Fish Pharmacology (Aquaculture Series 3)*. Kluwer Academic, Boston, 2000; p. 309.

69. Whaley, J. and Francis-Floyd, R. A comparison of metronidazole treatments of hexamitiasis in angelfish. *Proceedings of the International Association for Aquatic Animal Medicine*, 1991; pp. 110–114.

70. Whitaker, B.R. Preventative medicine programs for fish. In: *Zoo and Wild Animal Medicine: Current Therapy 4*. M.E. Fowler and R. Miller, eds. WB Saunders, Philadelphia, 1999; pp. 163–181.

71. Wildgoose, W.H. and Lewbart, G.A. Therapeutics. In: *Manual of Ornamental Fish*, 2nd ed. W.H. Wildgoose, ed. British Small Animal Veterinary Association, Gloucester, UK, 2001; pp. 237–258.

72. Willoughby, L.G. and Roberts, R.J. Towards strategic use of fungicides against *Saprolgenia parasiticia* in salmonid fish hatcheries. *Journal of Fish Diseases* 1992;15: 1–13.

73. Xu, D. and Rogers, W.A. Formaldehyde residue in striped bass muscle. *Journal of Aquatic Animal Health* 1995;5:306–312.

74. Xu, W., Zhu, X., Wang, X. et al. Residues of enrofloxacin, furazolidone, and their metabolites in Nile tilapia (*Oreochromis niloticus*). *Aquaculture* 2006;254:1–8.

75. Xu, N., Ai, X., Liu, Y. et al. Comparative pharmacokinetics of norfloxacin nicotinate in common carp (*Cyprinus carpio*) and crucian carp (*Carassius auratus*) after oral administration. *Journal of Veterinary Pharmacology and Therapeutics* 2015;38:309–331.

76. Yanong, R.P.E., Curtis, E.W., Simmons, R. et al. Pharmacokinetic studies of florfenicol in koi carp and three spot gourami *Trichogaster trichopterus* after oral and intramuscular treatment. *Journal of Aquatic Animal Health* 2005;17:129–137.

77. Yuan, J., Li, R.-Q., Shi, Y. et al. Pharmacokinetics of oxytetracycline in yellow catfish [*Pelteobagrus fulvidraco* (Richardson, 1846)] with a single and multiple-dose oral administration. *Journal of Applied Ichthyology* 2014;30:109–113.

78. Zhang, Q. and Li, X. Pharmacokinetics and residue elimination of oxytetracycline in grass carp, *Ctenopharyngodon idellus*. *Aquaculture* 2007;272:140–145.

79. Zhu, Y., Tan, Y., Wang, C. et al. Pharmacokinetics and tissue residues of marbofloxacin in crucian carp (*Carassius auratus*) after oral administration. *Aquaculture Research* 2009;40:696–709.

THERAPEUTICS FOR ORNAMENTAL, TROPICAL, BAIT AND OTHER NON-FOOD FISH: ANTIPARASITICIDES

JESSICA GASKINS AND SHANE M. BOYLAN

Statement: None of these therapeutic compounds are approved or available for extra-label use in food fish.

MEDICATION	DRUG CLASS	DOSE AND ROUTE	SPECIES	COMMENTS
Albendazole	Benzimidazole anthelmintic	5 mg/kg once[19]	Atlantic salmon	Caution: Bone marrow suppression and hepatic inflammation when used long term
		10 mg/kg once[29]	Atlantic salmon, rainbow trout, tilapia	
		10–50 mg/L every 2–6 hours[28]	Stickleback	
Chloroquine diphosphate	Aminoquinoline/ amebicidal	50 mg/kg PO once[17]	Red drum	Counseling Point: May use activated carbon to remove drug from system
		10 mg/L tank water, once[20]		Counseling Point: 10–20 ppm can affect the biofilter[21]
		10 mg/L once weekly; repeat weekly for 3 treatments for amyloodinium[21]		Clinical Note: Used for *Amyloodinium ocellatum*, monitor every 3 weeks
Closantel/ Mebendazole (50/75 mg/mL)	Salicylanilide antiparasitic with benzimidazole antiparasitic	1 mL/400 L once; may repeat in 3–7 days[39]	Koi	Counseling Point: Safe in koi but toxic in goldfish
Copper sulfate	Essential trace element	0.012 and 0.094 mg/L bath for 28 days[5]	European eel	Counseling Point: To assess true level will need a copper kit
		0.02 mg/L bath for 65 or 72 hours[6,7]	Rainbow trout	Caution: Extremely toxic to gill tissue and immunosuppressive
		0.15–0.2 mg/L tank water, until therapeutic effect[20,36]		Caution: Very toxic to invertebrates and plants
		0.2 mg/L tank water for 14–21 days[38]		Counseling Point: May be removed from system with activated carbon
		0.25 mg/L for 24–48 hour bath[9]		Counseling Point: May want to prepare stock solution of 1 mg/mL (1 gram CuSo4 · 5H2O in 250 mL distilled water)
		100 mg/L × 1–5 minute bath[3]		
		0.2 mg/L free copper ion for 90 days[21]		Counseling Point: *Benedeniella* in cownose rays only, possibly toxic to other elasmobranchs[21]

(*Continued*)

MEDICATION	DRUG CLASS	DOSE AND ROUTE	SPECIES	COMMENTS
Diflubenzuron	Benzoylphenyl urea (non-carcinogenic)	0.01 mg/L in tank water for 48 hours every 6 days for 3 treatments[31]	Fathead minnows, guppies	Clinical Note: Effective for ectoparasites; however, drug persists in water long term
Dimetridazole	Nitroimidazole	28 mg/kg in feed every 24 hours for 10 days[25]	Rainbow trout	Clinical Note: Used to treat *Ichthyophthirius multifiliis*
Emamectin	Avermectin insecticide	50 mcg/kg every 24 hours PO for 7 days[30]	Atlantic salmon, rainbow trout, brown trout	Clinical Note: Treats various sea lice species (*Lepeophtheirus salmonis*, *Caligus teres*, *C.elongatus*, and *C. rogercresseyi*)
Fenbendazole	Benzimidazole anthelmintic	1 mg/kg IV once[4]	Channel catfish	Caution: Species susceptibility that causes bone marrow suppression and death; do not use in elasmobranchs if at all possible[21]
		5 mg/kg PO once[14]	Channel catfish	
		6 mg/kg PO every 24 hours[12]	Rainbow trout	
		50 mg/kg PO every 24 hours for 2 days, repeat in 14 days[38]	Carp	
		40 mg/kg in feed every 4 days for 2 treatments[36]	Rainbow trout	
		1.5 mg/L for 12 hour bath[12]		
		2 mg/L tank water every 7 days for 3 treatments[20]		
		2.5 mg/g feed for 2–3 days, repeat in 14 days[38]		
		Medicated feed (brine shrimp in 4 mg/mL for 15–20 minutes) for 2 days, then repeat in 14 days[38]		
Formalin	Highly reactive aldehyde gas formed by oxidation of hydrocarbons In solution, it has a wide range of uses such as a disinfectant and as a laboratory fixative or preservative	0.015–0.025 mL/L tank water every 48 hours for 3 treatments (may do 50% water change on alternate days)[20] 0.125–0.25 mL/L up to 60 minute bath, repeat once every 24 hours for 2–3 days[20] Soft water: 0.4mL/L up to 60 minute bath every 3 days (max 3 treatments)[31] Hard water: 0.5 mL/L up to 60 minute bath every 3 days (max 3 treatments)[31] 25 ppm hardwater every other day for 3 doses[21] 100–200 ppm on oxygen bath for 1 hour[21]		Formulation Consideration: All doses based on 100% formalin, which is 37% formaldehyde Caution: Hazardous and carcinogenic, toxic to plants as well Counseling Point: Some species more sensitive than others so monitor closely for signs of respiratory distress (pale color, increased opercular movement, gasping) Clinical Note: Keep water well oxygenated

(Continued)

MEDICATION	DRUG CLASS	DOSE AND ROUTE	SPECIES	COMMENTS
Formalin with malachite green	(See individual descriptions)	0.025 mL/L Formalin + 0.1 mg/L malachite in tank water every 48 hours for 3 treatments[1,20]		Clinical Note: Combination is synergistic for *Ichthyophthirius* and is best to change water 50% on alternate days[1] Caution: Mutagenic and teratogenic, toxic to certain fish species
Freshwater	N/A	3–15 minute bath, repeat every 7 days as needed[20] 4–5 minute bath once[16]		Clinical Note: Useful for susceptible marine ectoparasites but be sure to aerate bath water well and monitor closely; small fish may not tolerate
Glacial acetic acid	Acetic acid is a product of the oxidation of ethanol and is used as a reagent or locally as a counterirritant and may be used topically to treat bacterial, fungal, or parasitic infections	1–2 mL/L for 30–45 second bath[20,39]		Counseling Point: Appears safe in goldfish but not for smaller tropical fish Clinical Note: Useful to treat monogeneans and crustacean ectoparasites
Furazolidone	Antibacterial and antiprotozoal nitrofuran	1 mg/kg PO, IV every 24 hours[23]	Channel catfish	Caution: Prohibited for use in food animals
		30 mg/kg PO[21]	Nile tilapia	
		67.5 mg/kg PO every 12 hours for 10 days[15]	Rainbow trout	
		25–35 mg/kg PO every 24 hours in feed for 20 days[9]	Rainbow trout, brown trout, brook trout, and cutthroat trout	
		50–100 mg/kg PO every 24 hours in feed for 10–15 days[20]	Salmonids	
		1–10 mg/L in tank water for ≥24 hours[20]		
Hydrogen peroxide 3%	Anti-infective and oxidizing agent	3.1 mg/L bath for 1 hour for external bacteria or 6.5 mg/L bath for 1 hour for *Ichthyobodo*[27]	Serpae tetra, tiger barb, blue gourami, suckermouth catfish, green swordtail	Clinical Note: Store in cool, dark place or will rapidly decompose Counseling Point: Concentration tolerated is species-dependent and may be harmful in smaller fish
		1–1.5 mg/L bath for 20 minutes[35]	Atlantic salmon	
		17.5 mL/L bath for 4–10 minutes[8]		

(Continued)

MEDICATION	DRUG CLASS	DOSE AND ROUTE	SPECIES	COMMENTS
Levamisole	Anthelmintic and immunomodulator	10 mg/kg PO every 7 days for 3 treatments[8]		Clinical Note: Appropriate for internal nematodes and external trematodes
		10 mg/kg IM days 1, 14, and 28[18]	Sandbar shark	
		11 mg/kg IM every 7 days for 2 treatments[8]	Eels	
		1 mg/L for 24 hour bath[33]		
		1–2 mg/L or 24 hour bath[8]		
		50 mg/L for 2 hour bath[8]		
		4 g/kg in feed every 7 days for 3 treatments[8]		
Malachite green	Organic compound that is a triarylmethane dye	0.1 mg/L in tank water every 3 days for 3 total treatments[20]		Caution: Mutagenic and teratogenic, toxic to certain fish species
		0.25 mg/L for 15 minute immersion every 24 hours[22]	Salmonids	Caution: Increased toxicity at higher temperatures and lower pH
		0.5 mg/L for 1 hour bath[20]	Salmonids	Counseling Point: Stains most objects, especially plastic aquarium decor or filtration equipment
		1 mg/L for a 30–60 minute bath[19]		
		1 mg/L for 1 hour immersion for fungal control on fish eggs[36]		
		2 mg/L for 15 minute bath for fungal control on fish eggs[36]		
		10 mg/L for 10–30 minute bath for fungal control on freshwater fish eggs[20]	Salmonids	
		50–60 mg/L for 10–30 second bath[19]		
		100 mg/L topically to skin lesions[20]		
Mebendazole	Benzimidazole anthelmintic	20 mg/kg PO for 7 days for 3 treatments[32]		Caution: As with all benzimidazoles, do not administer to brood fish (teratogenic)
		1 mg/mL for 24–72 hour bath[2,8,11]	European eel	
		10–50 mg/L for 2–6 hour immersion[28]	Stickleback	Clinical Note: Used to treat monogenean trematodes in eels
		100 mg/L for 10 min–2 hour bath[8]		

(*Continued*)

MEDICATION	DRUG CLASS	DOSE AND ROUTE	SPECIES	COMMENTS
Methylene blue	Thiazine dye	1–3 mg/L of tank water for treating ectoparasites in freshwater fish[20]		Caution: Toxic to nitrifying bacteria and plants Caution: Stains most objects, including aquarium decor and filtration equipment
Metronidazole	Antibiotic for anaerobes and antiprotozoal agent	25 mg/kg PO every 24 hours in feed for 5–10 days[20] 50 mg/kg PO every 24 hours for 5 days[8,37] 100 mg/kg PO in feed every 24 hours for 3 days[20] 6.6 mg/L in tank water every 24 hours for 3 days[20] 25 mg/L in tank water every 48 hours for 3 treatments[20] 6.25–18 mg/g PO in feed for 5 days[38] Medicated feed of brine shrimp (625 mg per 100 mL for 15–20 minutes prior to feed) given daily for 5 treatments[13]	 Koi	Counseling Point: Does not dissolve well in water so best to dissolve using properties of geometric dilution in small portions rather than adding directly into treatment tank
Niclosamide	Derivative of salicylamide anthelmintic	0.055 mg/L every 24 hours as bath[10]	Rainbow trout	
Piperazine	Various salt forms of the piperazine chemical family that are GABA agonist anthelmintics	10 mg/kg PO in feed every 24 hours for 3 days[20]		Clinical Note: Treats non-encysted gastrointestinal nematodes
Potassium permanganate	Highly oxidative, water-soluble potassium salt compound with purple crystals	5 mg/L bath for 30–60 minutes[20] 100 mg/L bath for 5–10 minutes[20] 1 g/L for 10–40 second bath[20]		Caution: Toxicity increases with increased pH Caution: Never mix with formalin Counseling Point: May prove toxic to goldfish species Counseling Point: Systems with high organic load will require higher doses Testing: Add KMnO4 to small sample of system water and red color should remain for at least 4 hours; continue adding KMnO4 until 4 hour test is adequate

(Continued)

MEDICATION	DRUG CLASS	DOSE AND ROUTE	SPECIES	COMMENTS
Praziquantel	Anticestodal anthelmintic	5 mg/kg PO every 24 hours for 3 treatments[36]		Counseling Point: Monitor patients for lethargy, incoordination, or loss of equilibrium
		5 mg/kg PO every 7 days in feed for 3 treatments[32]		Caution: Some marine fish are sensitive
		5 mg/kg PO, ICe once then repeat in 14–21 days[16]		Caution: May be toxic to *Corydoras* catfish
		50 mg/kg PO once[20]		Counseling Point: Water levels should be tested after repeat use because will be consumed by microbiota[34]
		2–10 mg/L for 2–4 hours as bath[24,38]		
		5–10 mg/L for 3–6 hour bath, repeat in 7 days[16]		
		5–12 mg/kg in feed for 3 days[38]		
Pyrantel pamoate	Pyrimidine anthelmintic	10 mg/kg in feed given once[32]		Clinical Note: Treatment of gastric nematodes
Sodium chloride	NaCl	1–5 g/L in tank water indefinitely for prophylaxis or treatment of ectoparasites[20]		Counseling Point: When adjusting amount of salt added, note that normal salinity is 30–35 g/L
		10–30 g/L up to 30 minutes as a bath[20]	Only for fish >100 grams	Counseling Point: Some species are highly sensitive to variability in salinity (catfish), so use with caution and lower doses in weak fish
		30 g/L for 10 minute bath[36]	Goldfish, koi	
		30–35 g/L for 4–5 minute bath[16]	Variety of marine species	Clinical Note: Modified salinity reduces monogenean reproductivity[21]
		20 ppt modified salinity for stenohaline parasite adjunct therapy (Dr. Shane Matthew Boylan, DVM. Personal communication. SC Aquarium. 2012)	Bala shark and tiger barb	Clinical Note: Prophylactic sodium chloride levels can cause neurological behavior, abnormal swimming, and ultimately death if not removed in bala sharks, tiger barbs, and some South American pleco species[22]
		1.5–3 ppt prophylactic parasite control (Dr. Johnny Shelley, MS, DVM, CertAqV. Personal communication. Veterinary Medical Officer USDA ARS Aquatic Animal Health Research Unit)		
Thiabendazole	Benzimidazole and fungicide	10–25 mg/kg in feed then repeat in 10 days[32]	Rainbow trout	Counseling Point: Higher doses tend to cause anorexia
		66 mg/kg PO once[32]	Rainbow trout	

(Continued)

MEDICATION	DRUG CLASS	DOSE AND ROUTE	SPECIES	COMMENTS
Trichlorfon (dimethyl phosphonate)	Organophosphate insecticide	0.25 mg/L in tank water for 96 hour immersion for every 3 days for 2 treatments if *Dactylogyrus* and change to every 7 days for 4 treatments if *Argulus*[20,26]	Channel catfish	Caution: Organophosphate, neurotoxic, avoid inhalation and contact with skin
				Counseling Point: Freshwater fish if >80°F, then increase to 0.5 mg/L in tank
		0.5 mg/L tank water every 10 days for 3 treatments[16]		Clinical Note: Copepods (not sea lice), for monogeneans and leeches a single treatment will often suffice
		0.5–1 mg/L in tank for marine fish every 3 days × 2 treatments for monogeneans and 1 mg/L every 48 hours for 3 treatments appropriate for turbellarians[20]		Counseling Point: Medication is temperature- and pH-dependent; higher pH decreases longevity; example: Cold freshwater lasts 7 days, warm (75°F) saltwater only a few hours[21]

REFERENCES

1. Brown, L. Aquaculture in fish medicine. In: *Aquaculture for Veterinarians: Fish Husbandry and Medicine*. Pergamon Press, Terry Town, NY, 1993; p. 139.

2. Buchmann, K. and Bjerregaard, J. Mebendazole treatment of psuedodactylogyrosis in an intensive eel-culture system. *Aquaculture* 1992;86:139–153.

3. Callahan, H.A. and Noga, E.J. Tricaine dramatically reduces the ability to diagnose protozoan ectoparasite (*Ichthyobodo necator*) infections. *Journal of Fish Diseases* 2002;25:433–437.

4. Davis, L.E., Davis, C.A., Koritz, G.D. et al. Comparative studies of pharmacokinetics of fenbendazole in food-producing animals. *Veterinary and Human Toxicology* 1988;30(Suppl 1):9–11.

5. Grosell, M.H., Hansen, H.J.M. and Rosenkilde, P. Cu update, metabolism and elimination in fed and starved European eels (*Anguilla anguilla*) during adaptation to water borne Cu exposure. *Comparative Biochemistry & Physiology* 1998;120:295–305.

6. Grosell, M.H., Hogstrand, C. and Wood, C.M. Cu update and turnover in both Cu-acclimated and in non-acclimated rainbow trout (*Oncorhyncus mykiss*). *Aquatic Toxicology* 1997;38:257–276.

7. Grosell, M.H., Hogstrand, C. and Wood, C.M. Renal Cu and Na excretion and hepatic Cu metabolism in both Cu acclimated and non-acclimated rainbow trout (*Oncorhynchus mykiss*). *Aquatic Toxicology*. 1998;40:275–291.

8. Harms, C.A. Treatments for parasitic diseases of aquarium and ornamental fish. *Seminars in Avian and Exotic Pet Medicine* 1996;5:54–63.

9. Heaton, L.H. and Post, G. Tissue residue and oral safety of furazolidone in four species of trout. *The Progressive Fish-Culturist* 1968;30(4):208–215.

10. Hubert, T.D., Bernardy, J.A., Vue, C. et al. Residues of the lampricides 3-trifluoromethyl-4-nitrophenol and niclosamide in muscle tissue of rainbow trout. *Journal of Agricultural and Food Chemistry* 2005;53:5342–5346.

11. Iosifidou, E.G., Haagsm, N., Olling, M. et al. Residue study of mebendazole and its metabolites hydroxymebendazole and amino-mebendazole in eel (*Anguilla anguilla*) after bath treatment. *Drug Metabolism and Disposition* 1997;25:317–320.

12. Iosifidou, E.G., Haagsma, N., Tanck, M.W. et al. Depletion study of fenbendazole in rainbow trout (*Oncorhynchus mykiss*) after oral and bath treatment. *Aquaculture* 1997;154:191–199.

13. Johnson, E.L. *Koi Health and Disease*. *Johnson Veterinary Services*. Reade Printers, Athens, 2006.

14. Kitzman, J.V., Holley, J.H., Huber, W.G. et al. Pharmacokinetics and metabolism of fenbendazole in channel catfish. *Veterinary Research Communications* 1990;14:217–226.

15. Law, F.C.P. *Total metabolic depletion and residue profile of selected drugs in trout: furazolidone*. Final DFA Report (Contract 223–90-7016). 1994.

16. Lewbart, G.A. Emergency and critical care of fish. *Veterinary Clinics of North America: Exotic Animal Practice* 1998;1:233–249.

17. Lewis, D.H., Wenxing, W., Ayers, A. et al. Preliminary studies on the use of chloroquine as a systemic chemotherapeutic agent for amyloodinosis in red drum (*Sciaenops ocellatus*). *Marine Science* 1988;30(Suppl): 183–189.

18. MacLean, R.A., Fatzinger, M.H., Woolard, K.D. et al. Clearance of a dermal *Huffmanela* sp. in a sandbar shark (*Carcharhinus plumbeus*) using levamisole. *Diseases of Aquatic Organisms* 2006;73:83–88.

19. Nafstad, I., Ingebrigtsen, K., Langseth, W. et al. Benzimidazoles for antiparasite therapy in salmon. *Acta Veterinaria Scandinavica* 1991;87(Suppl):302–304.

20. Noga, E.J. *Fish Disease: Diagnosis and Treatment*, 2nd ed. Wiley-Blackwell, Ames, IA, 2010; p. 340.

21. Xu, W., Zhu, X., Wang, X. et al. Residues of enrofloxacin, furazolidone, and their metabolites in Nile tilapia (*Oreochromis niloticus*). *Aquaculture* 2006;254:1–8.

22. Willoughby, L.G. and Roberts, R.J. Towards strategic use of fungicides against *Saprolegnia parasitica* in salmonid fish hatcheries. *Journal of Fish Diseases* 1992;15:1–13.

23. Plakas, S.M., El Said, K.R. and Stehly, G.R. Furazolidone disposition after intravascular and oral dosing in the channel catfish. *Xenobiotica* 1994;24:1095–1105.

24. Plumb, J.A. and Rogers, W.A. Effect of Droncit (praziquantel) on yellow grubs *Clinostomum marginatum* and eye flukes of *Diplostomum spathaceum* in channel catfish. *Journal of Aquatic Animal Health* 1990;2:204–206.

25. Rapp, J. Treatment of rainbow trout (*Oncorhynchus mykiss* Walb.) fry infected with *Ichthyophthirius multifiliis* by oral administration of dimetridazole. *Bulletin-European Association of Fish Pathologists* 1995;15:67–69.

26. Reimschuessel, R., Stewart, L., Squibb, E. et al. Fish drug analysis—Phish-Pharm: A searchable database of pharmacokinetics data in fish. *American Association of Pharmaceutical Scientists* 2005;7(2):E288–E327.

27. Russo, R., Curtis, E.W. and Yanong, R.P. Preliminary investigations of hydrogen peroxide treatment of selected ornamental fishes and efficacy against external bacteria and parasites in green swordtails. *Journal of Aquatic Animal Health* 2007;19(2):121–127.

28. Schmahl, G. and Benini, J. Treatment of fish parasites 11. Effects of different benzimidazole derivatives (albendazole, mebendazole, fenbendazole) on *Glugea anomala*, Moniez, 1887 (Microsporidia): Ultrastructural aspects and efficacy studies. *Parasitology Research* 1998;60:41–49.

29. Shaikh, B., Rummel, N., Gieseker, C. et al. Metabolism and residue depletion of albendazole in rainbow trout, tilapia, and Atlantic salmon after oral administration. *Journal of Veterinary Pharmacology and Therapeutics* 2003;26:421–428.

30. Stone, J., Sutherland, I.H., Sommerville, C. et al. Commercial trials using emamectin benzoate to control sea lice *Lepeophtheirus salmonis* infestations in Atlantic salmon *Salmo salar*. *Diseases of Aquatic Organisms* 2000;41:141–149.

31. Stoskopf, M.K. Appendix V: Chemotherapeutics. In: *Fish Medicine*. M.K. Stoskopf, ed. WB Saunders, Philadelphia, 1993; pp. 832–839.

32. Stoskopf, M.K. Fish pharmacotherapeutics. In: *Zoo and Wild Animal Medicine: Current Therapy 4*. M.E. Fowler and R.E. Miller, eds. WB Saunders, Philadelphia, 1995; pp. 182–189.

33. Tarascheewski, H., Renner, C. and Melhorn, H. Treatment of fish parasites 3. Effects of Levamisole HCl, metrifonate, fenbendazole, mebendazole, and ivermectin in *Anguillicola crassus* (nematodes) pathogenic in the air bladder of eels. *Parasitology Research* 1988;74:281–289.

34. Thomas, A., Dawson, M.R., Ellis, H. et al. Praziquantel degradation in marine aquarium water. *Peer J* 2016;4:e1857.

35. Thomasen, J.M. Hydrogen peroxide as delousing agent for Atlantic salmon. In: *Pathogens of Wild and Farmed Fish: Sea Lice*. G.A. Boxshell and D. Defaye, eds. Ellis Horwood, Chichester, UK, 1993; pp. 290–295.

36. Treves-Brown, K.M. *Applied Fish Pharmacology (Aquaculture Series 3)*. Kluwer Academic, Boston, 2000.

37. Whaley, J. and Francis-Floyd, R. A comparison of metronidazole treatments of hexamitiasis in angelfish. *Proceedings of the International Association for Aquatic Animal Medicine*, 1991, pp. 110–114.

38. Whitaker, B.R. Preventative medicine programs for fish. In: *Zoo and Wild Animal Medicine: Current Therapy 4*. M.E. Fowler and R. Miller, eds. WB Saunders, Philadelphia, 1999; pp. 163–181.

39. Wildgoose, W.H. and Lewbart, G.A. Therapeutics. In: *Manual of Ornamental Fish*, 2nd ed. W.H. Wildgoose, ed. British Small Animal Veterinary Association, Gloucester, UK, 2001; pp. 237–258.

THERAPEUTICS FOR ORNAMENTAL FISH, TROPICAL, BAIT AND OTHER NON-FOOD FISH: SUPPORTIVE THERAPY AND CARE

JESSICA GASKINS AND SHANE M. BOYLAN

Statement: None of these therapeutic compounds are approved or available for extra-label use in food fish.

MEDICATION	DRUG CLASS	DOSE AND ROUTE	SPECIES	COMMENTS
Ascorbic acid	Nutritive agent (vitamin C)	3–5 mg/kg IM q 24 hours[18] 25–50 mg/kg IM, SC[16]	Koi Southern flounder, vermilion snapper, bonnethead shark, lined seahorse	Clinical Note: Dilute with appropriate fluid to decrease acidity and thus damage to tissue Clinical Note: Water-soluble vitamin
Atipamezole (Antisedan)	α-2 antagonist to reverse dexmedetomidine	IM dose volume dependent per previous dexmedetomidine injection[1,16,23]	Black sea bass, bonnethead shark, sandbar shark	Clinical Note: Reverses effects of dexmedetomidine 5–10 minutes after IM injection Clinical Note: Dose volume of administered atipamezole is the same as preceding dose volume of dexmedetomidine[23]
Atropine	Anticholinergic alkaloid and antimuscarinic agent that antagonizes actions of acetylcholine and other choline esters	0.1 mg/kg IM, IV, ICe[21]		Clinical Note: Treatment of cholinesterase inhibitors poisoning, organophosphorus and carbamate insecticide toxicities Clinical Note: Repeated doses may stop bradycardia and/or asystole
B-vitamin complex (B1, B2, B6, B12)	Thiamine, riboflavin, pyridoxine and cyanocobalamin	10 mg/kg SC[16]	Southern flounder, bonnethead shark	Clinical Note: Dose is based on thiamine component Clinical Note: All are water-soluble vitamins
Butorphanol	Partial agonist and antagonist activity at μ-opioid receptors and partial agonist activity at κ-opioid receptors	0.05–0.1 mg/kg IM once[21] 0.4 mg/kg IM once[7,8]	 Koi	Clinical Note: Used most often for postoperative anesthesia

(*Continued*)

MEDICATION	DRUG CLASS	DOSE AND ROUTE	SPECIES	COMMENTS
Dexamethasone	Corticosteroid	0.2 mg/kg IM or SC once[16] 1–2 mg/kg IM, ICe[21] 2 mg/kg IC, ICe q 12 hours for chlorine toxicity[10]	Squirrelfish	Clinical Note: Treatment of stress, shock, or trauma
Dexmedetomidine	Centrally acting α-2 adrenergic agonist	0.025–0.1 mg/kg IM once[16]	Bonnethead shark, sandbar shark	Clinical Note: Analgesia without respiratory depression noted in opioids
Dexmedetomidine + Ketamine + Midazolam	See individual descriptions for dexmedetomidine and ketamine Benzodiazepine presumed to interact with the gamma-Aminobutyric acid (GABA) receptor complex	0.05–0.1 mg/kg dexmedetomidine + 2–4 mg/kg ketamine + 0.2 mg/kg midazolam given IM[1]	Black sea bass, red porgy	Clinical Note: Sedation appropriate for black sea bass but potentially fatal for red porgy[1] Clinical Note: Midazolam typically given in combination for surgical procedures
Doxapram	Respiratory stimulant at peripheral carotid chemoreceptors stimulating catecholamine release	5 mg/kg dripped over gill arches[17]		Clinical Note: Repeat application until desired affect is achieved
Epinephrine (1:1000)	α- and β-adrenergic agonist	0.2–0.5 mg/kg IM, IV, ICe, IC[18]	Koi	
Eugenol	Clove oil	1–25 mg/L[18] 60 mg/L[4,14] 90 mg/L[4] 40–120 mg/L bath[10]	Koi Walleye, smallmouth bass, northern pike, lake sturgeon and banded cichlid Walleye, smallmouth bass, northern pike, lake sturgeon and banded cichlid Angelfish, cardinal tetra	Clinical Note: Doses are species-specific[9]
Furosemide	Loop diuretic	2–5 mg/kg IM, ICe q 12–72 hours[18]	Koi	Clinical Note: May be used for ascites even though most species lack a loop of Henle

(Continued)

MEDICATION	DRUG CLASS	DOSE AND ROUTE	SPECIES	COMMENTS
Hetastarch	Colloidal replacement fluid	0.5–1 cc/kg IV slowly[16]	Variety of marine or freshwater species	Clinical Note: Improves cardiovascular pressure
Hydromorphone	Centrally acting pure μ-opioid narcotic	0.2 mg/kg IM once for surgical procedure[16]	Unicorn leatherjacket and various other species	Clinical Note: Shorter duration of action and more potent than morphine
Isoflurane	Inhalation anesthetic	0.5–2 mL/L bath or bubbled into water[6]		Caution: Exposure risk to clinicians and risk of overdose limit its use
Ketamine	NMDA receptor antagonist	5–10 mg/kg IM or SC once[16] 66–88 mg/kg IM[21]	Sandbar shark	Clinical Note: Most often used in combination with other medications such as dexmedetomidine and/or midazolam
Ketamine + Medetomidine	NMDA receptor antagonist + synthetic α-2 adrenoreceptor agonist	6 mg/kg ketamine and 0.06 mg/kg medetomidine IM[2]	Gulf of Mexico sturgeon	
Marine Teleost Ringer's Solution	Lactate Ringer's solution (LRS) + 7.2% sodium chloride + 50% dextrose + saltwater	368 mOsm/kg H_2O with 964 mL of LRS with 50 mL of 7.2% NaCl and 3.6 mL of 50% dextrose ICe[16]	Moray eel	
Meloxicam	Nonsteroidal anti-inflammatory (more COX-2 selective)	1 mg/kg IM, IV once[3]	Nile tilapia	
MS-222 (Tricaine methane-sulfonate)	Sodium channel blocker	15–50 mg/L in treatment water for sedation[6]		Counseling Point: Stock solution must be light-protected and buffered 2:1 with bicarb
		25–50 ppm in treatment water as induction[16]	Mahi mahi, bonnethead shark and other ram ventilators	Clinical Note: Ram ventilator species are more susceptible to respiratory depression due to their respiratory functions; they need less drug due to increased respiratory functions
		50–100 mg/L bath induction; 50–60 mg/L maintenance[20]		
		100–200 mg/L bath induction; 50–100 mg/L maintenance for procedures[6]		Counseling Point: Narrow margin of safety in young or small fish and in soft, warm water; also very species-specific
		200 mg/L in bath[19]	Lumpfish	
		1 g/L spray[12,16]	Sandbar shark	

(Continued)

MEDICATION	DRUG CLASS	DOSE AND ROUTE	SPECIES	COMMENTS
Phenoxyethanol	Phenol ether organic compound	0.1–0.5 mL/L[22]		
		0.15 mL/L[15]	Elasmobranch sp.	
		0.6 mL/L[22]	Carp	
Propofol	Short-acting, lipophilic sedative-hypnotic anesthetic agent	2.5 mg/kg IV[11]	Spotted bamboo shark	Clinical Note: Immersions of koi longer than 20 minutes had prolonged recovery time and increased mortality
			Koi	
		2.5 mg/L immersion up to 20 minutes[13]		
		6.5 mg/kg IV[2]	Gulf of Mexico sturgeon	
		7 ppm immersion[5]	Goldfish	

REFERENCES

1. Christiansen, E., Mitchell, J.M., Harms, C.A. et al. Sedation of red porgy (*Pagrus pagrus*) and black sea bass (*Centropristis striata*) using ketamine, dexmedetomidine and midazolam delivered via intramuscular injection. *Journal of Zoo and Aquarium Research* 2014;2(3):62–68.

2. Fleming, G.H., Heard, D.J., Francis-Floyd, R. et al. Evaluation of propofol and medetomidine-ketamine for short-term immobilization of Gulf of Mexico sturgeon (*Acipenser oxyrinchus De Soti*). *Journal of Zoo and Wildlife Medicine* 2003;34:153–158.

3. Fredholm, D.V., Mylniczenko, N.D. and KuKanich, B. Pharmacokinetic evaluation of meloxicam after intravenous and intramuscular administration in Nile tilapia (*Oreochromis niloticus*). *Journal of Zoo and Wildlife Medicine* 2016;47(3):736–742.

4. Fujimoto, R.Y., Pereira, D.M., Souza Silva, J.C. et al. Clove oil induces anaesthesia and blunts muscle contraction power in three Amazon fish species. *Fish Physiology and Biochemistry* 2018;44:245–256.

5. Gholipourkanan, H. and Ahadizadeh, S. Use of propofol as an anesthetic and its efficacy on some hematological values of ornamental fish *Carassius auratus*. *Springer Plus* 2013;2:76.

6. Harms, C.A. Anesthesia in fish. In: *Zoo and Wild Animal Medicine: Current Therapy*, vol. 4. M.E. Fowler and R.E. Miller, eds. WB Saunders, Philadelphia, 1995; pp. 158–163.

7. Harms, C.A. and Lewbart, G.A. Surgery in fish. *Veterinary Clinics of North America: Exotic Animal Practice* 2000;3:759–774.

8. Harms, C.A., Lewbart, G.A., Swanson, C.R. et al. Behavioral and clinical pathology changes in koi carp (*Cyprinus carpio*) subjected to anesthesia and surgery with and without intra-operative analgesics. *Comparative Medicine* 2005;55:221–226.

9. Javahery, S., Hamed, N. and Moradlu, A. Effect of anaesthesia with clove oil in fish (review). *Fish Physiology Biochemistry* 2012;38:1545–1552.

10. Lewbart, G.A. Emergency and critical care of fish. *Veterinary Clinics of North America: Exotic Animal Practice* 1998;1:233–249.

11. Miller, S.M. Mitchell, M.A., Heatley J.J. et al. Clinical and cardiorespiratory effects of propofol in the spotted bamboo shark (*Chylloscyllium plagiosum*). *Journal of Zoo and Aquarium Research* 2005;36(4):673–676.

12. Noga, E.J. *Fish Disease: Diagnosis and Treatment*, 2nd ed. Wiley-Blackwell, Ames, IA, 2010.

13. Oda, A., Bailey, K.M., Lewbart, G.A. et al. Physiologic and biochemical assessments of koi (*Cyprinus carpio*) following immersion in propofol. *JAVMA* 2014;245(11):1286–1291.

14. Peak, S. Sodium bicarbonate and clove oil as potential anesthetics for nonsalmonid fishes. *North American Journal of Fisheries Management*. 1998;18(4):919–924.

15. Penning, M.R., Vaughan, D.B., Fivaz, K. et al. Chemical Immobilization of elasmobranchs at uShaka Sea World in Durban, South Africa. *The Elasmobranch Husbandry Manual II: Captive Care of Sharks, Rays and Their Relatives*. M. Smith, D. Warmolts, D. Thoney, R. Heauter, M. Murray and J. Ezurra, eds. Ohio Biological Survey, 2016; pp. 331–338.

16. Shane M. Boylan, DVM (chief veterinarian, South Carolina Aquarium), personal communication, 2012.

17. Tonya Clauss, MS, DVM (senior director of Animal Health, Georgia Aquarium), personal communication, 2018.

18. Saint-Erne, N. Clinical procedures. In: *Advanced Koi Care*. N. Saint-Erne, ed. Erne Enterprises, Glendale, AZ, 2002; pp. 39–61.

19. Skar, M.W., Haugland, G.T., Powell, M.D. et al. Development of anaesthetic protocols for lumpfish (*Cyclopterus lumpus L.*): Effect of anaesthetic concentrations, sea water temperature and body weight. *PLOS ONE* 2017;12.7:e0179344.

20. Stoskopf, M.K. Anesthesia in pet fishes. In: *Kirk's Current Veterinary Therapy XII: Small Animal Practice.* J.D. Bonagura, ed. WB Saunders Co, Philadelphia, 1995; pp. 1365–1369.

21. Stoskopf, M.K. Fish pharmacotherapeutics. In: *Zoo and Wild Animal Medicine: Current Therapy*, vol. 4. M.E. Fowler, M.E and R.E. Miller, eds. WB Saunders, Philadelphia, 1999; 182–189.

22. Treves-Brown, K.M. *Applied Fish Pharmacology.* Kluwer Academic, Dordrecht, The Netherlands, 2000.

23. Zoetis. Antisedan package insert. www.zoetis.com/products/dogs/antisedan-_atipamezole_.aspx.

EXAMPLE OF CASCADE SYSTEM IN UNITED KINGDOM

RICHARD G. ENDRIS

If there is no suitable veterinary medicine authorized in the United Kingdom to treat a condition in a particular species, the veterinarian can treat an animal under their care in accordance with the Cascade. The Cascade is a risk-based decision tree that allows veterinarians to use their clinical judgment to treat an animal under their care by deciding which product to use when there is no authorized veterinary medicine available in the United Kingdom. As part of the Royal College of Veterinary Surgeons (RCVS) Code of Professional Conduct for Veterinary Surgeons, the veterinarian must obtain the owner's consent for their animal to be treated under the Cascade.

The veterinarian should balance the benefits against the risks of not following the clinical particulars on the Summary of Product Characteristics (SPC) and take responsibility for their decision. Risks could include those to:

- The animal
- The owner
- The person administering the medicine
- Consumers of food that may contain residues of the veterinary medicine
- The environment
- Wider public health (e.g., increased selection for antimicrobial resistance)

The veterinarian should think carefully about not following the SPC, as the advice and warnings given are there for good reason and based on assessed data. If the veterinarian ignores the advice and warnings in the SPC, the veterinarian may be open to litigation if something goes wrong with the treatment.

The steps under the Cascade, in descending order of suitability, are:

- A veterinary medicine authorized in the United Kingdom for use in another animal species, or for a different condition in the same species
- If there is no such product, either:
  o A medicine authorized in the United Kingdom for human use, or
  o A veterinary medicine not authorized in the United Kingdom, but authorized in another member state for use in any animal species in accordance with the Special Import Scheme; in the case of a food-producing animal the medicine must be authorized in a food-producing species
- A medicine prescribed by the veterinarian responsible for treating the animal and prepared especially on this occasion (known as an extemporaneous preparation or special) by a veterinarian, a pharmacist or a person holding an appropriate manufacturer's authorization (so-called specials manufacturers)
- In exceptional circumstances, medicines may be imported from outside Europe via the Special Import Scheme

The veterinarian or the person acting under their supervision may administer a product prescribed under the cascade; however, the prescription and use of the product remains the veterinarian's responsibility.

DISPENSING

Only veterinarians registered with the RCVS may prescribe medicines under the Cascade. A suitably qualified person (SQP) may dispense an authorized veterinary medicine, which falls within the scope of the qualification they hold, for use under the Cascade against a valid prescription from a veterinarian. A pharmacist may dispense authorized veterinary and human medicines and extemporaneous preparations they have prepared against a prescription from a veterinarian.

FOOD-PRODUCING SPECIES

The following conditions apply when prescribing a product under the Cascade for use in food-producing species:

- The pharmacologically active substances contained in the medicine must have an maximum residue limit (MRL), but not necessarily in the species for which it is intended to be used. For more information see EU Commission Regulation 37/2010.
- The veterinarian responsible for prescribing the medicine must specify an appropriate withdrawal period.
- The veterinarian responsible for prescribing the medicine must keep specified records.

SETTING WITHDRAWAL PERIODS

A withdrawal period is the length of time that must lapse between administration and the point the animal can be slaughtered to enter the food chain. The veterinarian is required to specify an appropriate withdrawal period to the animal producer when prescribing or administering a medicine to food-producing animals under the Cascade. When setting the withdrawal period, the veterinarian must take into account known information about the use of the product on the authorized species when prescribing for another species.

If a product is used as authorized, e.g., use of an imported product from another member state, the authorized withdrawal period should be followed.

The longer of the following two withdrawal periods should be applied when a medicine is given to an animal that it is not indicated for, or at a higher dose rate than recommended to an animal that the product is indicated for:

- The minimum statutory withdrawal period
- The withdrawal period stated on the product's SPC

The minimum statutory withdrawal periods are:

- 7 days for eggs and milk
- 28 days for meat from poultry and mammals
- 500 degree days for meat from fish

EXTEMPORANEOUS PREPARATIONS: SPECIALS

Any medicine tailored for a particular animal or herd prepared by a vet, a pharmacist, or a person who holds an appropriate manufacturing authorization is an extemporaneous preparation. A veterinary prescription is needed to use an extemporaneous preparation under the Cascade, but this may be written or oral. To prepare an extemporaneous preparation, the veterinarian should contact a holder of a Specials Manufacturing Authorization (ManSA), who is well prepared and equipped to prepare medicines of suitable quality.

STOCK OF MEDICINES

The veterinarian may keep human medicines, imported medicines and extemporaneous preparations in his/her possession for use under the Cascade. The amount held should be justified by the clinical need under the Cascade rules; these medicines should not be used as a first choice treatment in every situation. The veterinarian should keep up to date with new authorizations and change prescribing habits and stocking policies accordingly.

LABELING

The information that must be included on the label for products used under the Cascade is listed in the Veterinary Medicines Regulations (VMR). If all or part of the information cannot be included on the label, the veterinarian may include it on a separate sheet. It is the responsibility of the person supplying the medicine to ensure it is appropriately labeled.

RECORD KEEPING

As well as the normal record-keeping requirements, there are specific requirements for vets who administer or supply medicines under the Cascade. These must be kept for 5 years and made available upon request from a duly authorized person. The records that must be retained are listed in the VMR.

ADVERSE EVENTS

The veterinarian does not have to report adverse events to medicines prescribed under the Cascade, but the veterinarian is encourage to do so. Refer to guidance on reporting adverse events.

RESOURCES

http://www.epruma.eu/publications/factsheets/publication/24-factsheet-on-the-cascade-procedure.html

https://ec.europa.eu/health//sites/health/files/files/eudralex/vol-5/reg_2010_37/reg_2010_37_en.pdf

http://www.legislation.gov.uk/uksi/2013/2033/contents/made

https://www.gov.uk/guidance/record-keeping-requirements-for-veterinary-medicines

https://www.gov.uk/report-veterinary-medicine-problem/animal-reacts-medicine

REFERENCES FOR DRUGS USED IN AQUACULTURE IN OTHER COUNTRIES

RICHARD G. ENDRIS

SOUTHEAST ASIA

ASEAN countries

The ASEAN (Association of Southeast Asian Nations) includes Brunei, Indonesia, Malaysia, Myanmar, Philippines, Singapore, Thailand and Vietnam. The status of approved aquaculture drugs is discussed in the following websites.

http://www.asean.org/storage/images/Community/AEC/AMAF/UpdateApr2014/ASEAN%20Guideliness%20for%20Chemicals%20Final%20Draft%20Malaysia%20OK.pdf

http://journals.plos.org/plosone/article/file?id=10.1371/journal.pone.0124267&type=printable

Bangladesh

Drugs/chemicals used in aquaculture in Bangladesh are described in the following resources. Review of available documents indicates there is no requirement for veterinary prescriptions for use of aquaculture drugs/chemicals in Bangladesh.

Faruk, M.A.R., Ali, M.M.K. and Patwary, Z.P. Evaluation of the status of use of chemicals and antibiotics in freshwater aquaculture activities with special emphasis to fish health management. *Journal of the Bangladesh Agriculture University* 2008;6(2):381–390. http://ageconsearch.umn.edu/bitstream/208318/2/4838-17604-1-PB.pdf

Hossain, M.A., Hoq, M.E. and Mazid, M.A. Use of chemical and biological products in aquaculture in Bangladesh. *The Agriculturists* 2008;6(1&2):29–42.

India

Rao et al. (1992) discussed the use of chemotherapeutants in freshwater aquaculture and hatchery systems in India. A review of available documents indicates there is no requirement for veterinary prescriptions for use of aquaculture drugs/chemicals in India.

http://www.caa.gov.in/uploaded/doc/anitbiotics.pdf

Pathak, S.C., Ghosh, S.K. and Palanisamy, K. The use of chemicals in aquaculture in India. In: *Use of Chemicals in Aquaculture in Asia: Proceedings of the Meeting on the Use of Chemicals in Aquaculture in Asia* 20–22 May, 1996, Tigbauan, Iloilo, Philippines. J.R. Arthur, C.R. Lavilla-Pitogo and R.P. Subasinghe, eds. Tigbauan, Iloilo, Philippines: Aquaculture Department, Southeast Asian Fisheries Development Center. 2000; pp. 87–112.

Shariff, M., Subasinghe, R.P. and Arthur, J.R. eds. Diseases in Asian Aquaculture. 1992. http://www.fhs-afs.net/publications.htm

NORTHEAST ASIA

China

Many drugs and chemicals are in use in China for aquaculture. The major ones are listed in the first data source in the following list. As of 2000, no veterinary involvement was required for fish farmers to obtain aquaculture drugs/chemicals. The role of the administrative department of veterinary medicine at government department levels in the supervision and administration of veterinary drugs is discussed in the second data source.

Yulin, J. The use of chemicals in aquaculture in the People's Republic of China. In: *Use of Chemicals in Aquaculture in Asia: Proceedings of the Meeting on the Use of Chemicals in Aquaculture in Asia* 20–22 May, 1996, Tigbauan, Iloilo, Philippines. J.R. Arthur, C.R. Lavilla-Pitogo and R.P. Subasinghe, eds. Tigbauan, Iloilo, Philippines: Aquaculture Department, Southeast Asian Fisheries Development Center. 2000; pp. 141–153. https://repository.seafdec.org.ph/bitstream/handle/10862/600/9718511490_p141-153.pdf

http://www.fmprc.gov.cn/mfa_eng/wjb_663304/zzjg_663340/jks_665232/jkxw_665234/t209904.shtml

Japan

The major drugs used to treat cultured cold-water fish and shrimp in Japan are found in the following source. From a review of available documents, it is unclear whether veterinary prescriptions are required for use of aquaculture drugs/chemicals in Japan.

http://www.fao.org/docrep/003/w3594e/W3594E09.htm

Korea

Drugs are approved for use in aquaculture in Korea in the following fish species: snakehead, black sea bream, olive flounder, sea bass, convict grouper, catfish, mud loach, tilapia, yellowtail, eel, crucian carp, trout, mullet, red sea bream, sweet fish, atka mackerel, carp, horse mackerel, thread herring and filefish. A review of available documents indicates there is no requirement for veterinary prescriptions for use of aquaculture drugs/chemicals in Korea.

Kim, J.W., Cho, M.Y., Jee, B.-Y., Park, M.A. and Kim, N.Y. Administration and use of aquaculture drugs in Korea. *Journal of Fish Pathology* 2014;27(1):67–75. http://www.koreascience.or.kr/article/ArticleFullRecord.jsp?cn=HGOPB8_2014_v27n1_67

AUSTRALIA AND NEW ZEALAND

Australia

Aquaculture drugs are contained in the overall listing of veterinary drugs. Approved aquaculture drugs are listed on the following webpages. A review of available documents indicates there is no requirement for veterinary prescriptions for use of aquaculture drugs/chemicals in Australia, but veterinary involvement in treatment of fish is strongly implied. Drugs may be used off label. Default drug withdrawal time for aquaculture species is 35 days.

http://www.frdc.com.au/project/1996-314
http://www.pir.sa.gov.au/aquaculture/aquatic_animal_health/veterinary_medicine_use_in_aquaculture#toc1
https://www.ava.com.au/sites/default/files/documents/Other/Guidelines_for_prescribing_authorising_and_dispensing_veterinary_medicines.pdf
https://apvma.gov.au/node/10831

New Zealand

Approved drugs for aquaculture use in New Zealand are listed on the following website. Veterinary involvement in treatment of fish is strongly implied. Drugs may be used off label. The default aquaculture drug withdrawal is 35 days.

http://www.foodsafety.govt.nz/industry/acvm/vet-medicines/using/

LATIN/SOUTH AMERICA

Chile

Drugs approved for aquaculture use are listed on the following website. Data were compiled from several sources including various sponsor websites. Chilean requirements for veterinary prescriptions authorizing drug use for aquaculture generally follow those of the European Union.

http://www.fao.org/tempref/codex/Meetings/CCRVDF/ccrvdf21/rv21_11e.pdf

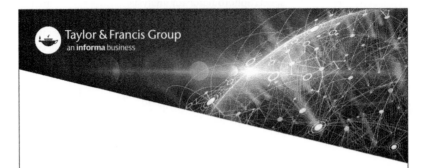

For Product Safety Concerns and Information please contact our EU
representative GPSR@taylorandfrancis.com Taylor & Francis Verlag GmbH,
Kaufingerstraße 24, 80331 München, Germany

Printed and bound by CPI Group (UK) Ltd, Croydon, CR0 4YY

01/05/2025

01858531-0001